Ghai's
Textbook of
PRACTICAL PHYSIOLOGY

Ghai's
Textbook of
PRACTICAL PHYSIOLOGY

As per the Competency-based Medical Education Curriculum (NMC)

Tenth Edition

Revised & Edited by

VP Varshney MBBS MD
Professor of Excellence and Head
Department of Physiology (FMS-Delhi University)
Ex-Head, Department of Physiology
Maulana Azad Medical College
New Delhi, India

Mona Bedi MBBS MD
Director-Professor
Department of Physiology
Maulana Azad Medical College
New Delhi, India

JAYPEE

JAYPEE BROTHERS MEDICAL PUBLISHERS
The Health Sciences Publisher
New Delhi | London

Jaypee Brothers Medical Publishers (P) Ltd

Headquarters
Jaypee Brothers Medical Publishers (P) Ltd
EMCA House, 23/23-B
Ansari Road, Daryaganj
New Delhi 110 002, India
Landline: +91-11-23272143, +91-11-23272703
+91-11-23282021, +91-11-23245672
Email: jaypee@jaypeebrothers.com

Corporate Office
Jaypee Brothers Medical Publishers (P) Ltd
4838/24, Ansari Road, Daryaganj
New Delhi 110 002, India
Phone: +91-11-43574357
Fax: +91-11-43574314
Email: jaypee@jaypeebrothers.com

Overseas Office
J.P. Medical Ltd
83 Victoria Street, London
SW1H 0HW (UK)
Phone: +44 20 3170 8910
Fax: +44 (0)20 3008 6180
Email: info@jpmedpub.com

Website: www.jaypeebrothers.com
Website: www.jaypeedigital.com

Ghai's Textbook of Practical Physiology

First Edition: 1983
Tenth Edition: **2023**

ISBN: 978-93-5465-895-2

Printed at: Samrat offset Pvt. Ltd.

Dedicated to

The Almighty, our students
and
our parents & families

—VP Varshney & Mona Bedi

Preface to the Tenth Edition

Ghai's Textbook of Practical Physiology has been considered as the most reliable book on the subject for medical students in India and abroad for many years. The *Ghai's Textbook of Practical Physiology* 10th edition, has been prepared for the benefit of medical students on the basis of our long teaching experience in physiology. Even though theoretical knowledge is important for the students, it becomes more important when used in practice, hence the importance of a detailed textbook of practical physiology.

The various sections of this book including those on hematology, human experiments and clinical physiology have been thoroughly revised as per the competency-based medical education curriculum (NMC) guidelines. We have attempted to familiarize the students with the clinical and experimental approach to human physiology. Well-labeled diagrams and flowcharts have been incorporated to improve the understanding. The book has been specially designed for step-by-step learning of practicals and experiments, which are essential for medical students seeking to develop expertise in physiology and clinical medicine. This tenth edition features numerous revised and redrawn illustrations to facilitate the easy assimilation of the practicals.

A basic format has been adhered to in each practical:

- Each experiment starts with STUDENT OBJECTIVES, which are basically learning objectives for the students. This is what the student is expected to learn at the end of each practical.
- This is followed by a brief INTRODUCTION of the practical.
- After explaining the PRINCIPLE, the APPARATUS required for the experiment is described.
- A detailed step by step PROCEDURE is then elaborated. The working instructions are simple so the average student can easily follow them.
- Next come the OBSERVATIONS and RESULTS.
- The PRECAUTIONS, which help to minimize the error in the practicals are listed after the RESULTS.
- As all experiments have a physiological and clinical importance, a separate heading has been ascribed for PHYSIOCLINICAL SIGNIFICANCE in each experiment wherever relevant.
- Each chapter ends with QUESTIONS along with their answers to help the student to prepare for their examination viva.
- Objective Structured Practical Examination (OSPE) is a reliable, valid and important method of assessing practical skills. These have been added at the end of each practical to acquaint the student with the mode of practical assessment.

We sincerely hope that this endeavor of ours, helps the students to comprehend the scientific basis of practicals in physiology and prepare for their examinations in a systematic manner.

We would always welcome suggestions and ideas from our students and friends for the betterment of this book in future. After all "The secret in education lies in respecting the students".

VP Varshney
Mona Bedi

Preface to the First Edition

The material included within the covers of this book conforms to the syllabi and courses of practical physiology laid down by the Medical Council of India (MCI), and followed by all the medical colleges. The book is divided into three main sections—amphibian, mammalian and human experiments. There is a separate section on electronic recorders and stimulators. If our students are not to be left behind the rapidly advancing field of medical electronics, they have to be introduced at the earliest to the use of some of these modern devices. The book also supplements the cyclostyled material provided by some physiology departments to their students.

In essence, each experiment begins with the PRINCIPLE on which it is based, and the APPARATUS required for it. Then follows the step-by-step PROCEDURES in which the working instructions are so framed that an average student will find no difficulty in tackling any experiment. Next, the OBSERVATIONS, RESULTS and CONCLUSION. The relevant theoretical aspects of each experiment that are needed for immediate reference, including deviations from the normal, are then described under the heading of DISCUSSION. This is intended to obviate the necessity for the student to refer to the textbooks again and again. Finally, the QUESTIONS generally asked from the students are grouped at the end of the each experiment. A student should be able to assess his/her comprehension of the relevant material in trying to answer these questions. The APPENDIX contains the units and measures employed in physiology, and the equivalents of metric, United States, and English (Imperial) measures. This is followed by some important reference values of clinical importance. These will certainly prove useful to the hurried and harried medical students for quick reference.

There is continuing controversy and divergence of opinion regarding the necessity of including amphibian experiments in the medical curriculum. Often, these experiments may appear to be time wasting and irrelevant to clinical medicine. However, they have to be included in a book meant primarily for the Indian medical student till such time the courses are revised by the MCI. In any case, they do serve a very useful purpose. They train the students to work with their hands in devising and setting up an experiment, making careful observations, critically analyzing the results and then drawing appropriate conclusions. These are the qualities that the students will depend on later in their clinical work. In fact, the ability to solve problems is the ultimate skill of the physician, and this ability will be honed if the above-mentioned qualities are suitably developed. A compromise can, however, be arrived at. The number of amphibian experiments to be done by the students themselves may be reduced while the rest are demonstrated to them in small groups by their tutors.

The chief aim of the book is to help the students in coping with the problems arising from the handling of various apparatuses during the practical work. If a student has a hazy notion of the purpose of an experiment and the correct technique of carrying it out, he/she will easily be disheartened and frustrated. We hope to help with a clear idea of what he/she is expected to do and a more definite plan of doing it.

It is a pleasure to acknowledge the valuable suggestions received from many friends and colleagues, especially Dr (Mrs) P Khetarpal, Dr (Mrs) Usha Nagpal, Dr Kanta Kumari, Dr RS Sidhu, Dr RS Sharma, Dr Ashok Kumar, Dr Parveen Gupta, Dr OP Mahajan, Dr S Mookerjee, Dr (Mrs) BK Maini, Dr SK Manchanda, Dr OP Tandon, Dr GM Shah, and Dr M Sayeed.

I must express my gratitude to my wife, Mrs Prem Ghai, for her understanding and unstinted support during the long months of collecting the material and the writing of the book.

I fail to find adequate words to thank my students who prompted and encouraged me in the first instance to write this book. We physiologists recognize the importance of the feedback systems of the body, and so too, is feedback essential for the development of a book. Criticism and suggestions from teachers and students for the further improvement of the book will be thankfully received and acknowledged.

I am indebted to Shri Jitendar P Vij (Chairman and Managing Director), M/s Jaypee Brothers Medical Publishers (P) Ltd, New Delhi, India, and his dedicated team, for their continued cooperation, enthusiasm and their excellent work in bringing out this book.

May this book act as an effective stimulus for the students to gain first-hand knowledge of experimental physiology, and ease their journey through a complex but fascinating science. As they gather experience, the path will become easier. The discipline of work will then become the most exciting and rewarding experience in their lives.

As they say, "When the going gets tough, the tough get going".

CL Ghai

Acknowledgments

First and foremost we would like to thank God, for giving us the power to believe in our passion and pursue our dreams. This could never have been possible without the faith we have in you, the Almighty.

We are deeply indebted to Dr Neha Jain, Assistant Professor, Physiology, World College of Medical Science and Research, Jhajjar, Haryana and Ex-Senior Resident, Department of Physiology, Maulana Azad Medical College (MAMC), New Delhi. This work would not have been possible without the continuous support and hard work provided by her.

Also, we extend our thanks to Dr Amina Sultan Zaidi, Assistant Professor, Department of Physiology, Hamdard Institute of Medical Sciences and Research (HIMSR), New Delhi and Ex-Senior Resident, Department of Physiology, MAMC, for extending assistance whenever required. Her innovative ideas helped in the betterment of the text. We are also thankful to Dr Aprajita Chaudhry, Ex-Assistant Professor, Department of Physiology, North DMC Medical College and Hindu Rao Hospital and Ex-Senior Resident, Department of Physiology, MAMC, for her help from time to time.

We are thankful to Mr Sunil Kumar, Ex Lab Attendant, Department of Physiology, MAMC, for his cooperation and active participation in the preparation of this manuscript.

Most importantly, we wish to thank all those who provided us unending inspiration...especially our students, who are our educators as well.

We are immensely appreciative to Shri Jitendar P Vij (Group Chairman) and Mr Ankit Vij (Managing Director) of M/s Jaypee Brothers Medical Publishers (P) Ltd, New Delhi, India, for believing in us and providing us with an opportunity to edit a book written by a renowned author. This was just like a big dream coming true. We are highly obliged to Mr MS Mani (Group President), Dr Madhu Choudhary (Director-Educational Publishing), Ms Pooja Bhandari (Production Head), Dr Sakshi Sanjeevani (Development Editor), Mr Rajesh Sharma (Production Coordinator), Ms Seema Dogra (Cover Visualizer), Mr Rahul Jadli (Proofreader), Mr Deepak Saxena (Typesetter), Mr Radhe Shyam (Graphic Designer), and all the staff of Jaypee Brothers Medical Publishers (P) Ltd, New Delhi, India.

Last but not least, we would like to thank our families. Nobody has been more important to us in the pursuit of this project than them. Their unending support has been immensely helpful in focusing on what has been an extremely enriching and fulfilling process.

Contents

Competency Table

Number	Competency The student should be able to:	Core (Y/N	Suggested Teaching Learning method	Suggested Assessment method	Chapter Number	Page Number
SECTION 1: Hematology						
PY2.11	Estimate Hb, RBC, TLC, RBC indices, DLC, Blood groups, BT/CT	Y	DOAP sessions	Practical/OSPE/ Viva voce	1.4, 1.5, 1.6, 1.7, 1.9, 1.10, 1.11	21, 27, 32, 40, 57, 60, 71
PY2.12	Describe test for ESR, Osmotic fragility, Hematocrit. Note the findings and interpret the test results, etc.	Y	Demonstration	Written/ Viva voce	1.8, 1.16	51, 90
PY2.13	Describe steps for reticulocyte and platelet count	Y	Demonstration sessions	Written/ Viva voce	1.12, 1.15	79, 88
SECTION 2: Human Experiments						
PY6.8	Demonstrate the correct technique to perform and interpret Spirometry	Y	DOAP sessions	Skill assessment/ Viva voce	2.2, 2.3	106, 115
PY11.14	Demonstrate basic life support in a simulated environment	Y	DOAP sessions	OSCE	2.4	119
PY5.16	Record arterial pulse tracing using finger plethysmography in a volunteer or simulated environment	N	DOAP sessions, Computer assisted learning methods	Practical/OSPE/ Viva voce	2.5	124
PY5.12	Record blood pressure and pulse at rest and in different grades of exercise and postures in a volunteer or simulated environment	Y	DOAP sessions	Practical/OSPE/ Viva voce	2.6, 2.7, 2.8	127, 137, 140
PY3.15	Demonstrate effect of mild, moderate and severe exercise and record changes in cardiorespiratory parameters	Y	DOAP sessions	Practical/OSPE/ Viva voce	2.8	140
PY5.13	Record and interpret normal ECG in a volunteer or simulated environment	Y	DOAP sessions	Practical/OSPE/ Viva voce	2.9	143
PY3.16	Demonstrate Harvard step test and describe the impact on induced physiologic parameters in a simulated environment	Y	DOAP sessions	Practical/OSPE/ Viva voce	2.10	151
PY10.20	Demonstrate (i) Testing of visual acuity, color and field of vision, and (ii) Hearing, (iii) Testing for smell, and (iv) Taste sensation in volunteer/simulated environment	Y	DOAP sessions	Skill assessment/ Viva voce	2.11, 2.13, 2.19, 2.20, 2.21, 2.22, 2.23, 2.24, 2.25	154, 158, 160, 163, 164, 169, 170, 171
PY10.12	Identify normal EEG forms	Y	Small group teaching	OSPE/Viva voce	2.26	172
PY9.9	Interpret a normal semen analysis report including (a) Sperm count, (b) Sperm morphology, and (c) Sperm motility, as per WHO guidelines and discuss the results	Y	Lecture, Small group discussion	OSPE/Viva voce	2.30	191

Contd...

Contd...

Number	Competency The student should be able to:	Core (Y/N	Suggested Teaching Learning method	Suggested Assessment method	Chapter Number	Page Number
PY9.10	Discuss the physiological basis of various pregnancy tests	Y	Lecture, Small group discussion	Written/ Viva voce	2.31	193
PY9.6	Enumerate the contraceptive methods for male and female. Discuss their advantages and disadvantages	Y	Lecture, Small group discussion	Written/ Viva voce	2.32	195
SECTION 3: Clinical Examination						
PY11.13	Obtain history and perform general examination in the volunteer / simulated environment	Y	DOAP sessions	Skill assessment/ Viva voce	3.1	199
PY6.9	Demonstrate the correct clinical examination of the respiratory system in a normal volunteer or simulated environment	Y	DOAP sessions	Skill assessment/ Viva voce/OSCE	3.2	203
PY5.15	Demonstrate the correct clinical examination of the cardiovascular system in a normal volunteer or simulated environment	Y	DOAP sessions	Practical/OSPE/ Viva voce	3.3	209
PY4.10	Demonstrate the correct clinical examination of the abdomen in a normal volunteer or simulated environment	Y	DOAP session	Skill assessment/ Viva voce/OSCE	3.4	214
PY10.11	Demonstrate the correct clinical examination of the nervous system: Higher functions, sensory system, motor system, reflexes, cranial nerves in a normal volunteer or simulated environment	Y	DOAP sessions	Skill assessment/ Viva voce/OSCE	3.5	218
SECTION 4: Experimental Physiology						
PY3.18	Observe with computer assisted learning (i) amphibian nerve—muscle experiments, (ii) amphibian cardiac experiments	Y	Demonstration, Computer assisted learning methods	Practical/ Viva voce	4.1–4.18	249–295

LIST OF PRACTICALS REQUIRING CERTIFICATION

Number	Competency The student should be able to:	Chapter Number	Page Number
PY5.12	Record pulse and blood pressure at rest in a volunteer	2.6	127
PY5.12	Record pulse and blood pressure in a volunteer in different grades of exercise.	2.8	140
PY5.12	Record pulse and blood pressure in a volunteer during change of posture	2.7	137
PY6.9	Demonstrate the correct clinical examination of respiratory system in a normal volunteer or simulated environment.	3.2	203
PY10.11	Demonstrate the correct clinical examination of higher function of nervous system in a normal volunteer or simulated environment.	3.5	218
PY10.11	Demonstrate the correct clinical examination of sensory system in a normal volunteer or simulated environment.	3.5	241
PY10.11	Demonstrate the correct clinical examination of motor system in a normal volunteer or simulated environment.	3.5	228

Contd...

Contd...

Number	Competency The student should be able to:	Chapter Number	Page Number
PY10.11	Demonstrate the correct clinical examination of reflexes in a normal volunteer or simulated environment.	3.5	233
PY10.11	Demonstrate the correct clinical examination of cranial nerves in a normal volunteer or simulated environment	3.5	219
PY10.20	Demonstrate the correct clinical examination of visual acuity, color and field of vision in a normal volunteer or simulated environment	2.11, 2.13, 2.19, 2.20	154, 158, 160, 163
PY10.20	Demonstrate hearing tests in a normal volunteer or simulated environment	2.21, 2.22, 2.23	164, 169, 169
PY10.20	Demonstrate test of smell in a normal volunteer or simulated environment	2.25	171
PY10.20	Demonstrate taste sensation in a normal volunteer or simulated environment	2.24	170

*OSCE:Objective Structured Clinical Examination
OSPE: Objective Structured Practical Examination
DOAP: Demonstrate, Observe, Assess, Perform.

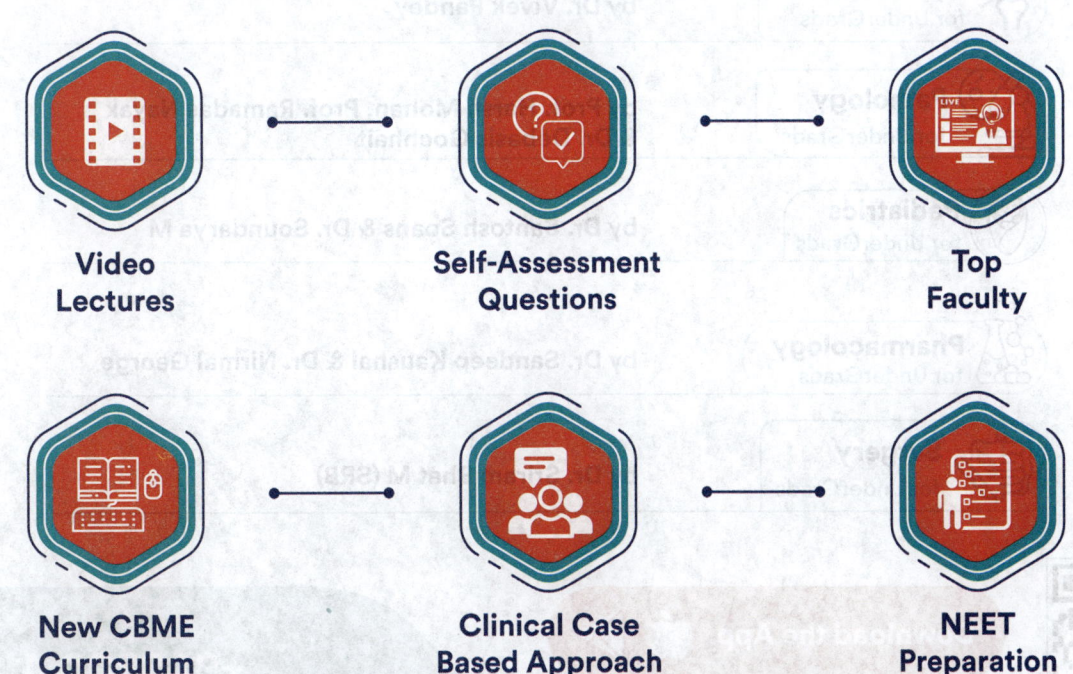

SECTION 1

Hematology

1.1: THE COMPOUND MICROSCOPE

STUDENT OBJECTIVES

After completing this experiment, the student should be able to:

- Name the different parts of the microscope and explain the functions of each.
- Explain the physical basis of microscopy and define the terms: magnification, resolution, and numerical aperture.
- Describe the mechanism of image formation and the type of image seen.
- Explain how to use low power (LP), high power (HP), oil immersion (OI) objective to obtain different magnifications.
- Describe the procedure (protocol) that must be followed every time while using a microscope.
- Name the precautions that must be observed during and after using the microscope.
- Explain the basic working of other types of microscopes.

INTRODUCTION

Antonie van Leeuwenhoek (1632–1723) was a Dutch tradesman and scientist, best known for his work on the development and improvement of the microscope and also for his subsequent contribution toward the study of microbiology.

The microscope is one of the most commonly used instruments in medical colleges and in clinical laboratories. Students of physiology use it in the study of morphology of blood cells and in counting their numbers. They will use it in histology, histopathology, and microbiology and later in various clinical disciplines.

Compound microscope: The compound microscope is so called because, in contrast to a single magnifying convex lens, it has two such lenses—the *objective* and the *eyepiece*. It magnifies the image of an object that is not visible to the naked eye to an extent where it can be seen clearly. The compound microscope can be *monocular* (has only one eyepiece **(Fig. 1A)**) or *binocular* (has two eyepieces to prevent eye strain) **(Fig. 1B)**.

Before using a microscope, the students must familiarize themselves with its different parts and how to use it and take its care. It will be discussed under the following heads:

- **Parts of the microscope**
  - The support system
  - The focusing system
  - The optical (magnifying) system
  - The illumination system.
- **Physical basis of microscopy**
  - Visual acuity
  - Resolving power
  - Magnification
  - Calculation of total magnification
  - Numerical aperture
  - Image formation
  - Working distance.
- **Protocol (procedure) for the use of microscope**
  - Focusing under low power (100x)
  - Focusing under high power (450x)
  - Focusing under oil immersion (1000x)
  - "Racking" the microscope.
- **Common difficulties faced by students**
- **Precautions and routine care**
- **Other types of microscopes.**

PARTS OF THE MICROSCOPE

The Support System

The support system acts as a framework to which various functional units are attached **(Fig. 2)**:

- **Base:** It is a heavy metallic, U-shaped or horseshoe shaped base or foot, which supports the microscope on the worktable to provide maximum stability.
- **Pillars:** Two upright pillars project up from the base and are attached to the C-shaped handle. The hinge joint allows the microscope to be tilted at a suitable angle for comfortable viewing.

> **Note:** The microscope is never tilted when counting cells in a chamber or when examining a blood film under oil immersion. It can be tilted for viewing histology slides.

- **Handle (the arm or limb):** The curved handle, which projects up from the hinge joint supports the focusing and magnifying systems.
- **Body tube:** Fitted at the upper end of the handle, either vertically or at an angle, the body tube is the part through which light passes to the eyepiece, thus conducting the image to the eye of the observer. It is 16–17 cm in length, and can be raised or lowered by the focusing system.
- **The stage:** It has two components: the **fixed stage** and the **mechanical stage.**
  - **Fixed stage:** It is a square platform with an aperture in its center, and fitted to the handle (limb) below the objective lenses. The slide is placed on it and centered over the aperture for viewing. The converging cone of light emerging from the condenser passes through the slide and the objective into the body tube.
  - **Mechanical stage:** It is a calibrated metal frame fitted on the right edge of the fixed stage. There is a spring-mounted clip to hold the slide or counting chamber in position while two screw heads move it from side to side and forward and backward. The vernier scale on the frame indicates the degree of movement. In

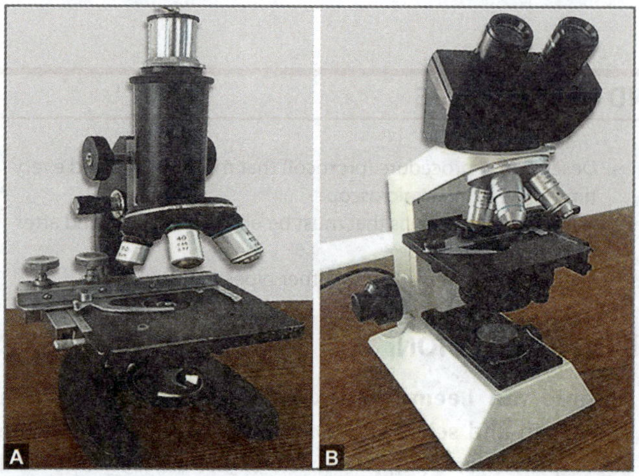

FIGS. 1A AND B: (A) Monocular microscope; (B) Binocular microscope.

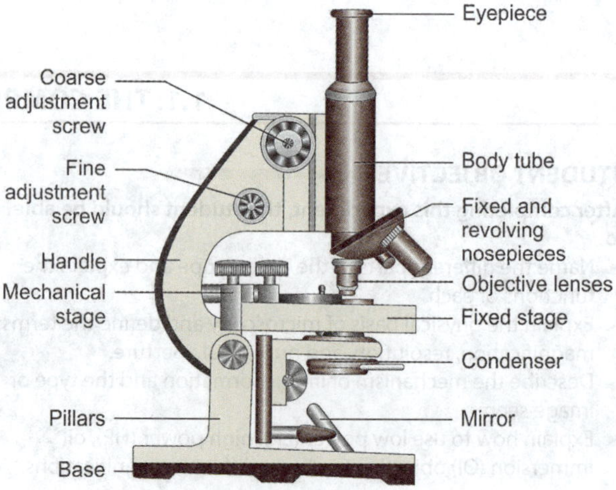

FIG. 2: Compound microscope.

some microscopes, the screw heads are mounted on a common spindle under the fixed stage.

Note: In some sophisticated and binocular microscopes, the entire stage, fixed and mechanical, can be raised or lowered (the aim in all microscopes is to bring the material under study and an objective lens at the proper working distance).

The Focusing System

The focusing system consists of **coarse** and **fine** adjustment screw heads. It is employed for raising or lowering the optical system with reference to the slide under study till it comes into focus. Thus, the adjustments place an objective lens at its optimal working distance, i.e. its focal length.

There are two coarse and two fine adjustment screws working on a double-sided micrometer mechanism, one pair (one coarse and one fine) on either side. If one coarse (or fine) adjustment is turned, its partner on the other side also rotates at the same time. It is, therefore, not sensible to use both hands on the coarse or the fine screws simultaneously.

The **coarse adjustment** moves the optical system up or down rapidly through a large distance via a rack and pinion arrangement. The **fine adjustment** works in the same way but several rotations of the screwhead are required to move the tube through a small distance, e.g. one rotation moves the tube by 0.1 mm or less. The fine adjustment is usually graduated in 1/50th of 0.1 mm, where each division corresponds to a movement of 0.002 mm of the tube. It is employed for accurate focusing.

Note: The left hand is used both for coarse and for fine focusing, while the right hand is used for the mechanical stage to move the slide in various directions. The student is advised to get into the habit of using the hands simultaneously for different purposes.

The Optical (Magnifying) System

The optical system consists of the body tube, the eyepiece, and the nosepiece that carries the objectives. It can be raised or lowered as desired.

- **The body tube:** The distance between the upper ends of the objectives and the eyepiece is called the tube length, which is 16–17 cm. The distance between the upper focal point of the eyepiece and the lower focal point of the objective is called **the optical tube length,** which is about 25 cm (A × 10 lens will produce an image 10 times the diameter of the object as it naturally appears when held at 25 cm from the eye).
- **The eyepiece:** The eyepiece fits into the top of the body tube. Most microscopes are provided with 5x, 8x, and 10x eyepieces, though 6x and 15x are also available. Each eyepiece has two lenses—one mounted at the top, the **"eye lens",** and the other, the **"field lens"** is fitted at the bottom. The field lens collects the divergent rays of the primary image and passes these to the eye lens, which further magnifies the image.

Note: The height of the eyepiece, when taken out of the body tube, is also variable. The 5x eyepiece is tallest, while 10x is shortest. A "pointer" eyepiece has a small pin mounted in it which is used to point out a particular cell or object in a field. A "demonstration" eyepiece, in which a teacher and a student can look through separate eyepieces mounted on a horizontal barrel, is a useful device (a short piece of hair gummed on the inside next to the eye lens can serve as a pointer).

- **The nosepiece:** It is fitted at the lower end of the body tube and has two parts: the **fixed** nosepiece, and the **revolving** nosepiece. The latter carries interchangeable objective lenses. Any lens can be rotated into position when desired, its correct position being indicated by a "click".
- **Objective lenses (also called objectives or simply "lenses"):** Three spring-loaded objectives of varying magnifying powers are usually provided with the student microscope. In some cases, there is a place provided for a "scanning" lens as well. Each objective has a cover glass which forms its outer covering and protects it. Though each lens can be unscrewed for cleaning, the students are not supposed to remove them.

Note: "x" is the sign of multiplication. The magnifying power of each objective, as that of the eyepiece, is etched on it.

The objective lenses (Fig. 3) are:

- **Low power (LP) objective (10x):** The LP objective in common use magnifies 10 times. It is used for initial focusing and viewing a large area of the specimen slide. The numerical aperture (NA) of this lens is always less than that of the condenser in most microscopes. In order to achieve focus, therefore, the NA has got to be closely matched by reducing the light reaching the specimen under study. This is achieved by lowering the condenser to the lowest position and by slightly opening the iris diaphragm.
- **High power (HP) objective (40x):** This lens magnifies the image 40 times. Because of its higher magnification, it is used for more detailed study of the material before switching to an oil immersion lens. The NA of HP lens is almost equal to, or slightly less than that of commonly used condenser. Therefore, the condenser has to be slightly

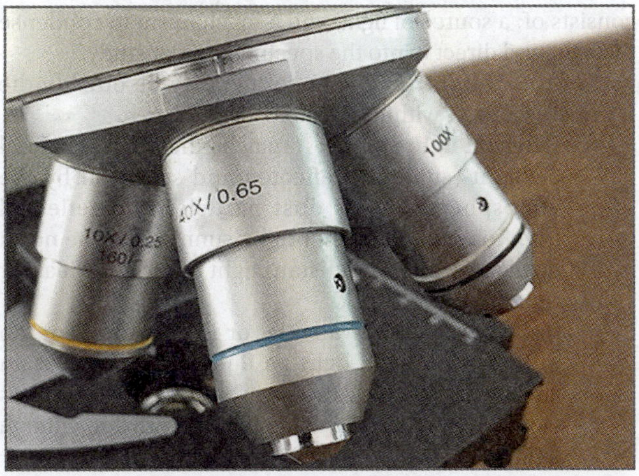

FIG. 3: Objective lenses.

Table 1: Important features of compound microscope.

Objective lens	*Numerical aperture*	*Mirror (simple microscope)*	*Position of condenser*	*Iris diaphragm*
Low power (LP) (10x)	0.25	Concave	Lowest position	Slightly open
High power (HP) (40x)	0.65	Concave	Midway	Half open
Oil immersion (OI) (100x)	1.25	Plane	Highest position	Fully open

raised midway and the iris diaphragm is also opened half to get more light and maximum clarity in focusing.

- **Oil immersion (OI) objective (100x):** The OI lens magnifies the image 100 times. Since the lens almost touches the slide, it has to be immersed in a special medium (most commonly cedar wood oil), a drop of which is first placed on the slide. The oil is used to increase the NA and thus the resolving power of the objective. Since the NA of the OI objective is always greater than that of the condenser. Thus the condenser has to be raised to its highest position and iris diaphragm should be fully opened. As this lens gives (with an eyepiece of 10x) a total magnification of 1,000 times, it is employed for detailed study of the morphology of blood cells and tissues **(Table 1)**.

Parfocal system: The objectives these days are so constructed that when one lens (LP, for example) is in focus, the others are more or less in focus. Thus switching from one lens to another (e.g. from LP to HP) requires only a little turn of fine adjustment to bring the image into sharp focus. This arrangement of lenses is called "parfocal system."

The Illumination System

No microscope can function optimally unless proper illumination (lighting) is provided. All the light that will reach the eye should come from the specimen under study. Light from any other part of the slide will tend to obscure the details. Such extra (extraneous) light is called glare. The illumination system must, therefore, provide uniform, soft, and bright illumination of the entire field of view. Two factors are involved in providing such uniform illumination:

- The construction and position of the condenser.
- The size of the iris diaphragm.

The **illumination system** of the bright-field microscope consists of: a source of light, and a mechanism to condense the light and direct it into the specimen under study.

- **Source of light:** The light source may be outside the microscope or within the microscope.
    - **External light source:** It may be the diffuse, natural daylight (sunlight) reflected and scattered by the atmosphere and its dust particles and reflected from the buildings. On bright, sunny days, the north daylight, which is a distant light source, is ideal for routine student work.
      If daylight is not available, or is not sufficient, an artificial source of light—a fluorescent tube, or an electric lamp housed in a lamp box with a frosted glass window, fitted on the worktable can provide enough light.
    - **Internal light source:** In most microscopes, there is a provision to remove the mirror and fit an electric microscope lamp in its place. This unit has frosted tungsten lamp to provide uniform white light.
- **The mirror:** A double-sided mirror, in fact two mirrors, one flat or planc and the other concave, fitted back to back in a metal frame is located below the condenser; it can be rotated in all directions.
    - The plane mirror is used with a distant source of light (natural, or daylight). The parallel rays of light are reflected parallel into the condenser.
    - The concave mirror, on the other hand, is employed when the light source is near the microscope. The divergent rays of light are reflected as parallel rays and directed into the condenser.
- **The condenser ("Substage" or "substage condenser"):** The condenser is a system of lenses fitted in a short cylinder that is mounted below the stage. It can be raised or lowered by a rack and pinion, and focuses the light rays into a solid cone of light onto the material under study. It also helps in resolving the image.
    - **The lens system:** The commonly used substage is Abbe-type condenser. It is composed of two lenses which should be corrected for spherical and chromatic aberrations.
      Since the condenser is a lens system, it has a fixed NA, which should be equal or less than that of the objective being used. Raising or lowering the condenser can vary its NA. And with the axes of the two being the same, all the light passing through the condenser is collected by the objective, thus allowing maximum clarity.

Note: It is clear from the above that the position of the condenser must always be adjusted with each objective to get best focus of light and resolving power of the microscope.

- **The iris diaphragm:** It is fitted within the condenser. A small lever on the side can adjust the size of the aperture of the diaphragm, thus allowing more or less light falling on the material under study. Reducing the size of the field of view (i.e. by narrowing the aperture) decreases the NA of the condenser. Thus, proper illumination includes a combination of position of light source, regulation of light intensity, position of condenser, and regulation of the size of field of view.
- **Filter:** A metal ring can accommodate a pale blue or green filter since monochromatic light is ideal for microscopy.

Generally, when viewing clear preparations under low power, we need less light, but more illumination is required when studying stained preparations under oil immersion lens.

PHYSICAL BASIS OF MICROSCOPY

Visual Acuity

The term visual acuity (VA) refers to the ability of the eye to resolve or recognize two very closely situated points of light or lines, which are not touching, as separate from each other rather than one. If the distance between the two points is less than a certain value, the two points are not resolved but appear as one (see Experiment 2.19 for details).

Resolving Power (Resolution)

The utility of a microscope depends not only on its magnifying power but also on its power of resolution, i.e. its ability to show closely located structures as separate and distinct from each other. This translates into the ability to improve the details of structures within a cell.

Generally, the resolving power of the unaided human eye is said to be between 0.15 mm and 0.25 mm. The resolving power of a lens depends on its NA as well as the wavelength of light. With the light microscope and OI lens of 100x, and NA of 1.30, its resolving power is about 0.25 µm (2,500 Angstroms) with white light, and about 0.19 µm with monochromatic green light (shortest wavelength: 5.5×10^{-5} cm). The electron microscope, however, gives very high magnifications and can separate dots that are about 0.5 nm apart or even less.

Note: 1 nanometer (nm) = 0.001 micrometer (µm) = 0.000001 mm

The resolving power of a microscope is expressed in terms of ***limit of resolution (LR),*** or the minimum separable distance. If this distance is less than LR, the two points appear as one. The formula for determining LR is: $LR = 0.61 \times W/NA$, where W = wavelength of light being used, and NA = the numerical aperture of the objective in use.

Magnification

In order to see clearly and distinctly, the details and contours of closely-located structures (say in a cell), and their image has to be magnified many times. How this is achieved is explained below.

Calculation of Total Magnification

Since the objective and eyepiece both magnify the image, it is easy to calculate the total magnification of any combination of objective lens and eyepiece. For example, with an eyepiece of 10x, the magnifications with the three objectives will be:

Low power objective (10x) = 10 × 10 = 100 times.
High power objective (45x) = 45 × 10 = 450 times.
Oil immersion objective (100x) = 100 × 10 = 1000 times.

Numerical Aperture

A powerful lens is made of glass of high refractive index, has a short focal length, and a small diameter. The small diameter allows only the central cone of light to pass through without getting too much refracted, while the peripheral rays that would be refracted more are cut off.

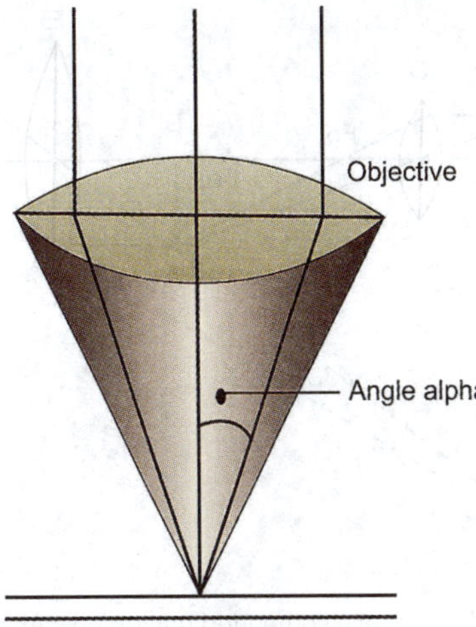

FIG. 4: Diagram to explain the numerical aperture. The angle alpha is shown.

The value "n sine alpha"—where "n" is the refractive index of glass, and "alpha" the angle subtended by it at the object is called the **numerical aperture,** as shown in **Figure 4**. Thus, the NA of a lens, which is an index of its power of resolution, is the ratio of its diameter to its focal length. As the NA increases, the resolving power of the lens increases.

The NA is also an index of light gathering power of a lens, i.e. the amount of light entering the objective. The NA can be decreased by decreasing the amount of light passing through the lens. Thus, as shown below, the illumination has to increase as the objectives are changed from LP to HP to OI. The magnifying power of each lens and its NA rather than its focal length, are etched on each objective lens.

- **Low power objective (10x; NA = 0.25; focal length = 16 mm)**
- **High power objective (40x; NA = 0.65; focal length = 4 mm)**
- **Oil immersion objective (100x; NA = 1.30; focal length = 2 mm).**

Image Formation in the Compound Microscope

It is the objective that starts the process of magnification. It forms a real, inverted, and enlarged image (primary image: A'-B') **(Fig. 5)** in the upper part of the body tube (A real image is that which can be received on screen). The field lens of the eyepiece collects the divergent rays of light of the primary image and passes these through the eye lens, which therefore the image seen by the eye is—virtual, inverted, and magnified, and appears to be further magnified the image. The light rays reaching the observer's eye are divergent and about 25 cm in front of the eye. **Figure 5** shows the ray diagram of a compound microscope.

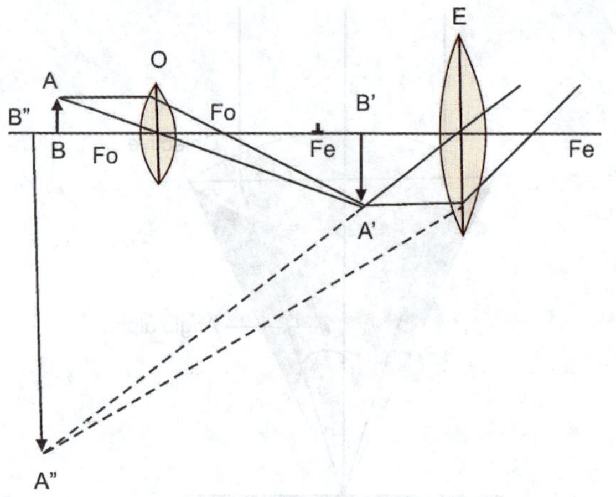

FIG. 5: The ray diagram of a compound microscope. AB = object; A' B' = real, inverted, magnified image; A" B" = virtual, inverted, magnified image; O = objective lens; E = eyepiece; Fo = focus of objective; Fe = focus of eyepiece.

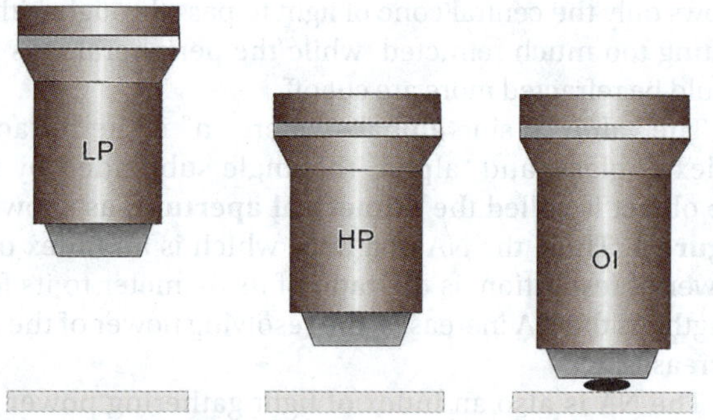

FIG. 6: Diagram to show the working distances of low power (LP), high power (HP) and oil immersion (OI) lenses.

Working Distance

The working distance is the distance between the objective and the slide under study. This distance decreases with increasing magnification. It is 8–13 mm in LP, 1–3 mm in HP, and 0.5–1.5 mm in OI lenses, respectively. **Figure 6** shows the approximate working distances for each lens. Note that the OI lens has to be immersed in a drop of oil.

PROTOCOL/PROCEDURES FOLLOWED WHILE USING THE MICROSCOPE

Principle

A focused beam of light passes through the material under study into the microscope. Parts of the specimen that are optically dense and having a high refractive index or are colored with a stain (dye), cast a potential shadow which is magnified in two main stages as it passes into the observer's eye.

Procedure

The student must avoid the bad habit of using objective lenses in a haphazard manner, starting with any lens at random and then switching over to another. A brief protocol (procedure) for using a microscope is given below:

Note:

1. Students using glasses should put on their glasses while using the microscope.
2. Although you will be using one eye with the monocular microscope, do not close the other eye as this will cause lot of strain on that eye. Practice keeping both the eyes open and, with practice, you will be able to ignore the unwanted image, and continue working for long hours.
3. Adjust adequate illumination to improve the contrast, according to the objective lens used.
4. After this step, the slide is viewed under low magnification to get a general view all over. One can then choose an area of interest for viewing it under higher magnifications.
5. First use the coarse adjustment screw to focus the slide till the object has become visible.
6. Do not use the fine focus screw until the object has become visible and brought into focus using the coarse adjustment screws.
7. Then use the fine adjustment to obtain the exact focus.
8. Use xylene swab to clean the objectives after using the microscope.

Important: A proper illumination of the specimen slide is very essential. However, the students often forget about its importance. The broad rule about illumination is described in **Table 2.**

This rule is not rigidly fixed. Depending on the source and strength of light, the condenser position and diaphragm size have to be combined to get optimal illumination.

Focusing Under Low Power

- Place the microscope on your worktable in an upright position, and raise the body tube 7–8 cm above the stage. Put the slide on the stage and, using the mechanical stage, bring the specimen over the central aperture.
- Select and adjust the mirror (plane or concave) so that the light shines on the specimen.
- **Under low power before focusing the object, the condenser is brought to the lowest position and the iris diaphragm is slightly opened to cut down excess light.**
- Looking from the side, and using the coarse adjustment, bring the body tube down so that the LP lens is about 1 cm above the slide. Now look into the eyepiece and gently raise the tube till the specimen comes into focus. But if it does not, i.e. if you have missed the focusing position, repeat the whole procedure. When the image comes into focus, scans the entire field, racking the fine adjustment all the time.

Caution: Do not bring the body tube down from any height while looking into the microscope. You might miss the focusing position and continue moving it down thereby breaking the slide or permanently scratching the objective lens.

Table 2: Characterization of illumination.

Objective	*Condenser position*	*Iris diaphragm*
Low power (10x)	Low	Partly open
High power (45x)	Midway	Half open
Oil immersion (100x)	High	Fully open

Focusing Under High Power

- For focusing under high magnification, simply rotate the nosepiece so that the HP lens clicks into position.
- **The condenser has to be slightly raised midway and the iris diaphragm is also opened half to get more light and maximum clarity in focusing:** Use fine adjustment as required.
- If the lens system is not parfocal, look from the side and bring the lens down to about 1–2 mm above the slide. Now look into the microscope and raise the tube slowly and gently till the image comes into focus.

Focusing Under Oil Immersion

This objective is the most frequently used in hematology because of its high magnification and resolution (It can also be used for mounted histology and pathology slides). *The two features of this objective are its very small aperture through which light enters it, and its deep focusing position that is about 1 mm from the slide.*

- The condenser has to be raised to its highest position and iris diaphragm should be fully opened.
- **Oil immersion lens is immersed in oil:** There is a thin layer of air between this objective and the glass slide when the lens is in focus (without the oil the image can be seen but it is very faint and blurred). When light passes from a denser medium (glass of the slide) into a rarer medium (the thin layer of air), they are refracted away from the normal. As a result, when light rays emerge from the slide, many of them are refracted away from the aperture of the objective and very few enter it, and a faint image results. Cedar wood oil, which has the same refractive index as that of glass, i.e. 1.55 (air = 1.00; water = 1.33), removes this layer of air so that the glass of the slide and the objective lens become a continuous column (thus avoiding refraction) and allow enough light to enter the objective. **Other mediums that can be used are glycerin and paraffin, their refractive index being 1.35–1.40. However, cedar wood oil, though costly, gives best results.**
- Raise the body tube so that the OI lens is about 8–10 cm above the slide. Place a drop of cedar wood oil on the slide, and looking from the side, slowly bring the objective down till it just enters the oil drop. The oil will spread out in the capillary space between the slide and the lens (thus effectively removing the thin layer of air).
- While looking into the eyepiece, slowly and very carefully raise the objective with coarse adjustment (without taking it out of the oil) till the cells come into view (if no cells are seen, repeat the whole process). Use the fine adjustment for fine tuning. When you move the slide, the oil will move with it. It is therefore a bad habit to cover the entire slide with oil to begin with.

"Racking the Microscope"

The cells and their constituents are three-dimensional structures and lie at different levels. Therefore, it is important not to keep a fixed focus but **to continuously "rack" the microscope** by using fine adjustment after the specimen has been brought under focus under any magnification. By turning the fine adjustment screw this way and that, various structures come into and go out of focus alternately.

COMMON DIFFICULTIES ENCOUNTERED BY STUDENTS

The beginner is likely to face some difficulties when starting to use the microscope for the first time, but these can be minimized if the procedures are strictly followed and proper precautions taken. Some common problems are:

- **The material cannot be focused or the image is very faint:**
  - The slide may not be near the focus of the objective, or there may be no visible material under it (e.g. part of the blood film may be missing from this area). Check this out and start with coarse adjustment once again.
  - The slide bearing the material may have been placed upside down on the stage, a common mistake made by the students with a blood film. The thickness of the glass slide does not allow the OI lens to reach down to its working distance. Reversing the slide will solve the problem.
  - If focusing is achieved with LP and HP lenses but not with OI lens despite all efforts, the lens may have been damaged earlier. Seek the help of your tutor.
- **There may be a dark shadow in the field:** If the shadow rotates when the eyepiece is rotated, remove it and clean it. Or there may be an air bubble in the cedar wood oil.
- **The field of view appears oval instead of round:** This problem arises when the objective has not been properly "clicked" into position.
- **The illumination of the image is poor:** Check the source of light, angle of the mirror, the position of the condenser, and iris diaphragm.
- **The image does not come into focus even when the objective is in the lowest position and the fine adjustment cannot move down any further:** This happens when the fine adjustment screw reaches the end of its thread (turn) before the image is brought to its focus. To overcome this problem, turn the adjustment screw in the opposite direction for several turns and then use the coarse adjustment screw to regain the focus once again (it is, therefore, best to keep the fine adjustment screw near the middle of its turning range).

PRECAUTIONS

1. Select a stool or chair of suitable height so that your eyes are at a level slightly above the eyepiece. This will ensure comfortable working for long periods.
2. Ensure that all the lenses are clean and free from dust and smudges. Do not touch them with your fingers, nor blow on them to remove dust.
3. Check the position of the objective, condenser, and diaphragm, to ensure optimal illumination.
4. Never lower any objective from any height while looking into the microscope.

5. Once a specimen has been focused, continuously "rack" the microscope.
6. Cleaning the microscope. Never leave cedar wood oil on the OI lens, because it may seep into the body of the objective and damage the lens permanently. Dried oil is difficult to remove. Remove oil with lens paper and then use xylene to clean the lens.
7. Cover the microscope with the plastic cover after use.

OTHER TYPES OF MICROSCOPES

Various types of microscopes have been especially introduced for particular purposes over the past many decades. They differ from the compound "bright-field" microscope in fundamental ways by employing different illumination and image-formation systems. Some of these are:

1. **Dissection microscope:** It is a binocular microscope used for microdissection under magnification.
2. **Dark-field microscope:** It employs a special condenser that causes light waves to cross on the material under study rather than passing through it. As a result, the field of view appears dark (hence called "dark-field" in contrast to "bright-field" microscopy) against which the object appears bright. It is used in microbiology to study spirochetes.
3. **Phase-contrast microscope:** Since the living cells are mostly transparent, they must be stained with vital stains, or they must be first fixed in alcohol and then stained with acid or basic dyes before they can be viewed under the microscope. In this microscope, a special phase plate is inserted into the condenser, which can retard the speed of some light waves. Since the tissue cells and organisms have different refractive indices, this microscope uses these differences to produce an image with good contrast of light and shade. Thus, unstained wet preparations can be studied (e.g. platelets). The interference microscope is based on similar principle.
4. **Interference-contrast microscope:** A special prism that can split a beam of light is added to the condenser. The two split beams are then polarized, but only one resultant beam passes through the specimen under study while the other (reference beam) does not. The two beams are then recombined to produce a three-dimensional image.
5. **Polarizing microscope:** It has a polarizer (filter), which is usually placed between the light source and the specimen, and an analyzer, which is located between the objective and the eyepiece. Such a system is used to study tissues that have the property of birefringence (e.g. muscle fibers).
6. **Fluorescence microscope:** A fluorescent dye is used to stain tissues which are then studied under this microscope.
7. **Transmission electron microscope (TEM):** Invented by Knoll and Ruska in 1940, the TEM uses a strong beam of electrons instead of light and electromagnetic fields in place of glass lenses. The electrons produce a wavelength of about 0.05 Å, and provide a practical resolution of about 5 Å (theoretically possible resolution is about 1 Å). The magnified image, which is visible on a fluorescent screen, can be recorded on a photographic film, and the negative further enlarged 6–8 times. Thus, the total magnification obtained can vary from one to several hundred thousand times.
8. **Scanning electron microscope (SEM):** This microscope, which achieves a resolution of about 30 Å, has been developed for three-dimensional study of surface topography of cells and object. Though similar to TEM, the SEM employs a different technique.

OBJECTIVE STRUCTURED PRACTICAL EXAMINATION

Aim: To focus a given slide of blood film under LP/HP/OI lens.

Procedural steps: See text above.

Checklist:

1. Raise the body tube, put the slide on the stage, and use mechanical stage to bring the object over the central aperture.
2. Choose the light source and correctly bring the objective lens into position:
   i. LP ii. HP iii. OI
3. Adjust the position of the condenser and iris diaphragm for:
   i. LP ii. HP iii. OI
4. Look from the side while lowering the body tube.
5. Adjust the light and use coarse and fine adjustment screws.
6. Rack the microscope constantly.

QUESTIONS

Q.1. Why is the microscope called a compound microscope? What type of image is produced by it?

A single convex lens works like a simple microscope. In the student microscope, there are two lens systems—the objective and the eyepiece which take part in the formation of the image—hence the term compound in contrast to simple. The image seen by the eye is a virtual, inverted and magnified image produced by the eyepiece from the real, inverted and magnified image (primary image) produced by the objective lens.

Q.2. When is a plane mirror used and when concave?

See text above.

Q.3. What is the total magnification and how will you calculate?

The total magnification obtained at any time depends on the combination of the objective and the eyepiece being used (See text above).

Q.4. What is meant by the term numerical aperture? What is its significance?

See text above.

Q.5. (a) How will you identify an oil-immersion objective lens? (b) Why is cedar wood oil used with this lens and not with others?

(a) It is identified by the magnification imprinted on the objective (100x). OI has a black rim around its lower end.
(b) See text above.

Q.6. Will you see any image with the oil immersion lens without the cedar wood oil?

The image will be visible but will be very faint because of the layer of air present between the slide and the lens. Removal of this air by the cedar wood oil clarifies the image.

Q.7. Why does the oil immersion lens have a pinhole sized aperture?

The aperture being very small, it allows only the central cone of light to pass through and form the image. Had the diameter been large, excessive refraction would have caused spherical and chromatic aberrations, thus making the image indistinct.

Q.8. Why should the position of the condenser be low with the LP lens and highest with oil immersion lens?

Since the aperture of the LP lens is wide, a high condenser would allow too much light to enter the microscope and cause glare. The position of the condenser with the oil immersion lens has to be highest to allow enough light to enter it through its pin-hole aperture.

Q.9. Why are different degrees of illumination required when using a microscope and why?

The clarity of an image depends on an optimal (ideal) amount of light available. The illumination (the process of providing light) can be altered by raising or lowering the condenser and opening or closing the diaphragm. A proper combination of the two has to be selected under different conditions. In general, we require less illumination when viewing a clear, unstained object, and greater illumination when viewing a stained preparation.

Q.10. What is meant by racking the microscope and what is its importance?

Since the cells and their components are three-dimensional entities, and situated at different levels, the focus has to be constantly changed to see all these structures.

Q.11. What are the other types of microscopes?

See text above

1.2: EXPERIMENTS ON BLOOD

STUDENT OBJECTIVES

After completing this experiment, the student should be able to:

- Explain what is a blood sample, what are its sources and what are its main constituents?
- Describe the purpose of collecting a blood sample.
- Indicate how to attain and maintain asepsis when collecting a blood sample.
- Collect capillary blood from a finger prick, heel-prick, and earlobe prick, and precautions to be taken during a skin-prick.
- Indicate the steps for obtaining a blood sample by venipuncture.
- Name the various anticoagulants employed in hematological studies and their mode of action.
- Provide samples of plasma and serum.

INTRODUCTION

Since blood is confined within the cardiovascular system, the skin has to be punctured before blood can be obtained. There are two common sources of blood for routine laboratory tests: ***blood from a superficial vein*** by puncturing it with a needle and syringe, or ***from skin capillaries*** by skin-prick. Arterial blood may be required for special tests. None of these samples can be called a representative sample because there are minor variations in their composition. But for routine hematological tests, however, these differences can safely be ignored.

- **Asepsis**
  - Sterilization of equipment
  - Cleaning/sterilizing of skin
  - Prevention of contamination.
- **Collection of blood sample**
  - Selection of site of puncture—capillary/venous blood
    - Containers for blood samples
    - Collection of blood samples.
- **Commonly used anticoagulants.**

ASEPSIS

The term asepsis refers to the condition of being free from septic or infectious material—bacteria, viruses, etc. The skin is a formidable barrier to the entry of foreign invaders and the first line of defense against bacteria and other disease-causing microorganisms which are present in abundance on the skin and in the air. Therefore, puncturing the skin always poses the danger of infection. In order to achieve asepsis, the following aspects need to be kept in mind.

Sterilization of Equipment

All the instruments to be used for collecting blood— syringes, needles, lancets, and cotton and gauze swabs— should preferably be sterilized in an autoclave. The old practice of boiling glass syringes and needles in tap water is now obsolete. Irradiated and sealed, single-use syringes, needles, lancets and blades are now freely available and are in common use.

Cleaning/Sterilization of Skin

Though it is impossible to completely sterilize the selected site for skin puncture, every aseptic precaution must be exercised. The selected area need not be washed and scrubbed unless grossly dirty. If washed, the area should be allowed to dry before applying the antiseptics because these agents do not act well on wet skin. At least 2–3 sterile cotton/gauze swabs soaked in 70% alcohol, methylated spirit, or ether should be used to clean and scrub the area. Cotton swabs are likely to leave fibers sticking to the skin and provide an undesirable contact, or they may appear as artifacts in a blood film. But if they are used, the final cleaning should be done with a gauze swab.

Note: After cleaning the skin, allow the alcohol to dry by evaporation (do not blow on it), because sterilization with alcohol is effective only after it has dried.

Prevention of Contamination

Any material used for skin puncture, or the operator's hands may cause contamination. Therefore, once the site has been cleaned and dried, it should not be touched again. Care must be taken to prevent contamination until the puncture wound has effectively closed/healed.

Physical Characteristics of Blood

Blood is a complex connective tissue in which living blood cells and the formed elements are suspended, which transports substances from one part of the body to another.

The various physical characteristics are as follows:

- *Color*: Depending on the amount of oxygen it is carrying, the color of blood varies from scarlet (oxygen-rich) to a dull red (oxygen-poor).
- *Viscosity*: Blood is about five times thicker or more viscous than water, largely because of its formed elements.
- *Specific gravity:* 3.5–5.4 times that of water
- *pH*: Blood is slightly alkaline, with a pH between 7.35 and 7.45.

Blood volume refers to the total amount of fluid circulating within the arteries, capillaries, veins, venules, and chambers of the heart at any time. The total blood volume is around 5–6 L, i.e 8% of body weight (assuming 70 kg as average body weight of a normal adult).

Composition of Blood

Blood consists of:

- Formed elements which account for 45%: These include red blood cells (erythrocytes), white blood cells (leukocytes) and platelets.
- Plasma makes up 55%: The fluid portion of blood is called plasma, which contains different types of proteins and other soluble molecules. It is approximately 91% water and 9% solids. It is the clear straw coloured portion of the blood and represents 5% of body weight.

COLLECTION OF BLOOD SAMPLE

The term "blood sample" refers to the small amount of blood—a few drops or a few milliliters—obtained from a person for the purpose of testing or investigations. These tests are carried out for aiding in diagnosis and/or prognosis of the disease or disorder.

Selection of Site for Skin Prick

Sources and Amount of Blood Sample

1. **Capillary blood:** The skin and other tissues are richly supplied with capillaries, so when a drop or a few drops of blood are required, as for estimation of Hb, cell counts, bleeding time (BT) and CT, blood films, microchemical tests, etc., blood from a skin puncture (skin-prick) with a lancet or needle is adequate. Capillary blood is also called **"peripheral blood"** as it comes out of the peripheral vessels (capillaries) in contrast to venous blood **(Table 3)**.

Table 3: Differences between venous and capillary blood.

Venous blood	*Capillary blood*
It is obtained from a superficial vein by venepuncture	It is obtained from a skin puncture, usually over a finger, ear lobe/or the heel of a foot
A clean venipuncture provides blood without any contamination with tissue fluid	Blood from a skin prick comes from punctured capillaries and from smallest arterioles and venules
There is less risk of contamination since sterile syringe and needle are used	There is greater risk of contamination and transmission of disease as one may be careless about sterilization since skin prick is considered a harmless procedure
Cell counts, Hb, and PCV values are generally higher	These values are likely to be on the lower side since some tissue fluid is bound to dilute the blood even when it is free-flowing
Venous blood is preferable when normal blood standards are to be established, or when two samples from the same person are to be compared at different times	Capillary blood is not suitable for these purposes

In adults and older children, capillary blood is generally obtained from a skin puncture made on the tip of the middle or ring finger, or on the lobe of the ear. In infants and young children in whom the fingers are too small for a prick, the medial or lateral side of the pad of the big toe or heel is used. The site for skin-prick should be clean and free from edema, infection, skin disease, callus, or circulatory defects.

2. **Venous blood:** When larger amounts (say, a few milliliters that cannot be obtained from a skin puncture) are needed for complete hematological and biochemical investigations, venous blood is obtained with a syringe and needle by puncturing a superficial vein. In infants, venous blood may have to be taken from the femoral vein, or the frontal venous sinus.

Note: Venous blood is always preferred for clinical tests.

3. **Arterial blood:** When arterial blood is needed for special tests such as blood pH, gas levels, etc., an artery such as radial or femoral is punctured with a syringe and needle. This, however, is not a routine procedure.
4. **Cardiac catheterization:** Blood from a heart chamber, taken through a cardiac catheter, may be required for special tests. Such local sampling offers a unique way of assessing the local cardiac milieu, this may prove useful in the monitoring of both local/systemic drug therapies and interventional technologies.

Containers for Blood Sample

A container is a receptacle into which blood is transferred from the syringe before sending it to the laboratory. Clean and dry 10 mL glass test tubes, collection bottles such as clean and dry 10 mL discarded medicine vials, glass bulbs, etc., are the usual ones in use. A container may or may not contain an anticoagulant depending on whether a sample of blood/plasma, or serum is required.

For a sample of whole blood or plasma: The blood is transferred to a container containing a suitable anticoagulant. This is to prevent clotting of blood.

For a sample of serum: No anticoagulant is used. The blood is allowed to clot in the container and serum is collected. Obviously, capillary blood does not require a container or anticoagulant.

Collection of Blood Samples

Collection of Capillary Blood (Skin-prick Method)

A single bold prick is given on the finger under aseptic conditions (**Fig. 7**). **Never squeeze the pricked finger** as this will expel tissue fluid along with blood to come out of the puncture site. The dilution of blood will, thus, nullify the results. *Hence for clinical work, venous blood is always preferred.* Skin-prick may be used on the bedside of a patient, or in an emergency when it is not convenient to take a venous sample.

Note: The thumb and little finger are never pricked because the underlying palmar fascia (venous bursae) from these digits are continuous with those of the forearms. Any accidental injury to these fasciae may cause the infection to spread into the forearm. Thus finger prick is given on the distal digit on the palmar surface of the 3rd/4th finger.

Remember that one deep puncture, which will give you free flowing blood, is less painful than 3 or 4 superficial pricks.

Apparatus

- **Blood lancet/pricking needle:** Disposable, sterile, one-time use, blood lancets (flat, thin metal pieces with 3–4 mm deep penetrating sharp points) are commercially available and should be preferred.

  Ordinary, narrow-bore **injection needles** are useless since they only make shallow cuts rather than deep punctures. However, wide-bore (22 gauge) needles may be used in an emergency or if blood lancets are not available.

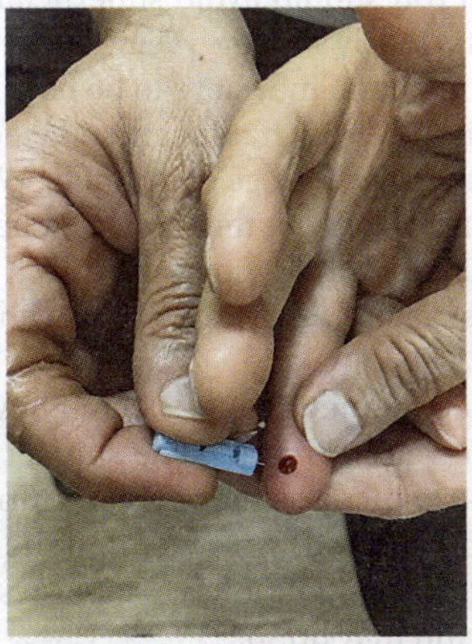

FIG. 7: Finger prick method.

  Cutting needles with three-sided cutting points (used by surgeons) can serve the purpose well.

  Pricking gun: A spring-loaded pricking gun that has a disposable, three-sided sharp point, and a loading and releasing mechanism, is ideal because the depth of the puncture can be preselected.
- Sterile gauze/cotton, moist with 70% alcohol/methylated spirit.
- Glass slides, pipettes, etc., according to requirements.

Note: The students should bring their own lancets. These may be reused two to three times, if required, after passing their points through a flame. Spirit does not kill the hepatitis virus which can be killed on heating. However, too much heating, however, is likely to blunt the pricking points.

Procedures

All aseptic precautions must be taken. The person giving the prick should wash his/her hands with soap and water, and wear gloves if possible.

Note: Keep all the equipment ready before getting a prick. If the finger to be pricked appears cold and bloodless, especially in winter, immerse it in warm water for 2–3 minutes.

- Clean and vigorously rub the ball of the finger with the spirit swab, followed by a final cleaning with dry gauze (Scrubbing increases local blood flow).
- Allow the alcohol to dry by evaporation for the following reasons:
  - Sterilization with alcohol/spirit is effective only after it has dried by evaporation.
  - The thin film of alcohol can cause the blood drop to spread sideways along with alcohol so that it will not form a satisfactory round drop.
  - The alcohol may cause hemolysis of blood.
- Steadying the finger to be pricked in your left hand, apply a gentle pressure on the sides of the ball of the finger with your thumb and forefinger to raise a thick, broad ridge of skin (do not touch the pricking area).
- Hold the lancet between the thumb and fingers of your right hand, and keeping it directed along the axis of the finger, but slightly "off" center so as to miss the tip of the phalanx (i.e. not too far down or too far near the top of the nail bed), prick the skin with a sharp and quick vertical stab to a depth of 3–4 mm and release the pressure. The blood should start to flow slowly, spontaneously and freely (without any squeezing)—if a good prick has been given.

Important: Do not squeeze or press the finger as the tissue fluid squeezed out will dilute the blood and give false low values. The squeeze also tends to close the wound edges. You may exert a slight tension on either side of the puncture with your thumbs in order to open up the wound more widely (a plug of epithelial cells tends to block the puncture especially if the wound is shallow, as often happens if a narrow-bore injection needle is used). The forearm or the hand may be squeezed or milked toward the fingers to facilitate blood flow. If all efforts fail, a fresh prick may be required.

- Wipe away the first two drops of blood with dry, sterile gauze as it may be contaminated not only with tissue fluid, but also with epithelial and endothelial cells which will appear as artifacts in the blood film.
- Allow a fresh drop of blood of sufficiently large size (about 3–4 mm diameter) to well up from the wound, and make a blood smear, or fill a pipette as the case may be.
- Clean the area of the prick with a fresh swab and ask the subject to keep the swab pressed on the wound with his/her thumb till the bleeding stops, which occurs in a minute or so.

Earlobe Prick

With the use of a sterile needle or corner edge of a sterile blade give a 2-mm deep prick (the skin here is usually thinner than at the fingertip). Wipe away the first drop and allow a new one to form).

Note: The BT and CT tests give better results here than at the finger prick.

Pricking the Heel

In infants and young children, blood can be collected from the cleaned and warmed medial or lateral areas of the heel.

Note: The central plantar and the posterior curvature areas of the heel should be avoided as the prick may cause injury to the underlying tarsal bones which lie near the surface.

Precautions

1. Keep the equipment for the test ready before getting/giving a finger prick.
2. The selected site should be clean, free from infection, edema, or skin disease.
3. The site should be vigorously cleaned and scrubbed with sterile gauze and alcohol. Scrubbing increases local blood flow.
4. The lancet/needle should be sterile, and if it is to be reused, it should be passed through a flame.
5. The puncture should be deep enough to give free flowing blood but not so very deep that it takes inordinately long time for the bleeding to stop.
6. Do not press or squeeze the finger to increase the blood flow from the skin-prick, though the arm or the hand may be milked toward the fingers.

Collection of Venous Blood

The blood sample from a vein must be collected by a medically qualified staff member who should screen the volunteer for any communicable diseases/especially viral hepatitis, and AIDS. Do not touch blood other than your own. Puncturing a vein and withdrawing blood from it needs assistance and complete aseptic precautions.

The following samples are not suitable for hematological tests:

1. *Clotted samples*: Even tiny clots in the anticoagulated blood can negate the results.
2. *Hemolyzed samples*: The red cells may be damaged and ruptured during collection or handling of blood. The released Hb tinges the plasma or serum red, rendering the sample unfit for tests.

For a sample of whole blood or plasma: (Plasma = Blood minus all the blood cells). Draw blood from a vein as and transfer it from the syringe to a container containing a suitable anticoagulant. Mix the contents well without frothing. A sample of whole blood is now ready for tests.

If plasma is desired, centrifuge the anticoagulated blood for 20–30 minutes at 2,500 rpm. Collect the supernatant plasma with a pipette and transfer it to another container (The packed RBCs will be left behind).

For a sample of serum: (Serum = Plasma minus fibrinogen and all the clotting factors). Transfer the blood from the syringe to a container *without any anticoagulant* in it, and keep it undisturbed. After the blood has clotted in an hour or two and the clot shrunk in size, the serum will be expressed. Remove the supernatant serum with a pipette and transfer it to a centrifuge tube. Centrifuge it to remove whatever red cells may be present. Clear serum can now be collected with another pipette.

Apparatus

Keep the following equipment ready before venepuncture:

1. Disposable gloves.
2. Sterile, disposable, one-time use, 10 mL syringe with side nozzle.
3. 10 mL test tubes/vials with or without anticoagulant.
4. Sterile gauze pieces moist with 70% alcohol/methylated spirit.
5. Tourniquet: A 2–3 cm wide elastic bandage with Velcro strips to keep it securely in place can be used. An inflated BP cuff can also be used.

Procedures

- Seat the subject comfortably on a chair with an arm rest.
- Compress the upper arm with his hands to make the veins prominent. The antecubital (medial basilic) vein is embedded in subcutaneous fat and is usually sufficiently large to take a wide-bore needle. It also runs straight for about 3 cm, and is usually palpable— even in obese subjects. If the vein is neither visible nor palpable, try the other arm. (You should avoid superficial veins because they are notoriously slippery. Veins above the ankle or on the back of the hand may have to be used).
- Once a suitable vein has been selected, support the subject's arm over the edge of the table. Wash your hands with soap and water, dry them on a sterile towel, and put on gloves. Take out the syringe and attach the needle (it is attached/detached with a little twist), with its bevel facing you.
- Apply the tourniquet about 2–3 cm above the elbow to obstruct the venous return. The subject may open and close her fist to increase the venous return and make the veins engorged (filled) with blood. If the vein is still not sufficiently prominent, a few "slaps" with your fingers over the region may do so.
- Clean the skin over the selected vein with gauze and alcohol and allow it to dry.

- Hold the syringe with the plunger pushed in, between your fingers and thumb of the right hand.
- With the first finger placed near the butt of the needle, puncture the skin and push in the needle under the skin with a firm and smooth thrust to the skin. Insert the needle proximally (i.e., in the direction of venous blood flow), with the bevel facing up, along the midline of the vein at a shallow angle (about 10–30°) to the skin.
- Slightly pull the plunger back with your thumb and little finger to produce a little negative pressure in the syringe. Advance the needle gently along the vein and puncture it from the side, a few mm ahead of the skin puncture. This prevents counterpuncture of the far wall of the vein and formation of a hematoma (local leakage of blood).
- As the vein is punctured, all resistance will suddenly cease and blood will start to enter the syringe. Do not withdraw blood faster than the punctured veins are filling; as too much pressure applied to the plunger is likely to cause mechanical injury and hemolysis of red cells. The subject may open and close the fist to enhance venous return.
- When enough blood has been collected, release the tourniquet and press a fresh swab over the skin puncture. Withdraw the needle gently but keep the swab in position. Ask the subject to flex the arm and keep it so to maintain pressure on the puncture site till the bleeding stops.
- Expel the blood gently into the container; do not apply force as it may cause mechanical injury to red cells. Gently shake, or swirl the container between your palms so that the anticoagulant (if used) mixes well with the blood without frothing.

Important: Try to access the vein efficiently and collect the blood sample within 30 seconds after tourniquet placement. Do not leave the tourniquet on for > 1 minute. This is because stagnation of blood in the vein is likely to alter its composition—the cell counts usually increasing.

Precautions

1. All aseptic precautions must be observed and disposable gloves, syringe and needles must be used.
2. The tourniquet (or the BP cuff) must be removed before taking the needle out of the vein to avoid formation of hematoma.
3. The blood from the syringe should be transferred to the container without delay to prevent clotting.
4. Ask the subject to keep the swab in position till the bleeding from the puncture site stops.

COMMONLY USED ANTICOAGULANTS

Anticoagulants, also known as blood thinners, are chemical substances that prevent or reduce coagulation of blood, thus prolonging the clotting time.

Anticoagulants for In Vitro Use

1. **Ethylene diamine tetraacetic acid (EDTA):** Both the potassium and sodium salts of EDTA are strong anticoagulants. The dry (anhydrous) dipotassium salt of EDTA, being more readily soluble than the sodium salt, is the anticoagulant of choice. The tripotassium salt of EDTA causes some shrinkage of RBCs that results in 2–3% decrease in packed cell volume.
   Mode of action: EDTA prevents clotting by removing ionic calcium (which is an essential clotting factor) from the blood sample by **chelation**. The platelets appear clear and are neither aggregated nor destroyed.
   Preparation: EDTA is used in a concentration of 1 mg/mL of blood. 0.2 mL of 2.5% solution of the salt placed in a container and dried in gentle heat in an oven is sufficient for 5 mL of blood. This provides 1 mg of EDTA/mL of blood (A number of containers can be prepared from the stock solution at a time).

   Note: Excess of EDTA (more than 2 mg/mL blood) affects all blood cells. Red cells shrink, thus reducing PCV, while WBCs show degenerative changes. Platelets break up into large enough fragments to be counted as normal platelets. Care should, therefore, be taken to use the correct amount of EDTA, and blood should be thoroughly mixed with the anticoagulant.

   Uses: Except for coagulation studies EDTA is used for most hematological tests.
2. **Trisodium citrate ($Na_3C_6H_5O_2.2H_2O$):** Trisodium citrate is the anticoagulant of choice in blood tests for disorders of coagulation.
   Mode of action: Acts as a chelating agent (inactivates calcium ions)
   Preparation: 3.8% solution is prepared in distilled water and then sterilized.
   Uses: Citrated blood, citrate and blood in the ratio of 1:9, is used for coagulation studies, and for ESR test by the Westergren's method in the ratio of 1:3. Along with other components, sodium citrate is used for storing donated blood in blood banks, since it can be safely given intravenously. Oxalates are toxic and cannot be given intravenously.
3. **Double oxalate mixture:** This is a mixture of ammonium oxalate and potassium oxalate in the ratio of 3:2 is an effective anticoagulant. It is thus called double oxalate.
   Mode of action: Oxalates prevent clotting by forming insoluble calcium salts, thus removing ionic calcium.
   Preparation: A large number of containers can be prepared at a time by placing 0.2 mL of oxalate mixture (3.0 g of ammonium oxalate and 2.0 g of potassium oxalate in 100 mL of distilled water) in each container and drying in gentle heat in an oven. This amount is sufficient for 8–10 mL of blood. Too much oxalate is hypertonic and damages all blood cells, while too little will not prevent clotting.
   Uses: Though each oxalate by itself (also sodium and lithium oxalate) can prevent clotting, a mixture is used. Sodium oxalate should not be used since it causes crenation of red cells. Ammonium salt should not be used in urea and non-protein nitrogen tests. It is used in the tests where the cell volume should remain unaffected, e.g., ESR, PCV.
4. **Sodium fluoride:** A mixture of 10 mg of sodium fluoride and 1 mg thymol is an anticoagulant as well as a preservative when a blood sample has to be stored for a

few days. Since fluoride inhibits glycolytic enzymes (thus preventing loss of glucose), it is employed when plasma glucose is to be estimated.

5. **Heparin:** Heparin, a highly charged mixture of sulfated polysaccharides, and related to chondroitin, has a molecular weight ranging from 15,000–18,000 and is a naturally occurring powerful anticoagulant. It is normally secreted by mast cells that are present in many tissues, especially immediately outside many of the capillaries in the body. Both mast cells and basophils release heparin directly into blood. Heparin is also a cofactor for the lipoprotein lipase—the clearing factor.
   Commercial heparin is extracted from many different tissues and is available in almost pure form (it was first extracted from the liver—hence the name "heparin"). Low megawatt fragments (mw 5000) have been produced from unfractionated heparin and are being used clinically since they have a longer half-life and produce more predictable results.
   Mode of action and uses: Heparin by itself has no anticoagulant activity. However, when it combines with **antithrombin III,** the ability of the latter to remove thrombin (as soon as it is formed) increases hundreds of times. The complex of these two substances removes many other activated clotting factors—such as IX, X, XI, and XII.
   Preparation: Theoretically, heparin is an ideal anticoagulant since no foreign substance is introduced into the blood. The required amount of stock solution is taken in a number of containers and dried at low heat. At a concentration of 10–20 IU/mL blood, it does not change red cell size and their osmotic fragility. It is, however, inferior to EDTA for general use. It should not be used for leukocyte counts, as these cells tend to clump. It also imparts a blue tinge to the background of blood films.
   Uses: It is used for estimation of blood gases, pH assay, and osmotic fragility. Clinically, it is used to prevent intravascular clotting of blood.
6. **Acid-citrate-dextrose and citrate-phosphate dextrose-adenine:** Acid-citrate-dextrose (ACD) and citrate-phosphate-dextrose-adenine (CPD-A) are the anticoagulants of choice for storing donated blood in blood banks. The CPD-A mixture is preferred as it preserves 2–3 DPG better.

Anticoagulants for In Vivo Use

The two in vivo anticoagulants are heparin and coumarins. Patients at increased risk of forming blood clots in their blood vessels, e.g. leg veins during prolonged confinement to bed, or during long flights, are sometimes put on these drugs (e.g. warfarin) to prevent thromboembolism. Their BT, CT, and PT are checked from time to time to adjust the dosage of the drug.

1. **Dicoumarol and warfarin:** The coumarin derivatives are vitamin K antagonists and thus inhibit the action of this vitamin that is essential as a cofactor for the synthesis of six glutamic acid-containing proteins— namely, factors II (prothrombin), VII, IX, and X, protein C, and protein S. The action of this anticoagulant is, however, slower than that of heparin.
2. **Heparin** is particularly used during open-heart surgery in which the blood has to be passed through a heart-lung machine; or the dialysis machine during hemodialysis in kidney failure, and then back into the patient.

Important: Anticoagulant therapy should not be confused with thrombolytic agents employed for dissolving blood clots.

STUDY OF COMMON OBJECTS

The students should realize that common objects of interest in microscopy such as, dust particles, cotton/wool/silk/synthetic and other fibers, air bubbles, stain precipitate, etc. are the usual artifacts which may cause confusion to a beginner. Few such common objects have been shown as they appear under the microscope in **Figures 8A to H**.

1. **Dust particles:** Dust particles include inorganic and organic matter such as silica, graphite, mica, and carbon. These particulate matters are of different sizes, angular or irregularly polygonal; with sharp edges, and unevenly light or dark brown, black, or yellow in color **(Fig. 8A)**.
2. **Starch granules:** These granules are oval or pear shaped and usually have a hilum at their narrow ends. Concentric rings (lines) are seen, especially when stained blue with dilute iodine solution added to a watery suspension of starch powder **(Fig. 8B)**.
3. **Hairs:** These are the growths of epidermis composed of dead, keratinized cells. The human hairs (pili) are long, filamentous and cylindrical and cover most of the skin surfaces except palms and soles **(Fig. 8C)**. Each hair has two layers: (i) medulla and (ii) cortex.
4. **Cotton fibers:** These appear as long, ribbon-like, semi-transparent filaments which are spirally twisted at intervals **(Fig. 8D)**.
5. **Stain granules:** Place a drop of Leishman's stain on a slide, spread it out thickly with another slide, and allow it

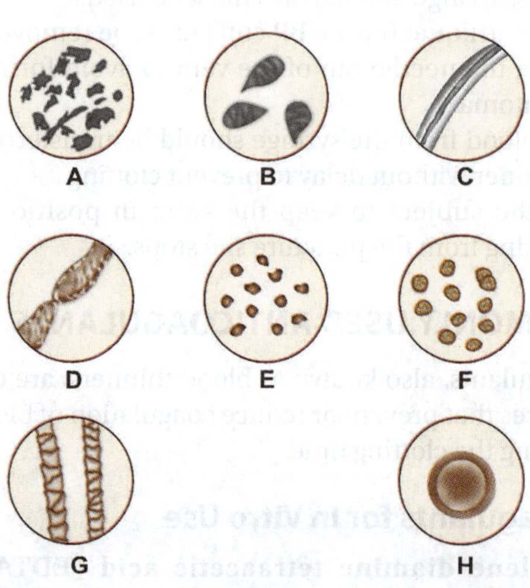

FIGS. 8A TO H: Common objects: (A) Dust particles; (B) Starch granules; (C) Human hair; (D) Cotton fiber; (E) Leishman's stain granules; (F) Fat globules of milk; (G) Woolen fiber; (H) Air bubble in water.

to dry at room temperature. Examine it under LP and HP lenses. Then put a drop of cedar wood oil and examine it under OI lens. The stain precipitate appears as round, uniformly dark blue-violet granules of uniform size (about 2 urn). The granules usually lie singly and do not form aggregates or clusters **(Fig. 8E)**.

6. **Fat globules:** A drop of diluted milk shows fat globules, most of which are round and of uniform size. A few may be found in clumps like a bunch of grapes **(Fig. 8F)**.
7. **Woolen fibers:** These are the body hairs of sheep, rabbit, or other animals. They appear as long, filamentous structures showing a cortex and medulla. Minute hairlets may be seen projecting from the surface **(Fig. 8G)**.
8. **Air bubbles:** Drop a cover-slip over a drop of water taken on a slide. This usually traps air bubbles of various sizes. They are usually round or oval due to surface tension of water around them. They appear as darkish rings with a clear area in the center **(Fig. 8H)**.

QUESTIONS

Q.1. What measures are taken to prevent infection during venepuncture and skin-pricking?

The instruments to be used should be properly sterilized. The site selected for puncturing should be clean and free from any disease. The area should be properly sterilized. The person withdrawing blood should wash his/her hands.

Q.2. What are the sources and main differences between venous blood and capillary blood? Why is capillary blood called peripheral blood?

See text above.

Q.3. What is the difference between plasma and serum? How will you get a sample of each?

See text above.

Q.4. What precautions will you observe to prevent hemolysis of venous blood samples?

The syringe, needle and the container should be clean and dry. The needle should be of wide bore, and the blood should be drawn slowly and without frothing. The needle should be removed from the syringe and blood should be expelled slowly into the container.

Q.5. What are anticoagulants? What is meant by in vivo and in vitro anticoagulants?

See text above.

Q.6. Why are the thumb and little finger not pricked for blood?

See text above.

Q.7. What are the sites for collecting capillary blood in infants?

See text above.

Q.8. Why should the pricked finger not be squeezed? What is meant by free-flowing blood and why should it be preferred over squeezed blood?

See text above.

1.3: HEMOCYTOMETRY

STUDENT OBJECTIVES

After completing this experiment, the student should be able to:

- Describe the principle underlying hemocytometry.
- Describe the counting chamber and the dimensions of different squares on the counting grid.
- Name the diluting fluids and their composition.
- Identify the red blood cell (RBC) and white blood cell (WBC) pipettes, name their parts, and the differences between them.
- Name the precautions to be observed during dilution of blood in a pipette.
- Calculate the dilution obtained with each pipette.
- Describe the possible sources of error during dilution of blood.
- Charge the Neubauer's chamber and name the precautions observed during charging.
- Focus the counting grid for RBC and WBC under low and high magnifications and identify and count the cells.
- Explain the possible sources of error for cell counting.

INTRODUCTION

Hemocytometry is the procedure of counting the number of cells in a sample of blood; the red cells, the white cells, and the platelets being counted separately. It is assumed that the cells are homogeneously mixed (suspended) in the plasma in all regions of the body. However, even under physiological conditions, there are slight differences (e.g. higher red cell counts in venous and capillary blood than in arterial blood) which, though minor, are accentuated by muscular exercise, changes in posture, meals, etc. Nevertheless, important clinical information can be obtained if cell counts are done carefully on a venous blood sample.

PRINCIPLE

Since the number of blood cells is very high, it is difficult to count them even under the microscope. This difficulty is partly overcome by diluting the blood to a known degree with suitable diluting fluids and then counting them. The sample of blood is diluted in a special pipette and is then placed in a capillary space of known capacity (volume) between a especially ruled glass slide (counting chamber) and a coverslip. The cells spread out in a single layer which makes their counting easy. Knowing the dilution employed, the number of cells in undiluted blood can then easily be calculated.

UNITS FOR CELL COUNTING

The result of cell counting is usually expressed as "so many cells per cubic millimeter (cmm; mm^3; µL) of blood". For example, RBC count—5.0 million/mm^3; WBC count—5,000 cells/mm^3.

The SI unit, however, is......cells per liter of blood.

$1\ mm^3 = 1\ \mu L = 10^{-6} L$, $1\ \mu L \times 10^{-6} = 1\ L$

APPARATUS

1. **The counting chamber (hemocytometer)**: It is a thick glass slide, appropriately ruled with a counting grid, i.e. squares of varying dimensions.
2. **The diluting pipettes:** Two different glass capillary pipettes, each having a bulb, are provided for counting RBCs and WBCs (these pipettes are sometimes called *cell pipettes* or blood pipettes. The third pipette that the students will be using is the hemoglobin pipette, which does not have a bulb).
3. **Coverslips:** Special coverslips having an optically plane and uniform surface should be preferred over ordinary coverslips.
4. **Red blood cell (RBC) and white blood cell (WBC)** diluting fluids.
5. Watch glasses, spirit swabs, blood lancet/needle, etc.

Counting Chamber: Improved Neubauer Chamber

The counting chamber was introduced by Crammer in 1805. Its modification by Thoma, and later by Neubauer remained in use for a long time. Improved Neubauer chamber is in current use.

The counting chamber **(Figs. 9A and B)** is a single, solid, and heavy glass slide. Extending across its middle third are three parallel platforms (pillars or flanges) separated from each other by shallow trenches (moats, gutters, or troughs). The central platform or "floorpiece" (sometimes also called the plateau) is wider, and exactly 0.1 mm (one-tenth of a mm) lower than the two lateral pillars. The floorpiece is divided into two equal parts by a short transverse trench in its middle as shown in **Figures 9A and B**. Thus, there is an H-shaped trench or trough enclosing the two floorpieces. The two lateral platforms can support a coverslip which, when in position, will span the trenches and provide a capillary space 0.1 mm deep between the undersurface of the coverslip and the upper surface of the floor pieces. Identically ruled areas, called "counting grids", consisting of squares of different sizes, are etched on each floorpiece. The two counting grids allow RBC and WBC counts to be made simultaneously if needed, or duplicate samples can be run.

Note: Hemocytometers with silver-coated floorpieces show the grids beautifully, which makes them easier to use by the students.

Thoma's Chamber

In this counting chamber, not used now, the central depressed platform is circular. The grid is only 1 mm^2, consisting of 25 groups of 16 smallest squares each. The dimensions of the smallest squares are the same, i.e., 1/20 mm × 1/20 mm. The 1 mm squares at the corners are absent.

Old Neubauer Chamber

There are nine 1 mm squares. The four corner groups of 16 squares each are for WBC counting, while the central 1 mm^2 area has 16 groups of 16 squares each for RBC counting (rather than 25 groups of 16 smallest squares as in improved Neubauer chamber). The medium squares are separated by triple lines.

The Counting Grid

The ruled area on each floorpiece, the counting grid, has the following dimensions:

- Each counting grid **(Fig. 10)** measures 9 mm^2 (3 mm × 3 mm). It is divided into nine large squares, each 1 mm^2 (1 mm × 1 mm).
- Of these nine squares, the four large corner squares are lightly etched, and each is divided by single lines into 16 medium-sized squares each of which has a side of 1/4 mm, and an area of 1/16 mm^2 (1/4 mm × 1/4 mm).

These four large corner squares are employed for counting leukocytes and are, therefore, called WBC squares **(Fig. 10)**.

- The central densely etched large square (1 mm × 1 mm), called the RBC square, is divided into 25 medium-sized squares, each of which has a side of 1/5 mm.
- Each of these medium squares is set off (separated) from its neighbors by very closely placed double lines (tram lines) or triple lines. These double or triple lines extend in

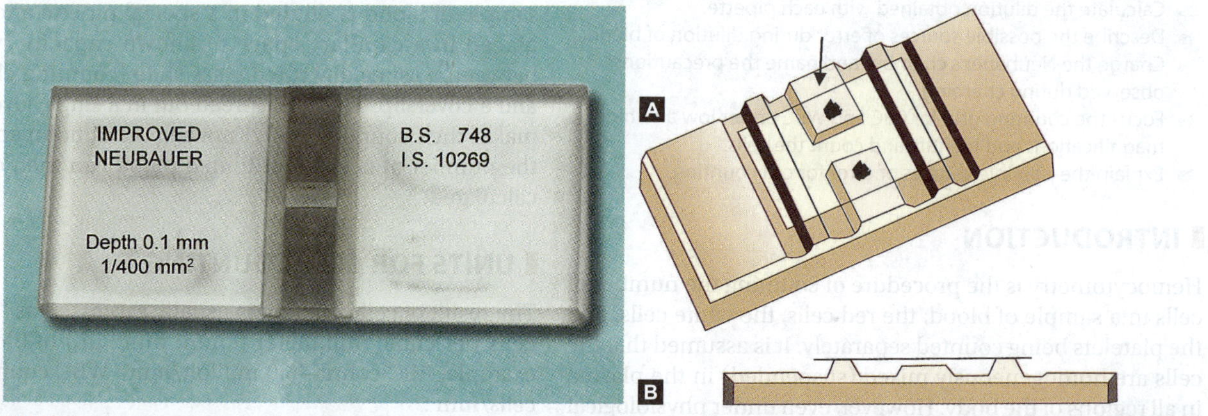

FIGS. 9A AND B: Hemocytometer, or counting chamber with improved Neubauer's ruling. (A) Surface view, with the coverslip in position. The locations of the counting grids on the two platforms (*floorpieces*) are indicated. The arrow indicates the place where the tip of the pipette should be placed for *charging* the chamber; (B) Side view with the coverslip in position. The space between the underside of the coverslip and the surface of the platform is 0.100 mm in depth. The depth and the area of the smallest square are etched on the surface of the chamber.

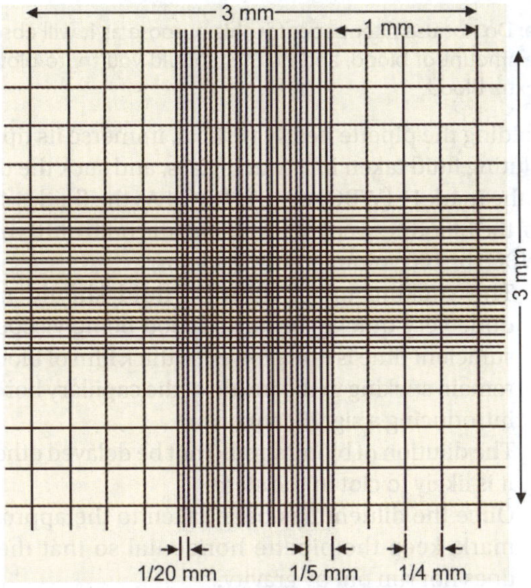

FIG. 10: The counting grid of improved Neubauer's ruling. The four corner groups of 16 squares (side = 0.25 mm) are used for counting WBCs. The RBCs are counted in five groups of 16 smallest squares each (side = 0.05 mm). The grid also provides a convenient scale for measuring the size of small objects like parasite eggs.
(RBCs: red blood cells; WBCs: white blood cells)

all directions beyond the boundaries of the 9 mm^2 ruling, i.e., in between all the WBC squares around the central RBC square.

- Each of the 25 medium squares (side = 1/5 mm), bounded by double lines (which are 0.01 mm apart) or triple lines, is further divided into 16 smallest squares by single lines. Thus, each smallest square has a side of 1/5 × 1/4 = 1/20 mm, and an area of 1/400 mm^2.

Note: Since each group of 16 smallest squares is demarcated from its neighbors by triple lines, the dimensions of the RBC square (largest central square) must be slightly larger than 1 mm × 1 mm, as indeed they are [the exact dimensions of the smallest squares (1/400 mm^2)] etched on the chamber surface.

Study of the Diluting Pipettes

1. Red blood cell pipette
2. White blood cell pipette.

Figures 11A and B shows the two glass capillary pipettes used for diluting the blood. Each pipette has a long narrow stem (for measuring the blood), which widens into a bulb (for diluting the blood/which in turn, leads to a short stem).

Parts of a Diluting Pipette

- **The stem:** The long narrow stem has a capillary bore and a well-grounded conical tip. It is divided into 10 equal parts (graduations) but has only two numbers etched on it—0.5 in the middle of the stem, and 1.0 (or 1) at the junction of stem and the bulb.
- **The bulb:** The stem widens into a bulb which contains a free-rolling bead—red in the RBC pipette, and white

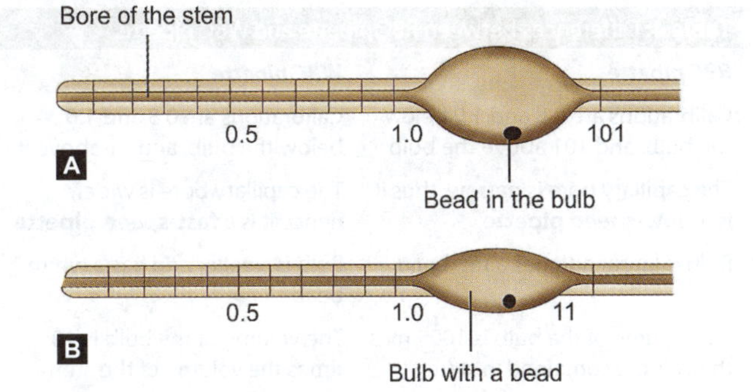

FIGS. 11A AND B: The diluting pipettes (blood pipettes). (A) RBC pipette: it has three markings—(1) 0.5, (2) 1.0, and (3) 101; (B) WBC pipette: it has three markings—(1) 0.5, (2) 1.0, and (3) 11.
(RBC: red blood cell; WBC: white blood cell)

in the WBC pipette. The bead helps in mixing the blood and the diluent and also helps in quick identification at a glance.

- **Rubber tube and mouthpiece:** The bulb narrows again into a short stem to which a long, narrow, and soft rubber tube bearing a mouthpiece (often red in RBC pipette, and white in WBC pipette) is attached. The rubber tube is 25–30 cm long to facilitate filling of the pipette by gentle suction. It also allows the pipette to be held horizontally so that one can comfortably watch the blood or diluting fluid entering the pipette.

Just beyond the bulb, the number 101 is etched on the RBC, and 11 on the WBC pipettes.

Principle Underlying the Use of Diluting Pipettes

It is important to understand that the numbers marked on the pipettes—0.5, 1.0, and 101 on the RBC pipette and 0.5, 1.0, and 11 on the WBC pipette—do not indicate absolute or definite amounts (or volumes) in terms of so many cubic millimeters (or μL), a mistake commonly made by the students. These figures only indicate relative volumes (parts)/or relative volumes in relation to each other. That is, half volume (from tip to mark 0.5), one volume (from the tip to mark 1.0) in both pipettes; and 11 volumes (from tip to mark 11 above the bulb in WBC pipette), and 101 volumes (from tip to mark 101 in RBC pipette). Of course, all these volumes will have certain definite volumes in terms of cubic millimeter, but we are not concerned with these but only the relative volumes or parts in relation to each other. It can be seen that the capillary bore in WBC pipette is wider than that in RBC pipette, and therefore, will hold more blood though the volume of the stem in both cases is 1.0 (one).

Differences between Red Blood Cell Pipette and White Blood Cell Pipette

The differences between RBC pipette and WBC pipette are described in **Table 4**.

Note: Though the dilution obtained with the RBC pipette is 10 times that obtained with WBC pipette, its bulb is not 10 times bigger. The reason is the much finer bore in the red cell pipette.

Table 4: Differences between RBC pipette and WBC pipette.

RBC pipette	*WBC pipette*
Calibrations are 0.5 and 1.0 below the bulb, and 101 above the bulb	Calibrations are 0.5 and 1.0 below the bulb, and 11 above it
The capillary bore is narrow, thus it is a **slow-speed pipette**	The capillary bore is wider, hence it is a **fast-speed pipette**
Bulb is larger and has a red bead	Bulb is smaller and has a white bead
The volume of the bulb is 100 times the volume contained in stem	The volume of the bulb is 10 times the volume of the stem

(RBC: red blood cell; WBC: white blood cell)

Filling the Pipette (Fig. 12)

- Place a drop of anticoagulated blood on a glass slide or get a fingerprick under aseptic conditions.
- Holding the mouthpiece of the pipette between your lips and keeping the pipette (with its graduations facing you) at an angle of about 40° to the horizontal, place its tip within the edge of the drop. Gently suck on the mouthpiece and draw blood until it is just above the mark 0.5 (capillary action cannot fill the pipette at this angle).
  - The blood drop should be of adequate size (say 3–4 mm in diameter). If it is too small or if the tip is lifted out of the drop, air will enter the pipette along with blood. If the tip presses against the skin, the bore at the tip will get blocked and no blood will enter the stem even if you suck hard at the mouthpiece.
  - Alternately, the pipette (after removing the rubber tube) may be filled with blood (without sucking/ by lowering its bulb end below the horizontal) and allowing the blood to flow down the stem by gravity.
- Remove the pipette from the blood drop and clean its outer surface with a cotton swab by wiping it toward the tip. Do not touch the bore at the tip otherwise some blood will be pulled out.
- Keeping the pipette horizontal all the time, bring the blood in the stem to the exact mark 0.5 by wiping the tip on your palm (or on a paper) a couple of times till the blood recedes to the exact mark.

Note: Do not use filter paper for this purpose as it will absorb a large amount of blood, and neither should you try to blow out the extra blood.

- Holding the pipette nearly vertical, immerse its tip in the diluting fluid taken in a watch glass, and suck the diluent to the mark 11 (WBC) or 101 (RBC). As the fluid is sucked up, the blood is swept before it into the bulb of 10 volumes (WBC) or 100 volumes (RBC pipette).
  - The sucking up of diluting fluid should not be done very quickly because blood being viscous, if a sufficient time is not allowed, a thick film of blood will remain sticking to the inside of the capillary bore, thus introducing a significant error.
  - The dilution of blood should not be delayed otherwise it is likely to clot in the stem.
  - Once the diluent has been taken to the appropriate mark, keep the pipette horizontal so that the fluid does not run out by gravity.
  - Do not place the pipette on the table, or delay the mixing because it becomes impossible to dislodge the cells from the walls of the bulb once they settle down.
- **Mixing the blood with the diluting fluid**: Once the diluting fluid has been sucked up, remove the rubber tube. Holding the short stem above the bulb between your thumb and first two fingers, and pressing the tip of the pipette against the palm of the other hand, rotate it to and fro for 3–4 minutes so that the blood and diluent get thoroughly mixed.

  Alternately, remove the rubber tube, close the pipette ends with thumb and forefinger of your right hand, and shake it vigorously with a figure of eight motion.

  Do not shake the pipette with an endwise motion as this will force the cells out of the bulb into the stem.
- **Charging the chamber:** Once the blood and the diluent have been mixed well, "charge" the chamber **(Fig. 13)**. Charging the chamber requires patience, practice, and understanding of how to correctly judge the size of the drop, the angle at which the pipette should be held on the floorpiece, and the time needed for filling (charging) the chamber. This is called the "speed of the pipette".

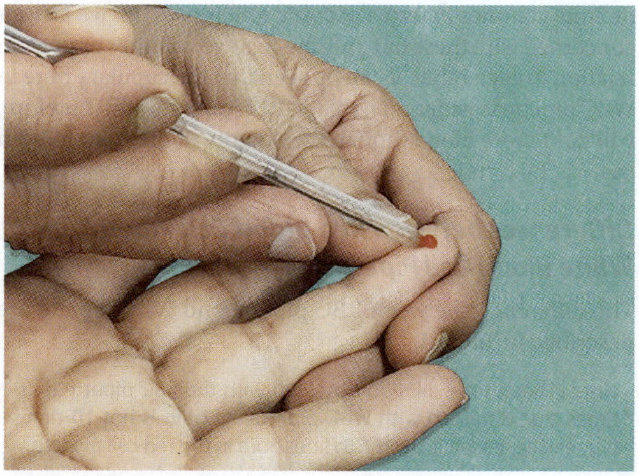

FIG. 12: Filling the pipette.

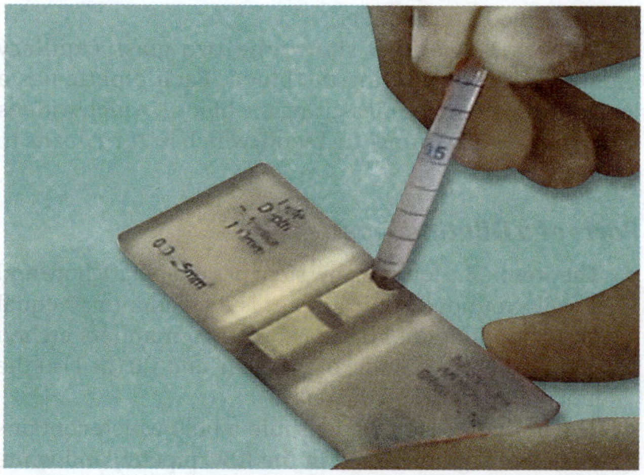

FIG. 13: Charging a chamber.

Obviously, it varies with the size of the capillary bore in the stem of the pipette.

- **High-speed pipette:** Since the bore of the WBC pipette is wider, a drop will form more quickly at its tip, and it will be larger, as compared to the RBC pipette. This requires that this pipette should be held more horizontally say, at an angle of 10–20° and for a shorter time.
- **Slow-speed pipette:** The bore of the RBC pipette being narrow, it will take a longer time for a suitable drop to form. It should, therefore, be held at a steeper angle—say, 60–70°.

It is for this reason that the students should first practice charging a chamber with the RBC pipette and then with the WBC pipette.

Calculation of Dilution Obtained (Dilution Factor)

When blood is sucked up to the mark 0.5 (half part or volume) and is followed by the diluting fluid, the blood enters the bulb first and is followed by the diluent to the mark 101 (RBC pipette), or mark 11 (WBC pipette). The stem in both pipettes contains only the diluent. Thus, *the dilution of the blood occurs in the bulb only.*

- **Red blood cell pipette:** Since the volume of the bulb is 100 (101 – 1.0 = 100), it means that 100 volumes (or parts) of diluted blood contain 0.5 (half) part of blood and 99.5 (100 – 0.5 = 99.5) parts or volumes of diluents. This gives a dilution of 0.5 in 100 (half in hundred), or 1 in 200 (one in 200), the dilution factor being 200 (the blood will be diluted 200 times). Similarly, if blood is taken to the mark 1.0 followed by diluted to mark 101, the dilution now would be 1 in 100.
- **White blood cell pipette:** In this case, the volume of the bulb is 10 (11 – 1 = 10). When blood is taken to the mark 0.5 (half part or volume) followed by diluent to the mark 11, the volume of the diluted blood is now 10, which contains 0.5 part of blood and 9.5 parts or volumes of the diluting fluid. This gives a dilution of 0.5 in 10 (half in ten), or 1 in 20 (one in 20), the dilution factor being 20 (the blood will be diluted 20 times). Similarly, if blood is taken to the mark 1.0 followed by diluted to mark 11, the dilution now would be 1 in 10.

For Red Blood Cell Counting

The red cells are counted in four corner groups and one central group of medium squares, each of which has 16 smallest squares, i.e. in a total of 80 smallest squares.

Area of smallest square = $1/20$ mm × $1/20$ mm = $1/400$ mm^2.

Since the depth of the chamber is $1/10$ mm, the volume of the smallest square = $1/400 \times 1/10 = 1/4{,}000$ mm^3.

For White Blood Cell (Total Leukocyte) Counting

This count is done in the four corner groups of large squares, each of which has 16 medium squares.

Area of one medium = $1/4$ mm × $1/4$ mm square = $1/16$ mm^2. Volume of this square = $1/16$ $mm^2 \times 1/10$ mm = $1/160$ mm^3.

Focusing the Counting Grid

Examine the grid on each floorpiece, without the coverslip, under low and high magnifications. Rack the condenser up and down, closing/adjusting the diaphragm at the same time. Find out the best combination of these two that shows the grid lines and squares clearly. When properly focused, the rulings (lines) appear as translucent darkish lines.

- With low magnification of 100 times, one large square, 1 mm × 1 mm is visible in one field, i.e. a group of 16 medium squares (for WBC counting), or a groups of 25 medium squares (for RBC counting).
- Examine the squares under high magnification.

PROCEDURE

1. Assuming that the blood and the diluent have been properly mixed, the next step is to charge the chamber. Place a coverslip on the chamber so that it spans the floor pieces and the trenches around them—a process called "centering" the coverslip.
2. Roll the pipette once more between your palms to mix the contents of the bulb. If this precaution is not taken, the counts are bound to be unreliable.
3. Keeping your finger over the top of the pipette and releasing it in a controlled manner, allow the first two drops to drain by gravity. This fluid contains cell-free diluting fluid in the stem which has not taken any part in the dilution of blood.
4. Hold the pipette at an appropriate angle (depending on the speed of the pipette) and watching carefully, allow a drop of diluted blood to form at its tip. Then quickly place the tip of the pipette on the floorpiece in gentle contact with the edge of the coverslip. As the surface of the drop touches the coverslip, the fluid will run under it by capillarity and form a uniform film. Lift the pipette as soon as the floorpiece is covered with diluted blood.
   - The chamber should be charged at one go and not in parts. For this, one needs a drop of proper size. Try to achieve an ideally-charged chamber.

   Before placing the chamber on the microscope stage, wait for 2–3 minutes for allowing the cells to settle down.

   Ideally-charged chamber: An ideally-charged chamber is completely filled with diluted blood. If any blood flows into the trenches, it is called "overcharging". If the fluid is insufficient to cover the floorpiece, or if there are air bubbles, it is called "undercharging" (air bubbles are formed if the coverslip or the floorpiece is dirty with grease or is moist).

   Effects of overcharging: When the chamber is overcharged the fluid will overflow into the gutters. This may give false low results as the cells will enter the gutter and settle there.

   Effects of undercharging: In an undercharged chamber fluid does not cover the entire central platform. There may be no cells in the peripheral squares thus giving the false low results.

   If there is over or undercharging, wash the chamber and coverslip in soap and water, dry them, and recharge the chamber.

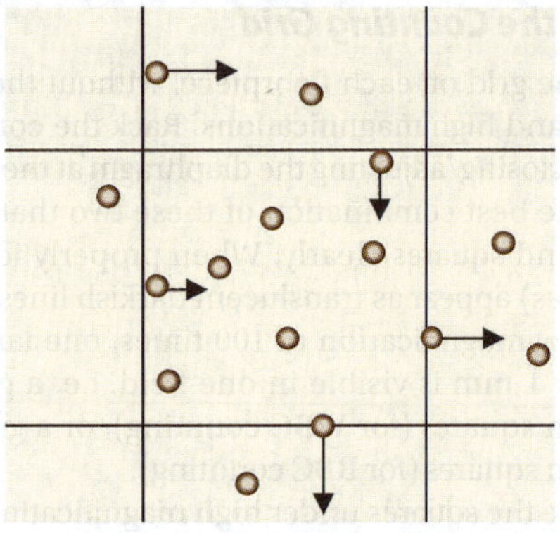

FIG. 14: Counting of cells. Arrows indicate the squares to which the cells belong.

5. Once the chamber has been properly charged, move it to the microscope. Wait for 2–3 minutes so that the cells settle down. Counting cannot be started when the cells are moving and changing places due to currents in the fluid. *Counting the cells*: Focus the appropriate squares under the required magnification and start counting as described in **Figure 14.**

Rules of counting **(Fig. 14)**:

1. Care should be taken not to count the same cells again.
2. Count the cells lying within a square and those lying on or touching its upper horizontal and left vertical line and those cells on its right and lower lines are ignored as they will be counted in the adjacent squares. This is called **"inverted L pattern"**. Arrows indicate the squares to which the cells belong.
3. Cells lying on or touching its lower horizontal and right vertical lines are to be omitted from that square because they will be counted with the adjacent squares. In this way, you will avoid counting a cell twice (you may omit cells lying on the upper horizontal and left vertical lines and count those lying on its lower and right lines. But whichever method is chosen, it is best to follow it for all cell counts).
4. In squares bound by triple lines, the *middle line* is considered the boundary of that square, and the same rules of counting apply.
5. While counting the cells, continuously "rack", the fine adjustment up and down so that cells sticking to the underside of the coverslip are not missed.
6. Only one pattern should be followed for the entire counting.

Sources of error in cell counting:

1. Pipette error
2. Dilution error
3. Chamber
4. Statistical
5. Field error.

Note: Three important sources of error: (1) pipette error, (2) chamber error, and (3) field error can produce a variation of as much as 10–15%, or even more in the hands of a student. On the other hand, hemoglobin and packed cell volume are easy to determine and give enough information about the blood picture.

PRECAUTIONS

1. The pipette should be clean and dry and the bead should roll freely.
2. The pipette should not be lifted out of the blood drop while filling it with blood, otherwise air will enter it.
3. The drawing up of diluent, after blood has been taken in the stem, should not be delayed, otherwise it will clot in it.
4. The pipette should be cleaned soon after the experiment is over.
5. Do not touch blood other than your own.
6. Ensure that the counting chamber and the coverslip are absolutely clean, grease-free, and dry.
7. While charging the chamber ensures that it is neither under nor overcharged.
8. Never bring the objective lens down while looking into the microscope as the chamber is likely to be scratched or broken.

Note: Automatic Electronic Cell Counters

The electronic cell counter uses a volumetric impedance method. An electrolyte solution (diluent) containing suspended blood cells is aspirated through the aperture. Two electrodes are located close to the aperture and constant current flows between them. When a blood cell passes through the aperture, the resistance between the electrodes momentarily increases and a very small voltage change occur corresponding to the resistance. The voltage signal is amplified and sent to the electronic circuit. The data is then corrected by the CPU and displayed on the screen.

QUESTIONS

Q.1. What is the principle underlying the use of a counting chamber?

See text above.

Q.2. What are the dimensions of WBC and RBC squares?

See text above.

Q.3. What are the features of an ideally-charged chamber?

See text above.

Q.4. How does the improved Neubauer chamber differ from the older variety of Neubauer chamber?

See text above.

Q.5. How will you identify a red cell pipette and a white cell pipette?

See text above.

Q.6. What is the function of the bead in the bulb?

The bead helps to mix the blood with its diluent. It tells whether the pipette is dry or not (it rolls freely if it is dry). It also helps to identify the pipette by just glancing at it.

Q.7. What are the units of markings on the pipettes?

There are no absolute units of volume marked on the pipette. They only denote relative volumes or parts in relation to each other.

Q.8. What is the function of the bulb in a diluting pipette?

The dilution of the blood occurs in the bulb only, and since the volume of the bulb is known, it is possible to dilute the blood with a diluent in accurately known proportions.

Q.9. Why is it important to discard the first two drops of diluted blood from the pipette before charging the counting chamber?

After the blood has been diluted in the pipette, the stem contains only the cell-free diluent. This fluid has, therefore, to be discarded before the chamber can be filled.

Q.10. How will you clean a pipette when blood has clotted in the stem?

The pipette is kept in strong nitric acid for 24 hours. A flexible suitably thick metal wire is used to clean the capillary bore after washing the pipette in running water. The process may have to be repeated.

Q.11. What is the significance of the tenth graduations on the stem?

Instead of taking 0.5 or 1.0 volume of blood, we can take smaller volumes, say 0.2 or 0.3 to get higher dilutions.

Q.12. Can a pipette be used for any other purpose than cell counting?

The RBC pipette can be used for counting platelets, WBCs (when their number is very high, as in some leukemias), or spermatozoa in the semen.

Q.13. How is the entry of air bubbles prevented while diluting the blood?

The pipette is tapped with the tip of index finger to knock the bead down below the surface of the solution in the bulb to prevent formation of bubbles.

Q.14. If the blood is sucked above the 0.5 mark of the pipette how is it brought down?

If more than the required amount of blood is drawn, the pipette is gently tapped to the palm or the tip of the pipette is touched against a nonabsorbent material in order to bring the blood to desired mark.

1.4: THE RED CELL COUNT

STUDENT OBJECTIVES

After completing this experiment, the student should be able to:

- Describe the relevance of doing red cell count.
- Identify the red blood cell (RBC) pipette; fill it with blood and diluent.
- Charge the counting chamber and count the red cells.
- Describe the composition of diluting fluid and the function of each component.
- Give the normal RBC count in different age groups.
- Describe the site and stages of erythropoiesis, and factors that regulate it.
- Explain the causes of anemia and polycythemia.

INTRODUCTION

PY2.11: Estimate Hb, RBC, TLC, RBC indices, DLC, Blood groups, BT/CT.

Red blood cells are the most abundant cells in the peripheral blood. The human RBC is normally a circular, non-nucleated, biconcave disc containing hemoglobin. The biconcave shape aids in exchange of oxygen and carbon dioxide maximally and also helps it to withstand osmotic lysis and to easily pass through narrow capillaries (diapedesis).

Red cell dimensions:

- Shape: Biconcave disc
- Size: 7.4 (7–8) micron in diameter
- Thickness: 2.0 micron
- Surface area: 140 square micron.

The formation of red blood cells is known as erythropoiesis.

Sites of formation:

- Fetal life—spleen, liver, thymus, and bone marrow
- Soon after birth—red bone marrow
- Adult life—long bone cavities and femur.

STAGES OF ERYTHROPOIESIS

The whole process of maturation requires 3–5 days and is mediated by interleukins and GM-CSF that influence the secretion of erythropoietin **(Flowchart 1)**. Average lifespan of RBCs is 120 days.

Functions

- To help in exchange in oxygen and carbon dioxide between lungs and tissues.
- Breakdown products of RBC, e.g. globin maintain the protein storage pool of the body.
- Storage of iron is needed for hemoglobin synthesis.

Normal Values

Adults:

- Males: 5.2 (4.5–6) million per mm^3 of blood.
- Females: 4.7 (4.0–5.0) million per mm^3 of blood.
- Newborns: 6–8 million per mm^3 of blood.

Methods of Counting

- Manual
- Automated

Manual Method

Principle

The blood is diluted 200 times in a red cell pipette and the cells are counted in the counting chamber.

Knowing the dilution employed, their number in undiluted blood can easily be calculated.

Apparatus

1. **RBC pipette:** It should be clean and dry and the bead should roll freely **(Figs. 15 and 16)**.
2. **Improved Neubauer chamber with coverslip:** These should be clean and dust free.
3. Microscope with LP and HP objectives and 10x eyepiece.
4. Disposable blood lancet/pricking needle:
   - Sterile cotton/gauze swabs.
   - 70% alcohol/methylated spirit.

FLOWCHART 1: Hematopoiesis—development of blood cells. Cells above dotted line: Development and maturation in bone marrow. Cells below dotted line: Cells present in blood.

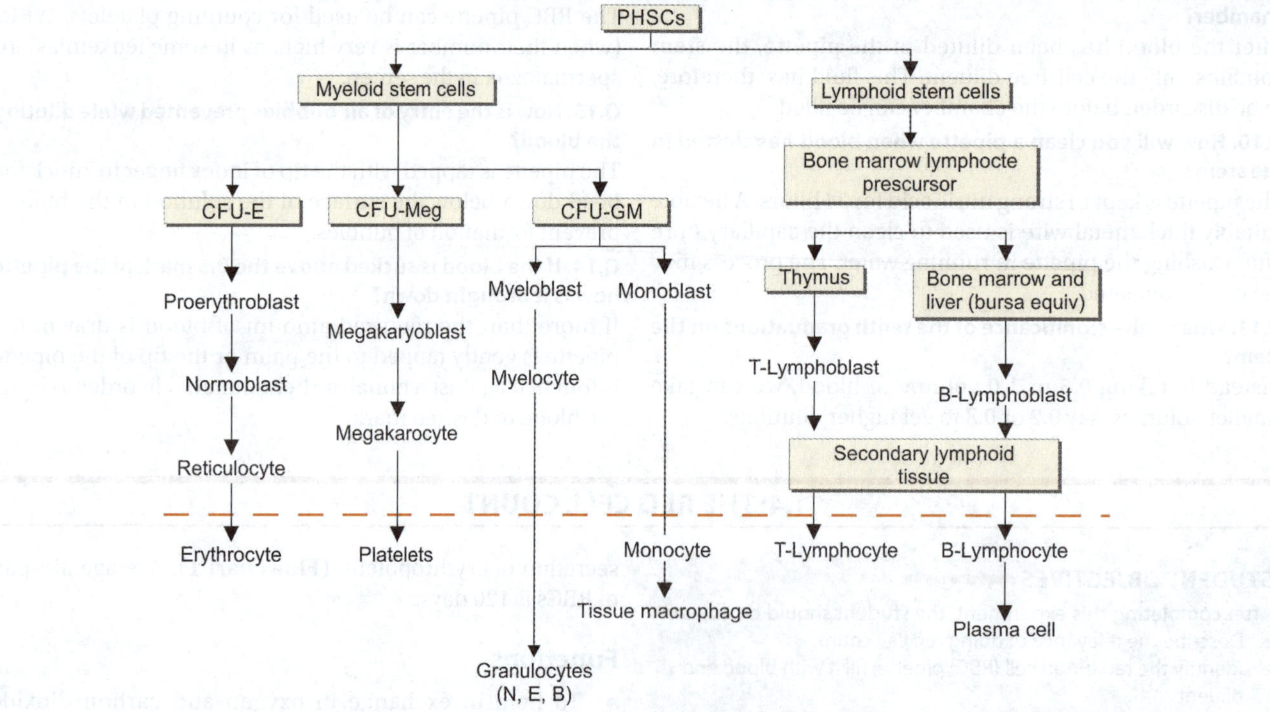

(CFUs: Colony forming units are committed (progenitor) cells; PHSCs: Pluripotent hematopoietic stem cells)

Hayem's fluid (RBC diluting fluid): The ideal fluid for diluting the blood should be isotonic and neither cause hemolysis nor crenation of red cells. It should have a fixative to preserve the shape of RBCs and also prevent their autolysis.

Composition of Hayem's fluid:

Sodium chloride (NaCl): 0.50 g

Sodium sulfate (Na_2SO_4): 2.50 g

Mercuric chloride ($Hg\ Cl_2$): 0.25 g

Distilled water: 100 mL

- Sodium chloride and sodium sulfate provide isotonicity so that the red cells remain suspended in diluted blood without changing their shape and size.
- Sodium sulfate also acts as an anticoagulant, and as a fixative to preserve their shape and to prevent rouleaux formation (piling together of red cells).

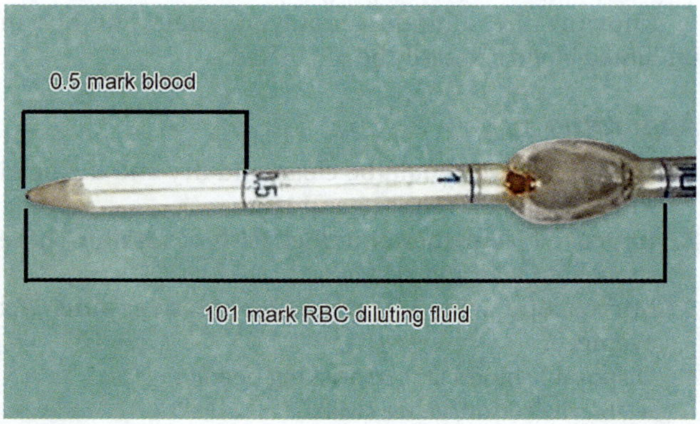

FIG. 15: RBC pipette.

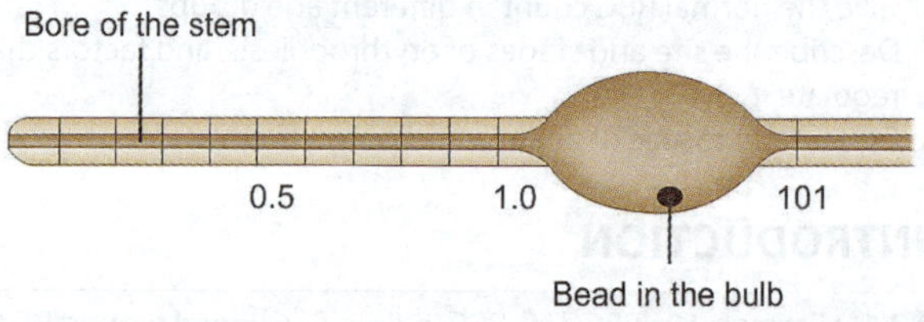

FIG. 16: The RBC pipette. It has 3 markings—0.5, 1.0, and 101.

- Mercuric chloride acts as an antifungal and antimicrobial agent, prevents contamination and growth of microorganisms.

Note:

- **Dacie's solution:** This diluting fluid is an alternative to Hayem's solution. It is simple to prepare and keep for a long time. It contains 3.13 g of trisodium citrate, 1.0 mL of 37% formalin (commercial formaldehyde), and distilled water to 100 mL.
- **Normal saline:** 0.9% sodium chloride solution can be used if Hayem's or Dacie's fluids are not available. However, the red cells have to be counted within an hour or so of filling the pipette. Also the RBCs are likely to form rouleaux. Further, a stock solution of normal saline cannot be kept for this purpose.

Procedure

- Place about 2 mL of Hayem's fluid in a watch glass.
- Examine the chamber with the coverslip "centered" on it, under low magnification. Adjust the illumination and focus the central 1 mm square (RBC square on

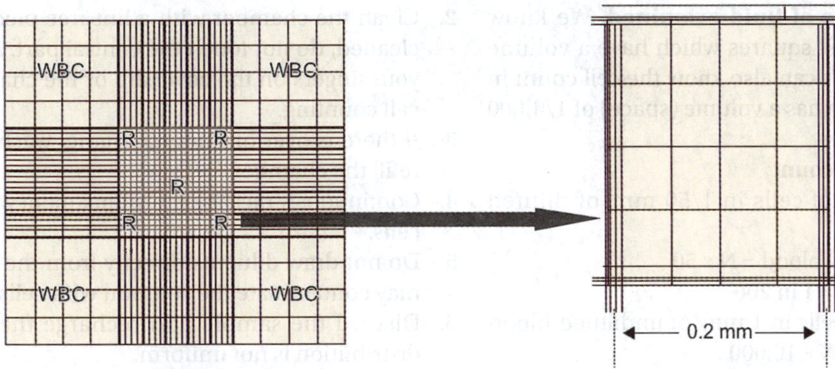

FIG. 17: Neubauer's chamber showing RBC squares under low power (10X). On right is RBC square as seen under high power (40X).

the counting grid) containing 25 groups of 16 smallest squares each **(Fig. 17)**. All these squares will be visible in one field. Do not change the focus or the field. Admitting too much light is a common cause of the inability to see the grid lines and squares clearly.

- Move the chamber to your worktable for charging it with diluted blood (it can be charged while on the stage, but it is more convenient to charge it on the table).
- **Filling the pipette with blood and diluting it:** Get a fingerprick. Wipe the first two drops of blood and fill the pipette from a fresh drop of blood up to the mark 0.5. Suck Hayem's fluid to the mark 101 and mix the contents of the bulb for 3–4 minutes as described earlier.
- **Charging the chamber:** Observing all the precautions, fill the chamber with diluted blood. Since the RBC pipette is a slow-speed pipette, it will need to be kept at an angle of 70–80° while charging the chamber. Move the chamber to the microscope and focus the grid once again to see the central 1 mm square with the red cells distributed all over. Wait for 3–4 minutes for the cells to settle down because they cannot be counted when they are moving and changing their positions due to currents in the fluid. During this time draw a diagram once again showing the RBC square. Then draw five groups of 16 square each, showing their relative positions—the four corner groups and one central group for entering your counts.
- **Counting the cells:** Switch over to high magnification (HP lens) and check the distribution of cells. If they are unevenly distributed, i.e. bunched at some places and scanty at others, the chamber has to be washed, dried, and recharged.
- Move the chamber carefully and bring the left upper corner block of 16 smallest squares in the field of view (There are no smallest squares above and to its left).

Rules for Counting (Figs. 18A and B)

See chapter on hemocytometry for details.

An occasional WBC (may be 1 in 600–700 RBCs) may be seen appearing grayish and granular but it is not to be counted with the red cells.

The counting will have been done in 80 smallest squares, i.e. in 5 blocks of 16 squares each.

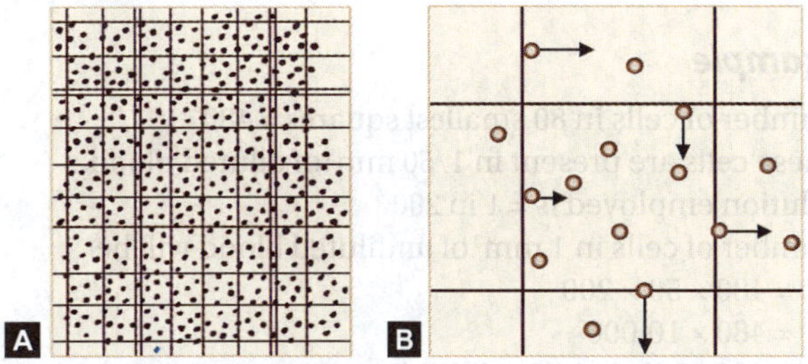

FIGS. 18A AND B: (A) Microscopic view of a charged chamber showing even distribution of red cells. A group of 16 smallest squares is shown in the middle; (B) Rules of counting: Count the cells lying within a square and those lying on or touching its upper horizontal and left vertical line cells lying or touching its lower horizontal and right vertical lines are to be omitted as they will be counted in the adjacent squares. Arrows indicate the squares to which the red cells belong.

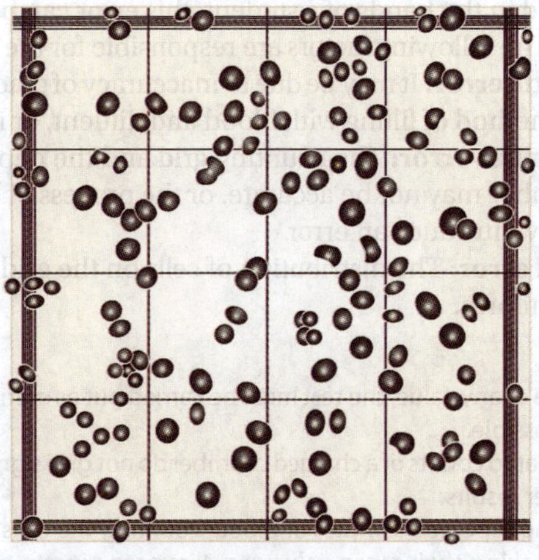

FIG. 19: Red blood cells in the RBC square.

Observations and Results

RBC in the RBC square under high power (Fig. 19). Add up the number of cells in each of the 5 blocks of 16 smallest squares. A difference of more than 20 between any 2 blocks indicates uneven distribution.

- **Calculation of dilution obtained (dilution factor).** Refer **Experiment 1.3**. Recall that the dilution with this pipette is **1 in 200** as blood is taken to mark 0.5.

$$\text{Thus, the dilution factor is} = \frac{\text{Final volume attained (100 parts)}}{\text{Volume of blood taken (0.5 part)}}$$

- **Calculation of volume of fluid examined.** We know the count in 80 smallest squares which have a volume (space) of 1/50 mm^3. We can also know the cell count in 1 smallest square which has a volume (space) of 1/4,000 mm^3.
- **Calculation of red cell count**
  Let N be the number of cells in 1/50 mm^3 of diluted blood.
  Cells in 1 mm^3 of diluted blood = N × 50
  Dilution employed was = 1 in 200
  Therefore, number of cells in 1 mm^3 of undiluted blood will be = N × 50 × 200 = N × 10,000.
  Thus, adding, 4 zeros in front of N will give the RBC count per 1 mm^3 of undiluted blood.

Example

Number of cells in 80 smallest squares = 480
These cells are present in 1/50 mm^3 of diluted blood.
Dilution employed is = 1 in 200
Number of cells in 1 mm^3 of undiluted blood will be:
= 480 × 50 × 200
= 480 × 10,000
= 480,0000, i.e. 4.8 million/mm^3.

Sources of Error

As mentioned in **Experiment 1.3**, despite all precautions in the procedures the degree of error with this method is said to be about ± 15%. Thus, with a count of 5.0 million/mm^3, the technical error of a single count comes to about ± 0.75 million/mm^3. And in the hands of a student, this error can be as high as 20%. The following factors are responsible for the error:

- **Pipette error:** It may be due to inaccuracy of graduations, the method of filling with blood and diluent, or mixing.
- **Chamber error:** The counting grid and the depth of the chamber may not be accurate, or the process of charging it may introduce an error.
- **Field error:** The distribution of cells on the grid may not be uniform.

Notes:
- To be of any value, the test must be carried out as meticulously as possible.
- Repeated counts of a charged chamber do not give significantly better results.
- Taking repeated samples of blood, counting the cells in each, and taking their mean value can eliminate pipette error. But this has hardly any practical value.

Normal Red Cell Count

- Express your result as..... million/mm^3
- The average cell counts and their ranges are:
  - *Males* = 5.0 million/mm^3 (4.75–6.0 million/mm^3)
  - *Females* = 4.5 million/mm^3 (4.0–5.5 million/mm^3).

Precautions

1. Observe all precautions described for getting a finger prick, filling the pipette with blood and diluent, and charging the chamber.
2. Clean the chamber with a lint-free piece of cloth. Once cleaned, do not touch the central part. Any oils left from your fingers on the coverslip or the chamber are fatal to cell counting.
3. If there is over or undercharging, wash, clean, dry, and refill the chamber.
4. Continuously rack the fine adjustment while counting the cells.
5. Do not draw diluents directly from the stock bottle as it may contaminate the solution with cells.
6. Discard the sample and recharge the chamber if the distribution is not uniform.
7. Follow the rules of counting to avoid the counting twice.

Physioclinical Significance

There are number of physiological and pathological conditions where RBC count can be altered.

1. **Decrease RBC count**
   - Physiological causes:
     - Pregnancy
     - RBC count is lower in children than adults
     - Females have lower RBC count than males.
   - Pathological: Anemia
     Hemodilution, e.g. excess ADH secretion as in posterior pituitary tumors.
2. **Increase in RBC count**
   - Physiological causes:
     - High altitude
     - Newborns
     - Hemoconcentration, e.g. excessive sweating.
   - Pathological:
     - Hemoconcentration, e.g. diarrhea, vomiting
     - Chronic hypoxia, e.g. congenital heart disease, chronic obstructive pulmonary disease
     - Polycythemia vera.

QUESTIONS

Q.1. Why is blood diluted 200 times for red cell count?
A high dilution is needed because the number of RBCs is very high.

Q.2. What is the function of the bead in the bulb?
The bead (red in this case) helps in mixing the contents of the bulb thoroughly. It helps in identifying the pipette at a distance. And, thirdly, it tells whether the bulb is dry or not (if it is not, the bead will not roll freely).

Q.3. Will the bead in the bulb affect the dilution?
The volume of the bead is taken into consideration during manufacturing of the pipette.

Q.4. How will you clean the pipette and the chamber after your experiment is over?
See text above.

Q.5. How will you clean a pipette/blocked with clotted blood?
See text above.

Q.6. What are the units of markings on the pipette?
These markings (0.5, 1.0, 101) do not represent any units but are relative volumes or parts in relation to each other.

Q.8. If Hayem's solution is not available, can you use any other solution?

See text above.

Q.9. Why should you discard the first few drops from the pipette before charging the chamber?

Even after thoroughly mixing the blood and the diluent, the stem contains only the diluent which is cell-free.

Q.10. What are the features of a properly charged chamber? How will over- or undercharging of the chamber affect the red cell count?

Refer to the chapter on hemocytometry for features of a properly charged chamber. When the chamber is overcharged, diluted blood flows into the trenches where the red cells, being heavier, sink down. This gives a false low count. Under charging, due to less blood in the chamber will also give a low count.

Q.11. What is the function of the coverslip?

Since the coverslip is absolutely flat and smooth, it ensures a uniformly deep capillary space between it and the floorpiece. Surface tension holds the diluted blood in place without its spilling into trenches unless the volume is more than the space available to it.

Q.12. Why should a chipped coverslip not be used?

A chipped or broken coverslip will not cover the floorpiece properly, thus resulting in uneven distribution of cells.

Q.13. Why should both sides of the chamber be charged?

- Charging on one side may lift the coverslip unevenly on that side. Charging the two sides keeps the cover slip uniformly placed.If the cover slip is not uniformly placed, the distance between the chamber and the cover slip will be higher than 0.1 mm, and the cell counts will not be accurate.
- Also both sides of the chamber need to be charged so as to reduce the error in counting.
- Both RBC and WBC counts can be done simultaneously by separately charging the two sides of the chamber.

Q.14. Why is it difficult to see the grid lines and cells clearly at the same focus?

Since the grid lines, the cells lying on the floorpiece, and those sticking to the underside of the coverslip are located at different levels in the 0.1 mm space, all of them may not be seen clearly at one focusing position. It is for this reason that 'racking' of fine adjustment is required.

Q.15. How will you differentiate red cells from dust particles?

Dust particles may be present on the objective, eyepiece, or in the diluent. They are irregular in size and shape. If they are on the eyepiece, they will rotate with the eyepiece. Red cells, on the other hand, are round discs, of uniform size, light pink in color which is lighter in the center.

Q.16. Can the red cells be counted with the low power objective?

Though the cells can be seen clearly under low power and can be counted by an experienced person, it is best for the student to count them under high power.

Q.17. Why is it necessary to follow the rules of counting?

The rules must be followed to avoid the error of missing some cells, and counting others more than once.

Q.18. What are the sources of error in this experiment?

See text above.

Q.19. What is the fate of leukocytes in this experiment?

An occasional leukocyte may be seen. It is larger than a red cell, appears refractile (shiny) and granular, it also contains a nucleus. Since the ratio of WBC to RBC is 1:600–700. Therefore, hardly any WBCs are counted. Since in healthy individuals, the total number of RBCs counted in 80 smallest squares (5 × 16) is approximately 600, WBCs do not affect the RBC count.

But if it is counted with the red cells, it will increase the count by 10,000/mm^3 since the multiplication factor is 10,000 for cells in 80 smallest squares.

Q.20. What is the site of formation of red cells during fetal life and after birth?

Sites of erythropoiesis:

- **Fetal life**—spleen, liver, thymus and bone marrow.
  - In the early weeks of embryonic life, primitive, nucleated red blood cells are produced in the yolk sac (mesoblastic phase).
  - During the middle trimester of gestation, the liver is the main organ for production of red blood cells, but reasonable numbers are also produced in the spleen and lymph nodes (hepatic phase).
  - During the last month or so of gestation and after birth, red blood cells are produced exclusively in the bone marrow (myeloid phase).
- **After birth till 5 years of age**—red bone marrow
- **Adult life**—long bone cavities and femur.

Q.21. What is the lifespan and fate of red cells?

The average lifespan of red cells as determined by radioac tive and agglutination methods is about 120 days (about 40 days in macrocytic anemia and spherocytosis). During their lifetime, they circuit the cardiovascular system some 300,000 times (their elastic framework, formed by the protein spectrin, permits them to regain their biconcave shape as they emerge through the capillaries). As they squeeze through 5–6 μm capillaries again, they are subjected to severe mechanical stress, wear and tear of their plasma membranes. Since there is no nucleus and other organelles, the red cells cannot synthesize new components to replace the damaged ones. The plasma membranes become more and more fragile with age; they are now more likely to burst particularly as they squeeze through the narrow trabecular spaces of the spleen.

About 10% of the worn-out RBCs fragment in the circulating blood. These fragments and old cells are removed from the blood and destroyed by the fixed phagocytic macrophages in the spleen, liver, etc. (The spleen has been called the graveyard of RBCs). The breakdown products, globin and iron of heme are recycled for reuse by the body.

Q.22. What is erythropoiesis? What are the stages of differentiation and maturation of red cells?

See text above.

Q.23. How is erythropoiesis regulated?

The proliferation and differentiation of various cells in the bone marrow is very accurately controlled by following factors:

Various hormones or factors (hemopoietic growth factors) that include: colony stimulating factors (CSFs), cytokines, interleukins (ILS), erythropoietin (EPO), etc. **Factors that regulate erythropoiesis:**

1. ***Erythropoietin (EPO):*** The critical balance between RBC production and destruction is maintained by adjustments in the circulating levels of EPO. Its blood level is greatly increased in anemia. The number of erythropoietin-sensitive stem cells in the bone marrow is greatly increased by EPO. These are then converted into RBC precursors and then to mature erythrocytes.

   Erythropoietin is a glycoprotein that contains 165 amino acid residues and 4 oligosaccharide chains. About 95% of EPO is secreted by the peritubular interstitial cells of the kidneys, and 15% from the perivenous hepatocytes of liver. Hypoxia is the most potent stimulator for EPO secretion. Cobalt salts and androgens also stimulate EPO secretion.
2. ***Grade I proteins:*** Proteins of animal origin, soya beans, etc.
3. ***Vitamins:*** B_{12}, folic acid, pyridoxine, other B complex vitamins, and vitamin C are needed for red cell formation.
4. ***Trace metals:*** Iron, copper, zinc, and cobalt are required in trace amounts.
5. ***Hormones:*** Androgens, thyroxin, growth hormone, and cortisol are required.

Q.24. Which physiological condition causes a decrease in RBC count?

See text above.

Q.25. What is anemia and what are its causes?

See chapter on Estimation of Hemoglobin.

Q.26. What is polycythemia and what are its causes?

Polycythemia: It refers to an increase in the number of red cells above the normal level. Erythrocytosis is a better term to describe an absolute increase in the total red cell mass.

1. **Polycythemia vera (erythremia, or primary polycythemia):** A gene abnormality in the early red cells causes them to form more and more cells. Erythropoietin production is not raised, but may be decreased.
2. **Secondary polycythemia:** Hypoxia due to lung diseases, congenital heart disease, and cardiac failure increases the RBC count.
3. **Polycythemia due to hemoconcentration:** Fluid loss during severe vomiting and diarrhea and loss of plasma in burns cause polycythemia. There is no increase in total red cell mass.

Physiological polycythemia is seen during residence at high altitudes, and in newborns. Emotional stress and severe exercise may cause a temporary increase in RBC count.

Q.27. What is meant by "Stem cell harvesting" and what is their practical value?

Transplantation of stem cells (confined mainly to red bone marrow) from normal persons to patients of certain leukemias and abnormal bone marrow, have been in use for many years. The abnormal bone marrow is first destroyed by drugs and whole body radiation, and bone marrow aspirated from the hip bone of a donor is then transfused into the patient. The normal stem cells (taken from the donor) then settle in the recipient bone marrow where they start to produce normal cells in due course of time.

The harvesting (collecting) of pluripotent stem cells (PHSCs) from the umbilical cord blood (where they are present in much larger numbers than in adult bone marrow) is now being employed. The PHSCs taken from the blastocysts of human embryos have been cultured and work on these cells may prove beneficial to currently incurable diseases like Parkinson's, Alzheimer's, diabetes mellitus, and repair of damaged heart muscle in coronary artery disease.

OBJECTIVE STRUCTURED PRACTICAL EXAMINATION-I

Aim: To dilute the given sample of blood 200 times using a pipette and diluent.

Procedural steps: See text above.

Checklist:

1. Selects the correct pipette and checks that it is clean, dry and patent. (Y/N)
2. Takes enough diluents in a watch glass and sucks blood to the exact 0.5 mark and sees that there are no air bubbles. (Y/N)
3. Wipes off blood sticking to the outside of the tip of the pipette. (Y/N)
4. Sucks diluting fluid exactly to the mark 101. (Y/N)
5. Holds the pipette horizontally between the palms and rolls it gently to mix the contents of the bulb. (Y/N)

OBJECTIVE STRUCTURED PRACTICAL EXAMINATION-II

Aim: To charge the Neubauer chamber with diluted blood provided to you in a RBC pipette.

Procedural steps: See text above.

Checklist:

1. Ensures that the chamber and coverslip are clean and dry. (Y/N)
2. Mixes the contents of the bulb between the palms. (Y/N)
3. Places the coverslip on the central plateau of the chamber to cover both the ruled areas. (Y/N)
4. Discards the first few drops from the pipette and allows a suitable-sized drop to form. (Y/N)
5. Places the tip of pipette on the chamber, touching the edge of the coverslip and allows the fluid to spread evenly over the counting grid without over- or under charging. Charges the other side also. (Y/N)

1.5: THE TOTAL LEUKOCYTE COUNT

STUDENT OBJECTIVES

After completing this experiment, the student should be able to:

- Indicate the importance of doing total leukocyte count (TLC) in a clinical setting and in practical physiology.
- Do the total leukocyte count by the manual method, and compare its degree of error with the error of RBC counting.
- Name the constituents of Turk's fluid and their functions.
- Indicate the precautions you will observe.
- Describe the normal TLC in different age groups.
- Name the different leukocytes, their site of formation, functions, and regulation of leukopoiesis.
- Define leukocytosis, leukopenia, and physiological and pathological conditions in which they are seen.

INTRODUCTION

PY2.11: Estimate Hb, RBC, TLC, RBC indices, DLC, Blood groups, BT/CT.

The white blood corpuscles (WBCs, leukocytes) constitute the major defense system of the body against invasion by bacteria, viruses, fungi, toxins, and other foreign invaders. Their number is kept remarkably constant in health, but it increases or decreases in many diseases particularly acute and chronic infections. A clinician generally wants this test done along with differential count, hemoglobin, etc. as part of "complete blood count" (CBC) in cases of fever, especially if the cause of fever is not immediately apparent (pyrexia of unknown origin or PUO).

STAGES OF LEUKOPOIESIS (FLOWCHART 2)

Normal count: 4,000–11,000 cells/mm^3 of blood in adults. The count after birth may be as high as 18,000–20,000/ mm^3, the normal levels being reached in a few years. In the adults, about 55–75% of the WBCs are granulocytes, while in young children, lymphocytes dominate. The count may be high in some physiological conditions such as heavy exercise, stress, etc.

TYPES OF LEUKOCYTES

The WBCs, unlike red cells contain nuclei but no hemoglobin. Depending on the presence or absence of clearly visible and conspicuous, chemical-filled granules (vesicles) in their cytoplasm (that are made visible by staining), they are grouped into two types: ***granular*** and ***agranular.***

- **Granulocytes:** There are three types of granulocytes that can be recognized under the compound microscope according to the coloration of their cytoplasmic granules—***neutrophils, eosinophils*** (eosin loving), ***and basophils*** (basic loving).
- **Agranulocytes:** In contrast to granulocytes whose nuclei are lobed, the nuclei of agranulocytes are not lobed but appear as a single mass. Although the cytoplasm contains chemical-filled granules, these are not visible under the light microscope due to their small size and poor staining with the usual dyes. The agranulocytes include—***monocytes*** and ***lymphocytes.***

FLOWCHART 2: Stages of leukopoiesis.

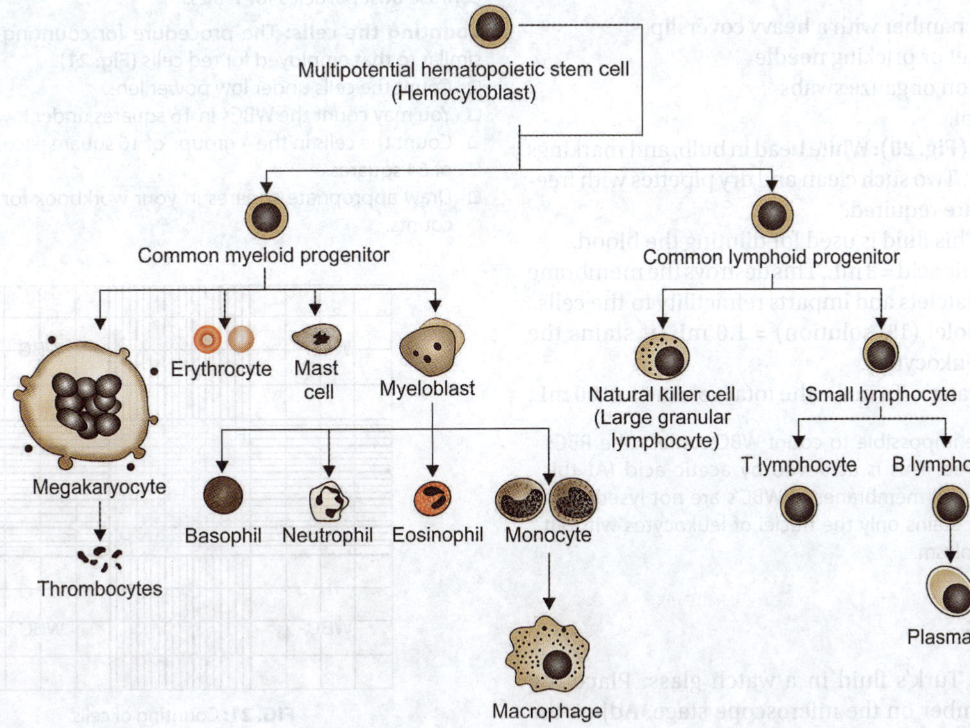

CHIEF FUNCTIONS OF LEUKOCYTES

- The chief function of leukocytes is to provide immunity (protection) against various invaders and thus constitute an important mechanism of survival by preserving health and fending off disease. The immune system consists of task-specific cells that are in a constant state of vigilance and readiness—like the branches of armed forces. They recognize the invaders as "foreign" to the body and engage them in combat at the site of invasion.
- The **tissue macrophages** (that develop from blood monocytes and act as the "sentinels"), and neutrophils (they act as the "infantry" and are transported by blood to the site of invasion), respond most quickly and destroy the invaders by phagocytosing them (both these cells move through the tissues by active amoeboid movements and are attracted to the inflamed area). Thus, these two types of WBCs along with antimicrobial proteins (interferons—alpha, beta, and gamma, and complement system and natural killer lymphocytes, form the ***second line of defense***). ***The first line of defense*** against infection are the surface barriers i.e. intact skin and mucous membranes, that prevent the entry of pathogens into the body.

PRINCIPLE

A sample of blood is diluted with a diluting fluid which destroys the red cells and stains the nuclei of the leukocytes. The cells are then counted in a counting chamber and their number in undiluted blood reported as leukocytes/mm^3.

APPARATUS

- **Microscope:**
  - Counting chamber with a heavy coverslip
  - Blood lancet or pricking needle
  - Sterile cotton or gauze swabs
  - 70% alcohol.
- **WBC pipettes (Fig. 20):** White bead in bulb, and markings 0.5, 1.0, and 11. Two such clean and dry pipettes with free-rolling beads are required.
- **Turk's fluid:** This fluid is used for diluting the blood.
  - Glacial acetic acid = 3 mL. This destroys the membrane of RBCs, platelets and imparts refractility to the cells.
  - Gentian violet (1% solution) = 1.0 mL (it stains the nuclei of leukocytes).
  - Distilled water = To make the total volume to 100 mL.

Note: It would be impossible to count WBCs unless the RBCs were first destroyed. This is achieved by acetic acid (At this concentration the cell membranes of WBC's are not lysed). The dye gentian violet stains only the nuclei of leukocytes without staining their cytoplasm.

PROCEDURE

- Take 1 mL of Turk's fluid in a watch glass. Place the counting chamber on the microscope stage. Adjust the illumination and focus the right upper group of 16 WBC squares. You will see all the squares in one field.

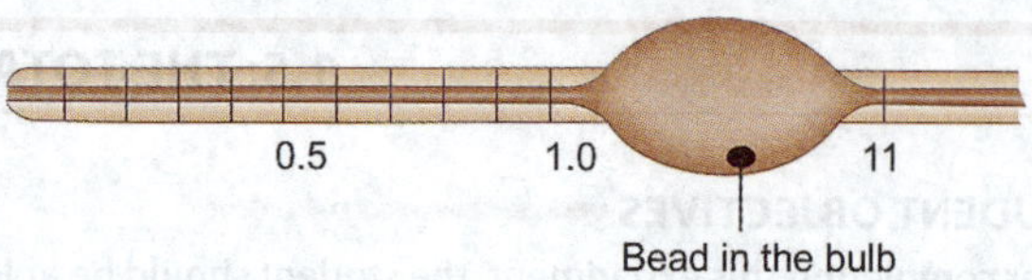

FIG. 20: The WBC pipette. It has 3 markings—0.5, 1.0, and 11.

- Observing all the aseptic precautions, get a fingerprick, discard the first two drops of blood, and let a good-sized drop to form.
- **Filling the pipette:** Dip the tip of the pipette in the edge of the drop, draw blood to the mark 0.5 and suck Turk's fluid to the mark 11. Mix the contents of the bulb thoroughly for 3–4 minutes.
- **Charging the chamber:** Discard the first two drops of fluid from the pipette so as to empty the fluid present in the stem. Charge the chamber on both sides. The chamber should neither be over-charged nor under-charged.
- Allow the cells to settle for 3–4 minutes, and then carefully transfer the chamber to the microscope. Use the fine adjustment again and try to identify the WBCs.

Under low magnification: The leukocytes appear as round, shiny (refractile), darkish dots, with a halo around them. These "dots" represent the nuclei, which have been stained by gentian violet. The cytoplasm is not stained.

Important: When examining cells or counting them, do not keep a fixed focus but continuously "rack" the microscope so that the cells and the lines come into and go out of focus. In this way, you will not miss cells sticking to the undersurface of the coverslip, or confuse dust particles for WBCs.

Counting the cells: The procedure for counting the WBCs is similar to that employed for red cells **(Fig. 21)**.
- Count the cells under low power lens.
- You may count the WBCs in 16 squares under low power.
- Count the cells in the 4 groups of 16 square each, i.e., in a total of 64 squares.
- Draw appropriate squares in your workbook for entering the counts.

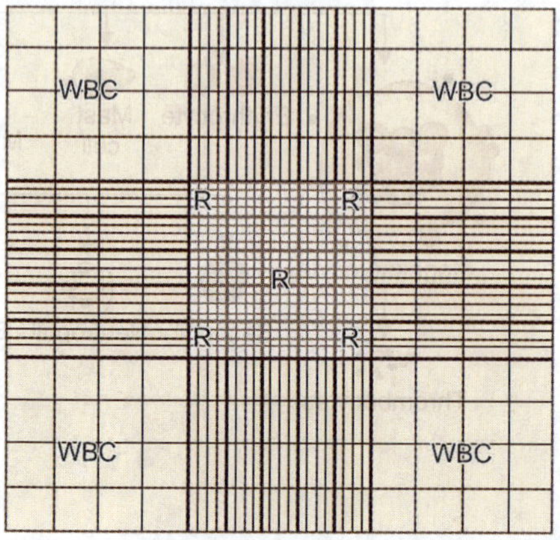

FIG. 21: Counting of cells.

OBSERVATIONS AND RESULTS

Calculations (Fig. 22)

Dilution factor = Final volume achieved (10 parts)/ Original volume taken (0.5 parts) = 20

Volume of fluid:

Area of 4 WBC squares = $4 \times 1 \times 1 = 4$ mm²

Depth of the chamber = 0.1 mm

Volume of fluid in the 4 WBC squares = $4 \times 0.1 = 0.4$ microliter

Calculation of TLC:

Let N be the total number of WBCs in 4 WBC squares Total no. of WBCs in 1 microliter of undiluted blood = N × Dilution factor (20)/0.4 = N × 50

Sources and Degrees of Error

The sources of errors are the same as described for RBC counting and include: Pipette error, chamber error, field error, and experimental error.

The degree of error which may be 30% or more in RBC counting is much less in TLC (about 5–10%) because of the low dilution employed (1 in 20) in this case. The error can be further reduced if counting is done on both platforms of the counting chamber. That the error in TLC counting is much less important than that in the RBC count is obvious from the following example: In a TLC of 8,000/mm³, even an error of 20% will give a count of 9,600/mm³ which is again well within the normal range.

Note: In case when the leukocyte count is very high, as in leukemia, the dilution has to be increased. For this purpose, the RBC pipette can be used in which the blood is sucked up to mark 1 and diluted 100 times. Further calculation is done accordingly.

PRECAUTIONS

- Observe all precautions described for a finger prick, filling the pipette, and charging the counting chamber.
- Keep all the equipment ready before getting a prick.
- When mixing the blood with the Turk's fluid, give sufficient time for complete hemolysis of red cells. However, ensure that the leukocytes are not centrifuged toward the ends of the pipette which can be avoided by keeping the pipette horizontal while mixing the contents of the bulb.
- Continuously "rack" the microscope while identifying and counting the cells.
- Though the condition of a charged chamber may remain stable for 80–90 minutes, the count is usually stable for 30–40 minutes. After that, the diluted blood starts receding due to drying and the count decreases. The counting of the cells should, therefore, not be delayed.

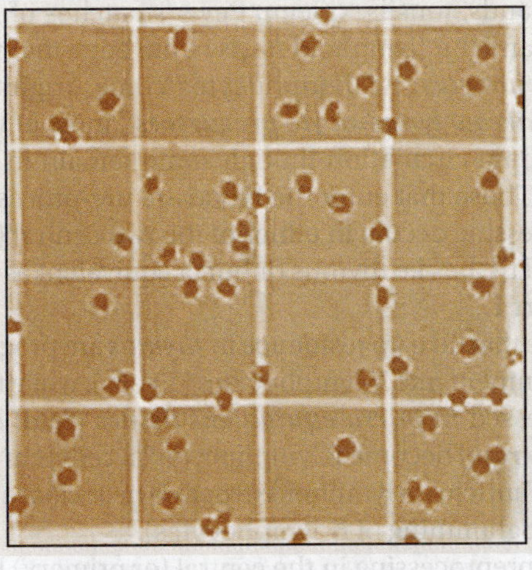

FIG. 22: White blood cells in WBC square.

PHYSIOCLINICAL SIGNIFICANCE

Conditions that increase TLC:

- **Physiological causes:** Physiological leukocytosis (i.e. in the absence of infection or tissue injury) has no clinical significance. There is no decrease or absence of eosinophils (eosinopenia) which is a feature of leukocytosis due to infection. Physiological leukocytosis is due to mobilization of WBCs from the marginal pool or bone marrow reserve ("Shift" leukocytosis). It is seen in the following conditions:
  - **Normal infants:** The count may be as high as 18–20,000/mm³ but it returns to normal level within 1–2 years.
  - **Food intake and digestion ("digestive leukocy tosis"):** There is a mild increase which returns to normal within an hour or so.
  - **Physical exercise**
  - **Mental stress**
  - **Pregnancy:** The count may be quite high especially during the first pregnancy.
  - **Parturition:** The high TLC is possibly due to tissue injury, pain, physical stress, and hemorrhage.
  - **Extremes of temperatures:** Exposure to sun, or to very low temperature can increase the WBC count.
- **Pathological causes:** A rise in TLC in disease is seen in:
  - **Acute infection with pyogenic (pus forming) bacteria:** The infection (due to cocci bacteria—*Streptococcus, Staphylococcus*) may be: (a) Localized, such as boils, abscess, tonsillitis, appendicitis, etc. (b) Generalized such as in septicemia and pyemia, bronchitis, pneumonia, peritonitis, meningitis, etc.
  - **Myocardial infarction:** The rise in TLC is due to tissue injury is not seen immediately after a heart attack but only after 4–5 days.
  - **Acute hemorrhage:** Maximum response occurs in 8–10 hours, the count returning to normal in 5–6 days.
  - **Burns:** Maximum response occurs in 5–15 hours, the count returning to normal in 2–3 days.
  - **Amebic hepatitis.**
  - **Malignancies:** High counts are seen in half the cases; secondary infection enhances the count.
  - **Surgical operations:** A postoperative rise is seen in all cases.

Conditions that decrease total leukocyte count:

- **Physiological causes:** A decrease in TLC under normal physiological conditions is unusual and rare. Exposure to acute extreme cold, may reduce the count to only slightly below the 4,000/mm³ level.

- **Pathological causes:** Leukopenia is due to disease, where TLC is abnormally low is never beneficial to the body. In fact, it may endanger the life of the patient. The condition is almost always due to a decrease in neutrophils (neutropenia) and may be caused by various drugs used in treatment, radiation, or certain infections as described here:
  - **Infection with nonpyogenic organisms:** Typhoid and paratyphoid fevers, and sometimes in protozoal infection like malaria.
  - **Viral infections:** Influenza, mumps, smallpox, acquired immunodeficiency syndrome (AIDS).
  - **Drugs:** Chloramphenicol, sulfonamides, aspirin, penicillins, cyclosporins, phenytoin, etc. Cytotoxic drugs used in treating malignancies may also cause leukopenia by depressing the bone marrow (other blood cells may also decrease).
  - **Repeated exposures to X-rays and radium:** These are used as radiotherapy in cancers, and cause bone marrow depression.
  - **Chemical poisons that depress bone marrow:** Arsenic, dinitrophenol, antimony, and others.
  - **Malnutrition:** Deficiency of vitamin B_{12} and folate, general malnutrition, starvation, extreme weakness and debility.
  - **Hypoplasia and aplasia:** Partial or complete depression of bone marrow, i.e. failure of stem cells, may occur as a result of autoimmunity, and other factors.
- **Preleukemic stage of leukemias** may show leukopenia.

QUESTIONS

Q.1. How will you differentiate a WBC pipette from a RBC pipette?

See **Table 4**.

Q.2. What do the three markings on the pipette indicate? How do you get a dilution of 1 in 20?

See text above.

Q.3. What is the volume of the bulb in the WBC pipette? Why is its bulb smaller than that of the RBC pipette?

The volume of the fluid in the bulb is 10 times the volume of fluid in the stem, which can give a dilution of 1 in 10 or 1 in 20. In the RBC pipette, the volume of the bulb is 100 times the volume of the stem, which can give a dilution of 1 in 100 or 1 in 200. Since the count of leukocytes is in thousands/ mm^3, the blood requires much less dilution as compared to red cell count which is in millions/mm^3.

Q.4. What is the function of the bead in the bulb?

The bead serves three purposes:

1. It aids mixing the blood with the diluent.
2. It helps in identifying the pipette by just looking at it.
3. It tells whether the pipette is dry or not. In a dry pipette, the bead rolls freely without sticking to the inside of the bulb which would happen if the bulb were wet.

Q.5. What are the other uses of WBC pipette?

The WBC pipette can be used for diluting the blood for counting RBCs in cases of severe anemia, or for counting platelets. It can also be used for counting sperms and bacteria.

Q.6. What is the composition of Turk's fluid? What is the function of each constituent?

The diluting fluid for TLC contains glacial acetic acid, gentian violet, and distilled water. The acid hemolyzes the red cells without affecting the WBCs at this concentration. The dye stains the nuclei of leukocytes.

Q.7. What is meant by the term "glacial"? Why should the acid in the Turk's fluid be glacial?

The term glacial means pure acetic acid. Only the glacial acid can give the typical "shine" (halo) or clear refractility around the WBCs due to swelling of nuclei. This differentiates them from dust particles which are opaque and of different shapes (It is called glacial because during its manufacture, it gives the appearance of a glacier at one stage).

Q.8. Why are the red cells not seen when counting the leukocytes?

The red cells are not seen because they are hemolyzed by the acid (they would, otherwise, not allow counting of leukocytes). The remnants of red cell membranes are faintly visible—the so-called ghost cells.

Q.9. Can any other agent be used to hemolyze the red cells?

No. Any weaker hemolytic agent would take an inordinately long time to lyse them. A strong agent, on the other hand, in addition to lysing the red cells will also damage the leukocytes.

Q.10. What is the normal total leukocyte count?

See text above.

Q.11. What is the difference between differential leukocyte count and absolute leukocyte count?

In differential leukocyte count (DLC), the percentages of various types of WBCs are determined, while in absolute leukocyte count, the number of different WBCs per mm^3 is calculated (This is done from TLC and DLC).

Q.12. What are the various types of leukocytes and what are their functions?

See text above.

Q.13. What is leukopoiesis? Where does it occur?

See Flowchart 2 above.

The granulocytes, monocytes, and ***"lymphocyte precursors"*** are formed in the bone marrow (as are RBCs and platelets), while ***"blood lymphocytes"*** (those seen in blood films) are formed mainly in the ***"peripheral (secondary) lymphoid tissue"*** scattered throughout the body such as lymph glands, tonsils, spleen, Peyer's patches of intestinal mucosa, and the "lymphoid nests in the bone marrow".

Lymphocytes: All lymphocytes come originally from ***"bone marrow lymphocyte precursors"***, most of which are released into circulation though some remain in the bone marrow. Those that enter the blood are pre-processed cells. The processing occurs in either of the two central (primary) lymphoid tissues i.e thymus or bursa equivalent as shown in **Flowchart 1**.

Those that take up residence in ***thymus*** are programed by its environment into T-lymphocytes (T cells), while those that are processed ***in bursa equivalent tissues (fetal liver and bone marrow)*** become B lymphocytes (B cells) (In birds, the bursa of Fabricius, a lymphoid structure near cloaca is the site of pre-programming of B-lymphocytes).

After preprocessing in the central (or primary) lymphoid tissue, both T and B cells take up residence in ***peripheral (or***

secondary) lymphoid tissue. From these locations, various types of lymphocytes continue to divide and redivide and enter circulation throughout life via the lymphatic channels.

Thus, after birth, most lymphocytes are being formed in the peripheral lymphoid tissue, thymus and spleen, though some are formed in the bone marrow.

Granulocytes and ***monocytes*** are continuously formed in the red bone marrow to replace those millions of cells that leave the blood and enter the tissues, or those that are destroyed. Similarly, lymphocytes are being formed continuously to replace those lost.

Note: With the exception of lymphocytes, the other cells of blood do not divide once they leave bone marrow.

Q.14. How is leukopoiesis regulated?

Over 70 billion WBCs pass from the blood into the tissues every day, and the same number enters the circulation from their sites of production. In spite of these huge numbers involved, the constancy of TLC suggests a very efficient feedback mechanism that controls their production and release.

The substances which stimulate or inhibit this process appear to be many and varied. They include **colony stimulating factors CSFs** (formed by monocytes and T-lymphocytes), ***interleukins*** (formed by monocytes, macrophages, and endothelial cells), ***prostaglandins*** (formed by monocytes), ***lactoferrin,*** and possibly other agents. All these substances were collectively called ***Leukocyte promoting factor*** (or ***leukopoietin).*** Thus, unlike RBCs, the products of dead and dying cells themselves control leukopoiesis. The ***CSF,*** a glycoprotein present in the body fluids, appears to play an important role in the physiological regulation of leukopoiesis. During tissue injury and infection, the bacterial toxins, products of injury, etc. cause great increase in the rate of production and release of leukocytes.

Q.15. What is meant by the terms leukocytosis and granulocytosis? Name the physiological and pathological conditions which cause leukocytosis.

While *granulocytosis* technically refers to an increase in the number of granulocytes (neutrophils, eosinophils and basophils), *leukocytosis* refers to an increase in the number of all white blood cells beyond 11,000/mm^3. Leukocytosis is a normal, protective response of the body to various types of stresses such as infections, severe exercise, surgery, tissue injury, etc.

The TLC may rise due to:

- **Redistribution within the blood:** The WBCs from the "marginal" pool are mobilized and poured into the circulating blood.
- **Release from bone marrow reserve:** This is another process by which the number of WBCs can be raised in a short time.

These two processes raise the TLC without increasing their rate of production. There are no immature cells in the blood.

Note: It is important to remember that leukopenia due to any cause makes a person more likely to get pyogenic and other infections.

Q.16. What is leukemia and what are its major types?

A malignant progressive disease of hematopoietic cells leading to abnormal proliferation of immature or abnormal leukocytes is called leukemia. There is an uncontrolled production and release of mature and immature WBCs into the circulation. The leukemias (commonly called blood cancers) may be **myeloid** (usually involving neutrophils) or **lymphatic** (involving lymphocytes), and acute or chronic.

In acute leukemia, there is accumulation of immature cells in the blood (acute lymphatic leukemia is the most common malignancy in children, while acute myeloid leukemia is common in adults). Chronic leukemia begins more slowly and may remain undetected for months. Mature cells accumulate in blood because they do not die at the end of their normal lifespan.

In most cases, the cause is not known. However, genetic factors, viruses (e.g. human T cell leukemia, lymphoma virus-1, HTLV-1), chemical factors, and ionizing radiations (accidents in atomic power plants, atomic blasts such as in Hiroshima and Nagasaki during World War II) are involved.

Q.17. What is the difference between leukocytosis, leukostasis, leukemoid reaction, and leukemia?

Leukocytosis: It is an increase in TLC count above 11,000/mm^3, irrespective of the types of cells involved. It may be physiological or pathological. The pathological causes include infection and tissue injury. The count usually does not exceed 20–25,000/mm^3 and there are no immature cells in the circulation.

Leukostasis: If the count is more than 100,000/mm^3, white cell thrombi may form in the brain, lung, and heart—a condition called leukostasis. Transfusion of blood before TLC is reduced, increases blood viscosity, thus increasing the risk of leukostasis.

Leukemoid reaction: It is an extreme elevation of TLC above 50,000/mm^3 as a result of the presence of mature and/or immature neutrophils. The causes include: Severe chronic infections, especially in children, severe hemolysis, malignant growths (cancer of breast, lung, and kidney). It is not leukemia, and can be distinguished from chronic myelogenous leukemia (CML) by estimating the leukocyte alkaline phosphatase (LAP level which is elevated in leukemoid reaction, but depressed in CML).

Leukoerythroblastic reaction is similar to leukemoid reaction but with the addition of nucleated red cells (normoblasts) on blood smear. The causes include: Marrow infiltration by malignancy, hypoxia, and severe anemia.

Leukemia: Leukemia is a cancerous growth of blood forming organs (bone marrow or lymphatic tissues). Due to uncontrolled production, both immature and mature WBCs are released into circulation. The TLC is generally above 40–50,000/mm^3 or even a few lakhs. Even when the count is moderately high, it is not called leukocytosis. Most cells are, however, functionally incompetent.

The term *aleukemic leukemia* is sometimes used for the preleukemic stage when blood picture is normal but the bone marrow study points to leukemia.

Bone marrow study is always undertaken when there is a doubt about diagnosis.

Q.18. What do you know about bone marrow transplantation? What are its indications?

Bone marrow transplantation is the intravenous transfusion of red bone marrow from a healthy donor (commonly taken from iliac crest) to a recipient. The purpose is to establish normal hemopoiesis and so, normal blood cell counts in the recipient. The procedure has been successfully used to treat certain types of leukemia, some cancers, severe combined immunodeficiency disease (SCID), some genetic disorders, hemolytic anemia, and so on. The patient's defective red bone marrow must first be destroyed by whole body irradiation and high doses of chemotherapy. The donor's marrow must, of course, be closely matched with that of the recipient to avoid rejection. The stem cells from the donor's marrow settle down and start to grow in the recipient's bone marrow cavities, where they begin to produce healthy cells of various types.

OBJECTIVE STRUCTURED PRACTICAL EXAMINATION-I

Aim: To dilute the given sample of blood 20 times for TLC by using diluent and a pipette provided.

Procedural steps: See text above.

Checklist:

1. Checks that the pipette is clean, dry, and patent. (Y/N)
2. Takes sufficient diluting fluid in a watch glass and sucks blood exactly to the mark 0.5 and confirms that there is no air bubble. (Y/N)
3. Wipes off blood sticking to the outside of the pipette tip. (Y/N)
4. Sucks diluting fluid to the mark 11. (Y/N)
5. Holds the pipette horizontally between the palms and rolls it gently. (Y/N)

OBJECTIVE STRUCTURED PRACTICAL EXAMINATION-II

Aim: To charge the counting chamber for TLC with diluted blood provided in a pipette.

Procedural steps: See text above.

Checklist:

1. Checks that the chamber and the pipette are clean and dry. (Y/N)
2. Places the coverslip on the floor piece and trenches. (Y/N)
3. Mixes the contents of the pipette by rolling it between the palms and discards the first two drops. (Y/N)
4. Charges the chamber by slow and controlled release of diluted blood at the edge of the coverslip. (Y/N)
5. Allows the diluted blood to spread under the coverslip to cover the ruled area. Allows the cells to settle down. (Y/N)

1.6: ESTIMATION OF HEMOGLOBIN

STUDENT OBJECTIVES

After completing this experiment, the student should be able to:

- Indicate the clinical significance of hemoglobin (Hb) estimation.
- List the characteristics of Hb important to estimate its concentration.
- Explain the absolute and relative Hb scales.
- Determine the Hb level by the Sahli's acid hematin method.
- List the sources and degree of error in this method.
- Name the advantages and disadvantages of Sahli's method.
- Name other methods of estimation of Hb.
- Indicate normal levels of Hb in different age groups and sexes.
- Describe the structure, synthesis, and functions of Hb.
- Name the varieties and derivatives of Hb.
- Name the common causes of increased and decreased levels of Hb.
- Classify anemias and mention the most common type of anemia in India.

INTRODUCTION

PY2.11: Estimate Hb, RBC, TLC, RBC indices, DLC, Blood groups, BT/CT.

Hemoglobin (Hb; molecular weight 64,450) is a chromo protein present in the red cells, and gives red color to the whole blood. It constitutes 95% of dry weight and 32–34% wet weight of red cells. It is a globular molecule consisting of four subunits. Each subunit consists of heme conjugated to a polypeptide chain. Two subunits contain alpha (α) chains (141 amino acid residues), while the other two subunits contain beta (β) chains (146 amino acid residues). The four polypeptide chains taken together make up the protein part called *globin* (globin constitutes 96% of the molecular mass of Hb). The *heme* is an iron containing porphyrin pigment called iron protoporphyrin IX. The porphyrin nucleus has four pyrrole rings synthesized from acetyl CoA and glycine. The synthesis of Hb begins in the proerythroblast, though it appears first in the intermediate normoblast, and continues till the reticulocyte stage. The materials required for Hb synthesis include: Grade 1 proteins, metals such as iron, copper, nickel, cobalt, and vitamins such as vitamin C, pyridoxine, riboflavin, nicotinic acid.

NORMAL VALUES

The levels of Hb in normal Indian adults especially in the economically deprived population are on the lower side of those reported from affluent countries. The reason may be the poor intake of grade 1 proteins and other nutrients. The average levels and their normal range are as follows:

Males: 14.5 g/dL (13.5–18 g/dL) of blood.
Females: 12.5 g/dL (11.5–16 g/dL) of blood.

TYPES OF HEMOGLOBIN

Normal Hemoglobin (Table 5)

The amino acid sequences of the polypeptide chains are determined by the globin genes. Slight variations in their composition can alter the properties of Hb.

- *Adult Hb (HbA):*
  - Hemoglobin A ($\alpha_2\beta_2$): About 95% of Hb in a normal adult is HbA.
  - Hemoglobin A2 (HbA2, or $\alpha_2\delta_2$): About 2–5% of Hb in an adult is HbA2.
- *Fetal Hb (HbF, or $\alpha_2\gamma_2$)*: During fetal life HbF predominates, in which two gamma chains replace the two beta chains. The gamma chains also contain 146 amino acid residues but have 37 that differ from those in beta chains. Since HbF has less affinity to 2,3-bisphosphoglycerate (2,3-BPG), it can accept greater amounts of O_2 from mother's blood at low PO_2.
- *Embryonic Hb*: This is a tetramer having two zeta (ζ_2) and two epsilon (ε_2) chains, forming Gower-1 Hb ($\zeta_2\varepsilon_2$) and Gower-2 Hb that contains two alpha and two epsilon chains ($\alpha_2\varepsilon_2$).
- HbA1c is characterized by α_2 and β_2 globin chains. It is formed by the covalent binding of glucose to HbA. The levels of HbA1c increase in poorly controlled diabetes mellitus.

Diffusion of CO_2 from fetal blood into mother's blood causes alkalinity of fetal blood and acidity of mother's blood. This causes an increase in the affinity of HbF for O_2, and release of O_2 from mother's Hb—this has been called *double Bohr effect*.

The differences between the two Hbs are shown in **Table 6**.

Abnormal Hemoglobin

Sometimes, abnormal polypeptide chains are synthesized due to mutant genes. These defects are widespread and over 1,000 abnormal Hbs have been described in humans. They are usually identified by letters.

In **HbS** (sickle cell anemia), the alpha chains are normal but in each beta chain, one glutamic acid residue has been replaced by a valine residue. HbS polymerizes at low O_2 tensions and forms elongated crystals (often 15 µm long) inside the red blood cells (RBCs) which assume sickle shapes. They pass through small capillaries with difficulty, and the spiked ends of the crystals cause rupture of these cells resulting in anemia.

Table 5: Types of normal hemoglobin.

Hemoglobin	*Composition*	*Adults*	*Newborns*
Hemoglobin A_{1c}	$\alpha_2\beta_2$	95%	20%
Hemoglobin A_2	$\alpha_2\beta_2$	<3.5%	
Hemoglobin F	$\alpha_2\delta_2$	<2.5%	<0.5%
Hemoglobin	$\alpha_2\gamma_2$	<1.0%	80%

Table 6: Differences between adult and fetal hemoglobin.

Adult hemoglobin	*Fetal hemoglobin*
Contains four polypeptide chains (two alpha and two beta chains)	The two beta chains replaced by gamma chains
Appears in red cells of the fetus in 5th month. At birth, 20% of total Hb is HbA	HbF at birth makes up 80% of total Hb. Disappears by 5th month after birth
Lifespan long—120 days	Lifespan short—about 2 weeks
It has the usual affinity for oxygen	It has greater affinity for oxygen as it binds 2,3-BPG less avidly
Percentage saturation at a PO_2 of 20 mm Hg = 30–35%	Percentage saturation at a PO_2 of 20 mm Hg = 70%

In **HbC,** there are two alpha and two beta chains. The glutamate of beta chains in 6th position is replaced by lysine residue. HbC disease occurs in black population. **HbD** has also two alpha and two beta chains. However, glutamine replaces glutamate in the 12th position of beta chains. **HbE, I, J, H, Bart's,** etc. are other abnormal Hbs. Many of these are harmless while some have abnormal O_2 equilibriums and cause anemia.

The abnormal Hbs are associated with two types of inherited anemias:

1. ***Hemoglobinopathies:*** These are due to abnormal chains e.g. HbS, HbC and HbE.
2. ***Thalassemias***: The chains are normal, but are less in amount or even absent. The α- and β-thalassemias are defined by decreased or even absent α- and β-polypeptides. The defects in the genes are in their regulatory proteins.

FUNCTIONS OF HEMOGLOBIN

- **Carriage of oxygen:** It carries O_2 from the lungs to all the tissues. Each iron atom loosely binds one molecule of O_2 at the 6th covalent or coordination bond. Each gram of Hb, when fully saturated, carries 1.34 mL of O_2 (1.39 mL by pure Hb). The affinity of Hb for O_2 is affected by pH, H^+, temperature, and 2,3-BPG.
- **Carriage of CO_2:** Hemoglobin carries about 23% of the total CO_2 carried by the blood from the tissues to the lungs. The CO_2 reacts with the amino radicals of the goblin to form carbaminohemoglobin—a reversible reaction that occurs with a loose bond.
- **Homeostasis of pH (buffer action of Hb):** Buffer systems convert strong acids and bases (which ionize easily and contribute H^+ or OH^-) into weak acids and bases that do not ionize as much to contribute H^+ or OH^-. As H^+ or OH^- are formed in red cells, or enter them, they are readily accepted by Hb (Hb + H = HbH) that gives up its oxygen. Hb is an excellent buffer and is responsible for 75% of the buffering power of blood. In fact, all proteins act as buffers because of the terminal carboxyl and amino groups.
- **Stabilization of tissue PO_2:** Hemoglobin is mainly responsible for stabilizing PO_2 in the tissues because sufficient amounts of O_2 are delivered between a PO_2 of 20 mm Hg and 40 mm Hg.

- **Regulation of blood flow and blood pressure:** In addition to the key role of Hb in carriage of O_2 and CO_2, Hb also plays a role in the regulation of local blood flow and blood pressure.

The iron ions of Hb have a strong affinity for ***nitric oxide*** (NO), a local vasodilator gas produced on demand by the vascular endothelium (NO was formerly called "endothelium-derived relaxing factor (EDRF)". The action of NO is immediate but very brief.

In the tissues, the reduced Hb, in addition to picking up CO_2 also picks up and removes excess of NO. The lack or removal of NO tends to cause vasoconstriction due to contraction of vascular smooth muscle. The result is decrease in blood flow and rise of blood pressure. In the lungs, the CO_2 is exhaled, and NO being a highly reactive free radical combines with O_2 and water to form inactive nitrates and nitrites. The Hb now picks another form of NO (along with fresh O_2) called ***super nitric oxide*** (SNO) formed in the lungs. In the tissues, Hb gives up O_2, while SNO causes vasodilatation of resistance vessels. (The Hb also picks up excess NO here). Thus, by transporting NO and SNO throughout the body, Hb helps to regulate peripheral resistance and, thus, blood flow and pressure.

Note: Blocking the synthesis of NO in experimental animals causes a prompt rise in blood pressure. This suggests that a tonic release of NO is essential for maintaining normal blood pressure. (Being a hormone and a neurotransmitter, NO has been shown to have a variety of other physiological functions).

FATE OF HEMOGLOBIN

Old and effete red cells and their fragments in the blood are ingested by the tissue macrophages largely in the spleen and liver. Here iron and globin are split apart and stored in their respective pools for reuse. The protoporphyrins from the breakdown of heme (this is the only reaction in the body where carbon monoxide is formed) are converted into biliverdin and bilirubin (the bile pigments) which are excreted in bile and then into urine and feces.

DERIVATIVES OF HEMOGLOBIN

- ***Oxyhemoglobin (oxyHb):*** There is a loose and reversible binding of oxygen with one of the coordination bonds of the iron atom. Since Hb contains four iron atoms, each molecule of Hb carries four molecules of oxygen.
- ***Reduced Hb:*** It results from release of O_2 from oxyHb.
- ***Carbaminohemoglobin:*** In this, CO_2 is attached to the globin part of Hb. The affinity of Hb for CO_2 is about 20 times that for oxygen.
- ***Carboxyhemoglobin (carboxyHb):*** Carbon monoxide is attached to Hb where O_2 is normally attached. The affinity of Hb for CO is 200–300 times that for O_2. It is normally present in small amounts, but in large amount in smokers in whom it impairs O_2 transport.
- ***Methemoglobin (MetHb):*** When blood is exposed to some drugs, or oxidizing agents in vitro or in vivo, the ferrous iron of Hb is converted into ferric iron forming metHb which is dark in color. When present in large amounts, it gives a dusky appearance to the skin. Small amounts of metHb are formed normally but an enzyme system converts it back to Hb.
- ***Sulfhemoglobin:*** It is formed by the action of some drugs and chemicals (e.g. sulfonamides), the reaction being irreversible.
- ***Cyanmethemoglobin (cyanmetHb; hemiglobincyanide):*** It is formed by the action of cyanide on Hb (Hb is metHb).

HEMOGLOBINOMETRY

The term refers to measurement of the concentration (amount) of Hb in the blood. For this purpose, advantage is taken of the following characteristics of Hb:

- Ability to combine with oxygen
- Presence of known amount of iron in each gram of Hb.
- Ability of a solution of a derivative of Hb to refract specific wavelengths of light, thus giving typical absorption bands.

Based on these features of Hb, the various methods can be grouped into the following categories:

1. **Visual color comparison:** This group includes Sahli's acid hematin, Haldane, and Tallquist methods. The Sahli's method is the most acceptable since the golden brown color of acid hematin is much easier to match with the standard than the red color of oxyHb.
2. **Gasometric method:** The Hb is fully saturated with oxygen and its amount is then measured with Van Slyke apparatus. Though very accurate, the method is time-consuming and tedious.
3. **Spectrophotometric methods:** The Hb is converted to other compounds (e.g. cyanmetHb, carboxyHb, alkaline hematin), and by using definite wavelengths of light; each of the derivatives can be measured.
4. **Electronic hematology analyzer:** The electronic analyzer, along with cell counts, can also provide Hb concentration automatically. A hemolyzing agent is added to the diluted blood to release the Hb which reacts with potassium ferricyanide and potassium cyanide in the solution to produce cyanmetHb. The cyanmetHb is then measured by spectrophotometry.
5. **Other methods:** These include: Estimation of iron content of blood, and the copper sulfate specific gravity method.

Note: Since many of the above methods are unsuitable for routine use, indirect methods based on color comparison are used. However, a standard solution of a derivative (e.g. acid hematin) cannot be used as its color will fade with time. Also there are personal errors in preparing standard solutions. To overcome these drawbacks, permanent colored glass rods, exactly matching the color of standard solution are provided with the apparatus. Though these glass rods or strips maintain their color for a long time, they can be tested from the National Standards Institute.

ABSOLUTE AND RELATIVE HEMOGLOBIN SCALES

In the past, when deciding the color density of the standard solutions in different methods, the same amount of blood was not taken. And since the earlier Hb tubes were calibrated only in percentage of normal, one had to know how much Hb was represented by 100% in each case. For example, a sample of blood containing 14.5 g/dL Hb would report 87% Hb by Sahli, 108% by Haldane, and 100% by Wintrobe methods, and so on. The values for 100% Hb by these methods are given as follows:

- Sahli = 17.0%
- Haldane = 13.8%
- Wintrobe = 14.5%
- Sahli-Adams = 14.5%
- Dare = 16.0%

To avoid this confusion, the practice of expressing Hb in "percentage" has been discarded and the Hb tubes are now graduated directly in g%. However, most manufacturers needlessly continue to indicate percentages in addition to readings in gram percent (g%) on the Hb tubes.

SAHLI'S ACID HEMATIN METHOD

Principle

The Hb present in a measured amount of blood is converted by dilute hydrochloric acid into acid hematin, which in dilution is golden brown in color. The intensity of color depends on the concentration of acid hematin which, in turn, depends on the concentration of Hb. The color of the solution (i.e. its hue and depth), after dilution with water, is matched against golden brown-tinted glass rods by direct vision. The readings are obtained in g%.

Apparatus

A. **Sahli (Sahli-Adams) hemoglobinometer (hemometer):** The set consists of **(Figs. 23A and B)**:

1. **Comparator:** It is a rectangular plastic box with a slot in the middle which accommodates the calibrated Hb tube. Nonfading, standardized, golden brown glass rods are fitted on each side of the slot for matching the color. An opaque white glass (or plastic) is fitted behind the slot to provide uniform illumination during direct visual color matching.
2. **Hemoglobin tube:** The square or round glass tube is calibrated in grams percent (2–24 g%) in yellow color on one side, and in percentage Hb (20–160%) in red color on the other side. There is a brush to clean the tube **(Fig. 23C)**.
3. **Hemoglobin pipette:** It is a glass capillary pipette with only a single calibration mark—0.02 mL (20 mm³, or 20 µL) **(Fig. 23D)**. There is no bulb in this pipette (as compared to cell pipettes) as no dilution of blood is done.

Note: The calibration mark 20 mm³ indicates a definite, measured volume and not an arbitrary volume, as is the case with diluting pipettes.

4. **Stirrer:** It is a thin glass rod with a flattened end which is used for stirring and mixing the blood and dilute acid.
5. **Pasteur pipette:** It is an 8–10 inch glass tube drawn to a long thin nozzle, and has a rubber teat. Ordinary glass droppers with a rubber teat also serve the purpose.
6. Distilled water.

B. **Decinormal (N/10) hydrochloric acid (0.1 N HCl) solution:** Mixing 36 g HCl in distilled water to 1 L gives "Normal" HCl; and diluting it 10 times will give N/10 HCl solution.

C. **Materials for skin prick:**

- Sterile lancet/needle
- Sterile gauze and cotton swabs
- Methylated spirit/70% alcohol.

Procedure

1. Using a dropper, place 8–10 drops of N/10 HCl in the Hb tube, or up to the mark 20% or 3 g, or a little more till the tip of the pipette will submerge, and set it aside.

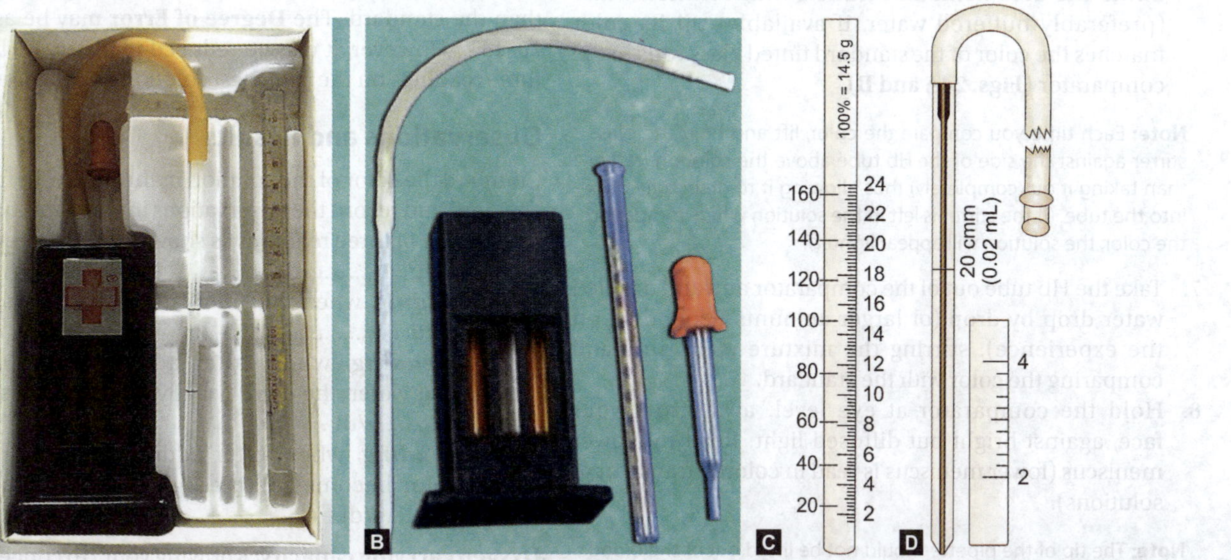

FIGS. 23A TO D: (A and B) Sahli-Adams hemoglobinometer; (C) Hemoglobin tube. It has graduations in g% on one side, and in percentage on the other. In this tube, 100% is equal to 14.5 g Hb/100 mL blood; (D) Hemoglobin pipette. It has only one marking, indicating 20 mm³ (0.02 mL, or 20 µL). Each division represents 0.2 g of Hb).

2. Get a fingerprick under aseptic conditions, wipe away the first 2 drops of blood. When a large drop of free flowing blood has formed again, draw blood up to the 20 mm^3 mark (0.02 mL). Carefully wipe the blood sticking to the tip of the pipette with a cotton swab, but avoid touching the bore or else blood will be drawn out by capillarity.

Note: If any blood remains sticking to the outside of the pipette, it will be that much extra blood in addition to 20 mm^3.

3. Without any waiting, immerse the tip of the pipette to the bottom of the acid solution and expel the blood gently. Rinse the pipette three to four times by drawing up and blowing out the clear upper part of the acid solution till all the blood has been washed out from it. Avoid frothing of the mixture. Note the time.
4. Withdraw the pipette from the tube, touching it to the side of the tube, thus ensuring that no mixture is carried out of the tube. Mix the blood with the acid solution with the flat end of the stirrer by rotating and gently moving it up and down.
5. Put the Hb tube back in the comparator and let it stand for 6–8 minutes (or as advised by the manufacturer). During this time, the acid ruptures the red cells, releasing their Hbs into the solution (hemolysis). The acid acts on the Hb and converts it into acid hematin which is deep golden brown in color.
   - The color of acid hematin does not develop fully immediately, but its intensity increases with time, reaching a maximum, after which it starts to decrease. An adequate time usually 6–8 minutes must be allowed before its dilution is started. Too little time and all Hbs may not be converted into acid hematin. And, waiting too long may result in fading of color. In either case, the result will be falsely low.
6. **Diluting and matching the color:** The next step is to dilute the acid hematin solution with distilled water (preferably buffered water, if available) till its color matches the color of the standard tinted glass rods in the comparator **(Figs. 24A and B)**.

Note: Each time you compare the color, lift and hold the glass stirrer against the side of the Hb tube above the solution (rather than taking it out completely) thus allowing it to drain fully back into the tube. (If the stirrer is left in the solution when comparing the color, the solution will appear lighter).

7. Take the Hb tube out of the comparator and add distilled water drop by drop (or larger amounts depending on the experience), stirring the mixture each time and comparing the color with the standard.
8. Hold the comparator at eye level, away from your face, against bright but diffused light. Read the lower meniscus (lower meniscus is read in colored transparent solutions).

Note: The tip of the pipette should not be lifted out of the blood drop during pipetting. This is done to prevent air from entering the pipette.

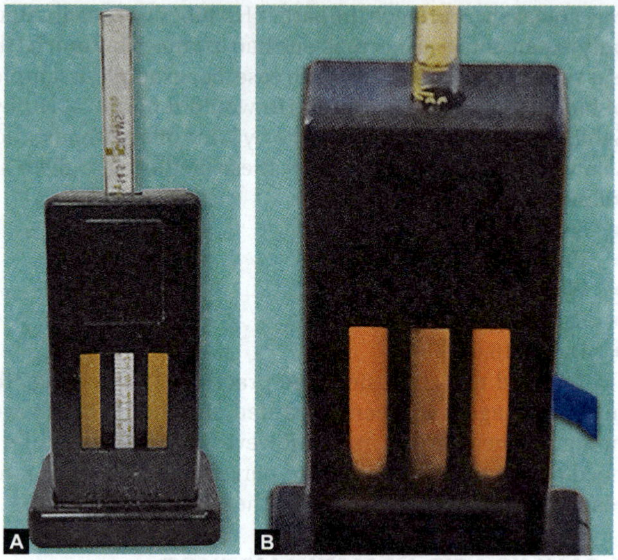

FIG. 24: Comparator.

Note: If the stirrer is left in the solution, it will lighten the color (since it is translucent) and thus matching will occur earlier. This will give a false low value. If, however, it is taken out every time the color is matched, it is bound to take away some of the solution out of the tube, thus, again giving a low value.

Sources and Degree of Error

False results with this method may be due to:

1. ***Technical error*:** It may be due to: Not taking exactly 20 mm^3 blood, or not giving enough time for formation of acid hematin, or using an old comparator that has faded glass rods.
2. ***Personal error*:** Generally, it is not difficult to match color but since it is a visual method, color matching may vary from person-to-person.

   For example, you may think that the color is matching, while your work-partner may consider it lighter or darker than the standard. The **Degree of Error** may be as high as 10–15%. However, it can be reduced to about 5% by taking three readings on the same test solution as described here.

Observations and Results

Compare the color of the solution in the tube with that of the standard and record the observations in your workbook. Take the average of three readings as shown here, and report your result as: Hb = ...g/dL.

- ***1st reading,*** when the color is slightly darker than the standard: ....g/dL.
- ***2nd reading,*** when, after adding a few drops of distilled water, the color exactly matches the standard: ....g/dL.
- ***3rd reading,*** when, after adding some more drops, the color becomes a little lighter than the standard: ....g/dL.

Oxygen carrying capacity: Knowing your Hb concentration, and that 1.34 mL of O_2 calculate its oxygen-carrying capacity as ....mL O_2/dL.

- **100% saturation:** When blood is equilibrated with pure (100%) oxygen at a PO_2 of 120 mm Hg, the Hb gets 100% saturated, i.e. it picks up as much O_2 as it possibly can.

For report:
- Oxygen-carrying capacity
- 100% saturation.

Advantages of Sahli's Method

The method is simple, fairly quick, and accurate. It does not require any costly apparatus, since it needs only direct color matching. Its running cost is minimal and can, therefore, be used in mass surveys.

Disadvantages of Sahli's Method

Since the acid hematin is not in true solution, some turbidity may occur. The method estimates only the oxyHb and reduced Hb, other forms, such as carboxyHb and metHb are not estimated. Also the degree of error may be high if proper precautions are not taken.

OTHER METHODS OF ESTIMATING HEMOGLOBIN

A. **Spectrophotometric methods:** In these methods, a photoelectric colorimeter is employed to measure the amount of light absorbed by a derivative of Hb.
   1. ***Cyanmethemoglobin method*:** All forms of Hb normally present in blood (i.e. oxyHb, reduced Hb, carboxyHb, and metHb) are converted into a stable compound—*cyanmetHb*. The sample of blood is treated with modified Drabkin's reagent (it contains potassium cyanide, potassium ferricyanide, and potassium phosphate—the last replacing sodium bicarbonate of Drabkin's reagent). The modified reagent speeds up the conversion, reduces turbidity, and enhances RBC lysis. The amount of light absorbed with yellow-green filters (peak at 450 nm) is compared with a standard solution in a photoelectric colorimeter. This method is the most accurate method of estimating Hb. Direct cyanmethemoglobin method has been the gold standard for hemoglobin estimation.
   2. ***Wu's alkaline hematin method*:** The blood is treated with N/10 NaOH, which converts all forms of Hb into alkaline hematin which is in true solution. There are two methods: (1) the standard method and (2) acid alkaline method.
   3. ***Haldane's carboxyhemoglobin method*:** The red cells are hemolyzed in distilled water to release Hb. Carbon monoxide is then passed through the solution to form carboxyHb that is bright red in color. The color is then compared with that of the standard.
   4. ***Oxyhemoglobin method*:** The blood is treated with ammonium hydroxide or sodium carbonate. The red cells are hemolyzed and the Hb is converted immediately and quickly into oxyHb. The solution is then compared with a standard gray screen in photoelectric colorimeter.

B. **Tallquist method:** A drop of blood absorbed on a white filter paper is allowed to spread over the paper to form an even spot. As soon as the blood spot loses its shine (gloss), but before it dries, it is matched against a scale of increasingly dark red-colored round spots printed on a card. The method, though quick is rather inaccurate due to personal error. It is sometimes used in mass surveys for anemia.

C. **Iron content:** The iron in blood is separated with sulfuric acid, and its amount measured. Since 1 g of Hb contains 3.35 mg iron, the amount of Hb can be calculated.

D. **Copper sulfate falling drop method:** It is a rapid method for estimating the approximate level of Hb, and is used in large surveys. It was used extensively during World War II where an indication of the necessity for blood transfusion was immediately required.

E. **Automated hemoglobin analyzer:** This is commonly used to analyze a variety of red and white blood cells as well as hematocrit and hemoglobin levels from the blood sample. These analyzers offer higher precision value at a fraction of the time when compared with manual methods.

Note: In resource poor settings where automated hematology analyzers are not available, the Cyanmethemoglobin method is often used. This method, though cheaper, takes more time. In blood donations, the semi-quantitative gravimetric copper sulfate method which is very easy and inexpensive may be used but does not provide an acceptable degree of accuracy.

PRECAUTIONS

1. All precautions mentioned for collecting fingerprick blood, and filling the pipette must be observed.
2. The finger should not be squeezed, and there should not be any blood sticking to the outside of the pipette tip.
3. Only the recommended time should be allowed for the formation of acid hematin by the action of acid on Hb.
4. When diluting the color of acid hematin solution, avoid over-dilution because the color cannot be concentrated.
5. When matching the color, the solution should be uniformly golden brown throughout the solution. Dark color near the bottom of the tube indicates poor mixing.
6. During color matching, three readings should be taken to reduce the personal error.

PHYSIOCLINICAL SIGNIFICANCE

The Hb concentration is always estimated as part of routine tests in outpatients department and also as a bedside test in indoor patients. It is indicated as part of complete hematological studies in all diseases of blood especially all types of anemias, leukemias, and in chronic diseases such as tuberculosis, chronic infections, malignancies, renal failure, etc.

A. **Increased level of Hb may be due to:**
   1. **Experimental error:**
      - Blood taken more than 20 mm^3 or blood sticking to the outside of the pipette tip
      - Fading of colored glass standards (rods).

2. **High red cell count:**
   - Physiological: Males, newborns, high altitude, etc.
   - Pathological: Polycythemia/hypoxia due to heart or lung diseases.

B. **Decreased level of Hb may be due to:**
- **Experimental error:**
   - Blood sample diluted with tissue fluid
   - Blood taken is less than 20 mm^3
   - Color of acid hematin not allowed to develop fully.

C. **Decreased red cell count:**
- **Physiological:** Females during pregnancy (hemodilution)
- All cases of anemia.

Note: Hemoglobin contributes to the red color of the erythrocytes. Normally, only a very small amount is present in the plasma, about 3 mg/dL, most of it being confined to red cells. If it was present in the plasma, it would increase the viscosity (thus raising blood pressure), and the osmotic pressure of blood (thus affecting fluid exchanges). It would also be excreted in the urine, besides being taken up and rapidly destroyed by the reticuloendothelial system.

Anemia

Anemia is a condition in which the oxygen-carrying capacity of blood is reduced. There are many kinds of anemia, and in all anemias there is a decreased concentration of Hb, usually below 11–12 g/dL as a result of decrease in red cell mass (RBC count below 4–4.5 million/mm^3).

Depending on Hb concentration, anemia may be:
- Mild: Hb = 10–12 g/dL
- Moderate: Hb = 7–9 g/dL
- Severe: Hb = Below 6 g/dL

The World Health Organization (WHO) criterion for anemia in adults is **a hemoglobin (Hb) value of less than 12.5 g/dL.** Children aged 6 months to 6 years are considered anemic at Hb levels less than 11 g/dL, and children aged 6-14 years are considered anemic when Hb levels are less than 12 g/dL.

The common causes of anemia in India are:
- Chronic loss of blood
- Deficiency of nutrients.

Normally, about 1% of RBCs are destroyed daily (cells present in about 50 mL of blood) and equal numbers (about 3 million/second) enter the circulation. It may be caused when more cells are lost, or when less cells are produced, or both.

It will develop if:
- Red cell production is normal but loss is increased.
- Red cell production is decreased but loss remains normal.
- Red cell production is decreased and loss is also increased.

Classification of anemia: The anemia may be classified on the basis of morphology of red cells, or the etiology (causes) of anemia:

A. **Morphological causes:** Anemia may be **microcytic, normocytic,** or **macrocytic,** and each type may be **hypochromic,** or **normochromic.** For example, iron deficiency anemia is usually microcytic hypochromic. B_{12} and folic acid deficiency anemia is macrocytic normochromic (there can be no hyperchromic anemia because the saturation of red cells with Hb cannot exceed the normal upper limit of 36%).

B. **Etiological causes:** Depending on the cause, the anemia may be grouped into:
- Excessive RBC loss or destruction.
- Inadequate RBC production.
- Excessive loss and decreased production of RBCs.

1. **Blood loss (hemorrhagic) anemia:** The loss of blood (i.e. RBCs) through bleeding may be mild or severe, internal or external, and acute or chronic (prolonged). The anemia is usually normocytic. The common causes include: Large wounds, bleeding piles, peptic ulcer, hookworm infestation, malarial parasites, or heavy menstruation. Enough iron cannot be absorbed to make up for the loss.
2. **Hemolytic anemias:** The red cell plasma membranes (cell membranes) rupture prematurely and pour their Hb into the plasma (hemolysis).
   It may be inherited or acquired:
   - **Inherited:** This can be due to **structural abnormalities** (hereditary spherocytosis and hereditary elliptocytosis), **defects in hemoglobin production** (thalassemia, sickle cell anemia) and **defective enzyme production.**
   - **Acquired:** The hemolysis of red cells may result from parasites (malaria), bacterial toxins, snake venom, adverse drug reactions (aspirin), autoimmunity, etc.
3. **Nutritional (deficiency) anemias:** These are due to lack of essential nutrients such as iron, vitamin B_{12}, folic acid, etc.
   - **Iron deficiency anemia:** This is **the most common type of anemia.** It may be caused by insufficient intake, inadequate absorption from gastrointestinal (GI) tract, increased iron requirements, or excessive loss of iron. Women are more likely to get it because of menstrual blood losses and increased iron demands of growing fetus during pregnancy.
   - **Deficiency of vitamins B_{12} and folic acid (folate):** Both of these vitamins are required for normal erythropoiesis. Deficiency of either causes anemia. There is a derangement of DNA synthesis (DNA is required by dividing cells). As a result, large immature, nucleated red cell precursors (megaloblasts) appear in the circulating blood; their lifespan is also short about 40 days (red cell production cannot keep pace with their destruction, hence anemia). The large mature red cells (macrocytes) are fully saturated with Hb.

   Deficiency of B_{12} may be due to: (1) inadequate intake, as in pure vegetarians (vegans) because vegetables and fruits contain very little or no B_{12}; (2) lack of intrinsic factor (IF) which is a glycoprotein produced by gastric parietal cells that helps in the absorption of

B_{12}. The IF binds with B_{12} in food (in this bound state, B_{12} is protected from being digested by GI tract enzymes) and both are absorbed together in distal ileum. B_{12} then gets freed from the IF and is released into portal blood. The basic abnormality is the destruction of parietal cells by autoimmune antibodies in the disease called **atrophic gastritis** (total gastrectomy can also lead to B_{12} deficiency). The result is that the patient develops a type of anemia called **pernicious anemia,** or **Addison's anemia.** Nervous lesions occur ultimately.

Deficiency of folic acid is a nutritional disease and is more common than B_{12} deficiency. Like B_{12} deficiency, folic acid deficiency is characterized by macrocytic anemia. Production of IF and HCl is normal. In patients with intestinal malabsorption (e.g. sprue), there is a serious difficulty in absorbing folic acid (and B_{12}).

4. **Aplastic anemia:** There is suppression or destruction of red bone marrow due to overexposure to ionizing radiations (gamma-rays, X-rays); adverse drug reactions that inhibit enzymes needed for erythropoiesis (drugs such as chloramphenicol, sulfonamides, and cytotoxic drugs used in treatment of cancers may cause this anemia). Certain poisons and severe infection may also produce aplastic anemia. The anemia is usually normocytic.
5. **Anemias due to chronic diseases:** Tuberculosis, chronic infections, cancers, lung diseases, etc. frequently cause anemia. The mechanism of causation is complex. The tissue macrophages are believed to become activated so that red cells are removed from the blood faster than they can be produced by the bone marrow.

This type of anemia is diagnosed by determining various blood indices and absolute corpuscular values. Estimation of levels of iron, vitamins, IF, etc. are also done.

QUESTIONS

Q.1. What is the principle on which the Sahli's method is based?

See text above.

Q.2. Why is Sahli's method most frequently employed as a routine test?

See text above.

Q.3. What is meant by the term "normality" of a solution? What is N/10 HCl and how will you prepare it?

The normality (N) of a solution is the number of gram equivalents in 1 L of water. A 1 N solution of HCl contains 1 + 35 = 36 g of HCl in water made to 1 L. Diluting this solution 10 times will give N/10 HCl.

Q.4. Can strong acids (such as nitric, sulfuric, and hydrochloric acids) or alkalis be used in place of decinormal HCl?

The strong acids which are very strong oxidizing agents and alkalis will cause disruption of Hb and thus cannot be used. Only N/10 HCl is used because standardization has been done for acid hematin.

Q.5. How would estimation of hemoglobin be affected if less or more than 8–10 drops of N/10 HCl is taken in the hemoglobin tube?

If less (3–4 drops) acid is taken, the blood may not mix well and/or may clot. All the Hb will not be converted into acid hematin. This will result in false low value. If much more acid is taken (say up to the level of 10 g), the final color developed in a case of anemia (Hb 6–8 g%) would be much lighter than the standard. Color matching will then not be possible, because the color of the solution cannot be concentrated.

Q.6. Can tap water be used for diluting and color matching?

No, it cannot be used because its salt content may cause turbidity which will interfere with color matching.

Q.7. Can N/10 HCl be used (if distilled water is not available) for diluting and color matching?

Yes, it can be used because it being transparent, it cannot further deepen the color once all the Hb has been converted into acid hematin.

Q.8. Why is it necessary to wait for 6–8 minutes after adding blood to N/10 HCl solution?

See text above.

Q.9. While matching the color, why is it important to lift the stirrer above the solution and not leave it there or take it out?

If the stirrer is left in the solution, it will lighten the color (since it is translucent) and thus matching will occur earlier. This will give a false low value. If, however, it is taken out every time the color is matched, it is bound to take away some of the solution out of the tube, thus, again giving a low value.

Q.10. Which of the two scales given on the hemoglobin tube are preferred and why?

The scale which gives the Hb concentration in a blood sample directly in gram percent is preferred. The scale in percentages is of no value as there is no standard single value of Hb which can be taken as 100%.

Q.11. What are the normal levels and ranges of hemoglobin at different ages?

- Newborns: 18–22 g/dL
- At 3 months: 14–16 g/dL
- 3 months to 1 year: 13–15 g/dL
- Adult males: 14.5 g/dL (13.5–17 g/dL)
- Adult females: 12.5 g/dL (11.5–15.5 g/dL).

There may be some decrease after age 60 years.

Q.12. Compared to males, why are the hemoglobin levels lower in females?

All other factors (age, body mass, etc.) being equal, the levels are lower in healthy females not because of menstrual loss of blood (20–30 mL). It is the estrogens in the females which have an inhibitory effect on the secretion of erythropoietin (EP) which is the main stimulant of red cell production. Also, the androgens (mainly testosterone) have a stimulatory effect on EP secretion. Both these factors tend to keep the red cell count higher in males.

Q.13. Why is the hemoglobin level high in the newborns?

The Hb may be as high as 20–22 g/dL at the time of birth due to the high red cell count (>6 million/mm³). The newborn has been living in state of relative hypoxia which is a very potent stimulus for the secretion of EP. As age advances, the Hb levels decrease, and adult levels are reached in a few years.

Q.14. What would happen if hemoglobin was present freely in the plasma instead of in the red cells?

- This would increase in viscosity of blood thereby increasing blood pressure.
- Free hemoglobin in the plasma might get excreted out by getting filtered through the kidney. This would cause severe damage to the kidneys.

Q.15. What are the common causes of increased and decreased hemoglobin readings?
See text above.

Q.16. What is the structure of hemoglobin, where is it synthesized, and what are the materials required for its synthesis?
See text above.

Q.17. Name some derivatives of hemoglobin.
See text above.

Q.18. What are the different varieties of hemoglobin and what is their significance?
See text above.

Q.19. What is the fate of hemoglobin?
See text above.

Q.20. What are the functions of hemoglobin?
See text above.

Q.21. What is anemia and how is it graded according to hemoglobin concentration? What are its common causes in India?
See text above.

Q.22. What are the common causes of anemia and how will you classify it?
See text above.

Q.23. Name some other methods for the estimation of hemoglobin. Which method is not accurate?
See text above.

OBJECTIVE STRUCTURED PRACTICAL EXAMINATION

Aim: To convert a known volume of blood sample into acid hematin using the apparatus provided.

Procedural steps: See text above.

Checklist:

1. Selects the Hb pipette and tube and checks that they are clean and dry. (Y/N)
2. Takes N/10 in the Hb tube up to the mark 20% or 3 g%. (Y/N)
3. Shakes the container of blood and draws blood into the pipette exactly to the mark 20 µL. (Y/N)
4. Wipes off blood from the tip of the pipette and blows out the blood into acid solution. (Y/N)
5. Rinses the pipette several times into acid solution. Notes the time. (Y/N)

1.7: EXAMINATION OF A PERIPHERAL BLOOD SMEAR AND DETERMINATION OF DIFFERENTIAL LEUKOCYTE COUNT

STUDENT OBJECTIVES

After completing this experiment, the student should be able to:

- Describe the relevance and special importance of preparing and staining a blood smear and doing the differential leukocyte count.
- Name the components of Leishman's stain and explain the function of each component.
- Prepare satisfactory blood films, fix and stain them, and describe the features of a well-stained film.
- Identify different blood cells in a film, and indicate the identifying features of each type of leukocyte.
- Differentiate between the different types of white blood cells.
- Carry out the differential leukocyte count and express the results in their percentages and absolute numbers.
- Describe the functions of each type of leukocyte.
- List the conditions in which their numbers increase and decrease.

INTRODUCTION

PY2.11: Estimate Hb, RBC, TLC, RBC indices, DLC, Blood groups, BT/CT

Many hematological and other disorders can be diagnosed by a careful examination of a stained blood film. A physician may order a differential leukocyte count (DLC) [always along with total leukocytes count (TLC)] to detect infection or inflammation, determine the effects of possible poisoning by chemicals, drugs, chemotherapy, radiation, etc. DLC is also done to monitor blood diseases like leukemia, or to detect allergy and parasitic infections. The determination of each type of white blood cell (WBC) helps in diagnosing the condition because a particular type may show an increase or decrease.

PRINCIPLE

A blood film is stained with Leishman stain and scanned under oil immersion, from one end to the other. As each WBC is encountered, it is identified until 100 leukocytes have been examined. The percentage distribution of each type of WBC is then calculated. *Knowing the TLC and the differential count, it is easy to determine the number of each type of cell per cubic millimeter of blood.*

Note: The special importance of a stained blood smear is that, unlike any other routine blood test, the smear can be retained and preserved as a permanent original record. The slide can be taken out and reassessed whenever required after days, weeks, months or even years. The slide can also be conveniently sent to specialists for their opinion in doubtful cases.

The stained smears can also provide information about the morphology and count of red cells and platelets, and hemoglobin (Hb) status, besides detecting the presence of various parasites (e.g. malaria).

APPARATUS

1. Microscope
2. Five to six clean glass slides

3. Sterile lancet
4. Cotton and gauze swabs
5. 70% alcohol
6. Glass dropper
7. Leishman stain
8. A wash bottle of distilled water (or buffered water, if available)
9. Fluff-free blotting paper
10. Disposable, sterile blood lancet/pricking needle.

Important: Once cleaned, do not touch the surfaces of the glass slides and coverslips.

Leishman stain: This stain is a simplification of Romanowsky group of stains. Romanowsky staining, also known as Romanowsky–Giemsa staining, is a prototypical staining technique that was the forerunner of several distinct but similar stains widely used in hematology (the study of blood) and cytopathology (the study of diseased cells). There are various Romanowsky staining types, the Leishman's stain is one of them.

Leishman's staining is probably one of the simplest and most precise methods of staining blood smear for diagnostic purposes. It contains a compound dye—**eosinate of methylene blue** dissolved in acetone-free methyl alcohol.

1. **Eosin:** It is an acidic dye (negatively charged) and stains the basic (positive) components of the cells such as granules of eosinophils, and cytoplasm of red blood cells (RBCs). It imparts a pink color.
2. **Methylene blue:** It is a basic dye (positively charged) and stains acidic (negatively charged) granules in the cytoplasm, nuclei of leukocytes, and the granules of basophils. It imparts a blue-violet color.
3. **Acetone-free and water-free absolute methyl alcohol:** The methyl alcohol is a fixative and must be free from acetone and water. It serves two functions:
   i. It fixes the blood smear to the glass slide. The alcohol precipitates the plasma proteins, which then act as a "glue" which attaches (fixes) the blood cells to the slide so that they are not washed away during staining.
   ii. The alcohol preserves the morphology and chemical status of the cells.
      - The alcohol must be free from acetone because acetone being a very strong lipid solvent, will, if present, cause crenation, shrinkage, or even destruction of cell membranes. This will make the identification of the cells difficult. (If acetone is present, the stain deteriorates quickly).
      - The alcohol must be free from water since the latter may result in rouleaux formation and even hemolysis. The water may even wash away the blood film from the slide.

PROCEDURE

Cleaning the Slides

Prepare acid-dichromate solution by mixing 1 part of concentrated sulfuric or nitric acid with 9 parts of 2–3% potassium dichromate solution.

- Wash the slides and coverslips with soap and water and rinse in running water. Then soak them overnight in the acid-dichromate solution. Follow this with a wash in running water, then in distilled water.
- Dip the slides in 90–95% alcohol and dry with a clean, lint-free cloth.
- Another method is to use a good detergent for overnight soak in place of acid-dichromate solution.
- The acid-dichromate solution is best kept in 1–2 L, wide-mouth jar. After washing the used slides, they are put in this jar.

Preparation of a Blood Film (Blood Smear) (Figs. 25A to D)

Blood films can be made from anticoagulated or fingerprick blood. Anticoagulated blood obtained from a student volunteer, or spare blood obtained from the clinical laboratory may be provided to the students to avoid skin pricks at (a drop of blood can be put on the slide without touching it). Students may also use their own blood from skin pricks.

1. Place three or four clean, grease free glass slides on a white sheet of paper on your work-table, one of these is to be used as a ***spreader***, the surface of which should be even and smooth.
2. Prick the finger under aseptic conditions.
3. Discard the first 2 drops and allow a medium-sized drop of blood to form on the fingertip.
4. Then touch the blood drop in the centerline of the slide, about 1 cm from the one end of the slide.
5. Place the narrow edge of the spreader on the first slide, at an angle of 45°, just in front of the blood drop.
6. Pull the spreader backward till the blood runs along the full width of the spreader at the line of junction.
7. Slowly and smoothly move the spreader to the other end of the slide.
8. Dry the smear by waving the slide in the air (do not try to blot-dry the film).
9. The smear should be spread in about half a second. Any hesitation will result in striations in the film.
10. Make as many trials as possible to get acceptable films, keeping in mind the features of an ideal blood smear. Dry the film by waving the slide in the air (do not try to blot-dry the film).

Fixing and Staining of Blood Films

Fixation is the process that makes the blood film and its cells adhere to the glass slide. It also preserves the shape and chemistry of blood cells as near living cells as possible. **Staining** is the process that stains (colors) the nuclei and cytoplasm of the cells. Both these purposes are achieved by the Leishman stain.

1. **Fixing the blood films:** Place the slides, smear side up, on a "staining rack" assembled over a sink (two glass rods placed across the sink, with the ends fitted into short pieces of rubber tubing). Ensure that they are horizontal.
2. Pour 8–10 drops of the stain on each unfixed slide by dripping it from a drop bottle or use a dropper. This

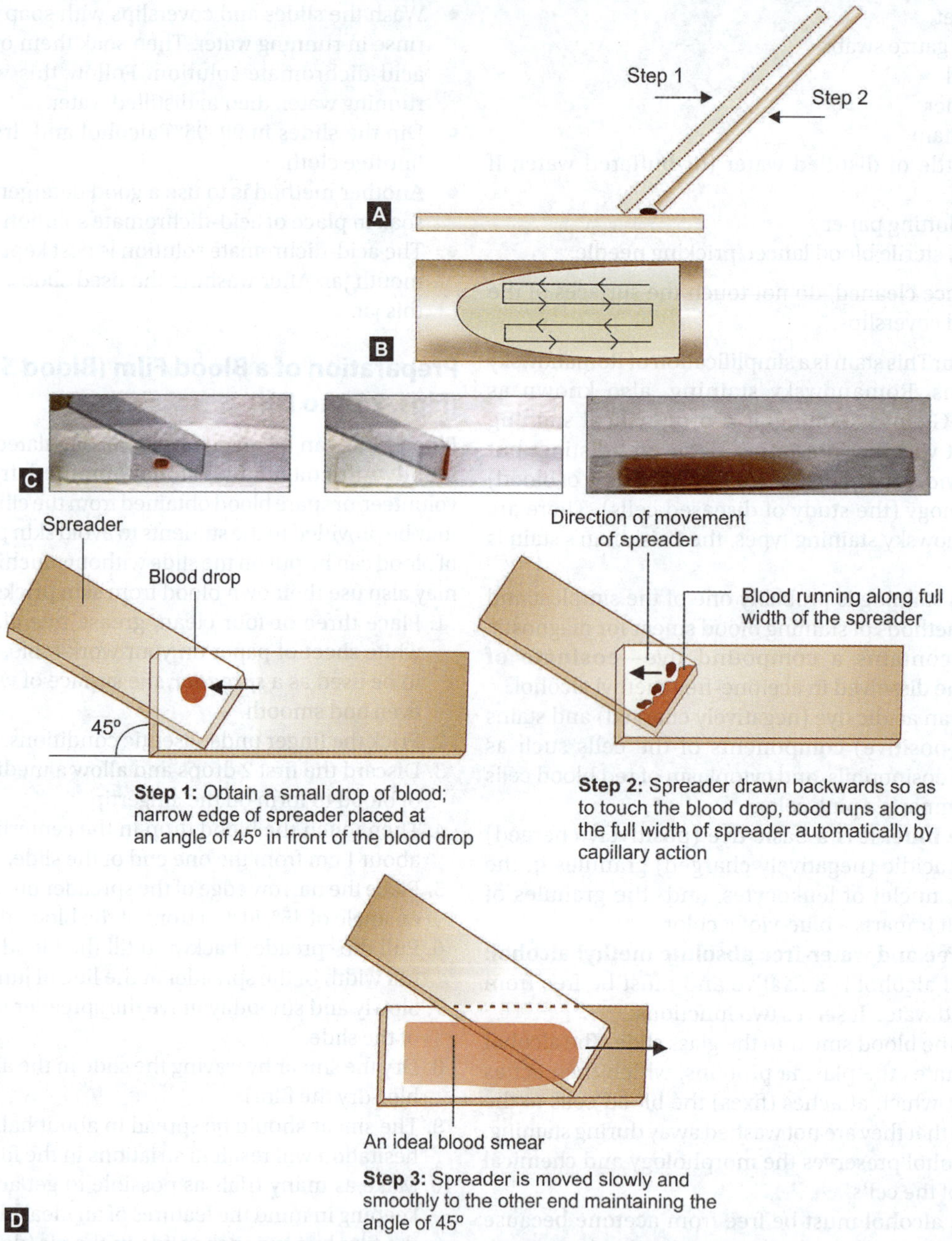

FIGS. 25A TO D: (A) Method of spreading a blood film. Step 1: The spreader is placed in front of the blood drop and pulled back till it touches the blood. Step 2: Spreader is pushed forward to spread the film; (B) The appearance of a well-prepared film, showing the movement of the objective over it; (C) Steps in preparation of a blood smear; (D) Schematic representation of steps in preparation of a blood smear.

amount of stain usually covers the entire surface and "stands up" from the edges of the slides without running off. Note the time.

3. Allow the stain to remain undisturbed for 1–2 minutes, as advised. During this time, watch the stain carefully, especially during hot weather, and see that it does not become syrupy (thick) due to evaporation of alcohol. If the stain dries, it will precipitate on the blood film and appear as round, blue granules.
   This can be prevented by pouring more stain on the slides as required.
4. **Staining the blood film:** After the fixing time is over, add an equal number of drops of distilled water (or buffered water, if available) to the stain. If the water is carefully dripped from a drop bottle or a dropper, the entire mixture will stand up from the edges of the slides (due to surface tension) without spilling over.
5. Mix the stain and water by gently blowing at different places on the slides through a dropper, without scratching the smear. A glossy greenish layer (scum) soon appears on the surface of the diluted stain. Allow the diluted stain to remain on the slide for 6–8 minutes, or as advised.
6. Flush off the diluted stain in a gentle stream of distilled water for about 30 seconds and leave the slides on the rack for about a minute with the last wash of water covering them. Drain the slides and put them in an

inclined position against a support, stained sides facing downward (to prevent dust particles settling on them) to drain and dry. The under sides of the slides may be blotted with filter paper.

Examination of Peripheral Blood Smear

- Examine the slides under low and high magnification. Describe what you see about the various cells and compare with what you saw in the drop preparation.
- Examine the slides against diffuse light, with naked eye. What is the color of the smear? Does it appear thick, thin, or granular? Are there any striations—longitudinal or transverse? Are there any vacant places in the film? Is it uniformly distributed in the middle two-thirds of the slide? Is its head—the starting point, straight and about 1 cm from the end? Are its edges about 2 mm from the long sides of the slide? Is there a tail? Try to answer all these questions.
- Note the degree of separation of cells. Do they lie in a single layer or in two, three or more layers? The red cells are non-nucleated, flat biconcave disks, round, oval or pear-shaped, thinner in the center and appear as colorless, or pale pink structures. (When stained with Leishman stain, they appear dull orange-pink). Note if there is any rouleaux formation (cells lying on top of each other like a pile of coins) and the number of cells in a rouleaux. Observe if any leukocytes are seen, and their types if possible. Do they show any ameboid movement? Do you see any platelets—in clumps, or showing disintegration? After a time you may see fibrin threads when clotting starts.

Features of an Ideal Blood Smear (Fig. 26)

1. The smear appears translucent and bluish-pink when seen against a white surface, its thickness being uniform throughout.
2. The blood film should occupy the middle two-thirds (about 5 cm) of the slide, with a clear margin of about 2 mm on either side.
3. It should be tongue-shaped, i.e. broad at the head (starting point), and taper toward the other end, but without any "tails".
4. The smear should be translucent, uniformly thick throughout, with no vacant areas, striations (longitudinal or transverse) or "granular" areas.
5. It should be neither very thick nor very thin (this can be learned only with practice). A thin film looks faintly pink against a white surface, while a thick smear appears red. An ideal film appears "buff" colored.

Note: A thick blood film results from taking too large a drop of blood, a faster movement, and a smaller angle of the spreader.

Microscopic Appearance of an Ideal Stained Smear

1. **Under low magnifications (10x):** The red cells appear as dots, uniformly spread out in a single layer. The WBCs cannot be differentiated.
2. **Under high magnification (45x):** The red cells are stained dull orange-pink and show a central pallor (due to biconcavity) which, if wide, may give the appearance of rings. The WBCs, with their nuclei deep blue-violet, lie unevenly here and there among the red cells. The platelets occur in small groups.
3. The red cells, as seen under the microscope, should lie separately from each other, without any crowding, or rouleaux formation.

Note: A thick blood film results from taking too large a drop of blood, a faster movement and a smaller angle of the spreader. At least one WBC can be seen per high-power field.

Staining defects:

1. **Presence of stain granules:** Occasionally, round, solid-looking, deep blue-violet particles of stain get precipitated all over a blood film. They appear if the Leishman stain is old, or if it has not been properly filtered, or if it was allowed to dry up on the slide during fixing. Finally, it may be due to insufficient washing of the greenish metallic scum that forms on the stain-water mixture during staining.
2. **Excessively blue appearance:** The RBCs appear deep blue or even bluish-black. The nuclei of WBCs are stained dark blue, with bluish cytoplasm in all cells; the PMNs cannot be differentiated. This appearance may be due to

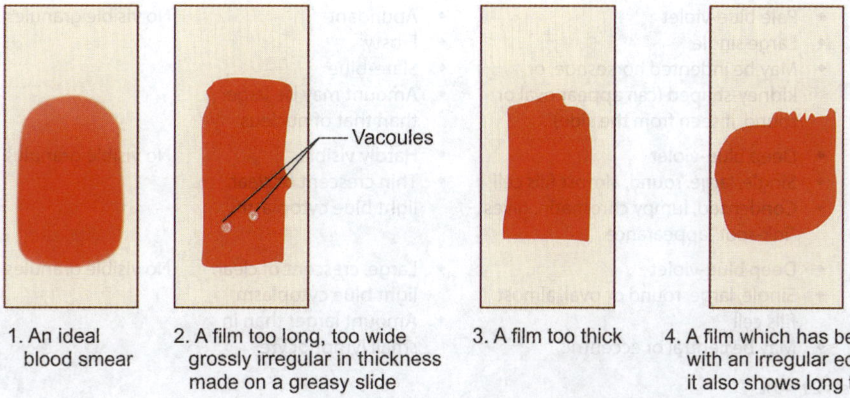
Vacoules
1. An ideal blood smear
2. A film too long, too wide grossly irregular in thickness made on a greasy slide
3. A film too thick
4. A film which has been spread with an irregular edged spreader; it also shows long tails

FIG. 26: Blood films made on glass slides.

over-staining, over-fixing, insufficient washing or the use of alkaline stain or water. It can be corrected by reducing the fixing and staining times, and proper washing under running water.

3. **Excessively reddish appearance:** In this case, the red cells appear pale pink. The WBCs show pale blue cytoplasm, while the nuclei typically appear lighter than the cytoplasm or even colorless. This appearance may be due to under-staining, over-washing or the use of more acidic stain or water. The defect may be rectified by restaining, if required.
4. **Faded appearance of blood cells:** This may result from the use of old stain, understaining or overwashing.

Identification of Leukocytes under Oil Immersion (100x)

- Place 2 drops of cedar wood oil in the center of the smear. Bring the oil immersion lens into position and focus the cells by keeping the condenser at the highest position and iris diaphragm fully opened.
- Examine the slide all over, at the head and tail ends, along the edges, and in between these areas. Identify each leukocyte, as you encounter it, from the description given in **Table 7**.

Important: Continuously "rack" the microscope as advised earlier, because it is impossible to identify the cells without doing so. All the cells of the blood, selectively stained and spread out in a single layer, are clearly seen. In the blood and tissues, the leukocytes show active ameboid movements. In a blood smear, however, they assume a round shape due to surface tension.

Cells Seen in a Blood Film

The following cells can be identified:

1. **Red cells:** Stained orange-pink, the red cells appear as numerous, evenly spread out, non-nucleated, biconcave disks of uniform size of 7.2–7.8 µm. Normally, the central paleness occupies the middle third of the cells but is wider in anemias. There may be some overcrowding and overlapping, or even rouleaux formation in the head end of the blood film.
2. **Leukocytes:** *Five main types of WBCs* are commonly seen in blood films. They are all larger than the red cells, nucleated, and unevenly distributed here and there among the red cells. They include three types of granulocytes i.e neutrophils, eosinophils and basophils, neutrophils being the most numerous. Also present are two types of agranulocytes (monocytes and lymphocytes). A sixth type of leukocyte, the plasma cell, is occasionally seen in the

Table 7: Appearance of white blood corpuscles in a stained blood film.

Cell type	Diameter (µm)	Nucleus	Cytoplasm	Cytoplasmic granules
Granulocytes				
Neutrophils (40–70%)	10–14	• Blue-violet • 2–6 lobes, connected by chromatin threads • Seen clearly through cytoplasm	Slate-blue in color	• Fine, closely-packed violet pink • Not seen separately • Give ground-glass appearance • Do not cover nucleus
Eosinophils (1–6%)	10–15	• Blue-violet • Bilobed, lobes connected by thick or thin chromatin band (spectacle shaped) • Seen clearly through cytoplasm	• Eosinophilic • Light pink-red • Granular	• Large, coarse • Uniform-sized • Brick-red to orange • Seen separately • Do not cover nucleus
Basophils (0–1%)	10–15	• Blue-violet • Irregular shape, may be S-shaped, rarely bilobed • Not clearly seen, because overlaid with granules	• Basophilic • Bluish • Granular	• Large, very coarse • Variable-sized • Deep purple • Seen separately • Completely fill the cell and cover the nucleus
Agranulocytes				
Monocytes (2–8%)	12–20	• Pale blue-violet • Large single • May be indented horseshoe, or kidney-shaped (can appear oval or round, if seen from the side)	• Abundant • Frosty • Slate-blue • Amount may be larger than that of nucleus	No visible granules
Small lymphocytes*	7–9	• Deep blue-violet • Single, large, round, almost fills cell • Condensed, lumpy chromatin, gives "ink-spot" appearance	• Hardly visible • Thin crescent of clear, light blue cytoplasm	No visible granules
Large lymphocytes*	10–15	• Deep blue-violet • Single, large, round or oval, almost fills cell • May be central or eccentric	• Large, crescent of clear, light blue cytoplasm • Amount larger than in small lymphocyte	No visible granules

*The total percentage of lymphocytes is 20–40%.

Large granular lymphocytes: These are part of the innate immune system, and are natural killer cells.

Small lymphocytes: These lymphocytes are the main agents of the acquired immune system. The two main types are: T and B cells.

blood films. The plasma cells are found in abundance in the lymphoid tissues. It is a specialized lymphocyte (B lymphocyte) that secretes antibodies. The chromatin of this cell gives a typical "cartwheel" appearance.

3. **Platelets:** They are membrane-bound round or oval bodies, with a diameter of 2–4 µm. They lie here and there in groups of 2–12, which is an in vitro effect, i.e. they do not form clumps in the circulating blood. They stain pink-purple, and being fragments of megakaryocytes, they do not possess nuclei.

Note: There are fewer and poorly-stained WBCs in the head end and the extreme tail; and some of these may be distorted. There appear to be more monocytes in the tail end, probably dragged thereby the spreader because of their larger size. Plenty of leukocytes are found along the edges though they may be poorly stained. *Population-wise, neutrophils are the most numerous leukocytes, then come the lymphocytes, monocytes, eosinophils, and basophils, in that order.*

Identifying a Leukocyte

A leukocyte is identified from its size, its nucleus, and the cytoplasm—its color, whether vesicles (granules) are visible or not, their color and size if visible, and the cytoplasm/nucleus ratio **(Figs. 27A and B)**.

The scheme of identification of cells in peripheral blood smear (PBS) is shown in the **Flowchart 3**.

1. **Size:** The size of a WBC is assessed by comparing it with that of the surrounding red cells which have a uniform size of 7.2–7.8 µm.
2. **Nucleus:** Note if the nucleus can be clearly seen through the cytoplasm and whether it is single or lobed. If single,

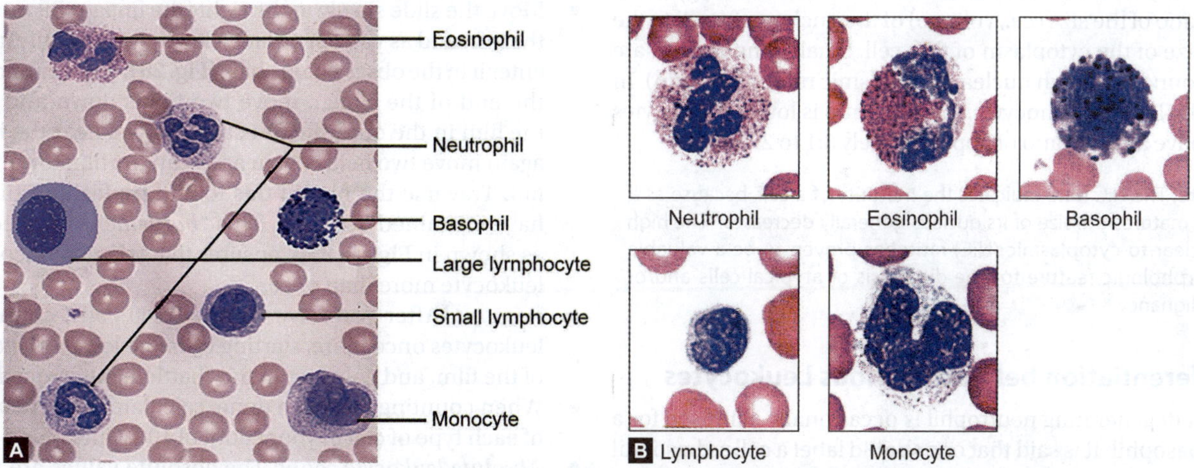

FIGS. 27A AND B: (A) Different types of blood cells in a blood film stained with Leishman stain. The size, shape of the nucleus and staining features of the cytoplasmic granules distinguish them from one another; (B) White blood cells under oil immersion.

FLOWCHART 3: Scheme of identification of cells in peripheral blood smear (PBS).

Observe the PBS under oil immersion (100x) after adding a drop of cedar wood oil
↓
RBCs are the most abundant cell size of about 7µm, appear pinkish in color
↓
Size of other cells is compared to that of RBC
↓
- Size of cell < Size of RBC (cells < 7 µm)
  - Thrombocytes (Platelets)
- Size of cell = Size of RBC (cells = 7 µm)
  - Small lymphocyte
- Size of cell > Size of RBC (cells > 7 µm)
  - Granulocyte
  - Agranulocyte

(Look for presence of granules in cytoplasm of cells)

- Granulocyte (Granules present)
  - Neutrophils
  - Basophils
  - Eosinophils
- Agranulocyte (Granules absent)
  - Lymphocyte
    - Large
    - Small
  - Monocyte

note its location—central or eccentric, its shape—round, oval, or horseshoe or kidney-shaped. Study its chromatin and whether condensed and lumpy or open and reticular. If lobed, count their number. Also note whether the lobes are connected by chromatin filaments or wider bands **(Figs. 27A and B)**.

3. **Cytoplasm and cytoplasmic granules:** The cytoplasm may or may not show "visible" granules, or they may be very fine and not visible separately. Note the color of the cytoplasm and the granules, whether neutral color (light violet-pink taking up both acid and basic stains), or large and coarse—brick-red or red-orange (eosinophils) or deep blue-violet (basophils).
4. **Cytoplasm-nucleus ratio:** Note the amount of cytoplasm in relation to the size of the cell and the nucleus. The nuclear-cytoplasmic ratio (also variously known as the nucleus:cytoplasm ratio, nucleus-cytoplasm ratio, N:C ratio, or N/C) is a measurement used in cell biology. It is a ratio of the size (i.e., volume) of the nucleus of a cell to the size of the cytoplasm of that cell. Small lymphocytes are round with high nuclear cytoplasmic ratio (N: C ratio). In the large lymphocytes, the N: C ratio is lower. Monocytes have an N:C ratio of approximately 3:1 to 2:1.

Note: The N:C ratio indicates the maturity of a cell, because as a cell matures the size of its nucleus generally decreases. The high nuclear-to-cytoplasmic (N:C) ratio has proven to be a valuable morphologic feature for the diagnosis of atypical cells and/or malignancy.

Differentiation between Various Leukocytes

- A degenerating neutrophil is occasionally confused for a basophil. It is said that one should label a cell as basophil only when one is absolutely certain of its identification.
- Occasionally, deep blue-violet, solid-looking granules of precipitated stain may appear on a blood film. These uniformly round artifacts, spread all over the film, should not be mistaken for cells, especially platelets.

Differential Counting of Leukocytes

- Draw 100 squares in your workbook for recording 100 WBCs as they are encountered and identified one after another. Enter these cells by using the letters "N" for neutrophils, "M" for monocytes, "LL" for large lymphocytes, "SL" for small lymphocytes, "E" for eosinophils, and "B" for basophils as shown in **Figure 28**.
- Alternative method (Tally bar method): You can also indicate these cells in a column and as you identify a cell, put a short vertical stroke for each cell identified. In this way, you can place different types of cells in groups of five, wherein four vertical lines representing four cells is crossed by a diagonal stroke representing the 5th cell.
- Place a drop of cedar wood oil on the right upper corner of the film, a few millimeters away from the head end. Bring the oil immersion lens into position till it enters the oil drop. Adjust the focus.
- Do not flood the entire surface of the slide with oil; as you move the slide, the oil will move with the objective lens.

N	N	SL	N	L	L	N	N	N	L
LL	E	N	N	N	N	L	M	N	L

FIG. 28: Differential counting of leukocytes. (Observation chart)

- Move the slide slowly to the right (the image will move to the left) and as you encounter a leukocyte, identify it, and enter it in the observation chart **(Fig. 28)**. As you approach the end of the smear, move two fields down and scan the film in the opposite direction. As you near the head, again move two fields down and scan the film toward the tail. Traverse the film in this to and fro fashion till you have examined 100 cells. This "*battlement*" procedure, as shown in **Figure 25B**, ensures that you do not count a leukocyte more than once.
- *Recount*: After you have counted 100 cells, count the leukocytes once more, starting from the lower left corner of the film, and going up in the "battlement" procedure.
- When counting has been done, calculate the percentage of each type of cell in your count of 100 white blood cells.
- *Absolute leukocyte count*: The absolute values are more significant than the DLC values alone. The reason is that the DLC may show only a relative increase or decrease of a particular type of cell with a corresponding change in the other cell types. For example, a neutrophil count of 85% may suggest neutrophilia, but if the TLC is, say, 8,000/mm^3, then the absolute neutrophil count of 6,800/mm^3 ($8{,}000 \times 85/100 = 6{,}800$) would be within the normal range.

$$\text{Absolute leukocyte count} = \frac{\text{Number of cells in DLC} \times \text{TLC count/mm}^3}{100}$$

- Normal values: The normal values for differential and absolute counts are given in **Table 8**.

Note: When counting the cells in a blood film, you can make a rough estimate of the TLC depending on whether the cells appear more frequently, or are sparsely populated amongst the red cells.

FUNCTIONS OF WHITE BLOOD CELLS

Neutrophils

The neutrophils (along with tissue macrophages) are the first to arrive at the site of invasion by microbes. The toxins from the bacteria and kinins from damaged tissues, and

Table 8: Normal values for differential and absolute leukocyte counts.

Differential count	*Percentage (%)*	*Absolute count (per mm³)*
Neutrophils	40–75	2,000–7,500
Lymphocytes (Large + small)	20–45	1,300–3,500
Monocytes	2–10	500–800
Eosinophils	1–6	4–440
Basophils	0–1	0–100

some of the CSFs attract more and more of these cells by chemoattraction (chemotaxis). The bacteria, which are made more "tasty" by a coating of opsonins (IgG, and a CSF), are then phagocytized by the neutrophils. Once the bacteria are ingested by a process of endocytosis, they get enclosed in membranous phagosomes within the neutrophils.

The neutrophil cytoplasmic granules contain various enzymes and chemicals that can kill bacteria and fungi within fractions of a second. These include three main groups of chemicals:

1. Lysozymes, proteases, and myeloperoxidases.
2. Proteins called "defensins" (α and β), form peptide "spears" that punch holes in bacterial membranes so that the resulting loss of cell contents kills the bacteria.
3. A group of strong oxidants, which kill the bacteria within fractions of a second, includes—superoxide (O_2^-, oxygen carrying an extra electron), hypochlorite (OCl^-) hydroxyl, halide, and hydrogen peroxide. The neutrophil granules fuse with the phagosome and discharge the above-mentioned chemicals. In this way, each neutrophil can kill 8–10 bacteria before itself is killed in the defense of the body.

The neutrophils also release leukotrienes, prostaglandins, thromboxanes, etc. that bring about the reactions of inflammation, like vasodilation and hyperemia, edema, redness, and pain. (All these are part of the body's defenses).

Note: The myeloperoxidases catalyze conversion of Cl^-, Br^-, and I^- to the corresponding acids, which are potent oxidants.

Eosinophils

Large numbers of eosinophils are present in the mucosa of lungs, and gastrointestinal and urinary tracts, where they provide "mucosal immunity". They play the following roles:

1. **Antiallergic role:** These cells are believed to release enzymes such as histaminase, leukotriene C_4, arylsulfatase, which neutralize the effects of histamine and other agents involved in allergic inflammation.
2. **Phagocytic function:** These cells are weakly phagocytic and so not of much use against the usual bacteria. However, they can ingest (phagocytose) and destroy antigen-antibody complexes; this prevents further spread of local allergic inflammation.
3. **Antiparasitic action:** The eosinophils are effective against certain parasites that are too big to be engulfed, e.g. larvae of trichinosis (pork worm), schistosomiasis, etc. These cells attach themselves to these parasites and their granules release hydrolytic enzymes, reactive form of oxygen (superoxide), and the larvicidal agent called "major basic protein" (MBP) which destroy the parasites.

Basophils

Like mast cells, the basophils liberate histamine, heparin and serotonin. Heparin prevents blood clotting and also removes fat particles from blood after a fatty meal.

Basophils collect where allergic reactions are taking place, e.g. lung in asthma, and connective tissue in skin allergy. Here they release histamine, serotonin (5-HT), bradykinin, eosinophil chemotactic factor, slow-reacting substance (SRS), and other chemicals. These agents promote and intensify the inflammatory reactions and are involved in immediate hypersensitivity reactions.

Thus, though eosinophils and basophils appear to have opposite effects in allergy, they act in a balanced manner to control the harmful effects of the offending antigens.

Monocytes (Monocyte-Macrophage System/ Reticuloendothelial System, RES)

The monocytes, after spending a day or two in the circulation (here they are immature), enter the tissue where they increase in size and become actively-phagocytic tissue macrophages. They guard all the possible points of entry of foreign invaders. They become activated by T lymphocytes.

The activated tissue macrophages migrate in response to chemotactic stimuli and engulf, and kill the bacteria by processes similar to those seen in neutrophils. Over 100 chemicals are secreted by these cells, including most of the bactericidal agents described for neutrophils. They also contain lipases which dissolve the lipid coating of bacteria like tuberculosis and leprosy. Each macrophage can kill up to 100 bacteria before itself is killed.

The macrophages also play an important role in immunity. They pass (present) the partly-digested antigens of the organisms directly to T and B cells, thus activating them to perform their specific functions in immunity.

Lymphocytes

They play a fundamental role in immune responses of the body.

***Types of lymphocytes*:** There are three primary lymphocyte populations: T-lymphocytes, B-lymphocytes, and non-T, non-B lymphocytes. The function of third-party cells is not clear, and unlike T and B cells, they do not contain antigen receptors in their plasma membranes.

PHYSIOCLINICAL SIGNIFICANCE

The suffix "-philia" means an increase in the number and the suffix "-penia" means a decrease in the number (of cells).

Neutrophilia: Increase in neutrophils in absolute and differential counts is called neutrophilia. (Leukocytosis or granulocytosis are a result of neutrophilia). It is the usual response to certain physiological and pathological stimuli. In the latter case, relatively younger cells appear in blood and cause "left shift". The causes include physiological and pathological.

- **Physiological neutrophilia:** It is seen in muscular exercise, physical and mental stress, after meals, and during pregnancy and after parturition. Neutrophils are mobilized from the "marginal" and "bone marrow" pools. There is no new formation of these cells.
- **Pathological neutrophilia (absolute count ≥ 10,000/mm³)** can be due to:
  1. Acute infections, especially localized due to pus-forming bacteria (streptococci and staphylococci), such as superficial or deep abscess, boils, tonsillitis, appendicitis, pneumonia, lung abscess.
  2. Surgery, trauma, burns, acute hemorrhage, hemolysis.
  3. Tissue necrosis (tissue death); myocardial, pulmonary, renal infarction, amebic hepatitis, malignancies.
  4. Drugs: Adrenaline, glucocorticoids (mobilization of marginal and "sequestered" cells in closed capillaries).

Neutropenia (absolute count ≤ 2,500/mm³): The terms leukopenia and granulocytopenia, usually mean neutropenia. Neutropenia is never beneficial. The major effect is a reduced ability of the patient to localize and confine infections (especially if the count is <1,000/mm³). The infection may spread to blood and cause septicemia, a serious emergency.

Infections with usual organisms, which rarely cause disease in normal persons (e.g. fungi, viruses like herpes simplex and herpes zoster), called **"opportunistic infections"**, may cause a serious condition if neutropenia is prolonged (>15 days).

- **Physiological neutropenia** is unusual and rare.
- **Pathological neutropenia.** The causes are:
  1. Typhoid and paratyphoid infections, viral influenza, kala-azar.
  2. Acquired immunodeficiency syndrome (AIDS).
  3. Depression of bone marrow due to drugs, chemicals, radiation, etc.
  4. Autoimmune disease—the neutrophils are destroyed by neutrophil antibodies: (The autoimmune diseases are due to immune responses against one's own "self" material, other examples are diabetes mellitus, rheumatoid arthritis, purpura, etc.).
  5. Severe overwhelming infection—the neutrophils are "used up" at a much faster rate than they are produced.

Eosinophilia (absolute count ≥ 500/mm³): The causes are:

1. **Allergic conditions:** Bronchial asthma, skin diseases like urticaria, eczema, and food sensitivity, etc.
2. **Parasitic infections:** Intestinal worms like hookworms, tapeworms, roundworms, especially those which invade tissues.

Eosinopenia (absolute count <50/mm³): The causes include: acute stressful illness, Cushing's syndrome (excess steroids), adrenocorticotropic hormone (ACTH), and glucosteroid treatment, and acute pyogenic infections.

Basophilia (absolute number ≥100/mm³): The condition is seen in viral infections (influenza), allergic diseases, smallpox, and chickenpox.

Basopenia: It is seen in acute pyogenic infections and during glucocorticoid treatment.

Monocytosis (absolute count ≥ 800/mm³): It is seen in:

1. Infectious mononucleosis (IM). It is a contagious viral disease caused by Epstein-Barr virus (EBV) and occurs mainly in children. Signs and symptoms include fever, fatigue, dizziness, enlargement of lymph glands, high TLC, especially large number of lymphocytes. There is no cure but the disease runs its course in a few weeks.
2. Malaria, kala-azar, subacute bacterial endocarditis, rheumatoid arthritis.
3. Leukemias, collagen diseases, malignancies.

Monocytopenia: It may be seen in bone marrow depression due to any cause.

Lymphocytosis (absolute count ≥5,000/mm³): High counts are seen in:

1. Healthy infants and young children. DLC may be about 60% though the TLC may be normal. This is sometimes called "relative lymphocytosis".
2. Viral infections: whooping cough, chickenpox, etc.; autoimmune disease.
3. Chronic infections like tuberculosis and hepatitis.
4. Chronic lymphocytic leukemia—this is the most common cause of lymphocyte count above 10,000/mm³.

Lymphocytopenia: The causes of decrease include:

1. Patients on steroid therapy.
2. Acquired immunodeficiency syndrome. The virus particularly attacks the helper/inducer (T4) cells.
3. Depression of bone marrow due to any cause.

PRECAUTIONS

1. The slides should be absolutely free from dust and grease, because blood will not stick to areas where oils from your fingers have been left. New slides should be preferred. But if old ones are to be used, they should be properly cleaned.
2. The edge of the spreader should be smooth and not chipped, otherwise the slide would leave striations along or across the smear. Leukocytes may also be caught in chipped places and be carried toward the tail.
3. When applying the slide to the blood drop from a fingerprick, do not touch the skin with the slide, but only the periphery (top) of the blood drop. This is to avoid taking up epidermal squames or sweat.
4. The blood should be spread immediately after taking it on the slide. Any delay will cause clumping of cells due to partial coagulation. This will give a "granular" appearance to the blood film, which is visible to the naked eye.
5. The angle of the spreader should be 35–45°. The more the angle of the spreader approaches the vertical, the thinner the film, and the lesser the angle, the thicker the film.
6. The pressure of the spreader on the slide should be slight and even and the pushing should be fairly quick while maintaining an uniform pressure throughout.
7. The film should be dried by waving it in the air immediately after spreading it. A delay can cause not only clumping,

but also crenation and distortion of red cells in a damp atmosphere (if water is allowed to slowly evaporate from the blood plasma on the slide, crenation occurs due to gradual increase in the concentration of salts).
8. By turning the spreader over, you can use it to make four blood films.
9. Do not allow Leishman's stain to become syrupy (thick) or dry up on the slide as this is likely to cause precipitation of the stain.
10. Avoid tap water for diluting the stain, and for washing off the diluted stain after "staining", because methylene blue components may not stain the cells properly.
11. The Leishman's stain should be kept in well-stoppered bottles. After use, the stopper should always be turned so as to keep out air from the solution. (The stain can be kept for months provided it is kept in airtight bottles).
12. Avoid bringing the stained film in contact with alcohol. If you do this, the stain will be extracted in a few seconds.
13. When counting the cells, use the "battlement" method. This is to avoid counting a cell twice.
14. Avoid counting the leukocytes in the extreme ends of the head or tail, and along the edges of the blood film.

QUESTIONS

Q.1. How are the glass slides cleaned?
See text above.

Q.2. What precautions will you take while preparing blood films? Why are four or five (or more) slides prepared at a time?
A number of slides are prepared for two reasons: (1) to get practice in the procedure and (2) the best-stained slide can be chosen for counting the cells.

Q.3. Why should the blood film be dried quickly soon after spreading it?
See text above.

Q.4. What are the features of an ideal blood film?
See text above.

Q.5. What is the composition of Leishman's stain and what is the function of each component? Why should the stain be acetone free?
See text above.

Q.6. What is buffered water? Why should it be preferred over distilled water?
Buffered water is phosphate buffer in which the pH is adjusted at 6.8. At this pH, there is optimal ionization of the stain particles so that they can penetrate the cells better. The buffer is prepared by dissolving 3.7 g of disodium hydrogen phosphate and 2.1 g of potassium dihydrogen phosphate in distilled water made to 1,000 mL. The pH is tested with a pH meter. If it is lower, the former is added; if it is higher than 6.8, the latter is added till the desired pH is reached.

Q.7. Why is Leishman's stain diluted after 1–2 minutes? What happens to the blood film during this period?
During the fixation period of 1–2 minutes, the pure absolute alcohol serves two purposes: (1) It precipitates the plasma proteins, which act as glue and attach (fix) the blood cells on to the glass slide and (2) It preserves the shape and chemistry of cells to as near the living state as possible.

The cells are not stained during this time, because the stain particles cannot enter the cells in their unionized state. Their ionization occurs only when water is added to the salts in the undiluted stain. (If diluted stain were added to start with, the blood smear itself would be washed away. Diluted Leishman's stain can be used if the blood film is first fixed in absolute alcohol).

> **Note:** The appearance of the glossy greenish scum (layer) floating on the surface of the diluted stain shows that the staining has been done properly. If the scum does not float, it means it has been deposited on the surface of the blood smear. The cells will now look hazy under the microscope.

Q.8. Can tap water be used for diluting the stain after fixation?
Tap water should not be used because the methylene blue components (methylene blue plus methylene azure formed from the former) may not stain the cells due to the unknown pH and salt content of this water. Also, tap water may contain impurities that may show up as artifact on the blood film.

Q.9. Can any other stain be used for blood films?
Yes. Giemsa's stain, like Leishman's stain, is a mixture of methylene blue, methylene azure, and eosin. Since it is an aqueous stain (i.e. containing water), the film is first fixed in absolute methyl or ethyl alcohol for 3–5 minutes. It is then stained in a staining jar containing the diluted stain. The staining is very similar to Leishman's stain.

Wright's blood stain is still another stain commonly used in some laboratories.

Q.10. What other information can be obtained from a blood film?
The other applications of blood film are:
1. Diagnosis of malaria, from malarial parasite seen in the red cells.
2. Diagnosis of leukemia from the type of blast cells.
3. Various parasitic infections, like filariasis, trypanosomiasis, etc.
4. Sex determination can be done from the presence of female sex chromatin which appears as a "drumstick" (Barr body) attached to a lobe of neutrophil nucleus.
5. Study of morphology of red cells in various types of anemias.
6. Estimation of platelet count by indirect method.

Q.11. Why is cedar wood oil used with oil immersion objective?
See chapter on Compound Microscope.

Q.12. Which part of the blood film should be avoided for counting the cells? Which is the best part?
The "head" (start) of the film and the extreme tail should be avoided because these areas contain fewer cells which are commonly distorted. They should also be avoided in the extreme edges. The area in between these regions is the most suitable for counting leukocytes.

Q.13. Which is the largest cell in the blood film? Which is the smallest? How do you assess the size of a cell?
The monocyte is the largest cell in a blood film. Its diameter is usually 15–18 µm, though a few may be somewhat smaller and others a little larger than these. The diameter of small lymphocytes varies between 7 and 9 µm. So, a few may be slightly smaller than the red cells.

Normally, the size of the red cells is unchanging—being 7.2–7.8 μm. Therefore, the size of a WBC can be estimated by assessing how many RBCs will span across a given leukocyte.

Q.14. What is a micrometer?

Micrometer is a measure of length in the SI system. The prefix "micro" means a millionth (10^{-6}). Thus, a micrometer is one millionth of a meter. A millimeter is one thousandth of a meter (milli = one thousandth, 10^{-3}). A micrometer would be one thousandth of a millimeter. (It is difficult to imagine how much a micrometer would be, because raising 10 to the power-6 does not tell us much. If it is remembered that a human hair is about 1/10 of a millimeter (100 μm) thick then one can imagine the diameter of a red cell, which will be about 1/13 of a hair thickness, i.e. about 13 red cells will span across the thickness of one hair.

Q.15. How are leukocytes classified and how can they be differentiated from each other?

See **Table 7**.

Q.16. What are the functions of various leukocytes?

See text above.

Q.17. What is the clinical importance of doing differential leukocyte count?

The differential count is done to find out if there is an increase or decrease of a particular type of WBC. Knowing the TLC, the absolute number of each type can be calculated. This information is important in detecting infection or inflammation, allergic and parasitic infections, and effects of chemotherapy and radiation therapy.

Q.18. What is absolute leukocyte count and what is its importance?

See text above.

Q.19. Can you get a rough idea of total leukocyte count while doing differential leukocyte count?

See text above.

Q.20. How does the differential leukocyte count of a child differ from that of an adult?

While granulocytes predominate in an adult where they form 50% to 70% of the TLC, the lymphocytes predominate in children where they form up to 40% to 50% of TLC.

Q.21. Is it possible to know the sex of a person from the blood film?

Yes. It is possible to do so. In females, the chromatin of the sex chromosome is seen as a "drumstick" (Barr body) extending from one lobe of the nucleus into the cytoplasm. However, it is not visible in all neutrophils.

Q.22. What is meant by the terms neutrophilia and neutropenia, and what are their causes?

See text above.

Q.23. Enumerate the conditions that cause eosinophilia and eosinopenia.

See text above.

Q.24. Name the conditions where basophils increase and decrease in number.

See text above.

Q.25. What is leukemoid reaction?

See chapter on Total Leukocyte Count.

Q.26. What are the causes of monocytosis and monocytopenia?

See text above.

Q.27. What are the causes of lymphocytosis and lymphocytopenia?

See text above.

Q.28. What is Cooke-Arneth count and what is its importance?

See chapter on Determination of Arneth Count.

Q.29. What is peroxidase reaction? Which types of leukocytes give a positive reaction?

Peroxidase reaction (peroxidase stain) for leukocytes: This test is carried out as follows—a dry blood film is first treated with a solution of benzidine and sodium nitroprusside dissolved in ethyl alcohol and then with hydrogen peroxide. After a thorough wash with water, the film is counter-stained with Leishman's stain in the usual manner.

The peroxidase reaction detects the presence of oxidizing enzymes in the cytoplasm of myeloid series of WBCs. Oxidase granules are seen in myelocytes and myeloblasts. Eosinophils show deeper blue granules, while basophils show no granules. Lymphoid series of cells are peroxidase negative. This reaction helps in distinguishing immature cells of the myeloid series from lymphoid series in cases of leukemia (the two series of immature cells look similar with Leishman's stain alone).

OBJECTIVE STRUCTURED PRACTICAL EXAMINATION-I

Aim: To prepare a blood film from a sample of blood provided.

Procedural steps: See text above.

Checklist:

1. Selects 3–4, clean, grease-free, dry slides and places these on a blotting paper. Mixes the provided sample of blood thoroughly without frothing. (Y/N)
2. Using a dropper, she places a small drop of blood near the end of a slide about 1 cm from the end. (Y/N)
3. Supporting the left end of the slide between thumb and middle finger of left hand, she places the spreader in front of the blood drop at an angle of 40°, and draws the spreader back and allows the blood to spread along its width. (Y/N)
4. Maintaining a light and even pressure and 40° angle, she moves the spreader forward, with a fairly fast and gliding motion, pulling the blood behind it in the form of a thin smear. (Y/N)
5. Makes 3–4 more such smears. (Y/N)

OBJECTIVE STRUCTURED PRACTICAL EXAMINATION-II

Aim: To stain the given blood film for differential count.

Procedural steps: See text above.

Checklist:

1. Places the blood film horizontally over the parallel glass rods assembled over the sink. (Y/N)
2. Pours 8–10 drops of Leishman's stain from a drop bottle to cover the blood film. (Y/N)

3. After 1–2 minutes (or as advised), then adds equal amount of buffered water, or double-distilled water, over the stain till the mixture stands from the edges of the slide. (Y/N)
4. Mixes the stain by blowing on it through a glass dropper for 8–10 minutes. Watches that at no stage the stain is allowed to dry on the blood film. (Y/N)
5. Then drains off the stain under a gentle stream of distilled/tap water. Then puts the slide against a support, stained side facing down. (Y/N)

OBJECTIVE STRUCTURED PRACTICAL EXAMINATION-III

Aim: To examine the provided stained blood film under oil immersion lens and focus any leukocyte.

Procedural steps: See text above.

Checklist:

1. Checks the stained slide to confirm the side on which the smear was made. Then examines it under low power and high power lenses by making suitable adjustments of light to check staining and cell distribution. (Y/N)
2. Raises the body tube, places a drop of cedar wood oil and swings the oil immersion lens into position. (Y/N)
3. Looking from the side, brings the oil immersion lens down slowly till it just enters the oil drop. (Y/N)
4. Raises the condenser and opens the iris diaphragm.(Y/N)
5. Looks into the microscope and scans the smear, "racking" the microscope all the time till she focuses a leukocyte. (Y/N)

1.8: DETERMINATION OF ERYTHROCYTE SEDIMENTATION RATE AND PACKED CELL VOLUME

STUDENT OBJECTIVES

After completing this experiment, the student should be able to:

- Describe the clinical importance of doing erythrocyte sedimentation rate (ESR).
- Explain why red cells settle down when blood is kept in a tube, and indicate the factors that affect their rate of settling.
- Name the methods employed for its determination.
- Describe the sources of error and precautions to be taken.
- Name the various conditions in which ESR increases or decreases and their physiological basis.
- Define hematocrit (Hct) and its clinical importance.
- Identify the Wintrobe tube and Westergren's pipette and explain how to fill them with blood.
- Indicate the conditions in which the Hct is increased and decreased.
- Explain whole body hematocrit.

DETERMINATION OF ESR

Introduction

PY2.12: Describe test for ESR, Osmotic fragility, Hematocrit. Note the findings and interpret the test results, etc.

Definition: The rate at which the red blood cells (RBCs) sediment when a sample of blood, to which an anticoagulant has been added, is allowed to stand in a narrow vertical tube for 1 hour is called **erythrocyte sedimentation rate (ESR)**. It is expressed in millimeters of clear plasma at the end of the 1st hour.

The determination of the rate at which the red cells settle or sediment is often required by a physician to rule out the presence of organic disease or to follow the progress of a disease. ESR is generally done as part of complete blood tests by following methods:

- Wintrobe's method
- Westergren's method.

Principle

In the circulating blood, the red cells remain uniformly suspended in the plasma. However, when a sample of blood, to which an anticoagulant has been added, is allowed to stand in a narrow vertical tube, the red cells (specific gravity = 1.095) being heavier (denser) than the colloid plasma (specific gravity = 1.032), settle or sediment gradually toward the bottom of the tube.

Sedimentation of Red Cells

The settling or sedimentation of red cells in a sample of anticoagulated blood occurs in three stages:

1. In the ***first stage,*** the RBCs pile up (like a stack of coins), and form rouleaux that become heavier during the first 10–15 minutes.
2. During the ***second stage,*** the rouleau being heavier sinks to the bottom. This stage lasts for 40–45 minutes.
3. In the ***third stage,*** there is packing of massed bunches of red cells at the bottom of the blood column. This stage lasts for about 10–12 minutes.

Thus, most of the settling of the red cells occurs in the 1st hour or so.

WINTROBE'S METHOD

Apparatus

- Pricking apparatus (disposable syringe and needle), sterile swabs moist with 70% alcohol, discarde penicillin bottles with powdered double oxalate mixture (6 mg ammonium oxalate and 4 mg potassium oxalate).
- **Wintrobe tube with stand (Fig. 29)**. Wintrobe tube is a 11 cm long, heavy, cylindrical glass tube, with a uniform bore diameter of 2.5 mm **(Fig. 30)**. Its lower end is closed and flat. The tube is calibrated in centimeters and millimeters from 0 to 10 cm from above downwards on one side of the scale (for ESR), and 10–0 cm on the other side (for PCV). Each centimeter is further divided into millimeters (mm). The mouth of the tube can be covered with a rubber cap to prevent loss of fluid by evaporation. A Wintrobe stand is provided for holding the tube upright when doing ESR. The Wintrobe stand can hold up to three (or six) tubes at a time.

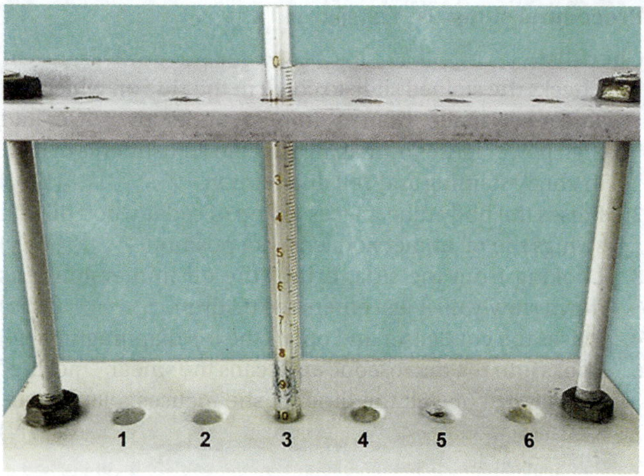

FIG. 29: Wintrobe's tube with a stand.

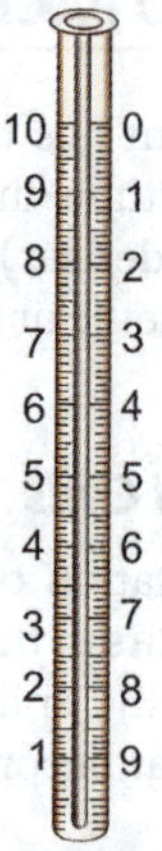

FIG. 30: Determination of erythrocyte sedimentation rate (ESR). Wintrobe tube.

- **Pasteur pipette:** It is a glass tubing drawn to a long thin nozzle about 14 cm long. A rubber teat is provided to suck blood into the pipette by a slight pressure. It is used for filling the Wintrobe tube **(Fig. 31)**.
- **Centrifuge machine:** It packs the red cells in the Hct tube by centrifugal force. The magnitude of force produced by rotation of the tube depends on:

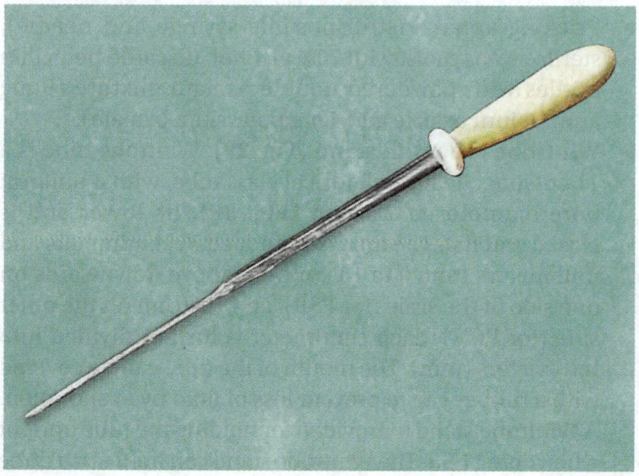

FIG. 31: Pasteur pipette.

- The radius, i.e. the distance between the center of the shaft and the bottom of the centrifuge tube when laid horizontally.
- The number of revolutions per minute (rpm).

In terms of gravitational force (G), the value of this force should be 2,260 units. This much force is created when the radius is 9 inches and the speed is 3,000 rpm.

Procedure

1. Draw 2.0 mL of venous blood and transfer it to a container of anticoagulant. Mix the contents gently but well by inverting the vial a few times, or by swirling it. Do not shake, as it will cause frothing.
2. Using the Pasteur pipette, fill the Wintrobe tube from below upwards. Ensure that there are no air bubbles.
3. Transfer the tube to its stand and adjust the screws, so that it will remain vertical. Leave the tube undisturbed in this position for 1 hour, at the end of which read the mm of clear plasma above the red cells.

Express your result as mm at the end of 1st hour (Wintrobe).

Normal values:

Males: 0–9 mm at the end of 1st hour

Females: 0–20 mm at the end of 1st hour.

WESTERGREN'S METHOD

Apparatus

- A 2 mL disposable syringe with needle, sterile cotton/gauze swabs moist with alcohol, discarded penicillin bottle.
- Sterile solution of 3.8% sodium citrate as the anticoagulant.
- **Westergren pipette and stand (Fig. 32)**. A Westergren pipette is 300 mm long, open from both the ends and has a bore diameter of 2.5 mm. It is calibrated in centimeters and millimeters from 0 to 200, from above downwards

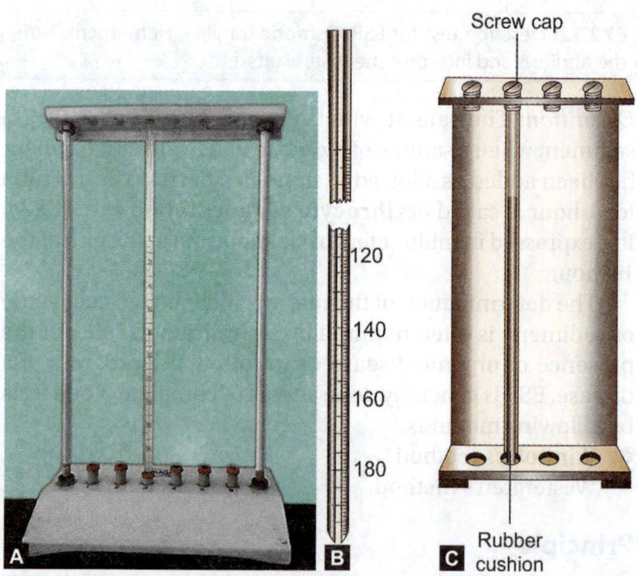

FIGS. 32A TO C: (A) Westergren pipette and stand; (B) Westergren pipette; (C) Westergren stand with the Westergren pipette in position.

in its lower two-thirds **(Fig. 32B)**. The Westergren stand can accommodate four to six tubes at a time. For each pipette, there is a screw cap that slips over its top, and, at its lower end, the pipette presses into a rubber pad or cushion. When the pipette is fixed in position, there is enough pressure of the screw cap to prevent leakage of blood from its lower end.

Procedure

1. Draw 2.0 mL of venous blood and transfer it into a vial containing 0.5 mL of 3.8% sodium citrate solution. This will give a blood:citrate ratio of 4:1. Mix the contents by inverting or swirling the vial. Do not shake, as it will cause frothing.
2. Fill the Westergren's pipette with blood–citrate mixture by sucking, after placing the tip of your finger over the top of the pipette to control the flow of blood into and out of it, or with a rubber bulb. Bring the blood column to exactly zero mark. (If there is a difference of 1–2 mm, it should be noted and taken into account before giving the final report at the end of 1 hour).
3. Keeping your finger (or the rubber bulb) over the pipette, transfer it to the Westergren stand by firmly pressing its lower end into the rubber cushion. Now slip the upper end of the pipette under the screw cap. Confirm that there is no leakage of blood and that the pipette will remain vertical.
4. Leave the pipette undisturbed for 1 hour at the end of which read the mm of clear plasma above the red cells.

Express your results as ....mm at the end of 1st hour (Westergren).

Normal values:
Males: 3–5 mm at the end of 1st hour
Females: 4–7 mm at the end of 1st hour.

Sources of Error

- Tilting of the tube and high temperature can lead to high values.
- Low temperature gives false low values.
- Hemolyzed blood may obscure the sharp line separating red cells and the plasma.

Precautions

1. All glass apparatus like tubes and pipettes should be absolutely dry.
2. To prevent hemolysis, detach the needle after venepuncture and then gently transfer the blood into the penicillin bottle.
3. Proper anticoagulant should be used for each method. It should be taken in a specific amount for a given method.
4. The blood should be collected in the fasting state.
5. There should be no air bubble while filling the Wintrobe tube or the Westergren pipette with blood.
6. The test should preferably be done within 2–3 hours of collecting the blood sample at room temperature.
7. The hematocrit (Hct) should be checked and correction factor should be applied in cases of anemia (nomograms are available for this purpose).
8. Clotted or hemolyzed blood must be discarded.
9. The Wintrobe tube or Westergren pipette should not be disturbed from the vertical position during the test.

Note: ESR estimation by Westergren method is more sensitive than the Wintrobe method.

MEASUREMENT OF PACKED CELL VOLUME

Measurement of Hct or packed cell volume (PCV) is the most accurate and simplest of all tests in clinical hematology for detecting the presence and degree of anemia or polycythemia. In comparison, hemoglobin (Hb) estimation is less accurate, and red blood cell (RBC) count far less accurate.

Also, if Hb, RBC count, and PCV are determined at the same time, various absolute corpuscular values (e.g. volume and Hb content of a single red cell) of a person can be determined. These values help in the laboratory diagnosis of the type of anemia in a person.

Procedure

1. Draw 5 mL of venous blood and transfer it to a container (penicillin vial or bulb) with anticoagulant. Rotate the bulb between your palms. This is done for the following reasons:
   a. To ensure proper mixing of cells and plasma (inaccurate results are likely, if this precaution is not taken).
   b. To oxygenate blood cells to remove CO_2 (red cells are larger when CO_2 is high, in venous blood).
2. Fill the Pasteur pipette with blood and take it's nozzle to the bottom of the Wintrobe tube. Expel the blood gently by pressing the rubber teat, and fill the tube from below upwards while withdrawing the pipette but always keeping its tip below the level of blood. Ensure that there is no air bubble trapped in the blood.

Note: Do not try to fill the tube from its top as blood will not flow down to its bottom because of air present in the tube.

3. Bring the blood column exactly to the mark 10 (or the mark 0 on the other side of the scale) at the top. There should not be any bubbles at the top of blood. If less blood is available, note the level.
4. Close the mouth of the tube with its rubber cap and centrifuge it at 3,000 rpm for 30 minutes (slower speed will not pack the red cells fully).
5. At the end of 30 minutes, take the reading of the upper level of packed red cells on the side of the scale where zero is at the bottom.

Observations and Results

Note that the blood has been separated into three layers **(Fig. 33)**:

- A tall upper layer of clear plasma—amber- or straw-colored. It should not be pink or red, which would indicate hemolysis of red cells in the sample or within the body (i.e. before withdrawal of venous blood) in hemolytic diseases. If there is hemolysis, the test must be repeated on a fresh sample.

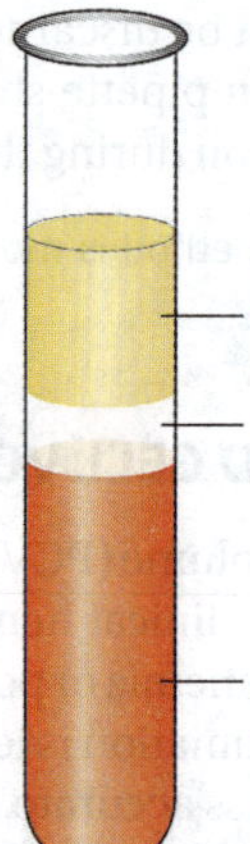

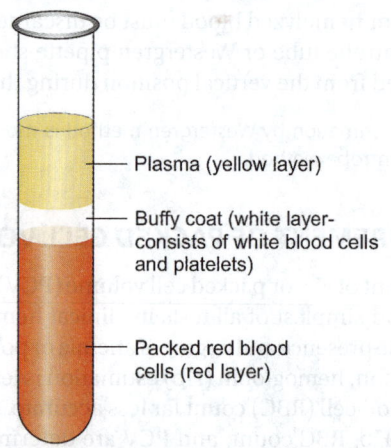

FIG. 33: Formation of three layers after centrifugation of blood.

- A grayish-white, thin layer (about 1 mm thick) the so-called **"buffy layer"**, consisting of platelets above and leukocytes below it.
- A tall bottom layer of red cells, which have been closely packed together. A grayish red line separates red cell layer from the layer of leukocytes above it. The line marks the upper limit of the red cell layer.

Note: Do not include the buffy coat while reading the height of the red cell column.

- The percentage of the volume of blood occupied by the red cells constitutes Hct or packed cell volume, i.e. the percentage of whole blood that is red cells.

  Hematocrit (Hct) =

$$\frac{\text{Height of packed red cells (mm)}}{\text{Height of packed RBCs and plasma (i.e., height of blood column)}} \times 100$$

  For example, if the height of packed red cells is 45 mm then

$$= \frac{45}{100} \times 100 = 45\%$$

- It also means that out of 100 volumes (or parts) of blood 45 volumes (or parts) are red cells and 55 volumes (or parts) are plasma. Thus, out of 1 liter of blood, 450 mL are red cells and 550 mL are plasma.

Normal values: The *average value of PCV is 42%* when the RBC count is 5 million/mm^3 and their size and shape are normal.

Adult males: 44% (38–50%)

Adult females: 42% (36–45%)

The PCV for *newborns* is about 50%.

"True" hematocrit [true cell volume (TCV)]: Even under optimum conditions, it is impossible to completely pack the red cells together, and about 2% plasma remains trapped in-between the red cells. This percentage is more (i.e. more plasma), if the red cells are abnormal in shape (e.g. spherocytosis and sickle cells). To compensate for the trapped plasma, the "true" cell volume (true Hct) can be obtained by multiplying the observed Hct value with 0.98.

Venous blood hematocrit: The Hct of venous blood is slightly higher than that of arterial blood, because as the pH changes from the arterial value of 7.41 to 7.37 in the venous blood, the red cells gain a little water.

Precautions

1. Use the recommended amount of ethylenediamine-tetraacetic acid (EDTA) as the anticoagulant. There should be no clotting or hemolysis of the blood.
2. The test should be done within 6–8 hours of collection of the sample.
3. The Wintrobe tube should be filled carefully using Pasteur pipette placing the tip of the pipette at the bottom of the tube.
4. The pipette should be gradually withdrawn as the blood fills in the Wintrobe's tube from below upwards, so that no air bubble is trapped in the tube.
5. The Hct should be checked and correction factor should be applied in cases of anemia (nomograms are available for this purpose).

PHYSIOCLINICAL SIGNIFICANCE

Erythrocyte Sedimentation Rate

Physiological Variations in ESR

- **Age:** ESR is low in infants (0.5 mm 1st hour Westergren) because of polycythemia. It gradually increases to adult levels in the next few years. However, it starts to increase after the age of 50 years.
- **Sex:** The ESR is somewhat higher in females, probably due to lower Hct (PCV).
- **High altitude:** People living at high altitudes have relatively higher ESR. (Polycythemia due to hypoxia actually should decrease ESR).
- **Pregnancy:** The ESR begins to rise after about 3rd month of pregnancy and returns to normal a few weeks after delivery. Hemodilution during pregnancy and increased fibrinogen: albumin ratio are probably the cause of increased rouleaux formation.
- **Body temperature:** Within limits, ESR varies with body temperature, which tends to affect viscosity.
- After a meal, ESR increases. Therefore ESR should be done in the fasting state.

Pathological Increase in ESR

The ESR is increased in any condition that is associated with inflammation and tissue damage. It is seen in:

- **All acute and chronic infections (localized or generalized),** e.g., pneumonia, tuberculosis, and acute episodes in chronic infections.
- **All anemias except** spherocytosis, sickle cell anemia, and pernicious anemia.
- **Bone diseases,** e.g., osteomyelitis.
- **Connective tissue diseases,** e.g., Systemic lupus erythematosis and rheumatoid arthritis.
- **All malignant diseases (cancers):** e.g. carcinoma of breast and leukemia, especially when they have spread to other parts of the body.

- **Acute noninfective inflammation,** e.g., gout.
- **Nephrotic syndrome:** Marked decrease in albumin level (due to loss in urine), and increase in fibrinogen and globulins raise the ESR.
- **Trauma, surgery,** etc.—any large-scale tissue injury raises ESR.

Pathological Decrease in ESR

- **Polycythemia:** Polycythemia (an increased number of red blood cells) will increase blood viscosity and can cause a reduced ESR. Too many red blood cells decrease the compactness of the rouleaux network also and thus lower the ESR. High red cell counts associated with hypoxia due to heart and lung diseases, such as congestive heart failure (CHF), congenital heart diseases, severe emphysema, etc. show a low ESR.
- Spherocytosis, pernicious anemia, and sickle cell anemia. In sickle cell disease, lower ESR occurs due to the abnormal shape of red blood cells that impairs rouleaux formation.
- **Afibrinogenemia:** Decrease or absence of fibrinogen in plasma, which is a genetic disorder, shows a low ESR.
- Severe allergic reactions.

Clinical Significance of ESR

1. **As an indicator of bodily reaction to tissue injury and inflammation:** The ESR values are not diagnostic. It is a sensitive indicator of inflammation and tissue damage, Thus, ESR is raised in all **pathological conditions.**
2. **Value of ESR as a prognostic tool:** ESR is a valuable prognostic test in following up the course of a disease, such as tuberculosis, rheumatoid arthritis, etc. and the response to treatment. If a weekly ESR shows a trend toward a decrease, it would indicate an improvement. But if the ESR shows an increase, it would mean that the disease is deteriorating.
3. **Since ESR increases with age,** the upper limit of normal can be calculated as:
   Males = Age ÷ 2
   Females = (Age + 10) ÷ 2.

Note: If the ESR is near the upper limit, the test is repeated after a month or so. Also, the correction factor to allow for anemia should be applied. The corrected Westergren ESR values is obtained applying the formula of Fabry (Corrected ESR = ESR measured × 15/55-Hct)

Physioclinical Significance of Hematocrit/PCV

- It is a simple but accurate test for determining the presence of anemia or polycythemia. It is also employed for determining various absolute and corpuscular values. Sometimes, it is used for screening for anemia. It is a very good indicator of RBC population and Hb content of the blood.
- Hct is an important factor that determines viscosity of blood.

Increased PCV is seen in:

1. Excessive sweating leads to hemoconcentration and thus increasing PCV.
2. All cases of polycythemia, *hypoxia* due to lung and heart diseases, etc.
3. Congestive heart failure, burns (loss of plasma), dehydration, after severe exercise and emotional stress.

Decreased PCV is seen in:

1. Hemodilution as in pregnancy and after ingestion of large amounts of water.
2. All types of anemia.
3. Bone marrow depression.

QUESTIONS

Q.1. Why do the red cells settle down in a sample of anticoagulated blood?
The red cells settle down because they are heavier (specific gravity = 1.095) than the plasma (specific gravity = 1.032) in which they are suspended.

Q.2. Can you use oxalate mixture in Westergren method and citrate in Wintrobe method?
No, the anticoagulants employed for each method cannot be interchanged because both methods have been standardized and employed in clinical practice for the last many years. (Sodium citrate cannot be used in the Wintrobe method because the blood will be too much diluted as compared to the height of the tube; and this will give high false values for ESR.)

Q.3. What are the advantages and disadvantages of the Wintrobe method?
The **advantage** of this method is that the same sample of oxalated blood can first be used for ESR and then, after 1 hour, for Hct (PCV) by centrifuging it. Thus, in cases of anemia, the appropriate correction factor can be applied.

The **disadvantage** is that this method is less sensitive because the column of blood is not as high as is desirable for good results, and chances of error are high, especially when the ESR is increased, say to over 50 mm.

Q.4. What are the advantages and disadvantages of Westergren method?
The **advantage** of this method is that it is more sensitive since the tube is sufficiently long and its diameter is also larger. The higher sensitivity and the longer tube are particularly important in cases where ESR is high (>80 mm).

The **disadvantage** is that the citrate solution dilutes the red cells, which by itself tends to raise the ESR. But the fibrinogen and globulins of plasma are also diluted which tends to lower the ESR. These two opposing effects, however, tend to neutralize each other.

Q.5. Why is ESR reading taken after 1 hour?
The reason for this is that more than 95–98% red cells settle down by the end of this time. After 1 hour, the rate of sedimentation does not significantly affect the ESR. Further, the method has been standardized for 1 hour and in clinical practice for long.

Q.6. What are the factors on which the rate of sedimentation of red cells depends?
Rate of settling of red cells depends on:

1. A downward gravitational force acting on the red cells due to their weight (mass).

2. An upward force due to viscosity of plasma, and the area of surface of red cells where viscous retardation occurs, i.e. the plasma–red cell interface.

Thus, the rate of settling of red cells will depend on a balance between these two opposing forces.

Factors affecting ESR

The factors that affect the ESR include the following:

1. **Technical and mechanical factors:** Factors like the length of the tube, diameter of the bore (if less than 2 mm), and the anticoagulant used affect the values of ESR obtained, e.g. liquid anticoagulant (sodium citrate) in the Westergren method changes red cell–plasma ratio, which increases the ESR.
2. **Physiological factors:** The red cell count, their size and their shape, raised body temperature, viscosity of plasma, and tendency to rouleaux formation, all affect the ESR.
3. **Viscosity of blood:** Increased viscosity of blood, whether due to increase in RBC count or plasma protein concentration, decreases ESR, while a decrease in viscosity increases ESR. (Viscosity of water:plasma:blood = 1:3:5).
4. **Nature of anticoagulant used:** Fluid anticoagulant e.g. sodium citrate in Westergren method changes red cell:plasma ratio, which increases the ESR.

Q.7. What is rouleaux formation? What are the factors that increase the rate of rouleaux formation and hence the ESR?

- *Rouleaux formation:*
  - In the circulating blood, the red cells remain separate from each other due to their constant movement and due to their mutual repulsion resulting from their negative electrostatic charges imparted by sialic acid moieties on the cell membranes. This repulsion force is known as ***zeta potential.*** However, fibrinogen neutralizes these charges and makes the RBCs sticky, so that they tend to adhere to each other and form larger rouleaux.
  - In health, the rouleaux (in a blood film or in a test tube) are small and settle slowly. But under certain conditions, rouleaux formation increases and thus it is the main factor that increases the ESR. **The importance of the size and the rate of rouleaux formation** is given below.
  - The surface area of a single red cell is about 150 μm², and 10 red cells would have a surface area of 1,500 μm²—when they do not form a pile. But when these 10 red cells form a rouleaux (pile), their surface area is only 600 μm², while their mass has increased 10 times. Thus, when the red cells form rouleaux, there is a greater increase in the masses of these red cells as compared to increase in their surface area. This decreases the retardation caused by plasma viscosity, which, in turn, increases the rate of settling of red cells, and thus the ESR.
- *Factors affecting rouleaux formation*
  - **Concentration of large, asymmetric molecules of fibrinogen, and globulins:** An increase in the concentration of these plasma proteins promotes rouleaux formation (and hence ESR); this is seen in almost all infections (acute and chronic, tissue destruction due to any cause, and wasting diseases).
  - **Bacterial proteins and toxins, and products of inflammation and tissue destruction** such as acute-phase reactants (e.g. C-reactive proteins of acute rheumatic fever), released into the blood neutralize the surface charges of red cells. This promotes stickiness of these cells, rouleaux formation, and faster settling.
  - **Number of red cells:** A decrease in RBC count promotes rouleaux formation, while an increase in count (e.g. polycythemia) decreases ESR.
  - **Size and shape of red cells:** Biconcave shape of red cells favors rouleaux formation, while red cells with an abnormal or irregular shape hinder rouleaux formation, which decreases the ESR. An increase in MCV, hereditary spherocytosis, and in sickle cell disease, ESR is decreased.

Q.8. Name the physiological and pathological variations in ESR.

See text above.

Q.9. What is the clinical significance of ESR?

See text above.

Q.10. What is the importance of determining hematocrit?

See text above.

Q.11. Which cells make up the buffy layer? How thick is it and when can it increase in thickness?

The buffy layer consists of packed platelets and leukocytes. Platelets being less dense, settle in a separate layer above the leukocytes. The buffy layer is about 1-mm thick but the thickness increases in cases of severe leukocytosis, leukemia, and thrombocytosis, especially primary thrombocytosis where the count may exceed 800,000/mm³.

Q.12. What is the effect of a high hematocrit?

Increase in Hct increases the viscosity of blood, which leads to an increase in peripheral resistance, and hence an increase in blood pressure.

Q.13. What is the difference between the PCV of arterial and venous blood?

The PCV of venous blood is a little higher than that of arterial blood because the red cells gain a little water due to *chloride shift.*

Q.14. Name the conditions where the PCV is increased and those where it is decreased?

See text above.

Q.15. What further information can be obtained from the buffy coat in a centrifuged tube of blood?

- The main reason to examine a buffy coat is to look for abnormal white blood cells that are circulating in the bloodstream. The most important cell to look for in a buffy coat is a mast cell which plays an important role in allergies and related conditions.
- A quantitative buffy coat is a standard laboratory test to detect infection with malaria or other blood parasites like trypanosomes, Leishmania, and Histoplasma.
- Buffy coats are important for DNA isolation from blood samples.

- Buffy coat preparation also allows the differentiation of white blood cells as they are more concentrated in the buffy coat than in the whole blood sample.

OBJECTIVE STRUCTURED PRACTICAL EXAMINATION-I

Aim: To fill the Wintrobe tube with the supplied anticoagulated blood for measuring ESR.

Procedural steps: See text above.

Checklist:

1. Selects the tube and sees that it is clean and dry. (Y/N)
2. Mixes the blood sample and draws blood into a Pasteur pipette or a dropper with a long nozzle. (Y/N)
3. Fills the tube with blood, starting from its bottom, and withdrawing the pipette till blood column reaches the zero mark. (Y/N)
4. Checks that there no bubbles; if there are, then removes them with a filter paper strip. (Y/N)
5. Places the tube vertically in the Wintrobe stand and notes the time. (Y/N)

OBJECTIVE STRUCTURED PRACTICAL EXAMINATION-II

Aim: To fill the Westergren tube with the supplied anticoagulated blood for measuring ESR.

Procedural steps: See text above.

Checklist:

1. Selects the Westergren tube and checks that it is dry and clean. (Y/N)
2. Mixes the blood sample. (Y/N)
3. Sucks blood into the tube and takes it to the zero mark, taking care to avoid any bubbles. (Y/N)
4. Presses the lower end of the tube into the rubber cushion of the stand and the upper end under the screw cap. (Y/N)
5. Confirms that it is vertical and notes the time. (Y/N)

OBJECTIVE STRUCTURED PRACTICAL EXAMINATION-III

Aim: To fill the Wintrobe tube with the supplied anticoagulated blood for measuring hematocrit.

Procedural steps: See text above.

Checklist:

1. Selects the Wintrobe's tube. (Y/N)
2. Mixes the blood sample. (Y/N)
3. Fill blood in the Wintrobe's tube properly using the Pasteur pipette till the 0 mark. (Y/N)
4. Places the Wintrobe's tube in the centrifuge machine. (Y/N)
5. Notes the final reading after adequate time. (Y/N)

1.9: DETERMINATION OF RED BLOOD CELL INDICES

STUDENT OBJECTIVES

After completing this experiment, the student should be able to:

- Explain the clinical significance of calculating the blood indices (also called red cell/corpuscular absolute values or erythrocyte indices).
- Describe the normal corpuscular values and how to obtain them.
- Describe the classification of anemia based on these standards.

INTRODUCTION

PY2.11: Estimate Hb, RBC, TLC, RBC indices, DLC, Blood groups, BT/CT.

The basic values of hemoglobin (Hb), red blood cell (RBC) count, and packed cell volume (PCV) [hematocrit (Hct)] give little information, if any about the condition of an average red cell, such as its volume, Hb content, or its percentage saturation with Hb. However, this information, in the form of absolute corpuscular values, especially if these are done electronically, can be calculated from three basic values of Hb, RBC count, and PCV.

Note: In addition to the indirect methods of calculating absolute corpuscular values from manually done Hb, Hct, and RBC, these values can be determined directly with automated electronic computers.

PHYSIOCLINICAL SIGNIFICANCE

It is helpful in morphological classification of anemias. The results of RBC indices are used to diagnose different types of anemia. There are several types of anemia, and each type has a different effect on the size, shape, and/or quality of red blood cells.

APPARATUS

The apparatus and materials required are those used for Hb, RBC count, and PCV.

PROCEDURE

1. Use the values of Hb, RBC count and PCV obtained during the previous experiment to calculate the RBC indices.
2. Calculate the absolute values for mean corpuscular volume (MCV), mean corpuscular hemoglobin (MCH), mean corpuscular hemoglobin concentration (MCHC), and color index (CI).

Mean Corpuscular Volume

Definition: The MCV is the average or mean volume of a single RBC expressed in cubic micrometers (μm^3 or femtoliters). It is calculated from the following two basic values:

1. Red cell count in million/mm^3
2. Packed cell volume in 100 mL blood.

Formula

$$\frac{PCV \times 10}{\text{RBC count in million/mm}^3} \text{ or } \frac{\text{PCV per liter}}{\text{RBC}(10^3/\text{mm})}$$

For example:

PCV = 45%, RBC count = 5.0 million/mm^3

$$MCV = \frac{45 \times 10}{5} = 90\ \mu m^3$$

(Normal range = 74–95 μm^3)

On the basis of MCV, the RBC can be normocytic, macrocytic, and microcytic.

- **Derivation of the formula:** In order to know the volume of one red cell from this formula, we have to determine either of the following two:
  1. The packed volume of RBCs in 1 mm^3 of blood, since we know their number (i.e. 5 million). or
  2. The number of RBCs in 100 mL blood, since we know their packed volume (e.g. 45 mL) in the same volume of blood.

  The calculations according to both the methods are described:
  1. Since PCV is 45%, the volume of packed cells in 1 mm^3 of blood = 0.45 mm^3

     Number of red cells in the same volume of blood (i.e. 1 mm^3) = 5 million

     Thus, there are 5,000,000 red cells in 0.45 mm^3 of blood.

     $$\text{Therefore, the volume of 1 red cell} = \frac{0.45\ mm^3}{5{,}000{,}000}$$

     Because 1 mm = 1,000 μm, the MCV is:

     $$MCV = \frac{0.45 \times 1{,}000 \times 1{,}000 \times 1{,}000}{5{,}000{,}000}$$

     $$= \frac{0.45 \times 1{,}000}{5} = 90\ \mu m^3$$

  2. The PCV of RBCs in 100 mL blood = 45 mL. Because 1 meter (100 cm) = 10^6 μm 1 cm = 10^4 μm. For volume, 1 cm^3 = $10^4 \times 10^4 \times 10^4 = 10^{12}$ μm (since the density of water at 4°C is taken as 1, for practical purposes, the density at room temperature may also be taken as 1)

     So, 1 cm^3 = 1 mL, and 1 mL = 10^{12} μm^3

     ∴ 45 mL = 45×10^{12} μm^3

     [We now have converted the volume of red cells (i.e. 45 mL) that are present in 100 mL blood into cubic microns (45 × 10^{12}), we now want to find out the number of RBCs in 100 mL blood, i.e. in 45 ml of packed red cells].

     Because 1 cm = 10 mm

     ∴ 1 cm^3 = 10 × 10 × 10 = 10^3 mm^3 (mm^3)

     : 1 mL = 10^3 mm^3 and, 100 mL = $10^3 \times 10^2 = 10^5$ mm^3

     Since, 1 mm^3 blood contains = 5 × 10^6 red cells

     100 mL will contain = 5 × 10^6 × 10^5 = 5 × 10^{11} red cells.

     Thus, the volume of 5 × 10^{11} RBCs in 100 mL blood = 45 × 10^{12} μm^3.

     $$\text{The volume of 1 red will be} = \frac{45 \times 10^{12}}{5 \times 10^{11}} = \frac{45 \times 10}{5} = 90\ \mu m^3 \text{ cell}$$

     $$\text{So, } MCV = \frac{PCV \times 10}{\text{RBC count in million/mm}^3}$$

Mean Corpuscular Hemoglobin

Definition: MCH quantifies the amount of hemoglobin per red blood cell. It is the average Hb content (weight of Hb) in a single RBC expressed in picograms (pg) (micro-microgram—μμg). It is calculated from the following basic values:

- RBC count in million/mm^3
- Hb in g%.

Formula

$$\frac{\text{Hb in g\%} \times 10}{\text{RBC count in million/mm}^3}$$

For example:

Hb = 15 g%, RBC count = 5 million/mm^3

$$MCH = \frac{15 \times 10}{5} = 30\ pg$$

(Normal range = 27–32 pg)

Derivation of the formula: The derivation of the formula is on the same lines as that for MCV. We want to convert the g Hb into pg.

Since, 1 g = 10^{12} pg

∴ 15 g = 15 × 10^{12} pg.

Thus, the Hb content of 5 × 10^{11} RBCs in 100 mL blood = 15 × 10^{12} pg

The Hb content of 1 red cell will be:

$$= \frac{15 \times 10^{12}}{5 \times 10^{11}} = \frac{15 \times 10}{5} = 30\ pg$$

(5 × 10^{11} red cells are present in 100 mL blood)

- The formula can also be expressed as

$$\frac{\text{Hb in g per liter}}{\text{RBC count in million/mm}^3}$$

- In macrocytic (large red cells) anemia, the MCH may be as high as 39 pg, because the cells are larger, but MCHC would be within normal range.

Mean Corpuscular Hemoglobin Concentration

Definition: MCHC indicates the amount of hemoglobin per unit volume. It represents the relationship between the red cell volume and its degree or percentage saturation with Hb, that is, how many parts or volumes of a red cell are occupied by Hb. The MCHC does not take into consideration the RBC count, but represents the actual Hb concentration in red cells only, (i.e. not in whole blood) expressed as saturation of these cells with Hb. So, it is a more reliable index as compared to other indices. **Note:** The Hb synthesizing machinery of red cells does not have the Hb concentrating capacity beyond a certain limit, i.e. RBCs cannot be, say 70% "filled" with Hb;

this upper limit is only 38%. MCHC is calculated from the following formula:

For example:
Hb = 15 g%, PCV = 45%

$$\text{MCHC} = \frac{\text{Hb in g per 100 mL blood}}{\text{PCV per 100 mL blood}} \times 100$$

$$= \left[\frac{\text{Hb g\%}}{\text{PCV\%}} \times 100\right]$$

$$\text{MCHC} = \frac{15}{45} \times 100 = 33.3\%$$

(Normal range = 30–38%)

- If the MCHC is within the normal range, the cell is *normochromic*, if it is below the range, the cell is *hypochromic*. However, *it cannot be hyperchromic* for the reason mentioned above. A large cell may contain more Hb, but its percentage saturation will not be more than 38%.
- **Derivation of the formula:** The derivation of the formula is as under:
  45 volumes of red cells contain = 15 g of Hb
  $$\text{1 volume of red cells contain} = \frac{15}{45}\text{g}$$
  $$\text{100 volumes of red cells will contain} = \frac{15}{45} \times 100 = 33.3$$
- Another way of expressing MCHC is as follows:
  $$\text{MCHC} = \frac{\text{MCH}}{\text{MCV}} \times 100$$
  (Because MCH is Hb concentration in 1 red cell, and MCV is the volume of one red cell)
  Taking MCH as 30 pg, and MCV as 90 cubic microns,
  $$\text{MCHC} = \frac{30}{90} \times 100 = 33.3\%$$

Mean Corpuscular Diameter

The MCD is determined by direct micrometric measurements of the red cells in a stained film. The **range is 6.9–8** μm, with an average of 7.5 μm. MCD can be used for measuring the mean corpuscular average thickness (MCAT).

Color Index

It is the ratio of Hb percentage to the RBC percentage.

$$\text{Color index} = \frac{\text{Hb concentration (percentage of normal)}}{\text{RBC count (percentage of normal)}}$$

$$= \frac{100}{100} = 1.0$$

(Normal range = 0.85–1.15)

$$\text{Color index} = \frac{\dfrac{\text{g\% Hb found}}{\text{Normal Hb (15 g\%)}}}{\dfrac{\text{RBC Count found}}{\text{Normal RBC count (5 milllion/mm}^3\text{)}}}$$

For the determination of CI, the results obtained in a particular case are compared with arbitrarily set "normal" values. The three traditional indices are—(1) color index, (2) volume index, and (3) saturation index, which are the relative measures of Hb, cell size, and Hb concentration of red cells as compared to "normal" values. Only the color index is mentioned above.

To establish a relation between Hb concentration and the RBC count, they are expressed in the same unit, i.e. "percentage of normal", it being assumed that a normal person has 100% Hb, and 100% RBC count. Traditionally, the normal 100% RBC count is fixed at 5 million/mm³, and the normal Hb at 15 g%, irrespective of age and sex.

For CI, we require the Hb concentration and the RBC count determined in an individual.

Note: The color index is low in iron-deficiency anemia and high in macrocytic anemias. But since both RBC count and Hb may decrease simultaneously in a way that the CI remains normal, the CI does not have much clinical value.

QUESTIONS

Q.1. Which are the common RBC indices?

The common RBC indices are as shown in the **Table 9** below.

Q.2. Which absolute corpuscular value is most useful?

MCHC is the most reliable and useful value for the following two reasons:

1. It does not take RBC count into consideration for its calculation. MCH and MCV, on the other hand, both depend on the RBC count, which has a high degree of error of ±15%.
2. MCHC tells us the actual Hb concentration in red cells only and not in whole blood.

Q.3. Why cannot the MCHC exceed the saturation limit of 38%?

The value of MCHC cannot exceed 38% because the Hb synthesizing and concentrating machinery does not have the capacity to saturate the cell beyond this limit. Thus, a cell can

Table 9: Common RBC indices.

Parameter	*Definition*	*Units*	*Formula*	*Example*
Mean cell volume (MCV)	Average volume of the red blood cell (RBC)	Femtoliters (fL) or 10^{-15} liter	$\text{MCV} = \frac{\text{Hematocrit (\%)} \times 10}{\text{RBC} (\times 10^{12}/\text{L})}$	$\text{MCV} = \frac{42 \times 10}{4.2} = 100\ \text{fL}$
Mean cell hemoglobin (MCH)	Average weight of hemoglobin (Hb) in the RBC	Picograms (pg) or 10^{-12} grams	$\text{MCH} = \frac{\text{Hb (g/dL)} \times 10}{\text{RBC} (\times 10^{12}/\text{L})}$	$\text{MCH} = \frac{12.5 \times 10}{4.1} = 30.5$
Mean cell hemoglobin concentration (MCHC)	Average concentration of Hb in the RBC volume	Grams/deciliter (g/dL)	$\text{MCHC} = \frac{\text{Hb (g/dL)} \times 100}{\text{Hematocrit (\%)}}$	$\text{MCHC} = \frac{12.5 \times 100}{37} = 34$

Table 10: Classification of anemias on the basis of MCV and MCHC.

	Normochromic	*Hypochromic*
Normocytic	After acute hemorrhage	After chronic blood loss
	Hemolytic anemias, except thalassemias	—
	Renal disease	—
	Aplastic anemia, chronic infection	—
Microcytic	—	Iron deficiency anemia
	—	Thalassemias (due to globin deficiency)
	—	Hypoproteinemia
Macrocytic	Deficiency of vitamins B_{12} and folic acid	Secondary to liver disease

have more MCV and MCH but the saturation will not exceed 38%.

Q.4. How will you classify anemias according to their cause?

See chapter on hemoglobin.

Q.5. How will you classify anemias on the basis of MCV and MCHC?

The anemias can be classified on this basis as given in **Table 10**.

1.10: BLOOD GROUPING (BLOOD TYPING)—ABO AND RH SYSTEM

STUDENT OBJECTIVES

After completing this experiment, the student should be able to:

- Define the terms blood "groups" and "blood types", and name the various blood group systems.
- Describe the physiological basis of blood grouping and its clinical significance.
- Describe the Landsteiner's law and explain the basis of the terms "universal" donor and "universal recipient".
- Describe the Rh factor and how it was discovered? What is its significance?
- Determine blood groups by using commercially available antisera and precautions to be observed.
- Explain how blood is stored in blood banks, and the changes that occur in blood during storage.
- List the indications for blood transfusion and the dangers associated with it.
- Explain why is essential to match donor and recipient blood groups before giving a transfusion.
- Describe the effects of mismatched blood transfusion.

INTRODUCTION

PY2.11: Estimate Hb, RBC, TLC, RBC indices, DLC, Blood groups, BT/CT.

The surfaces of human red cells contain a variety of genetically determined glycolipids and glycoproteins that act as antigens. The plasma contains antibodies that can react with these antigens when the two are mixed. Since the red cell antigens cause agglutination of RBCs in the presence of suitable antibodies, they are also called ***agglutinogens;*** the antibodies in the plasma are called ***agglutinins.***

BLOOD GROUP SYSTEMS

1. **ABO Blood Group (Classical)**
2. **Rh Blood Group (Rhesus)**
3. **Others, e.g. M or N.**

A group of related red cell antigens that show similar chemical, genetic, and reactivity properties constitutes a ***"blood group system".*** Within a blood group (e.g. ABO system), there may be two or more different ***"blood types"*** (e.g. A, B, O, and AB). However, the terms blood groups and blood types are often used synonymously.

There are at least 30 commonly occurring antigens and hundreds of rare antigens that have been found on the surfaces of human red cell membranes. Of different blood group systems, only two are of great clinical importance. These are the ***ABO system*** and the ***Rh system.*** Other blood group systems are—MN, Lutheran, Kell, Colton, Duffy, Kid, Diego, Lewis, Li, Yt, Xg, P, C, etc. These groups are of little importance because they are not antigenic, though they are of value in anthropological and genetic studies. Some of these function as cell recognition molecules.

Most Common Blood Groups in India

- O+ = 32.53%
- O- = 2.03%
- A+ = 21.8%
- A- = 1.36%
- B+ = 32.09%
- B- = 2.01%
- AB+ = 7.70%
- AB- = 0.48%

Physiological Basis of ABO System

The antigens A and B are complex oligosaccharides differing in their terminal sugars. Those found on red cells are glycolipids, while those found in tissues and body fluids are soluble glycoproteins. The fucose-containing **H antigen is the basic antigen and is found in all individuals.** In the case of antigen A, a transferase places N-acetylgalactosamine as the terminal sugar on antigen H. In antigen B, the terminal sugar is galactose. In AB persons, both transferases are present, while group O individuals have none of the enzymes, so that the **antigen H persists in them.** Normally, H antigen has no antigenic activity and, as a result, it is identified by the

Table 11: Results of reaction of different blood groups with different antibodies.

Blood group	Antigen on cell membrane	Antibodies in serum	Reaction with		
			Anti-serum A	Anti-serum B	Anti-serum Rh
A	A	anti-B	–	+	
B	B	anti-A	+	–	
AB	No antigen	anti-A, anti-B	+	+	
O	A, B	No antibodies	–	–	
Rh+	Rh	No antibodies			+
Rh–	No Rh antigen	No antibodies			–

("+": **Agglutination present**—RBCs are massed together in clumps and lose their outline; "–": **No agglutination**—RBCs remain separate and evenly distributed)

capital letter O. Since H antigen is not antigenic, there are no corresponding antibodies. (It seems that group O persons produce a protein that has no transferase activity; this results from single base deletion in the corresponding gene).

Genetic Basis of ABO System

The blood group of a person is determined by two genes, one on each of two paired chromosomes.

These genes can be any one of three types—A, B, or O, but only one type is present on each of the two chromosomes. The O gene is functionless and does not produce O antigen on red cells, while A and B genes produce strong antigens on red cells. Thus, there are six possible combinations of genes—AA, BB, AB, OA, OB, and OO—and each person is one of these six genotypes. A person with genotype O has no antigen on red cells and so the blood group is O. A person with genotype AA or OA is blood group A, while genotype BB or OB is blood group B.

Agglutinins of ABO System

The antibodies in the plasma are gamma globulins. The agglutinin reacting with antigen A is called anti-A (or alpha, α) and reacting with B antigen is called anti-B (or beta, β). Blood group O has no antigens, but both anti-A and anti-B antibodies in the plasma. Blood group AB has both A and B antigens, but no antibodies. *The immune system forms antibodies against whichever ABO blood group antigens are not found on the individual's RBCs.* Thus, a group A individual will have anti-B antibodies and a group B individual will have anti-A antibodies. *These antibodies are present without any specific red cell antigenic stimulus.* For example, they are absent in a newborn; the ABO antibodies start appearing in the plasma by the age of 3–4 months due to cross-reactivity of ABO antigens present in naturally occurring bacteria, viruses, pollen, etc. present in the environment.

Rh Factor

In addition to antigens of the ABO system, the red cells of 80–85% of humans also contain an additional antigen, called Rh antigen (or Rh factor) **(Table 9)**. The Rh factor is so named because this antigen was discovered in the rhesus monkey by Landsteiner and Wiener in 1940. They injected red blood cells of rhesus monkey (the common Indian variety with red ischial callosities) into rabbits. The rabbit's immune system

Table 12: Differences between ABO and Rh antibodies.

ABO system antibodies	Rh antibodies
The antibodies anti-A and anti-B are of the larger IgM type. They cannot cross the placenta.	Rh antibodies are of the IgG type. They can easily cross the placenta.
These antibodies react best with the antigens at low temperatures of 5–20°C. They are, therefore, called "cold" antibodies.	The antigen–antibody reactions occur best at body temperature. Hence, they are called "warm" antibodies.
ABO incompatibility between a mother and her fetus rarely causes any problems.	Rh incompatibility between a mother and her fetus may cause serious complications.

(Ig: immunoglobulin)

reacted by forming antibodies against rhesus red cells, and when the rabbit plasma was tested against human red cells, agglutination occurred in 80–85% of individuals.

Persons whose red cells contain this additional antigen are called **"Rh positive" (Rh +ve, Rh+)** while those who lack this antigen are called **"Rh negative" (Rh –ve, Rh–)**.

There are several varieties of Rh antigen—C, D, E, c, d, and e—but the *D antigen is the most common, and antigenically, the most potent.* Therefore, Rh +ve persons are also called RhD +ve and Rh –ve are called RhD –ve. The antibody of D antigen is called anti-D antibody (anti-Rh antibody). **However, there are no naturally occurring antibodies against Rh (D) antigen. The Rh (D) antigen is not present in body fluids and tissues, but only on red cells.** This antigen is a "warm" antigen and can cross the placenta easily. The differences between ABO and Rh antibodies are given in **Table 12**.

PRINCIPLE

The surface of the red cell membrane contains a variety of genetically determined antigens, called **iso-antigens** or **agglutinogens,** while the plasma contains antibodies **(agglutinins).** To determine the blood group of a person, his/her red cells are made to react with commercially available antisera containing known agglutinins. The slide is then examined under the microscope to detect the presence or absence of clumping and hemolysis (agglutination) of red cells, which occurs as a result of antigen–antibody reaction. There is a reciprocal relationship between antigens on the red blood cells and antibodies in the serum is known as Landsteiner's law.

The Landsteiner law (1900), which has two major components, states that:

1. If an agglutinogen is present on the red cells of an individual, the corresponding agglutinins must be absent in the plasma.
2. If an agglutinogen is absent in the red cells, the corresponding agglutinins must be present in the plasma.

Note: The exception to the second component of the law is that absence of Rh agglutinogen from the red cells in Rh –ve persons is not accompanied by the presence of anti-Rh agglutinins. Obviously, this component of the law was enunciated before the discovery of Rh factor in 1940 by Landsteiner and Wiener.

APPARATUS

1. Microscope, "glass dropper with a long nozzle", sterile blood lancet or needle, "sterile cotton/gauze swabs", alcohol, 5 mL test tube, toothpicks.
2. Clean, dry microscope slides. (A special porcelain tile with 12 depressions is available for this purpose and may be used in place of glass slides).
3. Normal saline (0.9%)
4. **Anti-A serum:** This contains monoclonal anti-A antibodies (against humans); these antibodies are also called anti-A or alpha (α) agglutinins. The anti-A serum can also be obtained from a person with blood group B.
5. **Anti-B serum:** This contains monoclonal anti-B antibodies (against humans); these antibodies are also called anti-B or beta (β) agglutinins. The anti-B serum can also be obtained from a person with blood group A.
6. **Anti-D (anti-Rh) serum:** This contains monoclonal anti-Rh (D) antibodies (against humans). These antibodies are also called anti-D agglutinins.

Note: The large volume requirements for high quality ABO and Rh(D) typing reagents can now be supplied by selected monoclonal antibodies.

Monoclonal antibodies are antibodies produced by a single clone of cells or cell line and consisting of identical antibody molecules. A monoclonal antibody is created by exposing a white blood cell to a particular antigen protein, which is then cloned to mass produce antibodies to target that antigen.

Note: The antisera are available commercially. For a quick identification, the anti-A serum is tinted blue, anti-B serum yellow, while the anti-D serum is colorless **(Fig. 34)**. The antibodies against Rh factor do not occur naturally.

Do not interchange the droppers provided with antisera bottles.

PROCEDURE

Preparation of red cell suspension: A suspension of red cells in saline should preferably be prepared and used instead of adding blood drops directly from the fingerpick to the antisera for the following reasons **(Fig. 36)**:

1. Dilution of blood permits easy detection of agglutination and hemolysis, if present. (Red cells in undiluted blood tend to form large rouleaux and masses. These may be difficult to disperse and may be mistaken for agglutination).
2. Plasma factors likely to interfere with agglutination are eliminated.

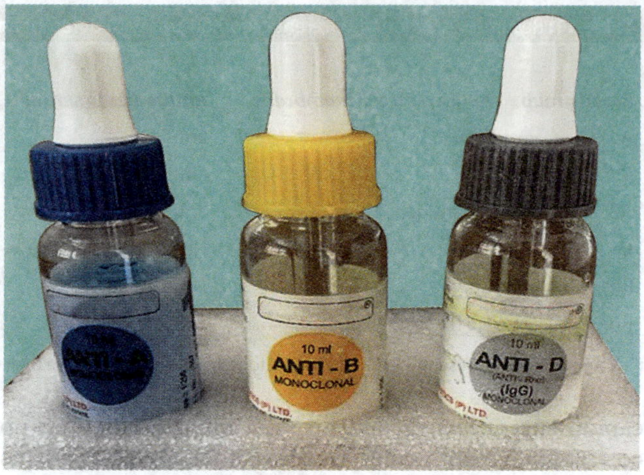

FIG. 34: Commercially available anti-A, anti-B, and anti-D serum.

Method: Put 2 mL of saline in a small (5 mL) test tube. Then get a finger pricked and allow a blood drop to form. Now place the pricked fingertip on top of the test tube and invert it. Mix the blood and saline by inverting the tube two or three times. A suspension of red cells is now ready.

Determination of Blood Groups

1. Mark the wells in blood group slides as A, B and D separately.
2. Put one drop of anti-A serum, anti-B serum and anti-D serum separately in the three wells marked as A, B and D on the blood group slide.
3. In addition, also take 1 drop of normal saline as control in a separate well.
4. Add a drop of red cell suspension drawn from the bottom of the test tube by a dropper on each of anti-A, anti-B and anti-D sera and one drop on the normal saline taken on the "control" side (The nozzle of the dropper should not touch any of the antisera) **(Figs. 35A and B)**.
   In this way, the red cells–saline mixture on the "control" side will act as a control to confirm agglutination or no agglutination on the corresponding test side **(Fig. 37)**.
5. Gently mix the antisera and red cells suspension, using three separate applicator sticks.
6. Wait for 8–10 minutes then inspect the three antisera—red cell mixtures and the "control" mixture, first with the naked eye to see whether agglutination (clumping of red cells) has taken place or not.
7. Then confirm under a low magnification microscope, comparing each "test mixture" with the "control mixture". **(Fig. 37)**
   - If there is no agglutination, the RBCs remain evenly distributed and separated from each other.

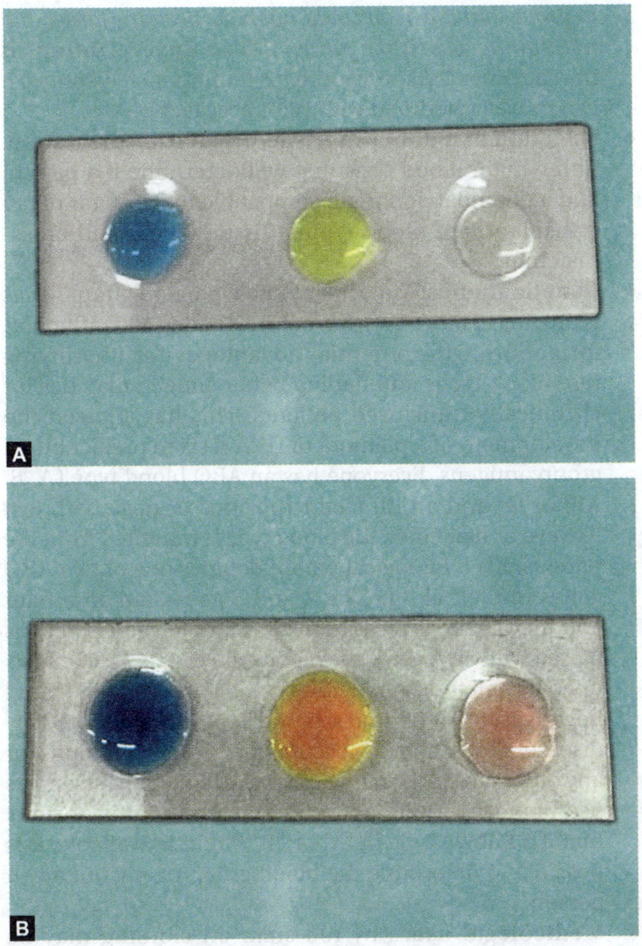

FIGS. 35A AND B: Marking of serum anti-A, anti-B, and anti-C.

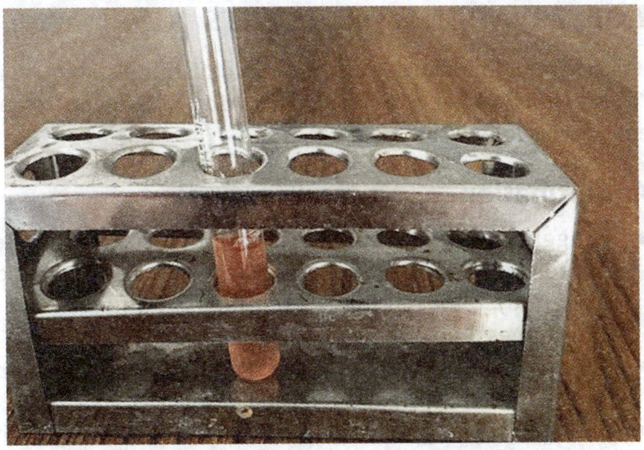

FIG. 36: Preparation of red cell suspension.

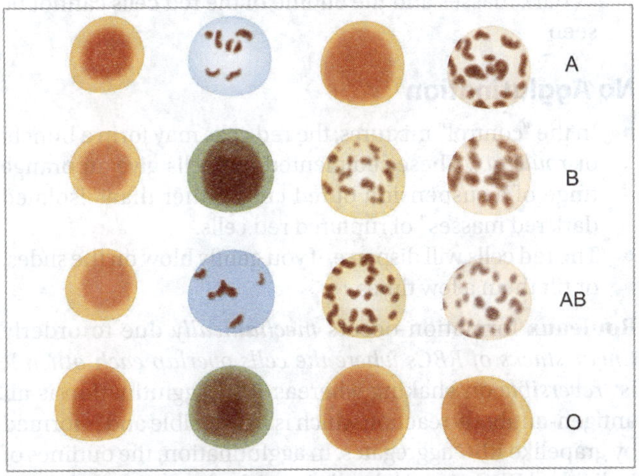

FIG. 37: Determination of blood groups (types) showing agglutination (hemolysis and clumping of red cells) and no agglutination (cells remain uniformly distributed). The reaction between anti-D serum and red cells is not shown. In **agglutination** RBC's are massed together in clumps and lose their outline. If there is no **agglutination** RBCs remain separate and evenly distributed.

- If there is agglutination, the RBCs are clumped together and lose their outline.

8. Reaction of different blood groups with different antibodies is given in **Tables 11 and 13**.

Table 13: Determination of blood groups.

(+) denotes agglutination		***(–) denotes no agglutination***			
Agglutination		***Your blood group is***	***Your RBCs contain agglutinogens***	***Your plasma contains agglutinins***	***Your plasma will agglutinate RBCs of group***
Anti-A serum	***Anti-B serum***				
+	–	A	A	Anti-B	B, AB
–	+	B	B	Anti-A	A, AB
+	+	AB	A, B	None	None
–	–	O	O	Both anti-A and anti-B	A, B, AB
Similarly, for Rh blood group:					
Agglutination	+ Your RBCs contain Rh(D) antigen. You are Rh +ve				
No agglutination	– No Rh(D) antigen in your red cells. You are Rh –ve				

Note:
- Agglutinin against agglutinogen not present in the red cells is present in the plasma of each type. There are no naturally occurring antibodies against Rh(D) antigen.
- It is obvious from the above that if a known type of "A" or "B" blood is available, it is possible to determine the blood group of any unknown person.
- False positive reaction: This can occur when the antisera are contaminated with bacterial growth.
- False negative reaction: It may occur due to improper storage of antisera leading to loss of its potency.

OBSERVATIONS AND RESULTS

It is essential that you should be able to distinguish between ***"agglutination"*** and ***"no agglutination"***. The features of each are as follows:

Agglutination

- If agglutination occurs, it is usually visible to the naked eye. The hemolyzed red cells appear as isolated (separate), dark-red masses (clumps) of different sizes and shapes.
- There is brick-red coloring of the serum by the hemoglobin (Hb) released from ruptured red cells.
- Tilting or rocking the slide a few times, or blowing on it does not break or disperse the clumps.
- Under the low power (LP) objective, the clumps are visible as dark masses and the outline of the red cells cannot be seen.

No Agglutination

- In the "control" mixtures, the red cells may form a bunch, or *rouleaux*. These sedimented red cells give an orange tinge of a suspension of red cells rather than "isolated dark red masses" of ruptured red cells.
- The red cells will disperse, if you gently blow on the slides, or tilt them a few times.

Rouleaux formation occurs *mechanically* due to orderly *linear stacks of RBCs where the cells overlap each other.* It is *reversible* on shaking whereas RBC agglutination is an antigen-antibody reaction which is irreversible and is formed by grapelike RBC aggregates. In agglutination, the outlines of individual RBCs cannot be distinguished.

Confirm all these features of "no agglutination" under the microscope.

Note: Since, similar agglutinogens and agglutinins (i.e. A and anti-A, B and anti-B, or D and anti-D) would react with each other, they cannot exist in the same individual. Therefore, the presence or absence of agglutination will indicate your blood group (blood type) as shown in **Table 13**, where the sign (+) denotes agglutination, and the sign (–) indicates no agglutination.

PHYSIOCLINICAL SIGNIFICANCE OF BLOOD GROUPING

Blood grouping/typing is important in:

- **Blood transfusion** for treatment purposes. Blood transfusion is a life-saving procedure in all cases of severe loss of blood and in life-threatening anemias. However, blood can only be given after blood grouping, which is an essential requirement before blood is given to any individual.
- **Determination of Rh incompatibility** between the mother and child.
- **Paternity disputes:** The ABO, Rh and MNS blood grouping is used to settle cases of disputed paternity. Antigens A and B are dominant, whereas O is recessive. *It is possible to prove that a person could not have been the father, but not that he was/is the father.* **("DNA fingerprinting"** is now a recognized procedure for settling such disputes. It can prove fatherhood with 100% accuracy).
- **Selection of a donor in tissue/organ transplantation.** Three main blood tests that will determine if a patient and a potential donor are compatible matches for organ transplant, are blood typing, tissue typing and cross-matching.
- **Genetic studies:** Molecular typing of blood group genes is proving to be a powerful tool, preventing alloantibodies formation, with potential advantages for identifying rare blood types and finding better antigen matches for chronically transfused patients. This has allowed the development of a plethora of DNA tests to predict blood group antigens. Everyone has an ABO blood type (A, B, AB, or O) and an Rh factor (positive or negative). Just like eye or hair color, the blood type is inherited from the parents. Each biological parent donates one of two ABO genes to their child. The A and B genes are dominant and the O gene is recessive. For example, if an O gene is paired with an A gene, the blood type will be A. Scientists often use methods to identify blood types (blood typing) because an individual's blood type isn't affected by disease, drugs, climate, occupation, living conditions, or any other physical circumstances. Additionally, scientists use blood-typing to determine paternity. It is obvious that if a known type of "A" or "B" blood is available, it is possible to determine the blood group of any unknown person.
- **Medicolegal use:** Any red stain on clothing may be claimed to be blood by a supposed victim. Therefore, it is first confirmed that it really is human blood. Blood grouping of the extracted sample can then prove or disprove the claim of the victim. In doubtful cases, the DNA fingerprinting can decide the claim one way or the other.
- **Susceptibility to disease:** The people of blood type O are more susceptible to peptic ulcer. Blood type A is more commonly seen in carcinoma of stomach, and to some extent in diabetes mellitus. A positive correlation has been shown between blood group A with chronic hepatitis-B infection and pancreatic cancer and blood group B with ovarian cancer. Protection against falciparum malaria can be achieved in blood group O people. Blood group O also increases the severity of infection in certain *Vibrio cholerae* strains.

PHYSIOCLINICAL SIGNIFICANCE OF RH FACTOR

Although there are no natural anti-Rh antibodies, and they never develop spontaneously, they can be produced only in Rh –ve persons. This can happen in either of two ways—one, when an Rh –ve person is given Rh +ve blood, and two, when an Rh –ve mother carries an Rh +ve fetus.

- ***In transfusions:*** When an Rh –ve person receives Rh +ve blood, there is no immediate reaction since there are no antibodies. But during the next few weeks/months, he/she may produce anti-Rh antibodies that will remain in the blood. (Even 0.5 mL of Rh +ve blood is enough to produce an immune response). However, if within a few weeks, or even years later, a second Rh +ve blood is injected, the newly donated red cells will be agglutinated and hemolyzed, thus resulting in a serious transfusion reaction.

- ***In pregnancy:*** The most common problem due to Rh incompatibility may arise when an Rh –ve mother (phenotype dd) carries an Rh +ve fetus (phenotype DD or Dd).

Normally, no direct contact occurs between maternal and fetal bloods. However, if a small amount of Rh +ve blood leaks from the fetus through the placenta into the mother's blood, the mother's immune system will start to make anti-Rh antibodies.

This happens at the time of delivery when small amounts of fetal blood leak into the mother as the placenta separates from the uterine wall. As a result, some mothers develop high concentrations of anti-Rh antibodies during the period following delivery. Therefore, the first-born baby will not be affected, unless the mother has previously received Rh +ve blood transfusion.

There are cases of fetal-placental bleeding during pregnancy itself when fetal blood may enter the mother's circulation. During the first pregnancy, however, the anti-Rh antibody levels do not reach high enough levels to cause complications. However, during the second and subsequent pregnancies, the mother's anti-Rh antibodies cross the placental membrane into the fetus where they cause agglutination and hemolysis. The clinical condition that develops in the fetus is called ***"hemolytic disease of the newborn (HDN)" or "erythroblastosis fetalis" chief clinical forms of HDN.*** The chief clinical forms (syndromes) of HDN are:

- ***Hydrops fetalis:*** If the hemolysis in the fetus is severe, it may die in the uterus, or the fetus may develop anemia, severe jaundice, and gross edema.
- ***Icterus gravis neonatorum (grave jaundice of the newborn):*** Though the infant is born at term, there is jaundice (hemolytic jaundice), or becomes so within a day or so. Anemia may be absent for a few days though reticulocyte count is high, and many nucleated red cells (erythroblasts) are present (hence the term "erythroblastosis fetalis").
- ***Kernicterus:*** In adults, the bile pigments cannot cross the blood-brain barrier (BBB) but in infants the BBB is not fully developed, so that these pigments may pass into the brain and get deposited in the basal ganglia, giving them a bright yellow color.

Note: The neurological syndrome of kernicterus is rarely a complication of "physiological jaundice of the newborn" because there is no hypoxic stimulus. Also the bilirubin level is not as high as in HDN. (The physiological jaundice is due to immaturity of the liver and disappears in a few days).

PRECAUTIONS

- The slides should be dry, dust-free, and grease-free.
- Identify and mark all slides, containers, and test tubes clearly and legibly. Double-check every step of the procedure.
- The droppers supplied with the antisera bottles should not be interchanged.
- Examine the slides with the naked eye and then under the microscope after 8–10 minutes but before the sera-blood mixtures dry up.
- Do not add undiluted blood from the fingerprick directly on to the antisera for two reasons, one, the sera may get intermixed, and two, false-positive reaction may develop. Sometimes, it is not possible to say with certainty whether agglutination has occurred or not. In such cases, the grouping must be repeated with diluted blood.
- A control should always be used to exclude false-positive results.

QUESTIONS

Q.1. What is a blood group system? What is the physiological and genetic basis of blood grouping?

See text above.

Q.2. What is meant by the terms "secretors" and "nonsecretors"?

The antigens A and B are present not only on red cells, but also in other tissues such as—liver, salivary glands, kidney, pancreas, etc. and body fluids such as, saliva, pancreatic juice, semen, and amniotic fluid of some persons. *Individuals who have high concentrations of these antigens in their body fluids are called "secretors"*. Those with low concentrations are called "nonsecretors".

Q.3. How can antibodies be present in a person when the corresponding antigens are absent? (i.e. why are anti-A antibodies present in a person whose blood group is B, while the antigen A is absent in that person).

The specific blood group antibodies are absent at birth. However, they are produced in the next few weeks/months, reaching a maximum by the age of 5-10 years. These antibodies are produced in response to A and/or B antigens (or antigens very similar to these), which are present in intestinal bacteria, or are taken in foods, such as seeds, plants, and in house dust. These antigens are absorbed into blood and stimulate the formation of antibodies against **antigens not present in the infants' red cells,** i.e. those antigens that are recognized as "non-self" by the body's immune system.

Q.4. What is Landsteiner law? How does it apply to all blood groups?

See above

Q.5. What are cold and warm antibodies?

The terms "cold" and "warm" antibodies are applied to the antibodies of the ABO and Rh systems of blood groups, respectively.

Q.6. How are antisera A and antisera B obtained?

The antisera can be obtained from the humans or from animals:

1. Antisera A, B and Rh are obtained by injecting their antigen into rabbit and collecting antibodies from their serum.
2. Antisera can be obtained from the clotted blood of individuals of blood group A (anti-B serum), and of blood group B (anti-A serum). However, since an antigen has many epitopes, a variety of antibodies against the antigen are produced. Also, since the titer (concentration) of antibodies is variable, monoclonal antibodies are used.
3. **Monoclonal antibodies:** If a single plasma cell could be isolated, it could be made to proliferate in a tissue culture and produce large quantities of identical antibodies. However, plasma cells and lymphocytes are difficult to grow in culture. The problem is solved as follows:
   - Animals are immunized with a particular antigen then they are sacrificed.
   - The antibody-producing plasma cells are extracted from the spleen and fused with myeloma cells. (The myeloma cells are B lymphocytes that are easy to grow and they proliferate endlessly).
   - The fused cells are separated by special techniques and each starts a clone of cells descended from a single cell. Thus, large amounts of antibodies can be obtained.

Q.7. What is the importance of using a control on each of the three test slides? What are false-positive and false-negative results?

The control in each case is only a suspension of red cells in saline. Its purpose is to avoid "false-positive" and "false-negative" results.

False-positive reaction: It means that though there is no actual agglutination, the reaction appears to be so. Formation of large rouleaux (this may happen, if undiluted blood is used) may give a false impression of agglutination, but the cells will quickly disperse on tilting the slide a few times. Bacterial contamination of an antiserum, or of normal saline, may show agglutination in all tests or in all controls.

False-negative reaction: It may occur due to loss of potency of the antisera because of faulty storage. All tests will come out negative with such an antiserum.

Note: In hospitals and blood banks where blood is to be collected for transfusion, the antisera are tested every day before using them for blood grouping/typing.

Q.8. What is the difference between agglutination and rouleaux formation? How will you confirm that agglutination has occurred on the microscope slide?

See above. The agglutination is always confirmed under the microscope.

Q.9. What is a zone phenomenon?

The phenomenon in which agglutination or precipitation does not take place in the zone having excess of either antigen or antibody is known as *zone phenomenon*. Maximum precipitation or agglutination occurs when both the reactants are in optimal proportion.

Q.10. Why should you wait for 8–10 minutes before checking for agglutination?

This much time is required for antigen–antibody reaction to occur.

Q.11. Why should the red cell–antiserum mixture be examined before it dries up?

If the mixture dries up, the dried red cells may form masses, which may be confused for agglutination.

Q.12. What is agglutination and what is its mechanism?

Agglutination, i.e. clumping and hemolysis of red cells, during antigen–antibody reaction occurs in two stages:

1. ***Sensitization:*** The antibodies bind (attach) to the antigens on the red cell surfaces without causing clumping and hemolysis. A single ABO antibody (IgM type) has 10 binding sites and can thus cross-link 10 red cells, while the Rh antibody (IgG type) has two binding sites and can link two red cells.
2. ***Agglutination:*** Immediately after sensitization, the red cells form clumps or lattices, which are followed by hemolysis. The antigen–antibody reaction also activates the complement system that releases proteolytic enzymes (the lytic complex), which ruptures the red cells and releases Hb. (The hemolysis in circulating blood is more severe due to larger amounts of complement system proteins, as compared to that occurring on the slides).

Q.13. What is cross-matching?

The red cells and the plasma of the donor and recipient blood are separated by centrifugation

1. **Direct (major) cross-matching**: The donor red cells are then tested with the recipient plasma. Since the reaction between donor red cells and recipient plasma is of prime importance, it is called "major cross-matching".
2. **Indirect (minor) cross-matching**: The donor plasma is tested against the red cells of the recipient. The whole process is called "cross-matching". This reaction is not very important and usually does not occur even in a mismatch, because the agglutinins are greatly diluted in the recipient plasma. Thus, the donor agglutinins can usually be ignored, if their potency is not too high. It is for these two reasons that this reaction is called "minor cross-match".

   If there is no agglutination in either case, the donor blood can safely be given to the recipient.

Note: Cross-matching must always be done before every blood transfusion.

Q.14. Why is the reaction between donor red cells and recipient plasma called "major cross-match" and what is its significance?

The donor red cells are tested against recipient plasma to ensure that the recipient plasma does not contain antibodies that would react with the antigens on the donor red cells. In the case of a mismatch, the donor red cells will start to hemolyze with serious consequences as soon as they enter the recipient's circulation during a transfusion. Since the reaction between donor red cells and recipient plasma is of prime importance, it is called "major side cross-match" or "major cross-match".

Q.15. Why is the reaction between donor plasma and recipient red cells called "minor cross-match"?

The donor plasma is tested against the recipient red cells to test the potency (strength; ability to cause a reaction) of donor agglutinins. This reaction is not very important and usually does not occur even in a mismatch, because the agglutinins are greatly diluted in the recipient plasma. For example, about 200 mL of plasma in one unit of O group donor blood (which contains both anti-A and anti-B agglutinins) gets diluted in about 3,000 mL of recipient plasma, and that also at a slow rate. Furthermore, the donor agglutinins are neutralized by the soluble antigens in the body fluids of the recipient. Thus, the donor agglutinins can usually be ignored, if their potency is not too high. It is for these two reasons that this reaction is called "minor cross-match".

Q.16. What is meant by the terms universal donor and universal recipient?

Since type O persons do not have either A or B antigens on their red cells, they are called *"universal donors"* because their blood can, theoretically, be given to all four blood types. Type AB persons are called *"universal recipients"* because they do not have circulating agglutinins in their plasma and can, therefore, receive blood of any type. (Recall that it is the reaction between donor red cells and recipient plasma that is important in transfusion of blood).

In practice, however, the use of these terms was found to be misleading and dangerous. Transfusion reactions were common until the discovery of Rh factor in 1940 by Landsteiner and Wiener. Then it was realized that the blood contains antigens and antibodies of blood groups other than the ABO system.

Note: Though it is a rule never to give blood without cross-matching, an exception could be made in a most extreme emergency, where group O Rh –ve blood may be given immediately.

Q.17. What is Rh factor and what is its clinical significance?

See text above.

Q.18. If an Rh –ve mother carries Rh +ve fetus, what are the complications that are likely to occur?

See text above.

Q.19. When an Rh +ve mother carries Rh –ve fetus, why are there no complications?

The Rh +ve red cells of the mother cannot cross the placenta into the fetus. But even if small amounts of maternal blood do leak into the fetus as a result of placental hemorrhage at any time during pregnancy, the fetus cannot respond by forming anti-Rh antibodies. The reason for this is that the ability to respond to foreign antigens develops after birth. However, when it does develop in later life, transfusion of Rh +ve blood will evoke anti-Rh antibody production.

Q.20. What is hemolytic disease of the newborn? What are the forms in which this condition may be manifested?

See text above.

Q.21. What is the probability of the occurrence of hemolytic disease of the newborn when the father is Rh +ve and the mother is Rh –ve?

The blood group antigens are a result of gene action. The gene related to **D** antigen is called **D.** When **D** is absent from a chromosome, its alternate form (allelomorph), called d, takes its place. The Rh genes of a person are inherited from both parents. If the genes carried by the sperm and ovum are identical, the offspring is homozygous **(DD or dd).** Thus, if both carry D gene, all the offspring will be DD (homozygous D+; Rh +ve). If one carries **D** and the other carries **d,** the offspring will be heterozygous D+ (Rh +ve). If both ovum and sperm carry **d,** the offspring will be dd (homozygous D –ve; Rh –ve).

Therefore, if the father's genotype is Dd, the offspring may be Rh +ve (Dd) or Rh –ve (dd), but if the genotype is DD, all offspring will be Rh +ve. Thus, the probability of HDN when the father is Rh +ve will depend on whether he is Dd or DD.

Q.22. How can hemolytic disease of the newborn be prevented? What is the treatment of severe hemolytic disease of the newborn (HDN)?

The hemolysis of red cells seen in HDN is due to the crossing over of anti-Rh antibodies from the Rh –ve mother (through the placenta) into the Rh +ve fetus. The condition can be prevented by desensitizing all Rh –ve mothers by giving them injections of **anti-Rh antibodies called anti-Rh gamma globulin (RhoGAM)** after every abortion, miscarriage, or delivery. These antibodies bind to and inactivate the fetal Rh antigens (on fetal red cells) present in maternal circulation. In this way, the Rh antigens from the mother's blood are cleared (removed) before they have had time to stimulate production of anti-Rh antibodies.

Treatment of severe HDN: The best treatment for a severe case of HDN is to successively withdraw small amounts of fetal blood and to replace them with equal amounts of **compatible Rh –ve blood.** Of course, this **exchange transfusion** does not change the inherited blood group of the infant. It only removes the red cells that are destined to be hemolyzed.

Note: Fetal Rh typing is now possible with samples of amniotic fluid or chorionic villi, and treatment with a small dose of Rh immune serum can prevent sensitization of mother during pregnancy. It is not known how this is achieved but one effect of anti-D antibody is to inhibit antigen-induced B lymphocyte antibody production. It also attaches to D antigen sites on fetal red cells in mother's blood.

Q.23. Why does the ABO-incompatibility rarely produce hemolytic disease in the newborn?

The ABO-incompatibility between the mother and fetus rarely causes HDN. The reason is that the anti-A and anti-B (anti-ABO) antibodies belong to IgM type of gamma globulins (cold antibodies) that do not cross the placenta.

Q.24. What is the incidence of blood types in various populations?

See Table 14 given below.

Table 14: Frequency distribution of blood groups in various populations.

	Caucasians	*African American*	*Hispanic*	*Asian*
O+	37%	47%	53%	39%
O–	8%	4%	4%	1%
A+	33%	24%	29%	27%
A–	7%	2%	2%	0.5%
B+	9%	18%	9%	25%
B–	2%	1%	1%	0.4%
AB+	3%	4%	2%	7%
AB–	1%	0.3%	0.2%	0.1%

Q.25. What is the importance of blood grouping?

See text above.

Q.26. How blood volume is restored in cases of severe hemorrhage, severe burns, prolonged vomiting or diarrhea or excessive sweating?

The total blood volume, plasma volume, or packed cell volume may be greatly reduced under certain circumstances. The blood volume can be supplemented by various solutions, plasma or whole blood (see Q/A 36).

Q.27. What are the indications for blood transfusion?

- **Acute hemorrhage:** Acute loss of blood resulting from accidents, during surgery, ruptured peptic ulcer and aortic aneurysm, ectopic pregnancy, etc. are some of the conditions, which may cause hemorrhagic shock, and therefore, need immediate blood transfusion. Cross-matched blood is always given, but if the situation is desperate, group O (Rh –ve) blood may be given to raise blood pressure. In burns, blood may be given though plasma is preferred.
- **Chronic anemias that cannot be treated with diet and drugs:** Packed red cells [hematocrit (Hct) about 70%] can be transfused when a quick restoration of Hb is required, as in pregnancy, emergency surgery, etc.
- **Exchange transfusion:** It is employed in hemolytic disease of the newborn (see Q/A 22).
- **Bleeding disorders:** Fresh blood or platelet concentrates are given in purpura. Fresh frozen plasma, or cryoprecipitate is given in hemophilia and other clotting factor deficiencies.
- **Granulocyte transfusion:** It is needed in cases of neutropenia (TLC <500/mm^3) with severe bacterial infection.
- ***Bone marrow depression*** due to any cause and infiltration by carcinoma cells.
- **Autologous transfusion** (see below; Q/A 28).

Q.28. What is autologous transfusion?

In addition to receiving blood from a donor, an individual may also receive one's own stored blood. The depositing of one or more units of packed RBCs for *autologous blood transfusion* before an anticipated need, e.g., elective surgery is called **predonation.** The popularity of this procedure is that it avoids the hazards of AIDS, hepatitis, etc. as well as risk of transfusion reaction.

It is also known as ***Preoperative autologous donation (PAD)*** in which blood is collected weeks before surgery. It is then stored in a blood bank and transfused back to the donor when needed. It is a form of autologous transfusion and is a common practice in some hospitals. After starting a course of iron tablets, two units of blood are collected, one 16 days before the operation, and the other 8 days later. An important technical innovation is the cell-saver machine **(Intraoperative cell salvage (ICS)**, which sucks up blood from the wound during the operation, recycles it, and returns it to the patient's body.

Q.29. What is blood doping? When is it employed?

Blood doping refers to a handful of techniques used to increase an individual's oxygen-carrying red blood cells, and in turn, improve athletic performance. The most commonly used types of blood doping include injections of erythropoietin (EPO), injections with synthetic chemicals that can carry oxygen, and blood transfusions. In this technique, some athletes were given a unit or two of their own blood (or red cells) which had been removed and stored for a few weeks. It was then reinjected in 2–3 sessions a few days before an athletic event. Since oxygen delivery to active muscles is the limiting factor, increased red cell count was expected to enhance their performance, especially in endurance events. The procedure was (and is) dangerous since it increases the load on the heart due to increased blood volume or viscosity.

The International Olympic Committee and World Anti-Doping Agency's (WADA) List of Prohibited Substances and Methods has banned blood doping.

Q.30. What are the dangers of blood transfusion?

The following are the dangers associated with blood transfusion:

- ***Transmission of disease*:** The donated blood has the potential of transmitting some serious diseases. It is, therefore, mandatory to test the blood for human immunodeficiency virus HIV antibodies (for AIDS), hepatitis B surface antigen, hepatitis C virus (HCV) antibodies, syphilis [Venereal Disease Research Laboratory (VDRL) test], and malarial parasite.
- ***Incompatibility due to mismatched transfusion*:** This is the most serious and potentially fatal complication. Whether the transfusion reactions are immediate or delayed, as well as their severity is determined by the speed and extent of hemolysis of donated red cells.
  - *Body aches and pains*: Within a short time of starting the transfusion, the patient complains of severe pain in the back, limbs, or chest, and a sense of suffocation and tightness in the chest. These symptoms are due to blockage of capillaries by clumps of agglutinated cells. Chills and fever generally accompany pains.
  - *Renal failure*: Acute renal failure (kidney shutdown) appears to result from three main causes:
    - Substance of immune reaction and toxic substances released from hemolyzing blood cause powerful renal vasoconstriction.
    - These substances and decrease in circulating red cells frequently cause circulatory shock. The arterial blood pressure falls to very low levels, and renal blood flow and urine output decrease.
    - If the amount of free Hb in plasma is small then whatever is filtered is reabsorbed. If this amount is large, it gets precipitated in and blocks many tubules. The result of all these factors is acute renal failure and death may occur in 8–10 days, if the shutdown is not resolved or treated with dialysis.
- ***Faulty technique of transfusion*:** *Cardiac arrhythmias, cardiac arrest, or circulatory overload* may occur, especially in elderly patients of chronic anemia, heart, or kidney diseases, if repeated transfusions are given, say, in 24 hours. *Thrombophlebitis* may occur, if the intravenous needle remains in the same site for many hours. *Air embolism,* i.e. entry of air into blood via the intravenous needle is much less likely to occur because of the use

of plastic bags (instead of glass bottles), which collapse down as they empty out of blood.

- ***Allergic reactions***: Reactions such as skin rashes and asthma may occur, if the donor blood contains substances to which the patient is sensitive.
- ***Pyrogenic reactions***: Reactions such as chills and fever are probably due to the presence of antibodies to leukocytes and platelets.
- ***Tetany***: With massive transfusions, the normal conversion of citrate to bicarbonate in the tissues may be delayed. This will result in fall in plasma ionic calcium and hence tetany.
- ***Iron overload***: Repeated transfusions in the absence of blood loss may lead to *hemochromatosis*.

Q.31. What precautions are taken while selecting a blood donor?

The following precautions are observed:

- The donor should be healthy, and aged between 18 years and 60 years. Pregnant and lactating women are excluded. Any healthy adult, both male and female, can donate every three months.
- The donor should be screened for communicable diseases such as AIDS, hepatitis, syphilis, malaria, etc.). The malarial parasite can survive at 4°C for 3 weeks.
- The donor's Hb should be within the normal range (usually above 12.5 gm%). Pulse—between 50 and 100/minute with no irregularities. Blood pressure—Systolic 100–180 mm Hg and Diastolic 50–100 mm Hg. Body weight—not less than 45 Kg.
- Professional donors must be discouraged.

Q.32. What are blood banks? How is donated blood stored? What is the fate of transfused citrate in the body?

With the modern surgical and medical procedures, the demand for blood has greatly increased. It is for this reason that blood banks were started where blood from voluntary donors could be stored, so that it was always available on demand. Most blood banks have lists of would-be donors, so that they may be contacted when required.

Storage of blood:

- After a donor has been screened for donation, one unit of whole blood (500 mL) is collected, under aseptic conditions, from the antecubital vein directly into a special plastic bag containing 63 mL of CPDA (citrate-phosphate-dextrose-adenine) mixture. The blood bag is suitably sealed, labeled, and stored at 4°C, where it can be kept for about 20 days (faulty storage, i.e. overheating or freezing can lead to gross infection and hemolysis).
- The *citrate* prevents clotting of blood, *sodium diphosphate* acts as a buffer to control decrease in pH, *dextrose* supports adenosine triphosphate (ATP) generation via glycolytic pathway and also provides energy for Na^+–K^+ pump that maintains the size and shape of red cells and increases their survival time, and *adenine* provides substrate for the synthesis of ATP, thus improving postdonation viability of red cells.
- Blood is stored at low temperatures for two reasons: one, it decreases bacterial growth, and two, it decreases the rate of glycolysis and thus prevents a quick fall in pH.

Table 15: Volume and contents of blood.

Component (volume)	*Contents*
Whole blood (1 unit = 500 mL)	RBCs, platelets, plasma
RBCs in additive solution (1 unit = 350 mL)	RBCs
FFP or other plasma product* (1 unit = 200 to 300 mL)	All soluble plasma proteins and clotting factors
Cryoprecipitate, also called "cryo" (1 unit = 10 to 20 mL)	Fibrinogen: factors VIII and XIII VWF
Platelets (derived from whole blood)	Platelets

*FFP: fresh frozen plasma

Changes in red cells during storage: Changes occur due to decreased metabolism, and include increase in their Na^+ and decrease in K^+ concentration due to reduced Na^+–K^+ pump activity, the result being a net increase in total base and water content of the cells that swell and become more spherocytic. The ATP content decreases and inorganic phosphate content increases.

Changes after transfusion: These changes occur within a day or so, the red cells lose sodium and gain potassium, with the volume, shape, and fragility returning to normal. Their survival time increases, if blood is given within a week of donation.

Fate of transfused citrate: The citrate (in the form of trisodium citrate) that is used to store blood can safely be injected intravenously (oxalates are toxic). Within a few minutes, the liver removes citrate from blood and polymerizes it into glucose, or metabolizes it directly for energy. But, if the liver is damaged or if large amounts of citrate are injected too quickly, the citrate may lower the calcium level in blood to result in tetany or even death from convulsions.

Blood substitutes: Separate components of blood—packed RBCs, whole plasma (fresh frozen plasma, FFP) to provide clotting factors, platelets, leukocytes, plasma, and plasma expanders are now available (See **Table 15**).

Q.33. What is the only certain way of avoiding blood incompatibility?

1. The slides and containers must be properly labeled.
2. Cross-matching is the only certain way of avoiding the dangers of mismatching.
3. Rh +ve blood should never be given to an Rh –ve female of any age before menopause.

Q.34. Name the precautions you will observe before and during blood transfusion.

- Blood should be transfused only when absolutely required.
- It should be confirmed that cross-matching has been done to exclude mismatching of groups other than ABO system.
- The blood bag should be checked for the blood type indicated on it.
- It should be confirmed that the blood has been checked for infections, especially AIDS.
- Rh +ve blood should never be given to an Rh –ve person.

- Blood should never be transfused at a fast rate—usually not more than 20–25 drops per minute, unless otherwise indicated (as in acute and severe loss of blood where blood may have to be pumped into the patient). A rapid transfusion, under normal conditions, may cause chelation of calcium ions and tetany.
- The condition of the recipient should be checked carefully for the first 10–15 minutes of starting the transfusion, and from time to time later on. The transfusion must be stopped, if there is a rapid rise of temperature, (>40°C), or any other reaction.

Q.35. What are the earliest effects of a mismatched transfusion?

Within a short time of starting the transfusion (i.e. when a few mL of blood have entered the recipient's body), there may be severe pain anywhere in the body, a sense of suffocation, and tightness in the chest. There may be chills and shivering, fever, etc. (see Q/A 30 for details).

Q.36. Which blood substitutes may be used to restore blood volume, if suitable donor blood is not available?

The blood volume may be reduced due to hemorrhage; plasma volume may be reduced due to burns, vomiting, or diarrhea. Therefore, the ideal treatment would depend on which body fluid needs replacement.

Whole blood: Though it is the ideal medium to replace lost blood because it replaces cells and plasma in physiological ratio, it may not be available. In such a situation, an intravenous drip of a crystalloid or colloid solution is immediately started. (This route is also available for any drug that may be needed, and of course, for later transfusions.)

Crystalloid solutions: A commonly used intravenous fluid is glucose saline (6% glucose in 0.9% sodium chloride). However, since crystalloids leave the circulation within a short time, this solution restores the blood volume temporarily.

Colloid solutions: Various colloid substitutes are available to increase the plasma volume. They are called plasma expanders, and include human albumin, dextrose, and dextrose with NaCl, and a polymer from degraded gelatin. Plasma separated from donated blood can be stored in a liquid form (FFP) for many months, and for a year, if it is dried (it is reconstituted with distilled water just before use).

Blood substitutes: Under certain conditions, instead of whole blood or plasma, a blood component may be required—say, to avoid circulatory overload, lower risk of transfusion, etc. These blood substitutes include— packed red cells, white blood cell (WBC) concentrates, immunoglobulins, and clotting factors concentrate.

Q.37. What is the Bombay blood group?

- The Bombay blood group is a rare blood group, phenotypes of this group lacking H antigen on the red cell membrane and have anti-H in the serum. It fails to express any A, B or H antigen on their red cells or other tissues. H antigen deficiency is known as the "Bombay phenotype" (h/h, also known as Oh) and is found in 1 of 10,000 individuals in India and 1 in a million people in Europe.
- Since there is no H antigen, there is no antigen A or antigen B on the red cells. However, the plasma contains anti-A, anti-B, and anti-H antibodies. As a result, such a person can receive blood only from a person having Bombay blood type.

Q.38. What is forward and reverse blood typing?

ABO testing is a *two-part process,* involving testing a person's red cells for A and/or B antigens as well as testing the person's serum/plasma for ABO antibodies.

The *first step* is blood grouping (typing) procedure, i.e. the blood cells are mixed with antibodies against type A and B blood, and the sample is checked to see whether the blood cells stick together (agglutinate). If blood cells stick together, it means the blood cells reacted with one of the antibodies. For example, if the blood cells agglutinate when mixed with antibodies against type B blood ("anti-B antibodies"), it is type B blood. This procedure is called "blood typing" or "**forward blood typing**".

The *second step* is called *"back typing" or "reverse blood typing or serum typing."* The liquid part of blood without red blood cells (plasma or serum) is mixed with blood cells containing known antigens, i.e. red cells from persons with blood types A, B, AB, and O. If agglutination occurs with A and AB red cells, the blood type is B; if agglutination occurs with B and AB red cells, the blood type is A; if agglutination occurs with A, B, and AB red cells, the blood type is O and if there is no agglutination in any RBCs, the blood type is AB. In AB blood type, there are no antibodies in the plasma (serum). Reverse typing can also be performed with commercial preparations of type A and B erythrocytes.

Thus, the forward grouping/typing suggests the presence or absence of A and B antigens in RBCs, whereas reverse grouping indicates the presence or absence of anti-A and anti-B in serum.

Unlike ABO typing, a "reverse" test is not performed for the Rh system, because a person does not have preformed antibodies to the D antigen, unless they have previously been alloimmunized to the D antigen through transfusion or pregnancy.

The *serum typing* is done along with *blood typing* as a precaution because in leukemias, the RBC antigens may become considerably weak. Also, in pseudomonas infection, the RBCs become agglutinated by all antisera due, probably, to unmasking of hidden antigens.

Note: Blood typing is the process of determining the blood type and Rh factor of a sample of blood. Cross-matching involves finding the best donor for a patient prior to blood transfusion. In addition to the blood type and Rh, minor blood groups are also evaluated. Blood typing focuses on the antigens on the surface of the red cell. Cross-matching focuses on antibodies in the plasma. In a cross-match, donor red cells are mixed with the plasma of the recipient. If antibodies exist in the recipient plasma to antigens on the red cells of the donor, transfusion reactions can occur.

1.11: DETERMINATION OF BLEEDING TIME AND CLOTTING TIME

STUDENT OBJECTIVES

After completing this experiment, the student should be able to:

- Indicate the physioclinical importance of doing bleeding time (BT) and clotting time (CT).
- Define hemostasis and describe how bleeding stops from a fingerprick.
- Determine BT by Duke's Method and CT by capillary tube method and give their normal values.
- Name the conditions in which BT and CT are increased.
- Describe the physiological basis of bleeding disorders.
- List the clotting factors and describe the steps in intrinsic and extrinsic pathways of clotting.
- Describe how clotting occurs in vivo and in vitro.
- Define the terms thrombosis and embolism.
- Indicate how clotting can be prevented in vivo and in vitro.

INTRODUCTION

PY2.11: Estimate Hb, RBC, TLC, RBC indices, DLC, Blood groups, BT/CT.

Bleeding after injury is a common experience for most of us. But bleeding stops automatically within a few minutes. However, suspicion of a disease arises when there is frequent and prolonged bleeding with minor injuries, such as during shaving, cutting of nails, or a fall on the knees. In others, there may be *spontaneous bleeding* (without any apparent trauma) in the skin, gums, or into joints, and muscles, etc. It is in all such cases that various tests are carried out.

HEMOSTASIS

Definition: The term hemostasis (Greek hema = blood; stasis = halt) refers to the **process of stoppage of bleeding after blood vessels are punctured, cut, or otherwise damaged.** Hemostasis which is a homeostatic mechanism to prevent loss of blood is a result of a complex, natural, physiological response. Thus, hemostasis has a high degree of survival value. It involves the following four interrelated steps:

1. Vasoconstriction (contraction of injured blood vessels)
2. Platelet plug formation
3. Formation of a blood clot
4. Fibrinolysis (dissolution of the clot).

PHYSIOLOGICAL BASIS OF BLEEDING DISORDERS

Excessive and prolonged bleeding with small injuries, or spontaneous bleeding may result from defects of:

- **Platelets:** Thrombocytopenic purpura, functional disorder of platelets.
- **Blood vessel walls:** Damage of capillary endothelium (Non-thrombocytopenic purpura)
- **Coagulation of blood:** Deficiency of clotting factors, vitamin K deficiency, anticoagulant overdose, disseminated intravascular clotting.

Defects of Platelets and Vessel Walls

Defects of platelets and vessel walls typically cause spontaneous bleeding from small vessels, or during cuts and bruises [e.g. pinpoint or petechial hemorrhages and purpuric lesions in the skin (blue-red patches)], and bleeding in the gums.

Defects of Clotting

Defects of clotting may lead to:

1. *Excessive bleeding into tissues* (muscles, joints, viscera, etc.) is usually due to injury to relatively large vessels. The delay in the formation of a clot fails to support the normal action of platelets in checking blood loss. *Deficiency of clotting factors*—inherited or in liver disease (hepatitis, cirrhosis, and vitamin K deficiency) are the usual causes.
2. *Thrombosis:* It is the clotting of blood that occurs within unbroken blood vessels. A *roughened endothelium* due to arteriosclerosis, infection, or injury is the common cause.

Note: Bleeding disorders may be *inherited or acquired*—the acquired defects being more common. Disorders due to platelet and vessel wall defects are more common than coagulation disorders that are due to deficiencies of clotting factors.

TESTS FOR HEMOSTASIS

1. Bleeding time (BT).
2. Capillary fragility test of Hess (tourniquet test).
3. Platelet count.
4. Clotting time (CT).
5. Clot retraction time (CRT).
6. Clot lysis time (CLT).
7. Prothrombin time (PT).

Other tests: These include: **Platelet aggregation and adhesiveness tests, prothrombin consumption test, partial thromboplastin test, thrombin time (TT), plasma recalcification time (PRT), activated partial thromboplastin time (APTT), Kaolin cephalin clotting time (KCCT)**, and special tests including assaying of clotting factors.

BLEEDING TIME

Bleeding time is the time interval between the skin puncture and spontaneous, unassisted (i.e. without pressure) stoppage of bleeding. The BT test is an *in vitro test of platelet function.* It is determined by two methods:

1. **Duke method**
2. **Ivy method.**

Note: The BT and CT are two simple tests that are used as a routine before every minor and major surgery (e.g. tooth extraction), biopsy procedures, and before and during anticoagulant therapy, whether or not there is a history of bleeding.

Bleeding Time by "Duke" Method (Fingertip; Earlobe)

Since the skin of the fingertip is quite thick in some persons, a small cut in the skin of the earlobe with the corner edge of a sterile blade gives better results. The earlobe method is the original "Duke" method for BT.

Apparatus

- Equipment for sterile fingerprick.
- Clean filter papers.
- Stopwatch.

Procedure

1. Get a deep fingerprick under aseptic conditions to get free-flowing blood. Start the stopwatch and note the time. The time of puncture of the finger is known as **Zero time.**
2. Blot the blood drops every 30 seconds by touching the puncture site with the filter paper along its edges, without pressing or squeezing the wound. Number the blood spots 1 onward.
3. Note the time when bleeding stops, i.e. when there is no trace of blood spot on the filter paper. Encircle this spot and number it as well. This is the end point **(Fig. 38)**. (Do not keep the filter paper on the table and then press your puncture site on it).
4. Count the number of blood spots and express your result in minutes and seconds.
5. You can also count the number of blood spots on the filter paper and multiply it by ½ to get the bleeding time in minutes.

Normal BT is 2–6 minutes.

The test is simple and quite reliable in spite of the fact that the depth of the wound cannot be controlled.

Precautions

- The skin site chosen for BT should be scrubbed well with alcohol to increase the blood flow.
- The skin should be dry and the puncture should be 3–4 mm deep to give free-flowing blood. Do not squeeze.
- Do not press the filter paper on the puncture site.

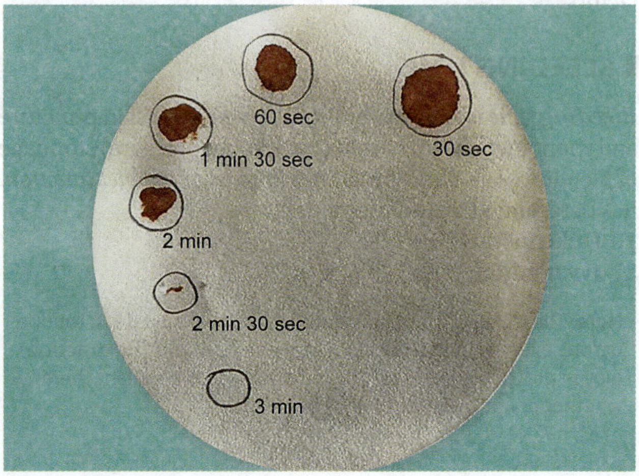

FIG. 38: Bleeding time (Duke's method).

- If bleeding continues for more than 10–12 minutes, stop the test and press a sterile gauze on the wound. Inform your teacher about the bleeding.

Bleeding Time by "Ivy" Method

This method is *more reliable* than the "Duke" method. However, it requires some practice to apply the blood pressure (BP) cuff and maintain the pressure.

Procedure

1. Clean the skin over the front of the forearm with 70% alcohol.
2. Apply a BP cuff on the upper arm, raise the pressure to 40 mm Hg and maintain it there till the end of the experiment.
3. Clean the skin area once again. Grasp the underside of the forearm tightly, make a 1–3 mm deep skin puncture, about 5–6 cm below the cubital fossa. Note the time.
4. Remove the blood every 30 seconds by absorbing it along the edges of a clean filter paper by gently touching the wound with it till the bleeding stops. This is the end point.

Normal BT with this method is up to 9 minutes.

Simplate Method

Though the "Duke" and "Ivy" BT methods are fairly reliable, it is not possible to control the depth of the wound made by a lancet or a blade. However, by careful standardization, it has become possible to do so. The most widely used technique uses a "template" or an *automated scalpel* to control the depth and length of the wound—usually 1 mm deep and 9 mm long—and a BP cuff inflated to 40 mm Hg to distend the capillary bed of the forearm.

Normal BT is less than 7 minutes.

Physioclinical Significance

- The BT is prolonged in purpura (platelet deficiency, or vessel wall defects) while it is usually normal in hemophilia.
- Lack of several clotting factors may prolong BT, though it is especially prolonged by lack of platelets.
- See Q6 also.

Note: Although a BT of over 10 minutes has a slightly increased risk of bleeding, the risk becomes great when the BT exceeds 15 or 20 minutes.

Comments: The BT test is an in vivo test of platelet function, and the "Ivy" method is probably the most reliable. However, a peripheral blood film is always examined for the number of platelets and their morphology. The students should note that platelets are involved both in BT and CT tests and one is normally affected without the other. If the BT is prolonged due to low platelet count (thrombocytopenic purpura), the platelets that are available are sufficient to give a normal CT.

CLOTTING TIME

Clotting time Clotting time is the time taken from the onset of bleeding to the formation of a fibrin thread.

It is determined by two methods:

1. **Wright's capillary glass tube method**
2. **Lee and White method.**

Capillary Blood Clotting Time (Wright's Capillary Glass Tube Method)

Apparatus

- Pricking sterile needle
- Chemically clean, 10–12 cm long, glass capillary tubes with a uniform bore diameter of 1–2 mm.
- Stopwatch.

Procedure

1. Give a sterile finger prick. Now dip one end of the capillary tube in the blood; the blood rises into the tube by capillary action **(Fig. 39)**. This can be enhanced by keeping its open end at a lower level.
2. Note the time of prick. This is called Zero **time.**
3. Hold the capillary tube between the palms of your hands to keep the blood near body temperature.
4. Gently break off 1 cm bits of glass tube from one end at intervals of 30 seconds, and look for the formation of fibrin threads between the broken ends. The endpoint is reached when fibrin threads span a gap of 5 mm between the broken ends ("fibrin thread formation"). Note the time **(Fig. 40)**.
5. The CT is taken as total time from the time of puncture (zero time) till there is formation of fibrin thread.

Normal CT is 3–8 minutes (at 37°C).

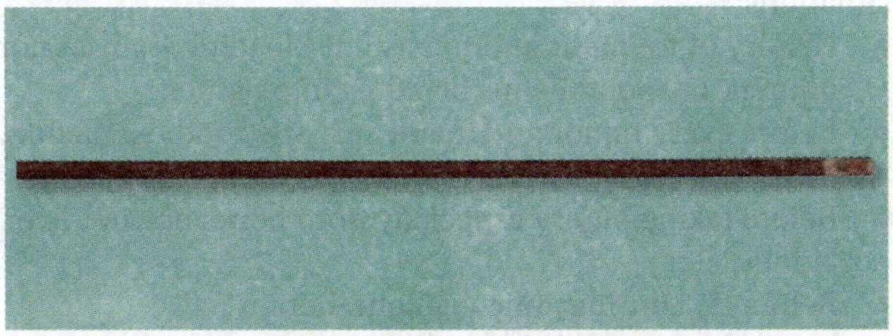

FIG. 39: Glass capillary tube filled with blood.

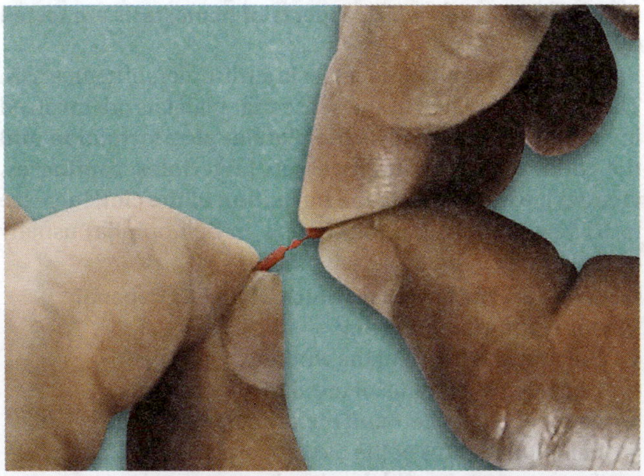

FIG. 40: Formation of fibrin thread.

Note: In capillary tube method clotting method involved is the intrinsic pathway. This is brought by exposure of the blood to electro negatively charged surface (glass tube).

Lee and White Test Tube Method

Single Test Tube Method

This method needs more arrangements than the capillary tube method but is a more sensitive and reliable method for the determination of CT.

1. Draw 2 mL venous blood by a clean, non-traumatic venepuncture. Note the time when blood starts to enter the syringe. This is the zero time. Transfer the blood to a chemically clean and dry test tube.
2. Holding the test tube in a water bath at 37°C, take it out at 30 second intervals and tilt it. The end point is when the tube can be tilted without spilling the blood.

Normal CT with this method in a glass tube is 5–10 minutes.

Multiple Test Tube Method

The CT can be determined more accurately by using 3 test tubes rather than 1 only.

1. Rinse 3 test tubes of 8 mm diameter with normal saline, drain them and place them in a metal rack kept in water at 37°C. Transfer 1.5 mL blood into each test tube.
2. Take out the first tube after 1 minute, tilt it to 45° and return it to the rack. Repeat every 30 seconds until clotting occurs, i.e. where the test tube can be tilted without spilling the blood. Note the time.
3. Repeat the tilting on the second test tube and note the time when clotting occurs (this happens a few seconds later because tilting the tube hastens clotting). The third tube acts as a control and a check on the end point in the second test tube.

Note: If a siliconized test tube is used at the same time, a delayed CT (40–70 minutes) can be shown.

Normal CT with this method is 5–10 minutes.

The CT depends on the condition of the glass itself, and even on the size of the test tube. Therefore, a high degree of standardization is needed.

Comments: This method is more reliable than the capillary blood CT method, because there is no admixture of blood with tissue fluid which contains tissue thromboplastin (extrinsic system). Thus, this method tests only the intrinsic system of blood clotting. However, this method is nonspecific because the CT can theoretically increase due to deficiency of any of the factors in the intrinsic system. But, in actual practice, a prolonged CT nearly always means hemophilia in which the CT may exceed 1 hour in severe cases.

Another method (drop method): This method is less accurate than the above method. Place a large drop of blood from a skin puncture on a clean and dry glass slide. Draw a pin through the drop every 30 seconds, and note the time when fibrin threads adhere to the pin and move with it out of the blood drop. The time elapsed between placing the blood drop on the slide and the formation of fibrin threads is the CT.

Normal CT with this method is 2–4 minutes.

In the original Duke's drop method for CT, two drops of 4–5 mm diameter are placed on a glass slide. The slide is tilted at 30 second intervals. The end point is the absence of change in the previous shape when the slide is held vertical.

Physioclinical Significance of Clotting Time

- The CT is prolonged in hemophilia and other clotting disorders, because thrombin cannot normally be generated. Yet, the BT which reflects platelet plug formation and vasoconstriction, independently of clot formation is normal.
- See Q.11 also.

CLOT RETRACTION TIME

Clot retraction time is the time required following withdrawal of blood for a clot to completely contract and express the serum entrapped within the fibrin net.

Transfer the test tube containing clotted blood to an incubator at 30°C. Normally, the clot starts to shrink (retract) in about 30 minutes (leaving behind straw-colored serum), becomes half its size in 2–3 hours, and becomes completely contracted in 24 hours. Note if there is any digestion of the clot or discoloration of serum.

Comments: Clot retraction time is directly proportional to the platelet count and inversely proportional to the fibrinogen concentration. Clot retraction (tightening or consolidation) depends on the release of many factors from the platelets, and so the CRT depends on the platelet count. The fibrin-stabilizing factor causes more and more cross-linking bonds between nearby fibrin fibers. Their spicules also release contractile proteins—actin, myosin, and thrombosthenin. The contraction (retraction) of the clot is activated by thrombin, and calcium ions stored in the endoplasmic reticulum, Golgi apparatus, and mitochondria.

In addition to forming a meshwork and entrapping blood cells and plasma, the fibrin fibers also adhere to the edges of the wound. When the clot contracts, it stitches the edges of the wound and thus prevents further loss of blood.

CLOT LYSIS TIME (CLT)

The dissolution (dissolving; also called fibrinolysis) of a clot is the process by which a clot becomes fluid so that the trapped red cells sink to the bottom of the test tube.

Normally, the CLT is about 72 hours. If it occurs within 24 hours, it is considered abnormal.

PROTHROMBIN TIME

The patient's blood is quickly oxalated (or citrated) to remove calcium ions so that prothrombin cannot be converted to thrombin. The sample is then centrifuged. Then to the oxalated plasma, a large excess of calcium ions (as calcium chloride solution) and rabbit brain suspension (to provide tissue thromboplastin; tissue factor, TF) is added. The excess calcium neutralizes the effect of oxalate and the TF converts prothrombin to thrombin via the extrinsic clotting pathway (i.e. factor VII).

The time required for clotting to occur is called the PT.

Normal PT is 15–20 seconds.

Clinical Significance

This test is used to monitor oral anticoagulant therapy. Since the potency of tissue thromboplastin (TF) may vary, blood from a normal person is used as a control when the test is used for controlling anticoagulant dose, or in a hemorrhagic disease. Bleeding tendency is present when the prothrombin level falls below 20% of normal (normal plasma prothrombin = 30–40 mg/dL). Prolonged PT suggests the possibility of deficiency of factors II (prothrombin), V, VII and X. Prothrombin level is low in vitamin K deficiency and various liver and biliary diseases.

TESTS FOR OTHER CLOTTING FACTORS

Tests similar to PT have been devised to estimate the quantities of other clotting factors. In each test, excess calcium ions and all the other factors, except the one being tested, are added to the oxalated blood (or plasma) all at once. The time required for clotting to occur is determined in the same way as for PT. The CT will be prolonged if the factor being tested is deficient. The time itself is used to quantitate the concentration of the factor.

QUESTIONS

Q.1. What is the clinical importance of doing BT and CT?

Bleeding time and CT are important in the following situations:

- History of frequent and persistent bleeding from minor injuries, or spontaneous bleeding into tissues.
- Before every minor and major surgery (tooth extraction, etc.).
- Before taking biopsy especially from bone marrow, liver, kidney, etc.
- Before and during anticoagulant therapy.
- Family history of bleeding disorders.

Q.2. How does BT differ from CT? What is the interrelation between them, and which aspects of hemostasis are tested by them?

Both BT and CT are done together in all disorders of hemostasis. They are interrelated in the sense that platelets are involved in both tests. **The BT tests the platelet plug formation and the condition of the microvessels (arterioles, capillaries, venules), while CT tests the formation of the clot.** Increase in BT (e.g. in purpura), or CT (e.g. in hemophilia) usually occurs independently of each other.

Q.3. What are the factors on which BT and CT depend?

Bleeding time depends on:

- Breadth and depth of the wound.
- Degree of hyperemia of the skin puncture site.
- Number of platelets and their functional status.
- Functional status of the blood vessels.
- Temperature: In cold weather, low temperature promotes vasoconstriction and thus shortens BT.

Clotting time depends on:
- Nature of contact surface (glass in this case; siliconized surface would prolong the CT).
- Presence or absence of clotting factors.
- Temperature: Low temperature may prolong the CT.

Q.4. What is meant by the term hemostasis? What are the steps by which it is brought about?

This term refers to the process of stoppage of bleeding from the injured blood vessels. Bleeding from small vessels stops automatically within a few minutes due to low pressure in these vessels besides other factors. But if a large artery is cut, surgical repair may be required.

Hemostasis involves the following interrelated steps:

1. **Contraction of injured blood vessels:** The immediate response of the injured vessels is the contraction (spasm) of the circular smooth muscle fibers in their walls. This spasm is due to:
   - Mechanical stimulation of smooth muscle fibers by the injury.
   - Local reflexes produced by stimulation of pain and other sensory receptors.
   - Release of potent vasoconstrictors from platelets (serotonin, epinephrine, thromboxane A2, prostaglandins, and from damaged endothelium (endothelins).

Note: The mechanical stimulation of smooth muscle of arteries (Even large arteries like the radial), arterioles, and venules may be so strong that bleeding stops for many minutes. Capillaries do not have smooth muscle in their walls; precapillary sphincters which, of course, can contract and relax, regulate the blood flow through them. During this time, the other factors go into action and further strengthen the vasoconstriction.

2. **Formation of platelet hemostatic plug:** The repair of the openings in the vessel walls depends on many important functions of platelets. Their initial reaction is adhesion followed by release reaction. As the injury exposes collagen fibers in the walls of blood vessels, receptors in the platelets interact with these fibers. They swell, become irregular in shape, and throw out many pseudopodia (spicules) and become more and more sticky. They adhere to each other and to collagen fibers in vessel walls. Therefore, at the site of injury, more and more platelets are activated and aggregated by platelet-activating factors (PAFs) (a cytokine secreted by platelets, monocytes, and neutrophils) and form a growing plug of platelets which is enough to effectively seal the openings in small vessels.

   The adhesiveness (stickiness) of platelets is promoted by ADP (released by them), and by von Willebrand factor (vWF).
3. **Formation of blood clot in the ruptured vessel:** If there is a large hole in the blood vessel, a blood clot is additionally required. The extrinsic and intrinsic pathways of coagulation form a meshwork of very sticky fibrin threads. They reinforce the platelet plug and stitch the wound edges together thus permanently sealing the ruptured vessel.
4. **Dissolution of clot by the fibrinolytic system:** A fibrin clot has a tendency to grow in size due to amplification and positive feedback cycles of the clotting factors. The fibrinolytic system does not allow the fibrin clot to grow and block a vessel which would cause serious complications. The dissolution of a clot called fibrinolysis (dissolving of fibrin fibers) is brought about by the formation of the active enzyme **plasmin** from **plasminogen** (a plasma protein) by the action of tissue *plasminogen activator* (tPA) released from injured issues.

Q.5. How does bleeding stop from a skin prick?

Bleeding from small vessels stops due to: (1) low pressure inside the vessels, and the natural elasticity of the tissues, (2) contraction of smooth muscle in the microvessels, (3) formation of platelet plugs, and (4) clotting of blood (if a larger vessel is cut).

Q.6. Name the conditions in which only the bleeding time is prolonged while the clotting time is normal.

Pronged BT with normal CT is seen in the following conditions:

1. **Low platelet count (thrombocytopenia):** It may be due to:
   - Decreased production of platelets
   - Increased destruction of platelets.
2. **Functional platelet defects:** Prolonged BT with normal platelet count suggests the following defects:
   - **Drugs:** Aspirin, large doses of penicillin, other drugs.
   - **Von Willebrand disease:** Inherited as an autosomal dominant trait, this condition is associated with a deficiency of a component of factor VIII called factor VIII-related antigen (VIII R: Ag; vWF) which acts as a carrier of factor VIII.

     The vWF in the injured vessel wall along with ADP released from platelets promotes platelet adhesion and plug formation. So when there is deficiency of vWF, the decreased platelet adhesion to connective tissue leads to traumatic and mucosal bleeding. The BT is prolonged, while platelet count is normal. Variants of this disease are also seen.
   - Other diseases: Uremia, cirrhosis, leukemia, etc.
3. **Vessel wall defects:** These defects are generally acquired, but may be inherited.
   - **Prolonged treatment with corticosteroids:** Also other drugs such as penicillin, sulfas, aspirin, etc. may damage vessel walls. There may be severe bleeding in a known case of purpura if aspirin is inadvertently administered.
   - **Allergic purpura:** There is damage to capillary walls by antibodies.
   - **Infections:** Infections such as typhus, bacterial endocarditis, hemolytic streptococci.
   - **Deficiency of vitamin C:** Petechiae, and bleeding from gums occur due to decreased intercellular substance and less stable capillary basement membrane.
   - **Senile purpura:** In the elderly, purpuric hemorrhages occur on the back of the hands and forearms due to prolonged pressure or mild trauma. Small vessels rupture due to increased mobility of skin

resulting from loss of elastic and connective tissues around blood vessels.

- **Connective tissue diseases:** Some of these diseases may be associated with purpuric bleeding.

Note: In all cases of purpura due to vessel wall defects, the platelet counts are normal, but BT is prolonged and the capillary fragility test is positive.

Q.7. What is the relation between the platelet count and the severity of bleeding?

Broadly speaking, the relation between the platelet count and the severity of bleeding is as follows:

- Above 100,000/mm^3: No clinical symptoms, bleeding is rare.
- 50,000–100,000/mm^3: Bleeding may occur after major surgery.
- 20,000–50,000/mm^3: Bleeding occurs with minor trauma of everyday life or gentle sports.
- Below 20,000 mm^3: Spontaneous hemorrhages in urinary and GI tract, nose bleeds, etc.
- At very low counts: Fatal hemorrhages may occur in the brain.

Q.8. What is meant by the term clotting of blood? Name the various clotting factors, their sources, and their role in clotting.

Clotting: Within the blood vessels, the blood remains in a fluid state. But when it is drawn out from the vessels, a series of chemical reactions occur. During the next few minutes, the blood thickens, and forms a gel called a clot. The clot consists of a network of insoluble threads called fibrin. The blood cells get entangled in this meshwork and give it a red color. Over a time, the clot retracts and serum is expelled out.

Clotting factors: The blood contains many inactive proteolytic enzymes also called "factors". **Surface contact or injury to blood (intrinsic system)** and/or **injury to the tissues (extrinsic system)** starts a chain of reactions in which an inactive enzyme precursor is converted into an active enzyme. The activated enzyme, in turn, acts on the next inactive enzyme to form the next active enzyme and so on in a fixed sequence—a process called **enzyme cascade.** Each clotting factor activates many molecules of the next and so on. Thus, the enzyme cascade is an amplifying system so that at the end of the process, i.e. when the cascade comes to an end, a large amount of the final product (fibrin) is formed.

Note: The activated enzyme is designated by the letter "a" after the numeral (e.g. factor XII to XIIa).

The Roman numerals (also called "factors") given to clotting substances in order of their discovery are given in **Table 16**, though some substances have not been given any such numerals.

Q.9. What is the mechanism of clotting of blood?

The clotting of blood involves the following four types of chemical substances:

1. Plasma clotting factors.
2. Platelet clotting factors.
3. Tissue factor—present on all the plasma membranes.
4. Calcium ions.

- 11 of the 12 known clotting factors are globulins.
- Prothrombinase [prothrombin activator, (PTA)] is a combination of factors V and X.
- Prekallikrein (Fletcher factor).
- High molecular weight kininogen (HMWK; Fitzgerald factor).

Note: Arabic numerals are sometimes used for platelet activities affecting clotting, for example, the terms:

- Platelet factor 3 (PF-3) is used for platelet phospholipid (PPL) procoagulant activity.
- Platelet factor 4 (PF-4) is used for heparin neutralizing activity of platelets.
- Though there are other Arabic numerals mentioned in literature, they are no longer used.

Table 16: Clotting factors.

Sl. No.	*Name/s*	*Source*	*Pathways of activation*
I	Fibrinogen	Liver	Common
II	Prothrombin	Liver	Common
III	Tissue thromboplastin (TPL) [tissue factor (TF)]	Damaged tissues and activated platelets	Extrinsic
IV	Calcium ions (Ca^{2+})	Diet, bones, platelets	All
V	Proaccelerin (accelerator globulin, AcG; labile factor)	Liver and platelets	Extrinsic and intrinsic
VI	There is no such factor		
VII	Proconvertin; stable factor; serum prothrombin conversion accelerator (SPCA)	Liver	Extrinsic
VIII	Antihemophilic factor (AHF); antihemophilic factor A; antihemophilic globulin (AHG)	Platelets and endothelial cells	Intrinsic
IX	Christmas factor (CF); antihemophilic factor B (AHF-B); plasma thromboplastin component (PTC)	Liver	Intrinsic
X	Stuart factor, Prower factor, Stuart-Prower factor; thrombokinase	Liver	Extrinsic and intrinsic
XI	Plasma thromboplastin antecedent; antihemophilic factor C	Liver	Intrinsic
XII	Hageman factor; glass contact factor; glass factor; contact factor	Liver	Intrinsic
XIII	Fibrin stabilizing factor (FSF); Laki-Lorand factor	Liver and platelets	Common

Basic Theory of Coagulation

More than 50 substances that cause or affect clotting of blood have been found in blood and in the tissues. Those that promote clotting are called ***procoagulants,*** and those that inhibit clotting are called ***anticoagulants.*** The balance between these two groups of substances decides whether blood will clot or not. Normally, the anticoagulants in the blood prevent blood from clotting as long as it is circulating in the undamaged blood vessels. However, when a blood vessel is ruptured, procoagulants in the damaged area become "activated" and clotting occurs—which is a homeostatic process to prevent further loss of blood.

Essential Stages of Blood Clotting

The three essential stages of the process of blood clotting are:

Stage 1—generation of prothrombin activator (PTA; prothrombinase): The PTA is a complex of Xa + Va + phospholipids + calcium ions. Its formation can begin in either or both of the following two pathways:

i. **Extrinsic pathway:** Injury to cells/tissues outside (extrinsic to) the blood vessels (e.g. skin, subcutaneous tissue, etc.).
ii. **Intrinsic pathway:** Injury to the blood, cells within the blood (e.g. platelets), or injury to cells in direct contact with blood (e.g. endothelial cells and underlying collagen fibers). Outside damage is not needed.

Stage 2—formation of thrombin from prothrombin: The PTA which is a proteolytic enzyme, splits prothrombin (an alpha-2 globulin present in the plasma) into the active enzyme thrombin.

Stage 3—formation of fibrin threads from fibrinogen: Thrombin acts as a proteolytic enzyme and splits off insoluble fibrin monomers from the soluble fibrinogen. The monomers polymerize to form fibrin thread which are stabilized (cross-linked) by factor XIII (Laki-Lorand factor) and calcium ions.

Stage 1: Generation of PTA **(Flowchart 4)**

- **Extrinsic pathway:** The extrinsic pathway (system) has fewer steps and is explosive, i.e. it occurs within 10–15 seconds of injury. It is so named because a tissue protein called **tissue factor (TF; tissue thromboplastin TPL; or factor III)** is released from the cells outside (extrinsic to) the blood vessels (e.g. cells of skin, subcutaneous tissue, etc.). It is a specific phospholipid-lipoprotein complex present on the surfaces of all cells including platelets. The TF which is released when cell membranes are damaged or perturbed (as by a cut, prick, or crush injury) activates factor VII to VIIa **(Flowchart 4)**. The complex of TF + VIIa + calcium ions activate factor X to Xa. Factor Xa combines with factor V and calcium ions to form the active enzyme PTA (prothrombinase). This pathway is inhibited by a TF pathway inhibitor that forms a quaternary structure with TPL, factor VIIa, and factor Xa.
- **Intrinsic pathway:** This pathway is more complex and occurs more slowly usually needing several minutes. It is so named because its activators are present either within (intrinsic to) the blood (e.g. platelets), or the cells in contact with blood (endothelial cells). Injury to blood such as by a contact with a "foreign" electro negatively

FLOWCHART 4: The intrinsic and extrinsic pathways for blood clotting.

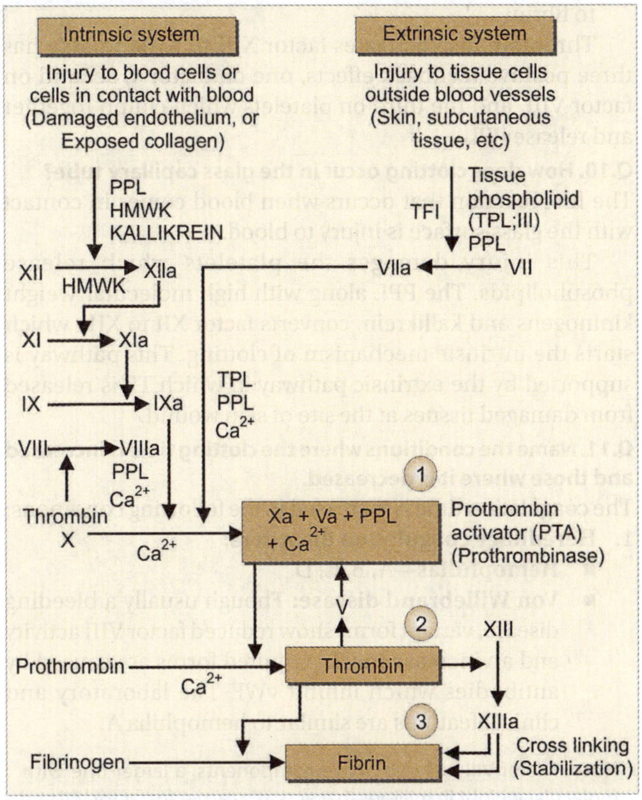

(Stage 1: Generation of prothrombin activator (PTA); Stage 2: Formation of thrombin from prothrombin; Stage 3: Formation of fibrin from fibrinogen; HMWK: high molecular weight kininogen; TFI: tissue factor pathway inhibitor; PPL: platelet phospholipid)

charged, water-wettable surface may occur when blood comes in contact with:

- Roughened or damaged endothelial cells and the exposed collagen fibers under them (injury in vivo)
- The slippery glass surface of a test tube or any other water-wettable surface (injury in vitro).

In both cases, the damaged platelets release phospholipids (PPL) which initiates the initial reaction of conversion of factor XII to XIIa. Factor XIIa converts XI to XIa and IX to IXa **(Flowchart 4)**. Factor IXa then forms a complex with VIIIa, PPL, and calcium ions. This complex activates factor X to Xa to form PTA.

- **Interaction between extrinsic and intrinsic factors:** It is clear from the above description that when a blood vessel is damaged/ruptured, coagulation involves both pathways at the same time. The TF starts the extrinsic system while contact of platelets and factor XII with collagen fibers in vessel walls starts the intrinsic system. The extrinsic system is explosive and with severe tissue injury, clotting can occur in 10–15 seconds. The intrinsic system requires 2–6 minutes to cause clotting.

Stages 2 and 3: Common Pathway

Once PTA (prothrombinase) is formed, the common pathway of blood clotting follows:

- ***In the 2nd stage,*** PTA + calcium converts prothrombin to thrombin.

- *In the 3rd stage,* thrombin + calcium converts fibrinogen to fibrin.

Thrombin also activates factor XIII to XIIIa. It also has three positive feedback effects, one on factor V, second on factor VIII, and the third on platelets which clump together and release PPL.

Q.10. How does clotting occur in the glass capillary tube?

The first reaction that occurs when blood comes in contact with the glass surface is injury to blood.

This injury damages the platelets which release phospholipids. The PPL along with high molecular weight kininogens and kallikrein, converts factor XII to XIIa which starts the intrinsic mechanism of clotting. This pathway is supported by the extrinsic pathway in which TF is released from damaged tissues at the site of skin wound.

Q.11. Name the conditions where the clotting time is increased and those where it is decreased.

The coagulation time is increased in the following conditions:

1. **Hereditary coagulation disorders:**
   - **Hemophilias**—A, B, C, D.
   - **Von Willebrand disease:** Though usually a bleeding disease, variant forms show reduced factor VIII activity and an increase in CT. Acquired forms are caused by antibodies which inhibit vWF. The laboratory and clinical features are similar to hemophilia A.

> **Note:** Factor VIII has two active components, a larger one with molecular weight in millions that acts as a carrier for factor VIII and is the vWF. Its deficiency leads to prolonged bleeding time. The smaller component has a molecular weight of 230,000; loss of this smaller component causes classic hemophilia.

   - **Afibrinogenemia and dysfibrinogenemia:** The concentration of fibrinogen may be greatly reduced (normal = 250–300 mg%) or absent or it may be chemically abnormal, though both may be present at the same time.
   - **Deficiency of factor XIII and defective cross-linking** is a rare disorder.
2. **Acquired coagulation disorders: These may develop in a variety of diseases as mentioned here.**
   - **Vitamin K deficiency:** Deficiency of vitamin K (major sources: Green vegetables, also gut bacteria) may be due to inadequate intake, intestinal malabsorption (obstructive jaundice), or loss of storage sites in liver. Since it acts a cofactor in the synthesis of prothrombin, and factors VII, IX and X, its deficiency leads to fall in their levels.
   - **Liver diseases:** There is a decrease of all clotting factors except VIII. There is also a reduced uptake of vitamin K, and abnormalities of platelet function.
   - **Intravascular clotting:** Clotting factors are used up and bleeding may occur.
   - **Anticoagulant therapy:** Patients receiving heparin or warfarin show an increased CT.
3. **Newborns:** Newborns, especially premature babies sometimes have a tendency to bleed because the plasma levels of certain factors are low, especially prothrombin. Usually, these levels reach normal by the 2nd or 3rd week after birth. Vitamin K is given if bleeding persists.

The CT is decreased in:

- ***Physiological conditions*:** Malnutrition, parturition.
- ***Pathological conditions*:** There is no pathological condition in which the CT is decreased.

Q.12. What is hemophilia?

Hemophilia (-philia = loving) is a group of bleeding disorders that result from deficiency of factors VIII, IX, X, or XII. The 4 types have been called hemophilia A, B, C, and D. All are inherited—A and B are sex-linked, being transmitted by females (they act as carriers of the disease) to males who suffer from the disease. (Females are protected by the second X chromosome which is usually normal).

Hemophilia A which is also called *classical hemophilia,* is the most common hereditary coagulation disorder. The clinical features of repeated bleeding from nose, into subcutaneous tissues, joints, muscles, etc. either spontaneously or on minor injuries, start early in life, or after surgery or injuries later in life. The severity of clinical features, however, depends on the severity of factor VIII deficiency.

Hemophilia B called Christmas disease was discovered in 1952 in a family with the surname Christmas. Hemophilias C and D are rare.

Hemophilia has been called a royal disease because some of the children of queen Victoria of England and Czar Nicholas II of Russia had this disease. (All hemophilias are treated with fresh blood transfusions, or concentrated clotting factors).

Q.13. Why does calcium deficiency not cause a bleeding disorder though it is essential for many steps of blood coagulation?

The reason why deficiency of calcium does not cause bleeding is that only minute amounts of ionic calcium are required for clotting. A condition of bleeding due to this deficiency is not compatible with life. However, tetany may result due to lack of this mineral.

> **Note:** Except for the first two stages in the intrinsic system of coagulation, calcium ions are required for the promotion of all blood clotting reactions.

Q.14. How is blood maintained in a fluid state within the body?

A balance between clotting and anticlotting mechanisms is required to prevent hemorrhage, and at the same time, to prevent intravascular clotting. Hemofluidity within the body is maintained by the following factors:

1. **Continuous motion (circulation) of blood** does not allow clotting factors to accumulate at one point.
2. **Endothelial surface factors:**
   - Smoothness of the endothelial surface prevents contact activation of factor XII of the intrinsic pathway (damage to endothelium causes this activation).
   - The glycocalyx layer on the endothelium repels clotting factors and platelets.
   - Thrombomodulin secreted by these cells removes thrombin as soon as it is formed. The complex of these two activates protein C which along with a cofactor inactivates factors V and VIII.
   - Prostacyclin secreted by endothelium counteracts platelet aggregation.
3. **Antithrombin action of antithrombin III-heparin complex and fibrin:** Antithrombin III, an alpha

globulin synthesized in the liver and normally present in plasma in a concentration of 15–30 mg/dL is called the *antithrombin-heparin cofactor.* A protease inhibitor of the intrinsic clotting system, it is one of the most important anticoagulants in the blood.

Heparin due to its low concentration in the blood has little or no anticoagulant activity. But when it combines with antithrombin III, it increases the effectiveness of antithrombin III in removing thrombin hundreds of times. This complex also removes activated factors IX, X, XI, and XII.

The fibrin fibers that are formed when a clot is forming adsorb 85–90% of thrombin that is formed. This reduces the local concentration of thrombin, thus preventing its spread into the remaining blood and spreading of the clot.

4. **Fibrinolytic system (the plasmin system):** Plasminogen (profibrinolysin), a plasma protein, when activated by tPA that is slowly released from injured tissues and endothelium is changed into plasmin. Plasmin, a strong proteolytic enzyme resembling trypsin, digests and dissolves fibrin fibers, fibrinogen, prothrombin, and factors V and VIII.

The activated protein C (APC), in addition to inactivating the two major clotting factors (V and VIII) not blocked by antithrombin III, also enhances the activity of tPA by inhibiting the activity of a tPA inhibitor. Thus, once the clot has formed and succeeded in stopping blood loss, the blocked vessel is reopened by the process of fibrinolysis over the next few days, and the blood flow is restored.

Note: Human plasminogen consists of a heavy chain of 500 amino acids and a light chain of 241 amino acids. Receptors of plasminogen are present on many cells, but especially on endothelial cells. When plasminogen binds to its receptors, it gets activated into plasmin that provides a mechanism that prevents clot formation in intact vessels.

Human tPA, produced by recombinant DNA methods, is commercially available and employed for dissolving clots in coronary arteries in early treatment of myocardial infarction. Streptokinase, a bacterial enzyme and a fibrinolytic agent is also used for the same purpose.

Q.15. What is the physiological importance of clotting of blood?

Coagulation of the blood is a homeostatic process, i.e. it maintains the integrity of the body including its internal environment.

1. Clotting prevents further loss of blood by sealing the injured vessels.
2. The wound edges are drawn together by the fibrin threads as the clot shrinks and retracts.
3. It provides a framework for repair of the wound. Scab formation protects against loss of body fluids and drying of tissues. Finally, it forms a scar.

Q.16. What is meant by the terms thrombosis and embolism? What are the dangers associated with these conditions?

Thrombosis: Though the anticoagulating and fibrinolytic systems keep the blood in a fluid state, clotting may occur spontaneously within an unbroken vessel—a process called thrombosis (thromb- = clot; osis = a condition of). The clot thus formed is called a thrombus, (pl = thrombi). Thrombosis must be distinguished from extravascular clotting that occurs in a test tube, wounds, or blood vessels after death. Generally, thrombosis can begin in either of the following two ways:

1. **Local damage or roughness of endothelial surfaces**, e.g. atheromatous patches in arteries (e.g. coronaries, carotid, cerebral), on damaged cardiac valves, or in veins of the lower limbs. Platelets are activated and start the intrinsic system of clotting.
2. **Slowing of blood flow (stasis)** in the pelvic and leg veins causes accumulation of clotting factors. This may happen as a complication of pregnancy, prolonged confinement to bed (fractures, surgery, severe burns), or during long flights in aeroplanes.

Embolism: The thrombus may dissolve spontaneously, or it or its fragments may get loosened and be carried away in the downstream blood. A blood clot, an air bubble, fat from broken bones, or a piece of tissue debris, transported by blood is called an embolus (em- = in; bolus = a mass). Emboli in arteries may get lodged in smaller arteries of any vital organ (e.g. brain), while emboli from the veins reach lungs and cause pulmonary embolism. Cases of thrombosis/embolism are treated with fibrinolytics and anticoagulant agents.

1.12: PLATELET COUNT

STUDENT OBJECTIVES

After completing this experiment, the student should be able to:

- Enlist the various methods of performing platelet count.
- Perform platelet count by ammonium oxalate method.
- Discuss the possible sources of error.
- Discuss the physioclinical significance of determining platelet count.
- State the normal value of platelet count.
- Discuss the functions of platelets.

INTRODUCTION

PY2.13: Describe steps for reticulocyte and platelet count.

Platelets play an important role in hemostasis. They are small in size (2–4 µm) and are non-nucleated. The platelets contain a wide variety of chemical substances that play an important role in:

1. Vasoconstriction
2. Hemostatic plug formation
3. Activation of factor X
4. Conversion of prothrombin to thrombin
5. It helps in clot retraction that results in permanent sealing of a ruptured vessel. Thus they take part in almost all stages of hemostasis.

Methods for platelet counting:

1. **Direct methods**
2. **Indirect method.**

DIRECT METHODS

Ammonium Oxalate Method

Apparatus

1. Microscope
2. Red blood cell (RBC) pipette
3. Improved Neubauer's counting chamber with coverslip
4. Equipment for finger-pick
5. Freshly prepared 1.0% ammonium oxalate solution.

Note: Platelet diluting fluid (1.0% ammonium oxalate) acts as an anticoagulant, preserves the platelets and destroys the RBC.

Principle

Blood is diluted with 1.0% ammonium oxalate which lyses the RBCs. Platelets are counted microscopically using an improved Neubauer's counting chamber. The total platelet count of undiluted sample is then calculated.

Procedure

1. Get a fingerprick and draw blood up to the mark 0.5. Suck the diluting fluid to the mark 101.
2. Mix the contents thoroughly and wait for 20 minutes. The red cells will be hemolyzed, leaving only the platelets. Mix the contents once again and discard the first few drops occupying the stem of the pipette) and charge the chamber on both sides. Place the charged chamber on wet filter paper and cover it with a petri dish to avoid evaporation.
3. Focus the RBC square under HP; adjust the diaphragm and position of condenser till you see the platelets - which appear as small, round or oval structures lying separately, highly refractile bodies with a silvery appearance.

Rack the microscope continuously and count the platelets in all the 25 RBC squares **(Fig. 41)**, as was done for red cell count. Record the observation in **Figure 42** given here.

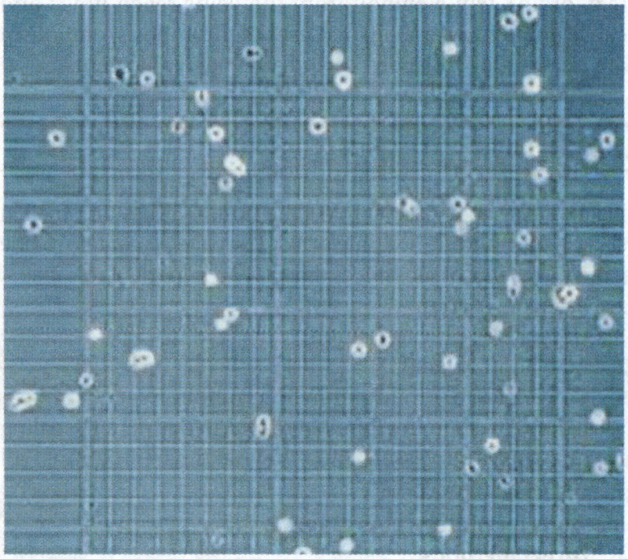

FIG. 41: Platelets as seen under high power.

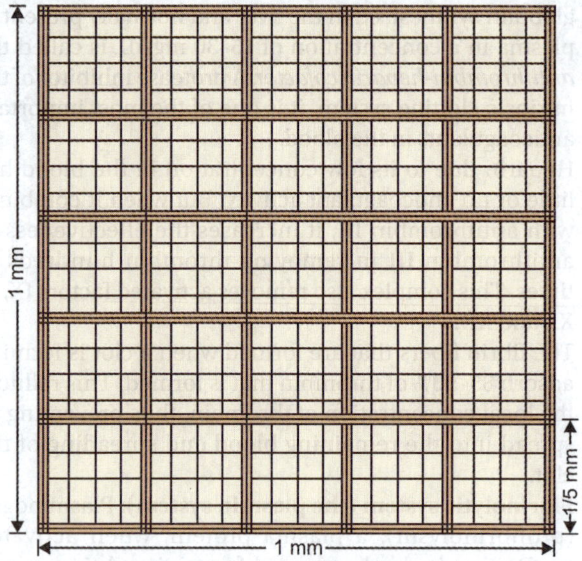

FIG. 42: Record the observation.

Knowing the dilution (1 in 200) employed and the dimensions of the squares, calculate the number of platelets in 1 mm^3 of undiluted blood.

Observations

Calculations

Dilution factor = 200

Volume of fluid = $1 \times 1 \times 0.1 = 0.1$ mm^3 or 0.1 µL

Let N be the total number of platelets in 25 RBC squares = 0.1 mm^3 of diluted blood

Therefore, number of platelets in 1 µL of undiluted blood

$$= \frac{N \times \text{Dilution factor (200)}}{0.1}$$

$N \times 10 \times 200 = N \times 2{,}000$.

Rees–Ecker Method

The Res-Ecker fluid contains the following:

- Brilliant cresyl blue 0.1 g–the dye stains the platelets
- Sodium citrate 3.8 g—to prevent clotting and makes the fluid isotonic
- Formalin (40% formaldehyde)—0.2 mL—prevents fungal growth and lyses red cells
- Distilled water—100 mL.

1. Draw freshly filtered diluent to the mark 0.5 in the RBC pipette. Get a finger-prick and draw blood in the pipette so that the diluent reaches the mark 1.0. Wipe the tip and fill the pipette with diluent once again to the mark 101. This gives a dilution of 1 in 200.
2. Roll the pipette gently between your palms for 3–4 minutes. (Taking the diluent first in the pipette prevents clumping and disintegration of platelets which occurs if blood is taken directly into the pipette).
3. Discard the first few drops occupying the stem of the pipette and charge both sides of the chamber in the usual manner. Place it on a wet filter paper and cover with a petri dish, and wait for 10 minutes to allow the platelets to settle.

4. Count the platelets (which appear as bluish, round or oval bodies, highly refractile on racking the microscope) in 5 groups of 16 squares each, as was done for red cells. Calculate their number in 1 mm^3 of undiluted blood.

Note: The chamber and the pipette must be cleaned with absolute alcohol to remove any dust particles, etc. to which platelets could adhere. Use a lint-free piece of cloth for final cleaning.

INDIRECT METHOD

1. Place a drop of 14% magnesium sulfate solution on your fingertip, and get a prick through this drop. Blood oozes directly into the solution which prevents clumping, and disintegration of platelets.
2. Spread a blood film with the diluted blood, dry it, and stain it with Leishman's stain.
3. Examine the stained film under oil immersion lens. Count the platelets and red cells in every 5th field until 1,000 red cells have been counted. Determine the **"platelet ratio"**, i.e. the ratio of platelets to red cells (usually, there is 1 platelet to 16–18 red cells).
4. Do the RBC count from a fresh finger-prick in a counting chamber, and calculate the count in 1 mm^3 of undiluted blood.

Calculation of platelet count: With the knowledge of platelet count, and the RBC count, the actual number of platelets per mm^3 blood can now be calculated.

(While doing DLC in a stained blood film, the platelets appear in groups of 3–15, and most of them show different degrees of disintegration. In the present case, however, the platelets lie separately from each other and their morphology can also be studied).

Normal platelet count is 150,000–400,000/mm^3.

Capillary fragility test of Hess (also called "tourniquet" test): This is an important test to assess the mechanical fragility of the capillaries (and formation of a platelet plug) by raising the pressure within them. It may reveal latent purpura.

1. Mark a 1 inch diameter circle on the front of the forearm, and using blue ink, mark any pink, purple, or yellow spots within the circle.
2. Apply a blood pressure cuff on the upper arm and note the systolic and diastolic pressures. Then, after a pause of about 2 minutes or so, raise the pressure to midway between systolic and diastolic levels and maintain it there for 15 minutes. Appearance of more than 10 new petechiae (pink or red spots in the skin) is a positive test, which may be seen in various types of purpura and vessel wall abnormalities.

AUTOMATED METHOD

It is a very accurate method. It is carried out on an electronic cell counter. The red cells and platelets in the diluted blood sample pass through an aperture. The particles between 2 μm^3 and 10 μm^3 (fL; femtoliter) are counted as platelets, the measuring range being 0–99.9 × 10^3/fL, and the coefficient of variation being within 1.5%. A platelet distribution graph can also be plotted.

QUESTIONS

Q.1. What is the normal platelet count? Describe briefly their site of formation, lifespan and platelet reaction.

Normal platelet count is 150,000–400,000/mm^3.

Site of formation: Under the influence of the hormone thrombopoietin (TPO), the platelets are formed in the red bone marrow. The myeloid stem cells develop into colony forming unit-granulocyte and macrophage (CFU-GM) which in turn develop into megakaryoblast and megakaryocytes. The platelets are formed by the pinching off of the cytoplasm of megakaryocytes (the largest cells of bone marrow—about 100 µm), each cell producing 2,000–3,000 fragments. Each fragment enclosed by a piece of cell membrane is a platelet (thrombocyte), disc-shaped and 2–4 µm in diameter.

Life span: About 60–70% of platelets formed in the bone marrow are in the circulating blood, while the rest are in the spleen. Their *lifespan is 7–10 days,* about 20% being consumed each day in the repair of microvessels. The aged and dead platelets are removed by tissue macrophages [reticuloendothelial system (RES)] mainly in the spleen, but also in the liver. Their number is kept remarkably constant, their production being regulated partly by the circulating platelets but mainly by TPO, and possibly interleukins 1, 3 and 6.

Platelet reactions: Though the circulating platelets are functionally inactive, they contain a variety of chemical substances. They contain two types of granules:

1. **Alpha granules**—which contain clotting factors, and platelet-derived growth factor (PDGF) which can repair damaged vessels by proliferation of endothelial cells, smooth muscle, and fibroblasts which lay down collagen fibers.
2. **Dense granules**—which contain ADP, ATP, serotonin, Ca^{2+}, etc. There are enzymes for the synthesis of thromboxane A2, fibrin-stabilizing factor, lysosomes; a few mitochondria, and membrane systems for storing calcium.

The earliest response of platelets is adhesive reaction and their aggregation. This may be followed by either dispersal of the collected platelets, or irreversible agglutination and release reaction.

1. **Adhesive reaction:** The platelets, because of ADP and [Von Willebrand factor (VWF)] (the later also produced by endothelium), stick to each other and to foreign surfaces (to form platelet plugs).
2. **Reversible agglutination:** After they have performed their function, their further aggregation is prevented by adrenalin, serotonin, and possibly other agents (e.g. prostacyclin from endothelial cells) which also promote their dispersion.
3. **Irreversible agglutination:** This is triggered by thrombin, ADP and exposure to foreign surfaces.

4. **Release phenomenon:** Irreversible agglutination is often followed by degranulation and release of many substances such as platelet factor 3, platelet factor 4 (it can inactivate heparin), etc. In addition to factor V, other factors especially factors VII, X and XII are also probably adsorbed on other platelets.

Q.2. How does aspirin act as an antiplatelet agglutinating agent and what is its clinical value?

Prostacyclin produced by endothelial and smooth muscle cells in the walls of blood vessels, and **thromboxane A2** formed in the platelets before they enter the circulation are both prostaglandins and synthesized from arachidonic acid (an essential fatty acid) via the enzyme cyclooxygenase.

Prostacyclin prevents platelet aggregation and causes vasodilation. On the other hand, thromboxane A2 promotes platelet aggregation and causes vasoconstriction. Normally, there is a balance between these two opposite effects and the blood vessels remain patent.

Small doses of aspirin irreversibly inhibit cyclo-oxygenase so that both prostacyclin and thromboxane A2 are reduced. However, endothelial cells form new enzyme in a few hours, while circulating platelets cannot do this. New platelets capable of forming thromboxane A2, have to enter circulation which is a slower process. Thus, the balance shifts in favor of prostacyclin for many hours so that platelets are prevented from aggregating at the sites of endothelial damage—a process which precedes formation of clots.

Aspirin is widely used on a long-term basis to prevent formation of clots in the coronary and cerebral vessels.

Q.3. Discuss in brief the functions of platelets.

The functions of platelets are:

1. **Hemostatic plug formation.**
2. **Role in blood coagulation:** Platelets are essential for clotting of blood. They release platelet phospholipid, which takes part in activating factors XII, XI, and X of the intrinsic system, and factor VII of the extrinsic system. Platelets also play an important role in *conversion of prothrombin to thrombin* because most of the prothrombin first attaches to prothrombin receptors on the platelets that are already bound to damaged tissues. The role of fibrin-stabilizing factor (factor XIII) released by platelets (Platelet- free plasma takes a long time to form a clot which is friable and does not retract normally).
3. **Clot retraction:** As already mentioned, the release of contractile proteins form platelets in a clot helps in clot retraction.
4. **Physiological function:** Even when there are no obvious injuries to blood vessels, minimal stress to capillaries and venules in the legs and feet by hydrostatic pressure of blood when we stand upright, or when these vessels are subjected to knocks and bumps, when we run or jump, opens up many gaps and holes in the endothelial cells hundreds of times a day. These multiple, small ruptures are sealed by platelet, which fuse with the injured endothelial cells and contribute their own cell membranes for repair. They also provide PDGF to help in the growth of new vessels to replace the damaged ones (about 20% of platelets are used up for repair purposes everyday. It can thus be visualized how platelet deficiency can lead to hemorrhages typical of purpura).
5. **Phagocytosis:** The platelets can ingest carbon particles, immune complexes, and viral particles.
6. **Transport:** They synthesize, store, and transport a number of substances. They can take up 5-HT against a concentration gradient and transport large amounts from the argentaffin cells of the intestinal glands.
7. **Role in local blood flow regulation:** Products of platelet aggregation (and many other stimuli) also cause the release of nitric oxide (NO), a powerful vasodilator from the intact endothelial cells. Thus, platelets may have a role in dilating the vessels in the vicinity of vasoconstriction and plug formation in microvessels.

Q.4. What are the physiological variations in the platelet count?

Variations in platelet count under physiological conditions are uncommon. However, minor variations occur as mentioned below:

1. Increased counts may be seen after severe exercise, and sometimes at high altitudes.
2. Decreased counts near the lower side of the normal may be seen in the newborns and in females, during menstruation.

Q.5. What is meant by the terms thrombocytosis and thrombocytopenia ? Enumerate the pathological variations in platelet count.

Thrombocytosis: This term refers to an increase in platelet count. It is of two types:

A. **Primary thrombocytosis:** Platelet count more than 800,000/mm^3—it is a myeloproliferative disease involving megakaryocytes. Bleeding and thrombosis may occur.

B. **Secondary (or reactive) thrombocytosis:** Platelet count more than 500,000/mm^3—this condition occurs after removal of spleen or after severe hemorrhage.

Thrombocytopenia refers to a decrease in platelet count. It may be due to decreased production or increased destruction of platelets.

A. **Decreased production:**
   1. **Bone marrow injury/depression/failure:** Drugs (sulfas, chloramphenicol, cytotoxic drugs); irradiation, acute septic fevers, toxemias, and aplastic anemia.
   2. **Bone marrow invasion:** By leukemias, and secondary deposits of malignant disease.
   3. **Periodic thrombocytopenic purpura (purpura hemorrhagica):** Cause not known.

B. **Increased destruction (i.e. decreased survival time):**
   1. **Drugs:** Thiazides, quinine, ethanol, estrogens, methyldopa, quinidine.
   2. **Immune thrombocytopenic purpura (ITP):** Autoimmune destruction of platelets. May be idiopathic, or associated with some disease, e.g. acquired immunodeficiency syndrome (AIDS).
   3. **Sequestration in spleen:** There is increased trapping and/or destruction by enlarged spleen.
   4. **Disseminated intravascular coagulation (DIC):** Platelets are depleted and coagulation factors

consumed during widespread clotting, e.g. severe infection (especially meningococcal, pneumococcal), severe and extensive burns, trauma (crush injuries), mismatched transfusion, and retained dead fetus. There may be severe bleeding in some cases.

5. **Hemorrhage with extensive transfusion.**

Q.6. What is purpura and what are its causes?

The term *purpura* is derived from the purple-colored petechial hemorrhages and bruises in the skin. The blood that leaks out from the capillaries, etc. changes color from red to purple to dark blue to green over a period of time. These colors are due to changes in the pigments derived from hemoglobin.

Causes of purpura: These include thrombocytopenia, functional platelet defects, vessel wall defects, allergy, and old age. Perhaps the most common cause of acquired platelet functional failure is ingestion of drugs, aspirin being the most common.

Purpura may be primary or secondary.

- **Primary purpura (idiopathic; cause not known):** In many cases, antibodies develop against platelets (ITP), causing their excessive destruction. The ITP may be acute or chronic. The acute variety is seen in children, commonly after infection. The onset is sudden, with fever, and purpuric lesions, epistaxis, etc. Steroids help in but some fresh blood has to be given (one unit raises the count by 10,000/mm^3). Splenectomy cures many.
- **Secondary purpura:** It is much more common than the primary form. The causes include: Drugs and chemicals, bone marrow depression/destruction, hypersplenism, etc.

Q.7. What do the platelets look like in a blood film stained with Leishman's stain?

The platelets appear as round or oval bodies, 2–4 μm in diameter. They lie here and there in clumps (aggregates) of 2–12 in number, which is an in vitro appearance. (They do not form clumps in the circulating blood). They stain pink-purple, somewhat darker in the center. But being fragments of cytoplasm, they do not contain nuclei. On careful study, granules may be seen.

Q.8. Which other diluting fluid may be used for counting platelets?

In "direct method", 1% ammonium oxalate solution is used, while the other fluid is "Rees-Ecker solution". In the case of "indirect method", 14% magnesium sulfate solution is used to prevent aggregation and disintegration of platelets before a blood film can be examined. It is not a diluting fluid.

1.13: DETERMINATION OF ARNETH COUNT (COOKE-ARNETH COUNT)

STUDENT OBJECTIVES

After completing this experiment, the student should be able to:

- Identify neutrophils of different ages.
- Determine their percentage distribution in various stages and express your results accordingly.
- Explain the terms left shift, right shift and their significance.
- Describe the function of neutrophils.

INTRODUCTION

Arneth count is the percentage distribution of neutrophils on the basis of the number of lobes in the nucleus. It indicates the maturity (stage of development) of the neutrophils. Arneth count is named after a scientist named *Joseph Arneth.*

The nuclei of young neutrophils have fewer lobes as compared to those of older neutrophils which have 5 or 6 lobes. A higher percentage of younger or older neutrophils in a blood film can provide useful information about the functional status of the bone marrow **(Figs. 43A and B)**.

APPARATUS

Same as that for differential leukocyte count (DLC).

PROCEDURE

1. Prepare and stain a fresh blood film in the usual manner. The blood film prepared during DLC can be utilized for Arneth Count.
2. Examine 100 neutrophils under high power (40X), noting the number of lobes in each cell **(Figs. 43A and B)**.
3. Enter the observations in the workbook. Use the tally bar method for this and calculate the percentages of each stage. Note the percentage distribution of various stages of neutrophils and plot a graph using these two parameters **(Fig. 44)**. Normal Percentage of each stage with description is given in **Table 17**.
4. These cells can be indicated in a column (instead of the 100 squares), and as the cell is identified a cell, put a short vertical stroke against that cell. In this way, you can place different types of cells in groups of 5, a horizontal stroke representing the 5th cell (Tally bar method).

Note: Occasionally it is not possible to do the staging of some neutrophils accurately especially when the lobes of the nuclei are folded. Two other factors may then be used:
1. The cell size decreases with aging.
2. The older cells contain fewer granules. In older cells (stages N_5, N_6), there may be no granules and the nucleus may show fragmentation.

PHYSIOCLINICAL SIGNIFICANCE

- The terms "left shift" and "right shift" refer to the appearance of younger neutrophils (shift to the left), or more mature cells (shift to the right) respectively in the blood **(Fig. 44)**.

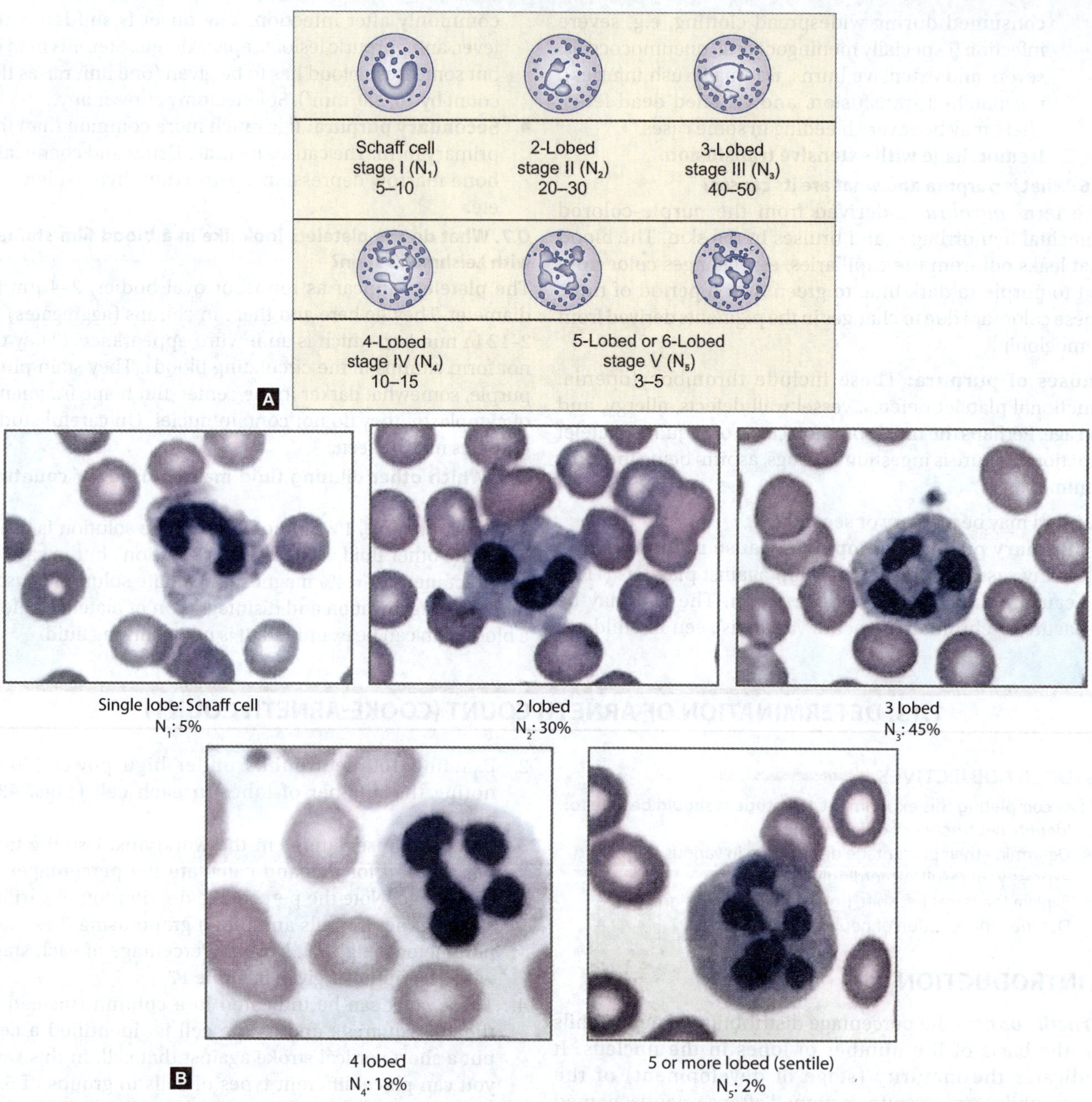

FIGS. 43A AND B: Cooke-Arneth count. The percent distribution of neutrophils in the circulation based on the number of their lobes.

Table 17: Percentages of each stage with description.

Stage		***Description***	***Percentage***
Stage I	(N_1)	Nucleus is C- or U-shaped, the two limbs being connected by a thick band of chromatin	5–10
Stage II	(N_2)	The two lobes are connected by a narrow band of chromatin	20–30
Stage III	(N_3)	Three lobes connected by chromatin filaments (Actively motile and functionally most effective)	40–50
Stage IV	(N_4)	Four lobes connected by chromatin filaments	10–15
Stage V	(N_5, N_6)	◆ Five lobes or more (N_6 = >6 lobes) ◆ Outline may be irregular ◆ Cytoplasmic granules poorly stained ◆ Functionally least motile and effective	3–5

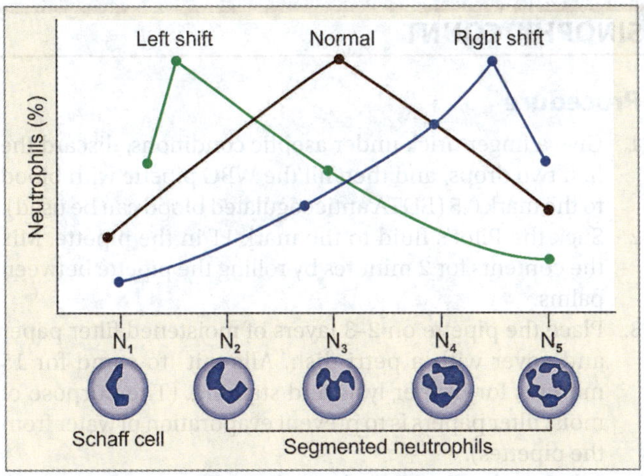

FIG. 44: Arneth curve showing right and left shift.

"Left shift" ("Regenerative shift")

$N_1 + N_2 + N_3 = >80\%$. This indicates a ***hyperactive bone marrow.***

Shift to left occurs in:

1. Acute pus-producing infections.
2. Tuberculosis: Though there is lymphocytosis, a shift to the left may be due to removal of older neutrophils from the blood.
3. Hemorrhage.
4. Low-dosage irradiation is said to stimulate bone marrow while heavy doses cause a shift to the right.

"Right shift" ("Degenerative shift")

$N_4 + N_5 + N_6 = >20\%$. This indicates a ***hypoactive bone marrow.***

Shift to right occurs in:

1. Bone marrow depression (hypoplasia and aplasia) due to any factor
2. Drugs, toxins, chemical poisons
3. Megaloblastic anemia, septicemia, uremia, etc.

- A shift of the count to one or the other side can provide important information about the functional status of bone marrow. It can tell us whether or not the bone marrow is actively forming and releasing neutrophils into the circulation.
- A shift to the left indicates that the bone marrow is actively forming and releasing neutrophils into the circulation. A shift to the right indicates decreased production and release of neutrophils.

PRECAUTIONS

- The smear should be one cell thick.
- Staining should be proper.
- Choose a stained slide that shows neutrophils clearly.
- Lobes of the neutrophils should be counted accurately. If the lobes cannot be seen, consider the size of the cell and the number of granules in the cytoplasm.
- At least 100 neutrophils should be counted.

QUESTIONS

Q.1. What is the relation between the number of lobes of the nucleus and the age of a neutrophil?

A newly formed neutrophil in the bone marrow is one-lobed and may be C- or U-shaped. Such cells are called *stab or Schaff* cells. They enter blood mostly as bilobed neutrophils. As their age increases, the number of lobes increases to 5 or 6 by the end of their lifespan of 8–10 hours.

Q.2. Which stage is most effective and least effective functionally?

A 3-lobed neutrophil is the most motile and functionally the most efficient in killing the bacteria. A senile neutrophil (stage V) is less motile and least effective.

Q.3. What is meant by the terms left shift and right shift? Is the Cooke-Arneth count of any clinical value?

See text above.

Q.4. If Cooke-Arneth count can provide such useful information about the functioning of bone marrow, why is it not used routinely in the labs?

There are two reasons for this test not being used as a routine:

1. Some physiological conditions cause shifting of neutrophils from various pools into the circulating blood. This is likely to cause confusion about left or right shift.
2. Better methods, e.g. bone marrow biopsy, are now available for assessing bone marrow function/activity.

Nevertheless, this count can provide some useful information from a blood film without bone marrow biopsy. It is also a good laboratory exercise.

Assignment

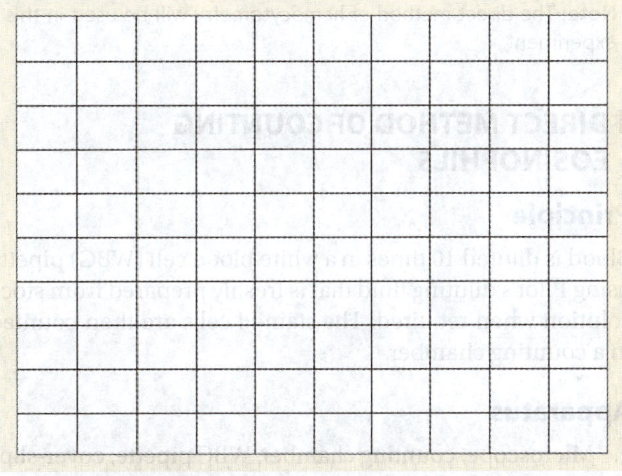

1. Express your values as a percentage of the total neutrophils counted.
   N_1: Single lobed.......................%
   N_2: Two lobed.........................%
   N_3: Three lobed.......................%
   N_4: Four lobed........................%
   N_5 and N_6: Five or more lobed.................%
2. Plot a graph of your own values with the neutrophil stages on the X-axis, and their percentage on the Y-axis. Draw another graph with the values given in the book and compare the two graphs.

1.14: ABSOLUTE EOSINOPHIL COUNT

STUDENT OBJECTIVES

After completing this experiment, the student should be able to:

- Describe the significance of doing absolute eosinophil count.
- Describe the morphology and functions of eosinophils.
- Carry out eosinophil count, and name the precautions.
- List the composition of Pilot's solution and the function of each component.
- Explain the physiological basis of changes in their count.

INTRODUCTION

Absolute Eosinophil Count (AEC) is a blood test that measures the number of eosinophils in 1 cmm of blood. It is required when the differential count shows a high percentage of these cells. This is especially true in cases of bronchial allergy, asthma, urticaria, intestinal parasites, pulmonary eosinophilia, etc.

COUNTING METHODS

The absolute count of eosinophils can be done by two methods:

1. ***Direct method***: The cells are counted directly by employing hemocytometer.
2. ***Indirect method***: The percentage of eosinophils is determined from a blood smear counting of leukocytes. If total leukocytes count (TLC) is done simultaneously, the absolute count can be calculated.

AEC= Differential count of eosinophil/100X TLC

Note: The direct method of hemocytometry will be used in this experiment.

DIRECT METHOD OF COUNTING EOSINOPHILS

Principle

Blood is diluted 10 times in a white blood cell (WBC) pipette using Pilot's diluting fluid that is freshly prepared from stock solution when required. The stained cells are then counted in a counting chamber.

Apparatus

1. Microscope, counting chamber, WBC pipette, cover-slips
2. Apparatus required for finger prick.
3. Pilot's diluting fluid

Composition of Pilot's Fluid

1. Propylene glycol (50 mL) lyses red blood cells and is a solvent for the stain.
2. **Phloxine (10 mL):** Stains only eosinophil granules
3. **Sodium carbonate (1 mL):** Lyses all leukocytes except eosinophils and enhances the staining of eosinophilic granules.
4. **Heparin:** 100 units (anticoagulant).
5. Distilled water to make 100 mL.

Procedure

1. Give a finger prick under aseptic conditions, discard the first two drops, and then fill the WBC pipette with blood to the mark 0.5 (EDTA anticoagulated blood can be used).
2. Suck the Pilot's fluid to the mark 11 in the pipette. Mix the contents for 2 minutes by rolling the pipette between palms.
3. Place the pipette on 2–3 layers of moistened filter paper and cover with a petri dish. Allow it to stand for 15 minutes for proper lysis and staining. (The purpose of moist filter papers is to prevent evaporation of water from the pipettes).
4. Take out the pipette and mix the contents once again for 30 seconds. Discard the fluid from the stem of the pipette and charge each side of the Neubauer's chamber.
5. Using the HP objective (40X), count the eosinophils (seen as pink cells with nuclei) in the 4 corner groups (WBC squares) of 16 squares each, i.e. in a total of 64 squares that were used for TLC. When the counting has been done, calculate the number of cells in 1 mm^3 of undiluted blood. Enter your observations in appropriate squares drawn here.

Observations (Fig. 45)

Calculate the number of cells in 1 mm^3 of undiluted blood.

Calculations (Figs. 46A to D)

- Determine the absolute eosinophil count of blood per mm^3 of blood by using the same calculation as was used while determining TLC.
- Normal absolute eosinophil count is 10–400/mm^3 (eosinophil count of capillary blood is usually 10–15% higher).

Normal absolute eosinophil count is 10–400/mm^3 (Eosinophil count of capillary blood is usually 10–15% higher).

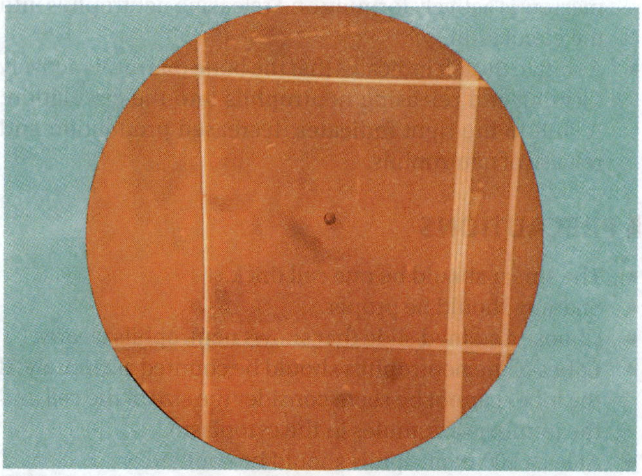

FIG. 45: An eosinophil as seen under high power (40X).

INDIRECT METHOD OF COUNTING EOSINOPHIL

For this both TLC and DLC are required. For example, if the TLC is 8,000/mm³ and eosinophils are 2% in DLC, then the absolute count would be = 2/100 × 8,000 = 160/mm³ of undiluted blood. This method can act as a check on the result of the direct method.

PHYSIOCLINICAL SIGNIFICANCE

The absolute count helps in diagnosing various allergic and parasitic conditions.

Eosinophilia is seen in:
- Allergic conditions,
- Parasitic infestations,
- Skin diseases,
- Pulmonary eosinophilia,
- Malignant neoplasia (eosinophilic leukemia, Hodgkin's disease),
- Addison's disease.

Eosinopenia is seen in:
- Cushing's syndrome,
- Acute pyogenic infections,
- Aplastic anemia.

> **Note:** Formerly, eosinophil count was considered as an index of adrenocorticotropic hormone (ACTH) activity in the blood. When ACTH is injected into a person with normal adrenocortical function, there is a drastic reduction in the absolute eosinophil count. This test called **"Thorn's test"** used to be employed to assess adrenocortical function. However, with better hormone assay tests, this test is no longer employed.

PRECAUTIONS

- Observe all precautions as for obtaining a blood sample, filling the pipette with blood, diluting it, charging the chamber, and counting the cells.
- Do the cell counting within 20–30 minutes of charging the chamber because the cells begin to disintegrate in the diluting fluid.
- The pipette should be placed on moist filter paper.
- If possible, use the indirect method to check on your results.

QUESTIONS

Q.1. What is the clinical significance of absolute eosinophil count?

See text above.

Q.2. Can any other diluting fluid be used for the count?

Yes. *Dunger's diluting fluid can be used. In this,* eosin replaces phloxine, and acetone replaces propylene glycol. This fluid contains: 5 mL of 1% aqueous solution of eosin, 5 mL of acetone (analytic), and distilled water to 90 mL.

In *Randolph's diluting fluid* which is similar to Pilot's solution, methylene blue is added to stain other leukocytes blue compared to red-orange eosinophils.

Q.3. Write briefly how the eosinophils are formed and what is their fate?

- Eosinophils are produced in the bone marrow from multipotent hematopoietic stem cells (HSC) in the red marrow. Hematopoietic differentiation involves the commitment of multipotent progenitors to a given lineage, followed by the maturation of the committed cells. Their production is regulated by (GM-CSF) granulocyte macrophage colony stimulating **factor**. Interleukins 3 and 5 and possibly by the products of dead and dying cells also help in their maturation.
- Although the eosinophil is a formed element of the peripheral circulation, it is primarily a tissue-dwelling cell. Once the eosinophil has entered the blood, it has a short half-life, ranging from 8 to 18 hours.
- In humans the tissue eosinophil/blood ratio is about 100:1. Furthermore, eosinophils tend to reside in those tissues where the epithelial surfaces are exposed to the external environment (gut); mast cells primarily reside in these tissues as well. Thus, eosinophils are considered merely to "pass through" the circulation en route to the tissues. The tissue lifespan of eosinophils ranges from 2 to 5 days.
- Their granules contain a variety of chemicals: **Major basic protein (MBP), eosinophil peroxidase, eosinophilic cationic proteins, arylsulfatase B, lysophospholipase, histaminase, cytokines, etc.**

Q.4. Name the conditions in which absolute eosinophil count increases and decreases.

See text above.

Q.5. Enumerate the functions of eosinophils.
- Defense against parasitic infections
- Defense against intracellular bacteria
- Participate in immediate allergic reactions
- Modulation of immediate hypersensitivity reactions
- They also act as the antigen-presenting cell to T- cell
- Produce cytokines, TNF and growth factors
- Involved in neoplasia and allograft rejection during raft transplantation.

Assignment

Enter your observations in appropriate squares.

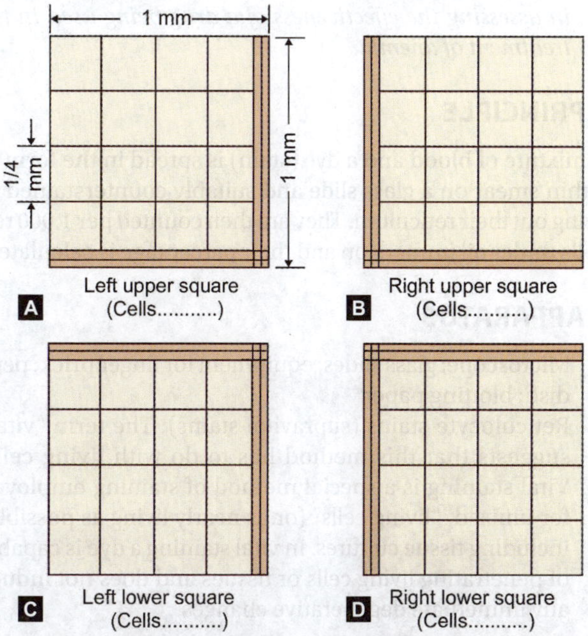

FIGS. 46A TO D: WBC squares.

1.15: RETICULOCYTE COUNT

STUDENT OBJECTIVES

After completing this experiment, the student should be able to:

- Indicate the significance of doing this count.
- Describe the theory of reticulocyte staining and the special stains that are used.
- Perform the relative and absolute reticulocyte counts.
- Define the terms reticulocyte response, reticulocytosis, and reticulocytopenia.
- Describe the electronic method of counting these cells.

INTRODUCTION

PY2.13: Describe steps for reticulocyte and platelet count.

- Reticulocytes are the non-nucleated *immediate precursors of red cells* that develop in the red marrow from the pluripotent hematopoietic stem cell (HSC). They contain large amounts of **the remnants of RNA and ribosomes.** Reticulocytes lose their mitochondria, ribosomes and basophilic tint to form mature erythrocytes. Reticulocytes stay in circulation for about 24 hours before they mature into erythrocytes.
- They are slightly larger (diameter = about 8.0 μm) than red blood cells (RBCs), and are present in large numbers in bone marrow and in small numbers in blood. Their cell membranes are sticky which plays an important role in their controlled release from the bone marrow. Most of them, because of their larger size and stickiness, are trapped in the trabeculae of the spleen. Here they ripen and mature in a day or two before entering the circulation once again.
- The reticulocyte count which is 1–2% of circulating red cells is an indicator of erythropoietic activity of red bone marrow. *It is indicated in all conditions where high counts are expected such as in hemolytic anemia. It can also help in assessing the effectiveness of a drug being used in the treatment of anemia.*

PRINCIPLE

A mixture of blood and a dye (stain) is spread in the form of a thin smear on a glass slide and suitably counterstained to bring out their reticulum. They are then counted per 1,000 red cells under oil immersion and their percentage is calculated.

APPARATUS

1. Microscope; glass slides; equipment for finger prick; petri dish; blotting paper.
2. Reticulocyte stains (supravital stains): The term "vital" suggests that this method has to do with living cells. Vital staining is a special method of staining employed for unfixed, "living cells" (or as nearly living as possible) including tissue cultures. In vital staining a dye is capable of penetrating living cells or tissues and does not induce any immediate degenerative changes.

Note: Vital staining are of two types: *Intravital staining* and *Supravital staining*:

- When the technique is applied *in vivo*, it is referred to as *intravital staining*, e.g., gastric mucosa and oral mucosa. In this method, a dye is injected into a living organism for selective staining.
- If the technique is applied *in vitro*, i.e. living cells outside the body it is known as *supravital staining*, e.g., Leukocytes, nerve fibres and nerve endings. Here, the living cells are stained by immersing them in a dye solution.

I. ***Brilliant cresyl blue:*** 1.0 g of this dye dissolved in 100 mL of citrate saline (1.0 volume of 3.8% sodium citrate and 4 volumes of normal saline). The dye stains the RNA of reticulocytes, citrate prevents clotting of blood, and normal saline provides tonicity (1.0% solution of the dye in methyl alcohol can also be used).

II. ***New methylene blue:*** While methylene blue does not stain the reticulum, new methylene blue (which is chemically different from methylene blue) stains this material more deeply and uniformly. 1.0 g of the dye is dissolved in 100 mL of citrate saline.

Reticulocyte Staining

The basophilic remnants of RNA and ribosomes in the cytoplasm of reticulocytes cannot be stained by the basic dye methylene blue which is a component of Leishman's stain. The material can only be stained with certain dyes such as brilliant cresyl blue. The dye enters the cells and stains the basophilic material to form bluish precipitates of dots, short strands, and filaments. This reaction can occur only in **supravitally (or vitally)** stained cells, i.e. in "unfixed" and "living" cells. The more the immature cells, greater is the amount of precipitable ribosomal material present in them.

PROCEDURE

- Take 1 mL of anticoagulated blood in a small test tube; add an equal amount of the supravital stain.
- Mix gently, and incubate at 37°C for 15-20 minutes to simulate the living conditions so that the stain may better penetrate the reticulocytes.
- Mix the mixture gently to re-suspend the blood cells and prepare 4-5 smears in the usual manner from this mixture.
- Choose the best stained smear for reticulocyte counting under oil immersion.

Alternate method:

1. Take 2–3 clean grease-free glass slides and place a drop of reticulocyte stain in the center of each slide about 1 cm from its end.
2. Get a fingerprick under aseptic precautions and add an equal-sized drop of blood to each drop of stain. Stir with a pin and put the slides on moist filter paper and cover with a petri dish. Allow the mixture to remain on the slides for 1 minute.

3. Make a smear of the blood-dye mixture on each slide, then counterstain with Leishman's stain in the usual manner. (This will stain all cells).

OBSERVATIONS AND RESULTS

1. ***Using an oil-immersion objective,*** bring the blood cells into focus and identify reticulocytes **(Fig. 47)**. The reticulocytes stain lighter than the red cells and also contain dots, strands, and filaments, etc. of bluish-stained material. They are non-nucleated cells that are slightly larger (diameter about 8 μm) than the red cells (average diameter = 7.5 μm).
2. Count 1,000 RBCs in a minimum of 10 fields under oil immersion, each containing 100-150 red cells. Count the reticulocytes and RBCs in different microscopic fields.
3. Record the number of reticulocytes encountered in this cell population **(Table 18)**.

CALCULATIONS

Reticulocyte percentage = (No. of reticulocytes/No. of RBCs) × 100

Normal Values

1. Newborns = 30–40%. Their number decreases to 1–2% during the first week of life
2. Infants = 2–6%
3. Children and adults:
   i. 0.2–2.0% (average = 1%)
   ii. Absolute count = 20,000–90,000/mm^3.

Absolute Reticulocyte Count

A direct reticulocyte counting by hemocytometer is not possible. An indirect absolute count can be obtained from the relative percentage by doing a total red cell count.

Absolute reticulocyte count = (Reticulocyte percentage × RBC count/microliter of blood)/100

Normal value = 25,000–100,000/mm^3.

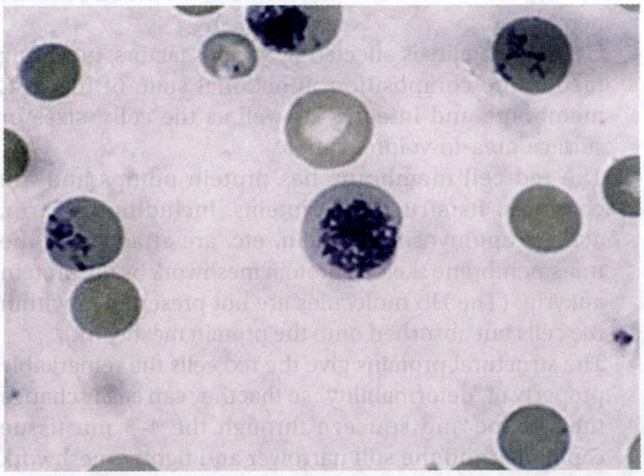

FIG. 47: Peripheral smear showing reticulocytes.

PHYSIOCLINICAL SIGNIFICANCE

1. **Reticulocytosis:** The term indicates an increase in the number of reticulocytes in the blood.
   A. **Physiological variations:** Increased count is seen in:
      - **Newborn infants:** The blood contains immature red cells, both nucleated and reticulocytes. After 1 year, there are no nucleated RBCs, and not more than 2% reticulocytes.
      - **High altitude:** Erythropoiesis is stimulated by the hypoxic stimuli via erythropoietin.
      - Reticulocyte count may be higher during **pregnancy.**
   B. **Pathological variations:** Increased count due to disease is seen in:
      - **Reticulocyte response during treatment of deficiency anemias:** There is increase in hemoglobin (Hb) and RBC count.
      - **After hemorrhage:** The count increases due to hypoxia.
      - **Chronic hemolytic anemias,** disorders of bone marrow (nucleated RBCs present), leukemias, secondary deposits in malignancies and miliary tuberculosis.
      - **Disorders of spleen and after splenectomy:** The response is irregular.
      - **Arsenic and foreign proteins**, etc. produce irregular response without increase in Hb and RBC count.
      - **Blood disorder in a fetus** or newborn (erythroblastosis fetalis).
      - **Kidney disease**, with increased production of a erythropoietin hormone.
2. **Reticulocytopenia:** Decrease in reticulocyte count may be seen in:
   - Bone marrow failure (for example, from a certain drug, tumor, radiation therapy, or infection)
   - Aplastic anemia
   - Cirrhosis of the liver
   - Anemia caused by low iron levels, or low levels of vitamin B12 or folate
   - Chronic kidney disease, with decreased production of erythropoietin
   - Hypopituitarism
   - Myxedema
   - After splenectomy

   There is no physiological situation in which their number decreases.

PRECAUTIONS

- Observe all precautions as for differential leukocyte count.
- The blood film should be thin so that the red cells lie separately from each other without any crowding or overlapping.
- There should be no rouleaux formation on the slide.

Assignment

Table 18: Count the number of reticulocytes and the number of RBCs in different microscopic fields.

Field No.	Number of reticulocytes	Number of RBCs
1.		
2.		
3.		
4.		
....		
10.		

QUESTIONS

Q.1. What are the indications for doing reticulocyte count?

Indications are:

1. Hemolytic anemia
2. To see response after treatment of anemia.

The reticulocyte count is used to estimate the degree of effective erythropoiesis and can help in the diagnosis of different types of anemia. A high reticulocyte count occurs due to increased EPO response which is seen in anemia due to hemolysis, blood loss, or response to treatment.

See text above.

Q.2. What are reticulocytes? Are they normally present in blood? Did you see these cells in the Leishman-stained blood films?

See text above.

Q.3. What is the chemical nature of reticular material?

It is the remnant of RNA and ribosomes.

Q.4. What is meant by the term "vital" staining? How does it differ from Leishman's staining you employed for blood films?

See text above

Q.5. How does a reticulocyte differ from a red cell?

See text above.

Q.6. What are the normal counts in newborns, infants, children and adults?

See text above.

Q.7. What is a reticulocyte response? Is its determination of any practical value?

Reticulocyte response is an increase in the number of reticulocytes in the circulating blood. It indicates a high rate of erythropoiesis. Its practical importance is as follows:

1. It is useful in assessing the erythroid activity of the red marrow.
2. It can be employed to check if the diagnosis and treatment of an anemic patient is proceeding on correct lines. For example, if iron deficiency is diagnosed, treatment with iron should produce a prompt reticulocyte response.
3. The potency of a particular drug can also be assessed. The response starts 2–8 days after the therapy is started and reaches a peak in the next 8–10 days. After that there is a gradual fall in the response, while the RBC count continues to rise steadily (it needs pointing out that reticulocyte response by itself must be interpreted very critically either as evidence of therapeutic efficacy of a drug, or as a prognostic sign, or for assessing the bone marrow efficiency).

Q.8. What is meant by the term reticulocytosis? Name the physiological and pathological conditions that cause an increase and decrease in the number of reticulocytes.

See text above.

Q.9. Is there any automated (electronic) method for counting reticulocytes?

Yes, there is a method in which the cells are stained with a fluorochrome dye that specifically stains RNA. The reticulocytes fluoresce when exposed to ultraviolet light and the cells can then be counted.

1.16: DETERMINATION OF OSMOTIC FRAGILITY OF RED BLOOD CELLS

STUDENT OBJECTIVES

After completing this experiment, the student should be able to:

- Define the osmotic fragility of red cells and describe the utility of this test.
- Explain how hemolysis of red blood cells occurs when they are exposed to hypotonic saline.
- Explain the effect of hypertonic saline on red cells.
- Name the conditions in which fragility of red cells is increased and decreased.

INTRODUCTION

PY2.12: Describe test for ESR, Osmotic fragility, Hematocrit. Note the findings and interpret the test results, etc.

- Osmotic fragility of red blood cells (RBCs) is defined as the erythrocyte resistance to hemolysis while being exposed to varying levels of dilution of a saline solution.
- Osmotic fragility test evaluates the ability of RBCs to withstand hypotonic saline without bursting. It is employed as a screening test for hemolytic anemias.
- Osmotic fragility is expressed as the concentration of the hypotonic solution in which the red blood cells are hemolyzed.
- Osmotic fragility is affected by various factors, including membrane composition, functional state of the RBC membrane and integrity as well as the cells' sizes or surface-area-to-volume ratios.
- The red cell membrane has protein pumps and ion channels. Its structural proteins, including spectrin, actin, tropomyosin, adducin, etc. are attached to the transmembrane skeletal protein meshwork by the protein ankyrin. (The Hb molecules are not present free within the cells but absorbed onto the protein meshwork).
- The structural proteins give the red cells the remarkable property of "deformability" so that they can easily change their shape and squeeze through the 4–5 µm tissue capillaries and the still narrower and tighter meshwork and trabeculae of the spleen (in the spleen, which is an important blood filter which detains large and abnormal-shaped and rigid cells, part of the blood flows through

the microvessels, while the rest "percolates" through the phagocytes and lymphocytes of the splenic pulp before entering the sinusoids).

PRINCIPLE

- The normal red cells can remain suspended in normal saline 0.9% NaCl; 5% glucose; 10% mannitol and 20% urea solution for hours without rupturing or any change in their size or shape. But when they are placed in decreasing strengths of hypotonic saline (<0.9% NaCl), they imbibe water (due to osmosis) and finally burst. The ability of RBCs to resist this type of hemolysis can be determined quantitatively.
- When RBCs are placed in isotonic saline, there is no change in the shape because fluid neither goes out of cells nor enters into it.
- In hypertonic saline (>0.9% NaCl), they shrink because the fluid goes out of the cells.

APPARATUS

- Test tube rack with 12 clean, dry, 7.5 cm × 1.0 cm glass test tubes.
- Glass marking pencil.
- Glass dropper with a rubber teat.
- Sterile swabs moist with alcohol.
- 2 mL syringe with needle.
- Freshly prepared 1% sodium chloride solution.
- Distilled water.

PROCEDURE

1. Number the test tubes from 1 to 12 with the glass marking pencil and put them in the rack **(Table 19)**.
2. Using the glass dropper, place the varying number of drops of 1% saline in each of the 12 test tubes as shown in **Table 19**. Then, after thorough rinsing of the same dropper with distilled water, add the number of drops of distilled water to each of the 12 tubes as shown in **Table 19.**
3. Mix the contents of each test tube by placing a thumb over it and inverting it a few times.
4. The saline solutions of increasing hypotonicity are thus prepared.
5. Mark the tonicity of saline on each of the test tubes. Note that tube no. 1 contains normal saline which is isotonic with plasma, while tube no. 12 contains only distilled water.
6. Draw 2 mL of blood from a suitable vein and gently eject one drop of blood into each of the 12 tubes. (The blood may be put into a container of anticoagulant, and a drop can be put into each tube with a pipette). Mix the contents gently by placing a thumb over it and inverting the tube only once.
7. Leave the test tubes undisturbed for 1 hour. Then observe the extent of hemolysis in each tube by holding the rack at eye level with a white paper sheet behind it **(Fig. 48)**.

OBSERVATIONS AND RESULTS

While judging the degree or extent of hemolysis from the depth of the red color of supernatant saline, tube no. 1 (normal saline), and tube no. 12 (distilled water) will act as controls, i.e. no hemolysis in normal saline (no. 1) and complete hemolysis in distilled water (no. 12).

1. The test tubes in which no hemolysis has occurred, the RBCs will settle down and form a red dot (mass) at the bottom of the tube, leaving the saline above clear.

Table 19: Preparation of saline solutions for testing the osmotic fragility of red cells.

Test tube number	***1***	***2***	***3***	***4***	***5***	***6***	***7***	***8***	***9***	***10***	***11***	***12***
No. of drops of 1% NaCl	22	16	15	14	13	12	11	10	9	8	7	0
No. of drops of distilled water	3	9	10	11	12	13	14	15	16	17	18	25
Tonicity strength of NaCl (in %)	0.88	0.64	0.60	0.56	0.52	0.48	0.44	0.40	0.36	0.32	0.28	0

Note: Use the same dropper, after thorough rinsing each time, for measuring saline and distilled water. This will ensure that the volume of all drops is equal for all test tubes.

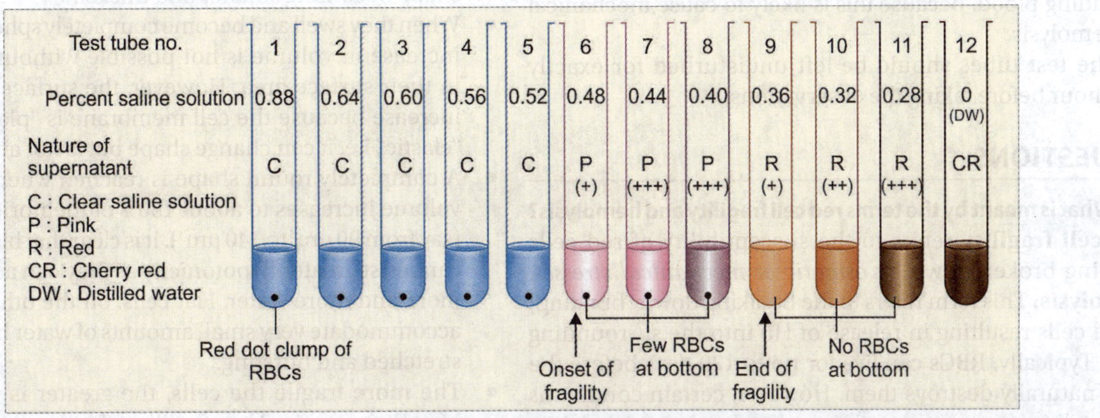

FIG. 48: Osmotic fragility test showing RBC suspension after 1 hour in increasing hypotonicity of NaCl solution and distilled water.

Note: When the test is done on a patient, it is always checked against a normal sample of blood which is tested on a separate series of saline solutions.

- When red cells become more fragile, hemolysis may begin at about 0.64% saline (second tube) and be complete at about 0.44% saline (seventh tube).
- When red cells are less fragile, hemolysis starts and is complete at lower strengths of saline.

2. If there is some hemolysis, the saline will be tinged red with Hb with the unruptured RBCs forming a red dot at the bottom. This marks the onset of fragility. Normally, this is seen in 0.48% NaCl solution (sixth tube).
3. The test tubes in which there is *complete hemolysis*, the saline will be *uniformly deep red* with no RBCs at the bottom of these tubes. This marks the end of fragility. It usually occurs in 0.36% NaCl solution (ninth tube).

Results: Carefully observe each tube for depth of red color of the supernatant and the mass of red cells at the bottom.

- Note the start of hemolysis (also called onset of fragility) and record the test tube number. Express your result in % saline.
- Note the start of complete hemolysis, i.e. the test tube in which there are no red cells at the bottom (hemolysis will be complete below this saline strength). Express your result in % saline.
- Hemolysis begins in .... % saline.
- Hemolysis is complete in .... % saline.
- Osmotic fragility of RBC in a given sample of blood ranges from .... % to .... % saline.

If there is doubt about the presence of intact RBCs at the bottom of a test tube, the solution can be centrifuged and the sediment examined under the microscope.

Normal Range of Fragility

Normally, hemolysis begins in about 0.48% saline. No cells hemolyze in solutions of 0.5% saline and above.

Hemolysis is complete at about 0.36% saline.

PRECAUTIONS

- Use the same dropper, after thorough rinsing each time, for measuring saline and distilled water.
- The test tubes should not be shaken vigorously after adding blood, because this is likely to cause mechanical hemolysis.
- The test tubes should be left undisturbed for exactly 1 hour before taking the observations.

QUESTIONS

Q.1. What is meant by the terms red cell fragility and hemolysis?

Red cell fragility refers to the susceptibility of red cells to being broken down by *osmotic or mechanical stresses.* **Hemolysis:** This term refers to the breaking down (bursting) of red cells resulting in release of Hb into the surrounding fluid. Typically, RBCs can live for up to 120 days before the body naturally destroys them. However, certain conditions and medications may cause them to break down quicker than usual.

Q.2. Define osmosis and osmotic pressure. How much osmotic pressure is exerted by the blood and what is its importance?

- **Osmosis:** It is the process of net movement of water from a weaker solution (of a solute and solvent) to a stronger solution through a selectively permeable membrane that is permeable only to water but not to solute (salts, proteins, etc.).
- **Osmotic pressure:** It is the pressure required to be applied to the stronger solution to prevent the movement of solute (water) from the weaker solution to the stronger solution. (It should be noted that the osmotic pressure does not produce the movement of water during osmosis).
- **Osmotic pressure of blood:** The total osmotic pressure of blood (or plasma) due to all crystalloids and colloids is about 5,000 mm Hg (6–7 atmospheres). But since the crystalloids (mainly NaCl) are equally distributed across (on the two sides) the capillary walls, it is only the *colloidal osmotic pressure* exerted by plasma proteins (about 25 mm Hg) that takes part in tissue fluid exchanges.
- **The colloid osmotic pressure:** It opposes hydrostatic pressure (blood pressure) within the capillaries about 32 mm Hg at their arterial ends and 12 mm Hg at the venous ends. As a result, filtration occurs at the arterial ends and reabsorption at the venous ends. Changes in these forces called starling forces can cause edema (accumulation of fluid in the tissues).

Q.3. What will be the effect of vigorous shaking of the test tubes after adding blood to each of them?

Vigorous shaking in an attempt to mix the contents of the test tubes is likely to cause mechanical rupture of RBCs with release of Hb into the saline.

Q.4. How do red cells behave in hypotonic and hypertonic saline solutions? How do they resist hemolysis in hypotonic saline?

- The red cell membrane is a selectively permeable membrane which allows water to pass through easily while the movement of various solutes is restricted to varying degrees.
- In hypertonic solutions, the RBCs, like other body cells, shrink (crenate) due to movement of water out of the cells **(exosmosis).**
- In hypotonic saline, water moves into the red cells **(endosmosis).** They swell up and lose their biconcave shape becoming smaller and thicker.
- When they swell and become completely spherical, further increase in volume is not possible without an increase in their surface area. However, the surface area cannot increase because the cell membrane is "plastic" but not "elastic", i.e. it can change shape but is not able to stretch.
- A completely round shape is reached when the red cell volume increases to about 150% of their original volume (say from 90 μm^3 to 140 μm^3). It is clear that biconcave cells can resist greater hypotonicity as they can accommodate more and more water. Flat cells, on the other hand, can accommodate very small amounts of water before getting stretched and bursting.
- The more fragile the cells, the greater is their degree of spherocytosis. Also, fragility of red cells is greater in venous blood.

Q.5. Give the normal range of fragility of red cells.

See text above.

Q.6. What will be the effect of waiting for 5–6 hours before observations are made on the test tubes?

If observations are made after, say, 5–6 hours, hemolysis is likely to occur in all hypotonic solutions. The reason is that without energy supply, various membrane pumps (especially Na^+-K^+ pump) will fail to function. Sodium chloride will enter the cells, they will swell up, and finally rupture.

Q.7. What is the clinical significance of doing an osmotic fragility test?

Though the test is not done routinely. It is employed as a *screening test in hereditary spherocytosis.*

Q.8. Name the conditions where osmotic fragility increases and those where it decreases?

A. **Increased red cell osmotic fragility:** It is seen in the following conditions:
   1. **Hereditary spherocytosis:** It is one of the most common causes of hemolytic anemias. A defect in the structural proteins causes them to become spherocytes (in normal plasma), and more fragile. Some red cells are trapped and broken up in the spleen, while others hemolyze in blood.
   2. **Autoimmune hemolytic anemia:** Autoimmune antibodies damage the structural proteins.
   3. **Toxic chemicals, poisons, infections, and some drugs (aspirin):** These agents make the red cells more fragile in some individuals.
   4. **Deficiency of glucose 6-phosphate dehydrogenase (G6PD):** This enzyme is required for glucose oxidation via hexose monophosphate pathway which generates NADPH. Normal red cells fragility is somehow dependent on NADPH. Deficiency of G6PD which is the most common human enzyme abnormality, increases the tendency of the red cells to hemolyze by antimalarial drugs and other agents.
   5. **The venom of cobra and some insects contains** lecithinase which dissolves lecithin from red cell membranes, thus making them more fragile.

B. **Decreased red cell fragility:** It is seen in acholuric jaundice and some anemias. The increase in red cell size in pernicious anemia makes them less osmotically fragile as compared to normal red cells. However, their mechanical fragility is greater than normal, as a result of which they hemolyze in blood and in spleen. Some of the conditions leading to decreased osmotic fragility are chronic liver disease, iron deficiency anemia, thalassemia, hyponatremia (Na < 130 mEq/L), polycythemia vera, and sickle cell anemia after splenectomy.

Q.9. What are the complications of hemolysis occurring in the circulating blood?

The Hb released from red cells will increase the osmotic pressure of blood thereby affecting tissue fluid exchanges. Further, if the tubular fluid is acidic, acid hematin crystals may be precipitated in the renal tubules and cause renal damage.

Q.10. Name some hemolytic agents.

Some of the hemolytic agents are:

- Hypotonic saline
- Incompatible blood transfusion
- Snake venom
- Severe infection
- Reaction to certain drugs. Aspirin is a common drug that may cause hemolysis at any time.

Q.11. What is the effect of 5% glucose, 10% glucose, urea solution of any strength, and urine on red cells?

- **5% glucose:** It is isotonic with blood (and plasma). The RBCs do not show any change in size or shape.
- **10% glucose:** Since it is hypertonic, the red cells will shrink due to exosmosis (water moving out). However, in the intact body, when 10% or even 20% glucose is given intravenously, the RBCs will shrink in the beginning. But later on, after some time, glucose gets metabolized and there are no harmful effects.
- **Urea solution:** As urea tends to move into the red cells, this is followed by water. The final result is hemolysis.
- **Urine:** Since urine is hypotonic, the red cells imbibe some water and swell up. In a highly concentrated urine sample, the red cells shrink to some extent.

Q.12. When does hemolysis occur in the body?

Hemolysis of red cells within the bloodstream may occur in many different ways. It may be due to *intrinsic causes* such as structural abnormalities (hereditary spherocytosis, sickle cells) or *extrinsic causes* e.g. mismatched blood transfusion, bacterial toxins, chemicals, adverse drug reactions, venom of snake and insects.

Q.13. Name some isotonic solutions.

Isotonic solutions of medical interest are:

- Sodium bromide: 1.5%
- Magnesium sulfate: 3.3%
- Sodium chloride: 0.9%
- Sodium nitrate: 2.5%
- Dextrose: 5%
- Sucrose: 10%
- Sodium bicarbonate: 0.9%.

Q.14. Do all the normal RBCs in a person or in a sample of blood have similar osmotic fragility?

The red cells in a person or in a sample of blood vary in their osmotic fragility because they belong to many generations. Younger cells are more resistant, while older cells are more osmotically and mechanically fragile (The old and worn out cells fragment in the circulation and are taken up by the Reticuloendothelial System). After removal of spleen, the cells become flat which decreases the volume to surface ratio, thereby decreasing osmotic fragility.

Q.15. Enumerate the physical factors affecting osmotic fragility test.

The physical factors affecting osmotic fragility test are:

1. Final *pH* of blood in saline: The fragility of RBCs increased by a fall in pH. A shift of 0.1 of a pH unit is equivalent to altering saline concentration by 0.01 g%.
2. The *relative volume* of blood in saline.
3. *Temperature:* A rise in temperature decreases the fragility, a rise of 0.5°C is equivalent to an increase in saline concentration of 0.01 g/dL.

1.17: DETERMINATION OF SPECIFIC GRAVITY OF BLOOD

STUDENT OBJECTIVES

After completing this experiment, the student should be able to:
- Define specific gravity and indicate the specific gravities of blood, plasma, and serum.
- Tell the clinical significance of this test.
- List the principle of determination of specific gravity of blood by Philips and Van Slyke's $CuSO_4$ method.
- List the factors and conditions affecting specific gravity of blood.

INTRODUCTION

- *Specific Gravity (SG)* is the ratio of the weight of a given volume of a fluid to the weight of the same volume of distilled water, measured at 25°C.
- The specific gravity of serum and plasma depends on the protein concentration. If water and plasma protein concentration are normal, the specific gravity of blood is dependent on the red cell volume (Hct), and therefore, the Hb concentration.
- The various methods used for determining the specific gravity of blood are:
  - **Direct method:** Equal volumes of blood and water taken in capillary tubes called pycnometers are weighed. The ratio of their weights determines the specific gravity of blood.
  - **Indirect method:** There are two methods:
    1. **Hammerschlag's method (chloroform-benzene mixture):** In this method, the densities of the two miscible (for example, chloroform—specific gravity 1.470 and benzene specific gravity 0.88) are equalized to match that of blood to determine the specific gravity.
    2. **Philips and Van Slyke's $CuSo_4$ method:** The procedure essentially involves comparing the specific gravity of blood, plasma, or serum against the specific gravity of a series of $CuSO_4$ solutions. After the specific gravity has been determined, line charts (or tables) are consulted to read off the concentration values.

PHILIPS AND VAN SLYKE'S $CuSO_4$ METHOD

This is the *most commonly used method.*

Principle

The specific gravity of blood is compared with the solutions of $CuSO_4$ with known specific gravity.

Apparatus

1. Well-stoppered bottles of 150 mL capacity—20 in number.
2. **Stock solution of copper sulfate** (specific gravity = 1.100) is prepared by dissolving 159.0 g of $CuSO_4.5H_2O$ in 1.0 liter of distilled water at 25°C. Its specific gravity can be checked by weighing 100 mL of the solution in a volumetric flask, against distilled water.
3. Syringe and needle "Pasteur pipette". Sterile swabs moist with alcohol.

Note: The procedure for estimation of plasma proteins and Hb concentrations is the same. Plasma or serum is obtained from a sample of venous blood. The "copper sulfate ($CuSO_4$) falling-drop method" is a rapid and accurate procedure for estimating plasma proteins and hemoglobin (Hb) concentrations, and hematocrit values in a large number of cases.

The test is useful in screening blood donors, and in handling emergency burn cases requiring plasma transfusions. The test is routinely done in many laboratories, and was used extensively during the Second World War.

4. **Standard copper sulfate solution for protein concentration. Table 20** shows the amounts of stock solution and distilled water to prepare 100 mL portions of the test solutions. The bottles are numbered 1 to 12, and the serial number, specific gravity, and protein concentration (g%) of each solution is indicated on the labels pasted on the bottles. Once prepared, the solutions can be used for 40–50 estimations.
5. **Standard copper sulfate solutions for hemoglobin concentration. Table 21** shows the amounts of stock solution and distilled water to prepare 100 mL portions of test solutions. The bottles are numbered 1 to 7, and the serial number, specific gravity, and Hb concentration of each solution are indicated on each bottle.

Procedure

1. Mix distilled water with the stock solution of $CuSO_4$, to prepare 10 mL of $CuSO_4$ solutions of specific gravity (SG) ranging from 1.050 to 1.066.
2. Mix each solution properly.
3. Allow a drop of blood to fall from a Pasteur pipette from a height of about 1 cm into each solution.
4. Observe the behavior of blood drop in the solution.
5. The blood drop will travel for some distance due to momentum:
   a. If the drop continues to sink, move to the next higher specific gravity solution.
   b. If it begins to rise, move to the lower specific gravity solution till you come to a solution where the drop remains stationary for about 15 seconds.

Note: When the plasma or blood drop falls into the solution, it becomes encased in a layer of copper proteinate and there is no change in its specific gravity for the next 15–20 seconds. This is the reason why the behavior of the drop is to be observed during this period. Within a short time, however, the drop becomes heavier and sinks to the bottom as a precipitate. In fact, the drops which initially float on the surface ultimately become heavier and settle down as shown in **Figure 49**.

Observation and Results

Note the SG of the solution in which the blood drop remains suspended for 15–20 secs. This gives the SG of the blood sample.

Table 20: Preparation of standard copper sulfate solutions for the determination of plasma protein concentration.

Bottle number	mL stock per 100 mL distilled water	Specific gravity	Protein concentration (g%)	Bottle number	mL stock per 100 mL distilled water	Specific gravity	Protein concentration (g%)
1	14.90	1.016	3.3	7	23.70	1.025	6.7
2	16.80	1.018	4.0	8	24.70	1.026	6.9
3	18.80	1.020	4.7	9	25.70	1.027	7.3
4	20.70	1.022	5.5	10	26.70	1.028	7.7
5	21.70	1.023	5.8	11	27.70	1.029	8.0
6	22.70	1.024	6.2	12	28.70	1.030	8.3

Table 21: Preparation of standard copper sulfate solutions for the determination of specific gravity of blood and hemoglobin concentration.

Bottle number	1	2	3	4	5	6	7
Stock solution (mL)	49	51	54	57	59	61	64
Distilled water (mL)	51	49	46	43	41	39	36
Specific gravity	1.050	1.052	1.055	1.058	1.060	1.062	1.065
Hb concentration (g%)	8.5	10.5	12.5	13.5	14.5	15.5	17

(Hb: hemoglobin)

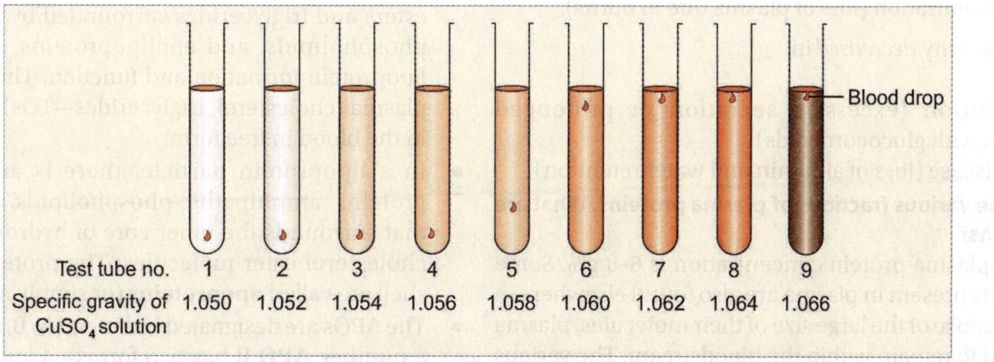

FIG. 49: Position of blood drop in $CuSO_4$ solutions ranging from SG 1.050 to 1.066.

Normal values:

The normal range of specific gravity of blood from 1.048 to 1.066.

Precautions

1. While preparing the stock solution, the ratio of water in copper sulphate must be measured accurately.
2. The reading should be taken within 15-20 seconds.
3. The drop of blood should fall from a Pasteur pipette from a height of about 1 cm into each solution.

QUESTIONS

Q.1. Define specific gravity. What is the specific gravity of serum, plasma, blood, and red blood corpuscles? What does the specific gravity of blood depend on?

- See text above
- The specific gravity of serum, plasma, blood and red cells is given in the **Table 22.**
- See text above

Q.2. What are the various methods of determining the specific gravity of blood?

See text above

Table 22: The specific gravity of serum, plasma, blood, and red cells.

	Specific gravity
Serum	1.22–1.024
Plasma	1.028–1.032
Blood	1.058–1.062
Red cells	1.092–1.095

Q.3. Why is copper sulfate method preferred over the other mixtures?

This method is chosen because the chemical is cheap, and it is not hygroscopic. Also, its temperature coefficient of expansion is about the same as that of blood. No correction factor for temperature is, therefore, required.

Q.4. What is the clinical significance of determining the specific gravity of serum, plasma, and blood?

- It is used to measure the hemoglobin content, PCV, blood proteins and degree of dehydration. It also gives an idea of hemoconcentration.
- The test is employed in the screening of blood donors, mass surveys for anemia and in handling emergency cases of burns requiring repeated transfusions of plasma, plasma expanders or blood.

Q.5. What are the physiological and pathological conditions in which the specific gravity of blood is increased and decreased?

The specific gravity of blood is affected by:

1. Red cell count
2. Hemoglobin concentration
3. Plasma (or serum) protein concentration
4. Water content of blood.

A. Physiological conditions:

It is *increased* in:

1. Newborns
2. At high altitude due to polycythemia.

It is *decreased* in:

1. Pregnancy (due to hemodilution)
2. After excess water intake.

B. Pathological conditions:

The specific gravity is *increased* in:

1. Polycythemia due to any disease (e.g. congenital heart disease, cardiac failure)
2. Polycythemia vera
3. Severe dehydration (diarrhea, vomiting)
4. Hemoconcentration (loss of plasma due to burns).

The specific gravity *decreased* in:

1. Anemias
2. Hemodilution (excessive secretion or prolonged treatment with glucocorticoids)
3. Kidney disease (loss of albumin and water retention)

Q.6. Name the various fractions of plasma proteins. What are their functions?

The normal plasma protein concentration is 6–8 g%. Some of the proteins present in plasma are also found elsewhere in the body. Because of the large size of their molecules, plasma proteins tend to remain within the bloodstream. The various fractions of plasma proteins are:

- Albumin = 4.0–5.5 g%
- Fibrinogen = 0.3–0.5 g%
- Globulins = 1.5–3.0 g%
- Prothrombin = 30–40 mg%.

Using filter paper electrophoresis, the patterns of serum proteins are:

- Albumin = 57%
- Alpha-1 globulin = 4.7%
- Alpha-2 globulin = 8.45%
- Beta-1 and beta-2 globulins = 11.33%
- Gamma globulins = 18.52%.

With the exception of gamma globulins which are synthesized in the plasma cells in lymphoid tissue, all the other proteins (albumin, fibrinogen, and some globulins) are synthesized in the liver.

Functions of plasma proteins: The proteins perform the following functions:

- **Osmotic pressure:** The osmotic pressure of plasma proteins called oncotic pressure is involved in tissue fluid exchanges.
- **Protein metabolic pool:** Though these proteins form part of the protein metabolic pool, they are not ordinarily used for providing energy.
- **Buffering function:** They exert about 15% of the buffering action of the blood (all proteins, including Hb are buffers). They function to convert strong acids or bases into weak acids or bases. Strong acid or bases ionize easily and can contribute many H^+ or OH^- ions, which can affect the pH to a great extent. Weak acids or bases do not ionize as much and thus contribute fewer H^+ or OH^- ions.
- **Viscosity of blood:** The plasma proteins contribute to the viscosity of blood and so affect the blood pressure.
- **Coagulation of blood:** Fibrinogen, prothrombin, and many clotting factors form part of the clotting mechanism.
- **Role as carriers:** They act as carriers in the transport of many substances, such as hormones, metals, calcium, ions, amino acids, bilirubin, vitamin B_{12}, drugs, etc. Binding these substances prevents their rapid clearance from the body by the kidneys. Major lipids do not circulate in the free form but in combination with plasma proteins.

Q.7. What are lipoproteins? What are their functions and clinical significance?

- **Definition:** A lipoprotein is a complex biochemical assembly with a central core containing cholesterol esters and triglycerides surrounded by free cholesterol, phospholipids, and apolipoproteins, which facilitate lipoprotein formation and function. The major lipids in plasma (cholesterol, triglycerides—TGs) do not circulate in the blood in free form.
- In a lipoprotein particle, there is an outer coat of proteins, amphipathic phospholipids, and cholesterol that surrounds the inner core of hydrophobic TGs and cholesterol ester molecules. The proteins in the outer shell are called **apoproteins** (or simply **APO).**
- The APOs are designated by letters (A, B, C, D, and E) plus a number. **APO B** has two forms—a low mw form, APO B-48 that transports ingested lipids, and a high mw form, APO B-100, which transports endogenous lipids. Their levels have clinical significance in atherosclerosis. APO E concentration greatly increases in nerve injuries and is concerned with the repair process.
- **Functions of lipoproteins:** There are several types of lipoproteins each having a different function. However, all are mainly transport vehicles functioning as a sort of pick-up and delivery service. They are classified on the basis of density that varies with the ratio of lipids (they have low density) to proteins (they have a high density). Thus, the lipoproteins are grouped in, from largest and lightest to smallest and heaviest, the following groups—**very low, low, intermediate, and high-density lipoproteins.**
- **Clinical significance:** Their clinical significance lies in relation to coronary artery disease, and atherosclerosis (a form of arteriosclerosis).
- The **low-density lipoproteins (LDLs)** carry about 50% of cholesterol. They transport cholesterol from the liver to body cells for use in repair of cell membranes and production of steroid hormones and bile salts. However, excess LDLs promote atherosclerosis, so that their cholesterol is called "bad cholesterol".

- The **high-density lipoproteins (HDLs)** contain about 20% cholesterol. They remove and carry excess cholesterol from body cells to the liver for elimination. Since, they lower blood cholesterol level, their cholesterol is called "good cholesterol".

The desirable levels of various lipoproteins **(Table 23)**.

Table 23: The desirable levels of various lipoproteins.

Lipid parameter	***Target***
LDL cholesterol	<100 mg/dL
In patients with overt CHD	<70 mg/dL
HDL cholesterol (men)	>40 mg/dL
HDL cholesterol (women)	>50 mg/dL
Triglycerides	<150 mg/dL
Total cholesterol	<200 mg/dL
Non-HDL cholesterol	<130 mg/dL
In patients with overt CHD	<100 mg/dL
Apolipoprotein B	<90 mg/dL
In patients with overt CHD	<80 mg/dL

1.18: DETERMINATION OF VISCOSITY OF BLOOD

VISCOSITY OF BLOOD

Viscosity which represents the mutual attraction between the particles of a fluid is the internal friction or "lack of slipperiness" between the adjacent layers especially between the outermost layer of the flowing blood and the walls. The shape of the molecules rather than their size determines the viscosity.

The viscosity of blood depends mostly on the ratio of red cells to plasma (fluid) volume and to a lesser extent on the plasma protein concentration. The viscosity of blood in vivo especially in the microvessels is about 1.2 (water = 0.695) because of axial streaming of red cells (Fahraeus-Lindqvist effect).

Apparatus

Viscosimeter (Viscometer) The viscosimeter is a U-shaped glass tube, one limb of which is wider with a bulb near its lower end. The other limb has a bulb near its upper end and a narrow capillary bore below it. There are two markings, 1 and 2, above and below the bulb in this limb.

PROCEDURE

The limb with the wide tube is filled with anticoagulated blood; the blood is then sucked up into the narrow limb to above the mark 1. The time taken by the blood to fall from mark 1 to mark 2 is noted. The procedure is then repeated with water and is compared with that of blood. The apparatus must be kept vertical throughout the experiment. **Normal viscosity of blood** = About 3–4 times that of water, i.e. its relative viscosity is 3–4.

Effect of Temperature on Viscosity

Temperature has an important effect on viscosity. Water has a viscosity of 1 cP [centipoise (after Poiseuille)—the unit of viscosity] at 20.3°C and about 1.8 cP at 0°C. The viscosity of plasma and blood is even more sensitive to changes in temperature. Thus, the temperature of skin and subcutaneous tissues exerts an important effect on the viscosity of blood.

Significance of Viscosity of Blood

The **viscosity** of blood is one of the three factors on which the resistance (i.e. the opposition) to flow of blood in the blood vessels depends, the other two being—**average radius of the blood vessels** and the **total blood vessel length.** Since resistance, in fact, peripheral resistance to blood flow is directly proportional to the viscosity of blood, any factor that affects viscosity will increase or decrease the blood pressure. In this way, variations in viscosity of blood influence the load to which the heart is subjected during contraction.

Increased viscosity is seen in polycythemia due to any cause, congestive heart failure, diabetes mellitus, multiple myeloma, icterus, profuse sweating when water intake is limited, severe vomiting and diarrhea, and leukemias.

Decreased viscosity is seen in anemias, edematous states, and sometimes in malaria.

Human Experiments

SECTION 2

UNIT I: RESPIRATORY SYSTEM

2.1: STETHOGRAPHY: RECORDING OF NORMAL AND MODIFIED MOVEMENTS OF RESPIRATION

STUDENT OBJECTIVES

After completing this experiment, the student should be able to:

- Define stethography.
- Explain how the movements of breathing can be recorded.
- Define various terms used in connection with respiratory movements.
- Give an account of the physiological basis of how normal breathing is maintained and controlled.
- Describe the effect of hyperventilation and breath-holding on respiration.
- Explain why ventilation increases during muscular exercise.
- List the factors that cause "breaking point" after voluntary breath-holding.

INTRODUCTION

- **Stethography** is the *process of recording respiratory movements with the help of a stethograph*. The respiratory movements, i.e. inspiration and expiration are brought about by the activity of respiratory neurons in the brainstem, which in turn controls the activity of the respiratory muscles.
- The discharge of brainstem is in turn modified by the various inputs converging on the brainstem neurons (e.g. speech, swallowing, coughing, biochemical alterations on blood, emotions, proprioceptive impulses, etc.).
- The recording of movements of the chest by stethography can be taken as an index of respiratory activity.

PRINCIPLE

Working of a stethograph: Because of the corrugation of the rubber tubing of the stethograph, the mean radius of the tube remains unchanged when it is stretched during chest expansion. This leads to an increase in its volume and a fall in pressure within it. This is transmitted to the tambour where the higher atmospheric pressure pushes the diaphragm, and along with it, the writing lever downward. Thus, the downstroke of the lever is inspiration, while upstroke is expiration.

APPARATUS AND MATERIALS

1. **Stethograph:** It consists of corrugated canvas-rubber tubing about 60 cm long and 3–4 cm in diameter. It has a hook and chain device for tying it across the chest wall. One end of the stethograph is closed while the other end can be connected via pressure rubber tubing to an air recording system, as shown in **Figures 1A and B**.
2. **Marey's or Brodie's tambour:** The tambour is a metallic cup or a small flat saucer with a rubber diaphragm stretched over its top. A light-metal capillary writing lever is mounted on a small metal disc that rests on the diaphragm. A rubber tube attached to an outlet connects the tambour to the stethograph.
3. **Kymograph:**
4. Stop watch, tap water in a cup, time marker, polythene bag of 5–6 liters capacity.

PROCEDURES

- Seat the patient on a stool with her/his back to the recording apparatus, and ask her to relax and breathe normally.
- Tie the stethograph around the patient's chest at a level where respiratory movements are maximum (usually midchest at 4th–5th intercostal space).
- Slightly stretch the stethograph so that respiratory movements can cause adequate pressure changes within the stethograph.
- Mount the tambour on the stand and connect the stethograph to it. Bring the writing point in contact with the drum surface at a tangent.
- Set the kymograph at a slow speed of 2.5 mm/sec, and record a few respiratory movements. Note that as the chest expands during inspiration, the stethograph gets stretched and its length increases.

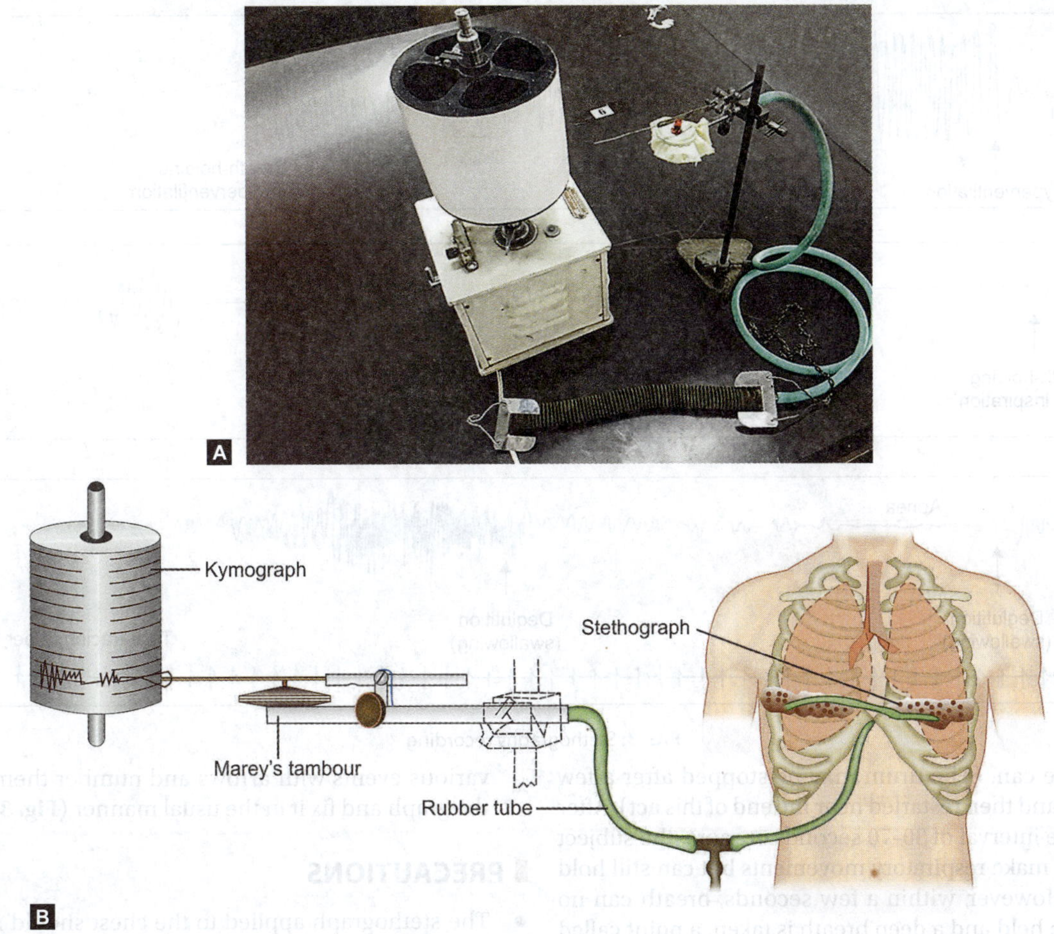

FIGS. 1A AND B: Stethograph.

Note the following:
i. Rate of breathing (this you will record after obtaining a time tracing)
ii. Relative duration of inspiration and expiration
iii. Presence or absence of a gap between one inspiration and the next expiration, and between one expiration and the next inspiration.

OBSERVATIONS

- **Effect of deglutition (swallowing):** Ask the subject to take a mouthful of water, and while movements are being recorded to swallow it. After a few respiratory movements, ask him/her to drink water from the cup in one go. Note that there is a temporary stoppage of breathing in both cases a condition is called **"deglutition apnea"** (apnea = temporary stoppage of respiration) **(Fig. 2).**
- **Effect of modified respiratory movements:** Record the effect of coughing, sneezing, talking, singing, laughing, yawning, sobbing, and Valsalva maneuver on respiratory movements giving a 2–3 minutes interval between each act.
- **Effect of breath-holding:** See next experiment on breath-holding time. Ask the subject to take a deep breath, close the nose and mouth, and then to hold breath for as long

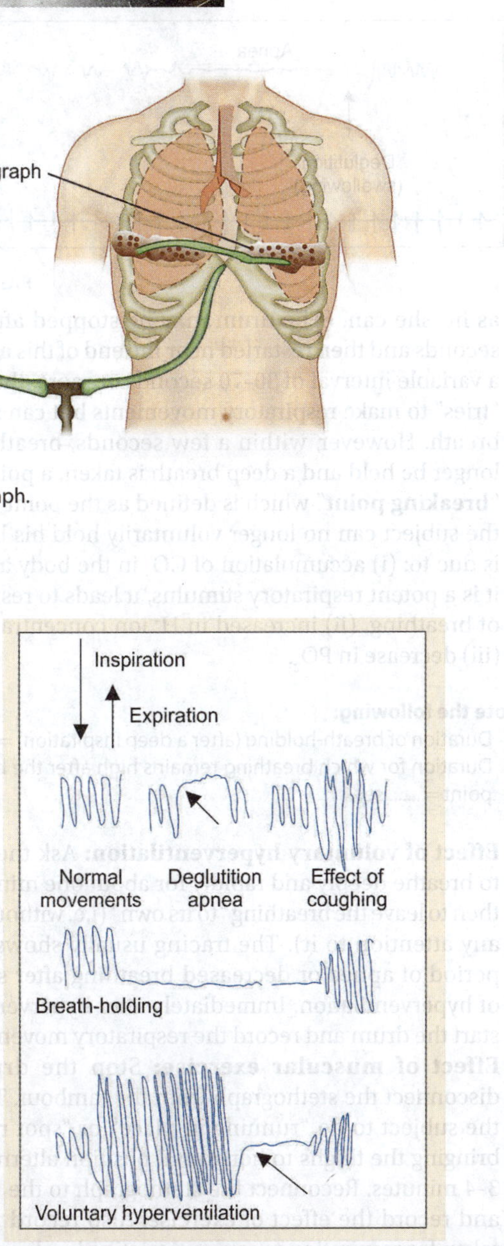

FIG. 2: Stethography. Recording of normal and modified movements of respiration.

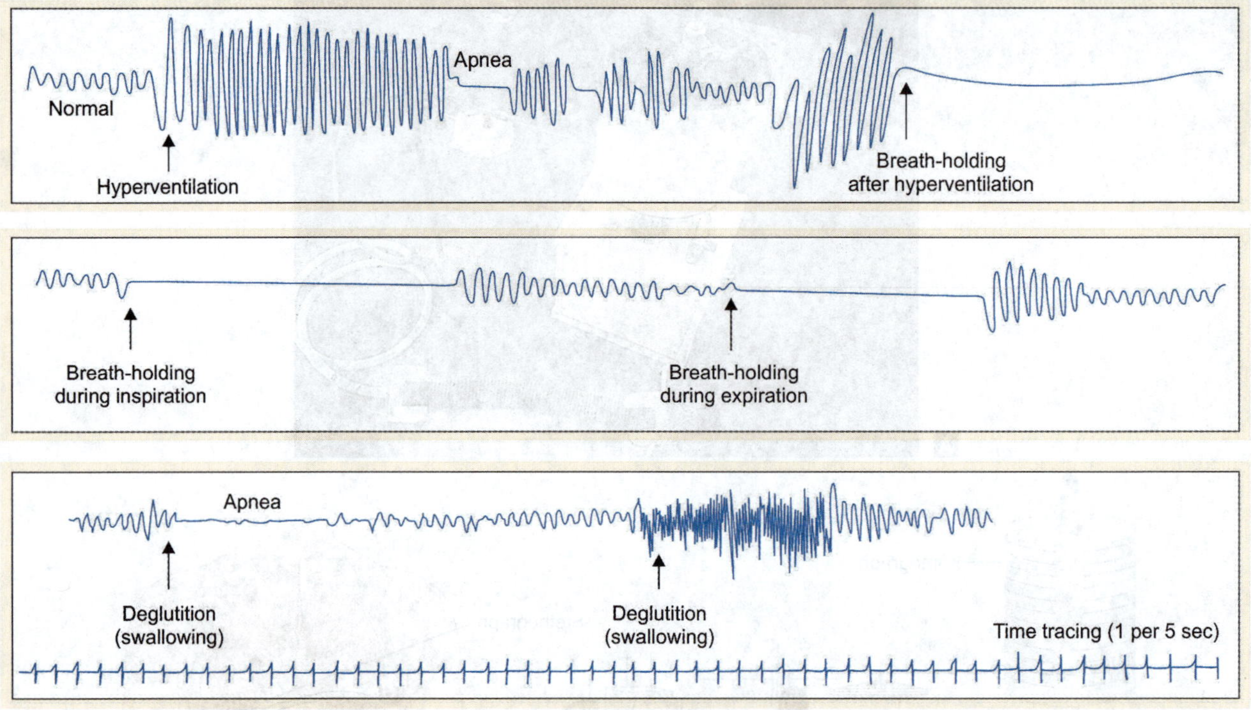

FIG. 3: Stethography recording.

as he/she can. (The drum may be stopped after a few seconds and then restarted near the end of this act). After a variable interval of 30–70 seconds or more, the subject "tries" to make respiratory movements but can still hold breath. However, within a few seconds, breath can no longer be held and a deep breath is taken, a point called **"breaking point"** which is defined as the point at which the subject can no longer voluntarily hold his breath. It is due to: (i) accumulation of CO_2 in the body and since it is a potent respiratory stimulus, it leads to resumption of breathing, (ii) increased in H^+ ion concentration and (iii) decrease in PO_2.

> **Note the following:**
> i. Duration of breath-holding (after a deep inspiration) = ... sec.
> ii. Duration for which breathing remains high after the breaking point = ... sec.

- **Effect of voluntary hyperventilation:** Ask the subject to breathe deeply and rapidly for about one minute, and then to leave the breathing "to its own" (i.e. without paying any attention to it). The tracing usually shows a short period of apnea or decreased breathing after stoppage of hyperventilation. Immediately after hyperventilation, start the drum and record the respiratory movements.
- **Effect of muscular exercise:** Stop the drum and disconnect the stethograph from the tambour. Then ask the subject to do "running in place" or "spot running", bringing the thighs to horizontal position alternately for 3–4 minutes. Reconnect the stethograph to the tambour and record the effect of exercise. Also record the time taken for respiration to return to resting levels.
- Record a 5 second time interval below the graph obtained, keeping the kymograph speed unchanged. Indicate various events with arrows and number them. Remove the graph and fix it in the usual manner **(Fig. 3)**.

PRECAUTIONS

- The stethograph applied to the chest should not be too tight nor too loose.
- Do not let the subject look at the tracings being obtained.
- Do not allow the subject to hyperventilate for more than 2 minutes or so. Record a few normal movements before each maneuver.
- Before and after each recording, normal tracings should be taken.
- The stethograph should be disconnected from the tambour during exercise.
- Recording should be taken immediately after exercise.

QUESTIONS

Q.1. What is meant by the terms—ventilation, eupnea, tachypnea, bradypnea, hyperpnea, hypercapnia and hypocapnia, hypoxia, and asphyxia?

- The term **ventilation** means movement of air into and out of the lungs.
- The term **eupnea** means normal breathing.
- **Apnea** is a temporary stoppage of respiration (breathing; the terms respiration and breathing refer to the process of breathing).
- **Tachypnea** and **bradypnea** refers to increased and decreased rate of respiration. The term **hyperpnea** refers to increased ventilation (above the resting value of 6–8 liters per minute) whether due to increased rate, or depth, or both rate and depth.

- The terms **hypercapnia** and **hypocapnia** refer to increased and decreased CO_2 in the body, i.e. retention or washing out of CO_2.
- **Hypoxia** refers to decreased oxygen supply at the tissue level, while **asphyxia** means excess of CO_2 and lack of oxygen in the body.
- **Asphyxia** is a lack of oxygen or excess of carbon dioxide in the body that results in unconsciousness and often death and is usually caused by interruption of breathing or inadequate oxygen supply.

Q.2. What is the working principle of a stethograph?
See text above.

Q.3. Is breathing (respiration) an automatic process or a voluntary act? How is normal respiration maintained and controlled?
Respiration is both a spontaneous (automatic) process (i.e. without any conscious effort or being aware of it), as well as a voluntary activity. When we are not/or do not become aware of our breathing (such as during sleep and while we are at our daily tasks), it goes on automatically and spontaneously. However, we can become aware of our breathing whenever we want to or think about it; then we can increase or decrease, or even stop our breathing at least for a short time.

- **Spontaneous or automatic breathing:** The alternate contraction and relaxation of respiratory muscles (diaphragm, intercostals, etc.) brings about changes in the size of the thorax; as a result of which air enters and leaves the lungs. These muscles which are striated, skeletal, or voluntary are rhythmically stimulated by impulses in their motor nerve supply (phrenics and intercostal nerves). These motor nerves have no activity of their own but are activated by a rhythmic discharge of impulses (depolarization and repolarization) from the **"medullary rhythmicity area"**, which is a part of the respiratory center in the brainstem. Thus, the medullary rhythmicity area sets up the basic rhythm of inspiration and expiration.
- **Voluntary control of respiration:** The voluntary control over breathing is exerted via the corticospinal (pyramidal) tracts that control voluntary muscle activity throughout the body. The axons of these tracts (upper motor neurons) descend from the cerebral motor cortex, bypass the brainstem respiratory center and end on phrenic and other neurons that innervate respiratory muscles.

Maintenance and control of respiration: Respiration is maintained by the rhythmic discharge of impulses from the medullary rhythmicity area. The activity of this center is controlled by a variety of inputs. These inputs include—cerebral cortex, hypothalamus (emotions affect our respiration), central and peripheral chemoreceptors, baroreceptors, stretch receptors in the lungs, and muscles, joints, and ligaments.

Q.4. Why should the subject not look at the tracings being obtained?
Respiratory movements are easily affected by our becoming aware of them—their rate, depth, rhythm, etc. If the subject looks at the record being obtained, he/she will become conscious (aware) of it so that the movements are bound to change and not represent the true effects of various maneuvers.

Q.5. What is deglutition apnea? Describe its mechanism and physiological significance.

- **Definition:** This term refers to a **temporary stoppage** of breathing when we swallow food or fluids. It is a reflex phenomenon, and occurs automatically whether we swallow a sip of a drink, or drink a cupful of water. During the pharyngeal stage of deglutition which may last for 0.5 second or more, the food or fluid stimulates the sensory nerve endings of touch in the mucosa of pharynx.
- **Mechanism:** Afferent nerve impulses are set up and relayed along the 5th, 9th, and 10th cranial nerves and cause via the deglutition center, inhibition of respiratory center. This stops the breathing **at any point of inspiration or expiration**. Simultaneously, there is a closure of glottis, the opening between vocal cords.
- **Physiological significance of deglutition apnea:** The stoppage of breathing and closure of glottis prevents the entry of food or fluid into the upper respiratory passages, which would cause aspiration pneumonia or other complications (it is a common experience that whenever a particle of food or fluid tends to enter our respiratory passages, there is a strong bout of coughing till the offending particle is expelled; all this happens reflexly).

Q.6. What is the "breaking point" and what is its cause?
See text above.

Q.7. What is hyperventilation, and what are its effects? Are there any harmful effects if it is carried on for long?

- Hyperventilation refers to increased volume of air moving into and out of the lungs per unit time—whether due to increase in rate, depth or both. It can result from:
  1. **Voluntary effort:** This is the most powerful stimulus for increasing the ventilation.
  2. **Muscular exercise:** It is the second most powerful respiratory stimulus.
  3. **Chemical stimuli:** High PCO_2, low PO_2 or increased H^+ ion concentration resulting from lung and heart diseases can increase the ventilation.
     - While the chemical stimuli increase the ventilation to about 80–90 liters/minute, (from the resting level of 6–8 liters/minute), voluntary hyperventilation can achieve rates of over 200 liters/minute at least for short periods.
- **Effects of voluntary hyperventilation:**
  - When a person hyperventilates for 1–2 minutes and then stops and allows respiration to continue on its own without exerting any control over it, there is a short period of apnea. This is followed by a few breaths and then a period of apnea once again followed by a few breaths. The cycle may last for a while before returning to normal rhythm.
  - The apnea is due to washing out of CO_2 (hypocapnia), but as CO_2 accumulates, the breathing starts again. (Though CO_2 is a "waste" product of metabolism, it is a "stimulus par excellence" for respiration. Thus, while a high PCO_2 stimulates breathing, a low PCO_2 inhibits it until the blood PCO_2 returns to normal).

- **Harmful effects of hyperventilation:**
  - Though a single bout of hyperventilation may have no ill effects, chronic hyperventilation as seen in neurotic patients may produce certain ill effects. The arterial PCO_2 may fall from the normal level of 40 mm Hg to 15–20 mmHg. This degree of hypocapnia produces vasoconstriction of cerebral blood vessels. (CO_2 is a very strong vasodilator, so its lack will result in vasoconstriction). The cerebral ischemia causes dizziness, lightheadedness, etc. Constriction of retinal blood vessels may cause blurring of vision.
  - A more serious effect of chronic hyperventilation and associated hypocapnia is alkalosis which causes precipitation of ionic calcium. If the serum calcium is already low, an attack of tetany may be precipitated. (Calcium stabilizes cell membranes; low ECF calcium increases membrane permeability to sodium ions which in turn cause spontaneous depolarizations.) As a result, there are extensive tetanic spasms of the skeletal muscles especially in limbs and larynx.

Q.8. What is the cause of increased ventilation during exercise?

A variety of factors are involved in increasing the ventilation during exercise.

1. **Psychic stimuli:** Ventilation often increases in anticipation of the exercise, i.e. before the exercise has started. Soon after the start of exercise, and before blood PCO_2, PO_2 and H^+ ions have time to change, there is a sudden and large increase in ventilation (mainly due to increase in depth) due to the next two factors mentioned below.
2. **Impulses from motor cerebral cortex:** As the motor cortex sends impulses via corticospinal tracts to the motor neurons of active muscles, it also sends via collaterals of the tracts, excitatory impulses to the respiratory center (as it does to vasomotor center). The result is a sudden increase in ventilation.
3. **Impulses from proprioceptors:** Body movements, especially those of the limbs, stimulate the proprioceptors (stretch receptors) in the active muscles, tendons, ligaments, joints, etc. These excitatory impulses are also relayed to the respiratory center (it is important to note that even passive movements of the limbs increase the ventilation).
4. **Chemical stimuli:** Normally, the increased ventilation is enough to supply the extra O_2 to the active muscles, as well as to remove the excess of CO_2 produced without any significant change in arterial PO_2 and PCO_2 especially in trained athletes. In fact, the PO_2 may be higher and PCO_2 lower than the normal. Thus, low PO_2 and high PCO_2 cannot explain respiratory stimulation during exercise. Sometimes, the neural signals may be too weak to stimulate the respiratory center; it is then that the chemical stimuli play a role. Also, in later stages of severe exercise, it is the chemical stimuli that increase the ventilation. (Even though there may be no gas changes, the sensitivity of the respiratory center to the normal levels may be involved).
5. **Other factors:** Increased body temperature, increased blood K^+, lactic acidosis, hypoxia in exercising muscles stimulating the sensory nerve endings, fluctuations in blood gases—all help in increasing the ventilation.

Q.9. Why does ventilation and oxygen utilization remain high after the end of exercise?

- During moderately severe and severe muscular exercise, the muscles obtain their energy from anaerobic (i.e. in the absence of O_2) metabolism of glucose which results in the formation of lactic acid. The buffering of lactate liberates more CO_2 which further stimulates respiration. After the end of exercise, however, ventilation and O_2 utilization remain high until the "oxygen debt" incurred during anaerobic glycolysis is repaid, i.e. the lactate is converted back to pyruvate when O_2 supply is restored after exercise.
- The cause of increased ventilation after exercise is, thus, not high PCO_2 (which is normal or low), or low PO_2 (which is normal or high) but the increased arterial H^+ ion concentration due to lactic acidemia.

Q.10. What is periodic breathing?

- Periodic breathing is a disturbance of respiratory control where periods of apnea alternate with periods of increased respiration. This waxing and waning of breathing begins with shallow breaths which gradually increase in depth, each phase lasting 20–30 seconds. This is called **Cheyne-Stokes breathing.**
- Various irregular forms such as **Biot's breathing** (also known as ataxic breathing—is a breathing pattern in patients with acute neurological disease), Kussmaul's breathing, sleep apnea syndrome, etc. are also seen. It is generally a sign of brain damage, increased intracranial pressure, congestive heart failure, uremia, etc.

Q.11. What is the Valsalva maneuver? Explain its significance, and effect on breathing.

- **Valsalva maneuver** is forced expiration against a closed glottis. Brief periods of straining and forced expiration, such as during defecation, urination, trying to lift a heavy weight, etc. are a common experience. A deep breath is taken, and the expiratory muscles of chest and abdomen are forcefully contracted while keeping glottis closed so that air cannot leave the lungs.
- The raised pressures have important effects on venous return and blood pressure.
- The record of respiratory movements shows a deeper inspiration than normal, and then stoppage of breathing during expiration. The tracing may show a downward shift.

OBJECTIVE STRUCTURED PRACTICAL EXAMINATION

Aim: To record the respiratory movements of the subject provided.

Procedural steps: See text above.

Checklist:

1. Checks out the apparatus. (Y/N)
2. Seats the subject on a stool with his back to the recording apparatus. Tells him to relax, and explains the procedure. (Y/N)

3. Ties the stethograph firmly around his mid-chest and connects it to the tambour. (Y/N)
4. Sets the kymograph at slow speed (1.2 mm/sec) and records a few respiratory movements. (Y/N)
5. Using a signal marker, records the time tracing below the graph. (Y/N)

DETERMINATION OF BREATH-HOLDING TIME

Different individuals can hold their breath for variable periods of time depending on the functional status of the lungs, development of respiratory muscles, practice, age and sex. Determination of breath-holding time (BHT) is a simple test which can provide useful information in health, and diseases of the lungs.

Procedures

1. The subject should sit quietly for a few minutes, breathing normally. The procedure should be explained to the subject in clear terms. Use a stopwatch and note the time for each determination.
2. Ask the subject to pinch his/her nostrils with the thumb and forefinger, and hold his/her breath after a quiet inspiration. Note the time for which the breath can be held. Make three observations at intervals of 5 minutes.
3. Using the same procedure, record the BHT after (a) a quiet expiration, (b) a deep inspiration, (c) a deep expiration, (d) hyperventilation (deep and fast breathing) for 1–2 minutes, (e) rebreathing from a polythene bag for 15–20 seconds with a nose clip on (discontinue if there is discomfort), and (f) 8–10 deep breaths of pure oxygen from Benedict-Roth apparatus.
4. Tabulate your results as shown here. The highest value for each determination is the BHT for that exercise.

Observations and Results

- Explain the results from the following data (**Table 1**).

Table 1: Observations and results of breath-holding.

Breath-holding after.......		***Readings (in sec)***
a.	Quiet inspiration	
b.	Quiet expiration	
c.	Deep inspiration	
d.	Deep expiration	
e.	Hyperventilation	

QUESTIONS

Q.1. Why cannot a person hold his/her breath for periods longer than a minute or so? What is the cause of the breaking point?

- The normal level of CO_2 in the body (arterial PCO_2 of 40 mm Hg) is just sufficient to maintain a resting ventilation of 6–8 liters/min. This degree of ventilation is enough to supply adequate amounts of O_2 to the tissues at rest. Any increase in ventilation by high PCO_2 (or low PO_2) or other stimuli shows that the "ventilatory drive" has increased (i.e. the medullary respiratory center has been stimulated). On the other hand, the cerebral cortex can temporarily allow voluntary breath-holding, and thus oppose the ventilatory drive.
- Thus, two opposing factors are operating during breath-holding: The **ventilatory drive, and voluntary stoppage of breathing**. Since the ability to hold breath remains unchanged in a normal person, the "breaking point", i.e. the point when a breath has to be taken is reached when the ventilatory drive is so strong that it overcomes the desire to continue to hold breath. (It is interesting to note that the world record for breath-holding is 5 min 13 sec). It is also obvious that a person cannot commit suicide by holding breath because breathing will begin even if that person losses consciousness.

Note: Usually, the breaking point is reached when the arterial (and alveolar) PCO_2 increases from the normal 40 mm Hg to about 60 mm Hg, and the PO_2 falls from the normal 100 mm Hg to about 50 mm Hg.

Q.2. What is the effect of prolonged hyperventilation on breath-holding time?

Hyperventilation washes out CO_2 from the body so that both PCO and H^+ ion concentration decrease. At the same time, there is some increase in PO_2. Therefore, it will take some more time for these chemical stimuli to increase the ventilatory drive so that it reaches the breaking point.

Q.3. What are the factors that increase and decrease the BHT?

- The normal BHT after a deep inspiration may vary from 40 sec to over a minute.
- It can be increased by practicing breathing exercises as part of yoga training. Breathing pure O_2 before holding breath delays the breaking point. Hyperventilation increases BHT as described above. Reflex or mechanical factors also affect BHT. Psychological factors such as motivation (e.g. telling the subject that his performance is improving, increases the BHT).
- Breath-holding time decreases in many diseases, e.g. chronic bronchitis, emphysema, congestive heart failure, and so on.

Q.4. What are breath-holding attacks?

- Breath-holding attacks occur in *infants and young children* and are generally precipitated by emotional distress such as fright, pain, anxiety, or frustration. The child starts crying, and suddenly holds his/her breath, becomes limp or stiff and may become blue and lose consciousness.
- The attack lasts briefly and recovery is rapid and complete. In some cases, there may be a rigid phase followed by tonic-clonic convulsions. These attacks are harmless and stop by the age of 3 years; they are not considered epileptic in origin.

2.2: PULMONARY FUNCTION TESTS

STUDENT OBJECTIVES

After completing this experiment, the student should be able to:

- Determine various lung volumes and capacities.
- Explain the difference between the lung capacities and volumes.
- Calculate maximum voluntary ventilation (MVV) and minute ventilation (MV) by spirometry.
- Indicate the differences between static and dynamic lung volumes and capacities.
- Define "timed vital capacity" and indicate its significance.
- Define peak expiratory flow rate and explain its clinical significance.

INTRODUCTION

PY6.8: Demonstrate the correct technique to perform and interpret Spirometry.

- Pulmonary function tests (PFTs) are noninvasive tests that show how well the lungs are working. The tests measure lung volume, capacity, and rate of flow and gas exchange. This information can help the healthcare provider to diagnose and decide treatment of certain lung disorders.
- Though a large number of PFTs are possible, many of them are highly sophisticated and are carried out in special cases for research work. A few comparatively simple tests can provide useful information in most cases of lung diseases.
- These tests help the physician to make a physiological assessment of lung function rather than a pathological diagnosis which the physician has in most cases already arrived at during clinical examination.

PHYSIOCLINICAL SIGNIFICANCE OF PULMONARY FUNCTION TESTS

Tests for pulmonary functions are employed to:

1. Assess the normal functioning of the lungs.
2. Evaluate the physical fitness and effects of physical training.
3. Reach a diagnosis when a patient complains of dyspnea (breathlessness) and to assess the degree of disability.
4. Follow the progress of disease and the effectiveness of treatment.
5. Assess respiratory status before anesthesia and cardiothoracic surgery especially if a lung is to be removed.
6. Determine the incidence of respiratory dysfunction in the community and workers in hazardous industries.
7. Obtain medico-legal information and opinion in certain situations, e.g. claim for lung damage in a hazardous occupation.

SIMPLE BEDSIDE TESTS TO ASSESS LUNG FUNCTION

1. **Chest expansion and respiratory rate:** Measure the chest expansion with a tape placed around the chest just below the level of nipples. The normal chest expands by 5–10 cm following a deep inspiration after a forceful expiration (See Experiment 3.2).
2. **Breath-holding time:** (See Experiment 2.1).
3. **Respiratory endurance test (40 mm Hg test):** A BP apparatus is required for this test. Disconnect the rubber tube leading from the mercury reservoir to the BP cuff. Ask the subject to take a deep breath, pinch his nostrils, and exhale into the tube, raising the mercury to 40 mm level and to hold it there for as long as possible. Normal = 40–70 seconds or more.
4. **Snider's test:** Hold a burning matchstick about 12 inches in front of the subject's face and ask him to blow it out with a single forceful expiration.

CLASSIFICATION OF PULMONARY FUNCTION TESTS

The PFTs are employed to assess the three basic processes involved in the supply of O_2 to and removal of CO_2 from the body—***ventilation, diffusion,*** and ***perfusion of lungs***. Thus they can be classified on the basis of these tests:

1. Tests of ventilatory function
2. Tests to assess gas exchange function
3. Tests to assess the perfusion of lungs.

Tests of Ventilatory Function

Assessment of ventilatory function can be accomplished by:

a. Measurement of lung volumes and capacities
b. Measurement of dead space
c. Measurement of compliance
d. Measurement of airway resistance.

Measurement of Lung Volumes and Capacities

Most of the lung volumes and capacities can be measured using a recording spirometer.

Spirometry

Spirometry is a simple and useful technique for assessing the ventilatory functions of the lungs. It refers to the recording of volume changes during various clearly defined breathing maneuvers. It can be performed using a recording spirometer or computerized spirometer. Although spirometry is the standard technique, plethysmography can also be used as it is more accurate.

Recording spirometer

The **recording spirometer** is electrically driven, and is used to provide a graphic record (called **spirogram)** of various lung volumes and capacities. It is used routinely to assess some of the pulmonary functions in health and disease in physiological and clinical studies **(Fig. 4)**. It consists of:

1. ***Double-walled cylindrical chamber:*** It contains water between its two walls (as in vitalograph or simple spirometer; **Consult Experiment 2.3)** to maintain an airtight seal. A 9-liter lightweight metal "gas bell" dips into the water from above and floats in it. A chain attached to the top of the bell passes over a frictionless pulley and carries **a counter-weight and a pen writer**. As the volume of air increases and decreases, the writing point moves down and up on the surface of the paper that passes under it. This provides a continuous record of the displacement of air in the bell with each inspiration and expiration.
2. ***Soda lime tower:*** It is fitted within the spirometer and removes (absorbs) CO_2 from the expired air so that one can continue to breathe into and out of the spirometer (color change of soda lime from white to pink indicates that is near the point of exhaustion).
3. ***Kymograph:*** There is an on/off switch and a pilot lamp on the front of the apparatus. The paper assembly carries ***mm graph paper*** calibrated for both *volume of air* and *time*. The paper speed regulator has three markings: 60—0–1,200.
   i. 60 mm/min speed is for normal recordings.
   ii. 1,200 mm/min is for recording timed vital capacity.
   iii. The "zero" mark is for the "neutral" position of the kymograph at which the paper does not move.
4. ***Chart paper:*** It is calibrated for time along the X-axis, where 1 mm = 1 sec at the slower speed, and 20 mm = 1 sec at the faster speed. The calibration along the Y-axis is for volume where 1 mm movement of the pen writer (1 mm on the chart paper) represents 30 mL at both speeds. A slot on the side of the unit allows exit of recorded paper.
5. ***Breathing assembly:*** The breathing assembly has a mouthpiece which is connected to the spirometer via a Y piece by two rubber-canvas corrugated tubes, one carrying a unidirectional valve for inspiring air from the bell and the other carries a unidirectional valve for expiring air into the atmosphere. The third component of the assembly is a free-breathing valve which has a directional tap. The tap can be turned to permit a person either to breathe room air, or air from the spirometer bell **(Fig. 5)**.
6. Also provided are: ***Inlet*** for filling the gas bell with oxygen or any other gas. A ***tap*** for draining water out of the apparatus. A ***chart reverse knob*** can rewind the recorded chart paper by turning the knob clockwise. A ***nose clip*** is provided for closing the nostrils during recording.

Procedure

- Fill three-fourth of the space between the two walls of the chamber with water. Dip the gas bell from above into the water. Connect the valve to the atmosphere and wash and fill the gas bell with fresh air by slowly raising and lowering it 3–4 times.
- Seat the subject facing the spirometer and instruct her/him about the procedures that will be carried out. Insert the mouthpiece between the teeth and lips and apply a nose clip on the nostrils. Tell the subject to breathe through the mouth for about a minute to familiarize her/him with mouth breathing.
- Connect the subject to the spirometer and allow her/him to breathe quietly for a short time. Then start the kymograph at the speed of 60 mm/min and record the excursions of the pen writer for about a minute. Note

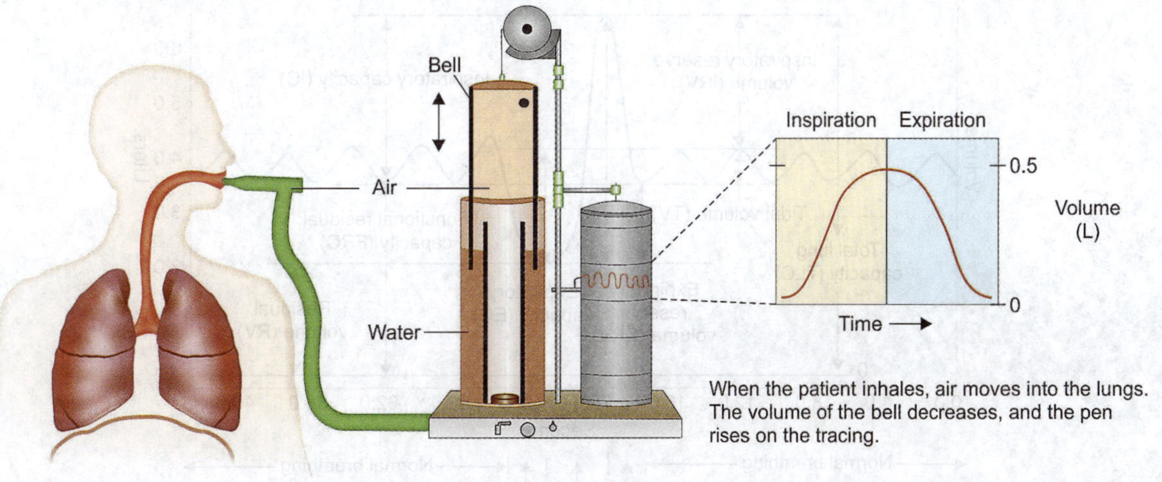

FIG. 4: Recording spirometer.

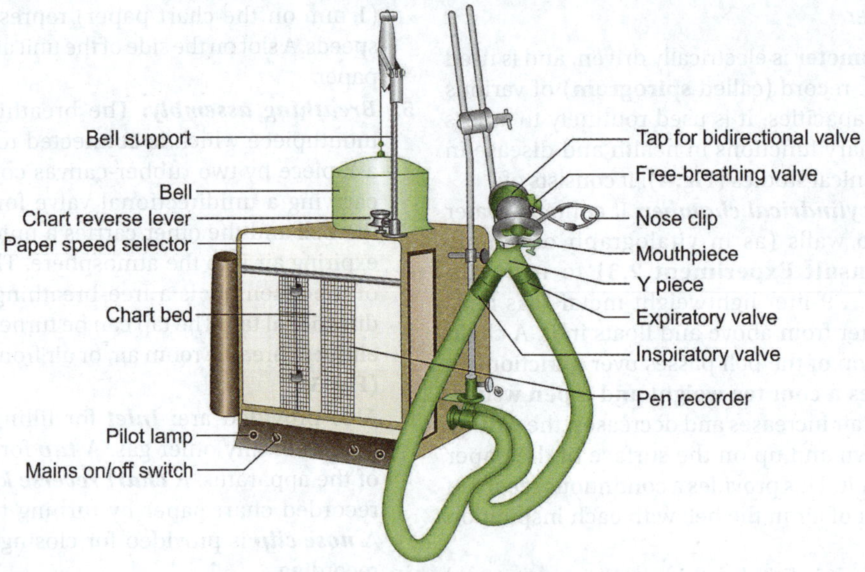

FIG. 5: Recording spirometer.

that the upstrokes are inspirations and downstrokes are expirations.

- The record of tidal breathing will be used for calculating the rate of respiration, tidal volume (TV) and minute ventilation (minute volume; MV).

To record IRV (**Fig. 6**), ask the subject to breathe in as deeply as possible after a quiet inspiration. IRV + TV will give IC. Record a few tidal breaths.

- To record ERV, ask the subject to breathe out as forcefully as possible after a quiet expiration.
- To record MVV (MBC) ask the subject to breathe quickly and deeply for 15 seconds. Convert the heights of all the excursions of the pen writer in 15 sec into volume per minute to obtain MVV.
- To record forced vital capacity (FVC), and timed vital capacity (FEV1), quickly change the kymograph speed to 1,200 mm/min, and ask the subject to first take a deep breath and then expel the air from the lungs as forcefully and as quickly as possible (as for VC). Take 3 readings at intervals of about 2 minutes.

Precautions

1. Subject should not be facing the recording spirometer during the recording.

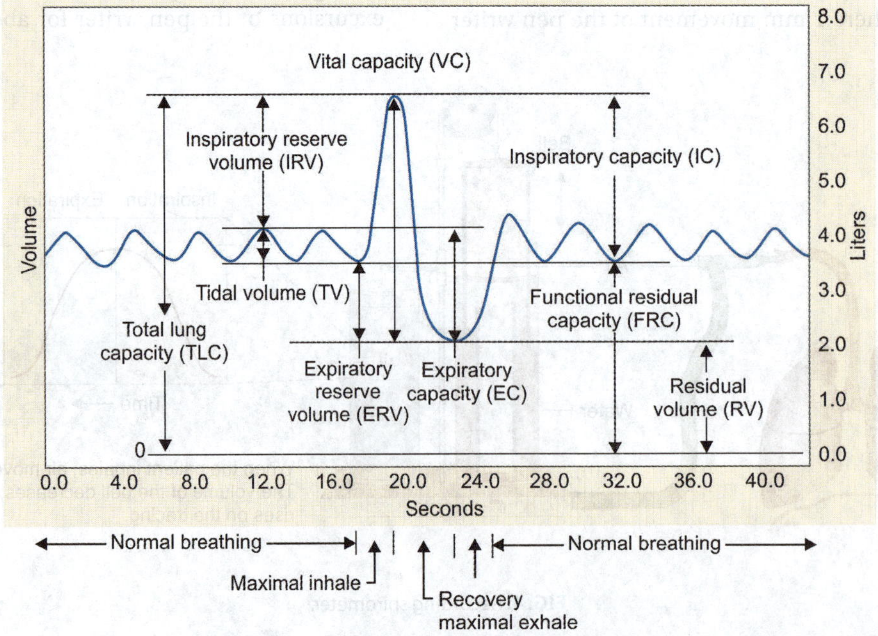

FIG. 6: Lung volumes and capacities (normal spirogram).

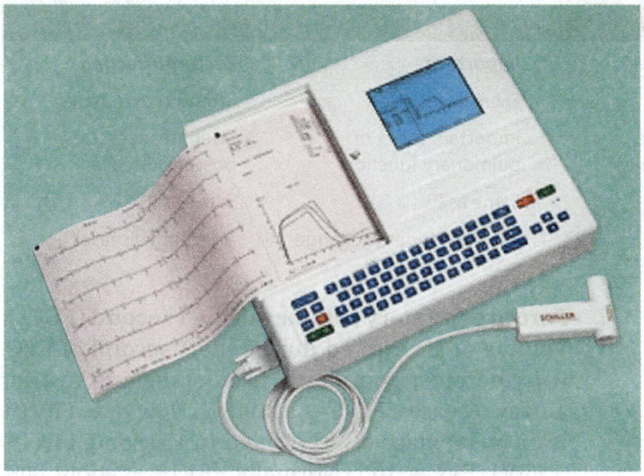

FIG. 7: Computerized spirometer.

2. All lung volume and capacities are measured from end that is expiratory position.
3. Look for the color of soda lime (change of color from white to pink indicates that is near the point of exhaustion).

Computerized spirometer

Nowadays portable computerized spirometers are used for the pulmonary functions tests. These are quick and easy to use and are accurate as well **(Fig. 7)**.

Static and Dynamic Lung Volumes and Capacities

The volume of air in the lungs changes considerably during a respiratory cycle. However, for convenience, four lung volumes and four lung capacities are distinguished as shown in **Figure 6**. The term **lung volumes** refer to the non overlapping subdivisions, or fractions of the total lung air, while the term **capacities** refer to the combination of two or more lung volumes. The lung volumes and capacities may either be **static** or **dynamic** depending on whether or not time factor has been taken into consideration.

- **Static volumes and capacities:** These measurements are those where time factor is not taken into consideration. They are expressed in milliliters or liters, and include:
  - **Static volumes:** Tidal volume (TV), inspiratory reserve volume (IRV), expiratory reserve volume (ERV), and residual volume (RV).
  - **Static capacities:** Inspiratory capacity (IC), vital capacity (VC), functional residual capacity (FRC), and total lung capacity (TLC).
- **Dynamic volumes and capacities:** These measurements are those where time factor is taken into account, that is, they are time-dependent. They are expressed in milliliters or liters per second or per minute and include:
  - **Dynamic volumes:** Minute ventilation (MV), maximum voluntary ventilation (MVV).
  - **Dynamic capacities: Capacities are a combination of volumes.** VC (timed vital capacity, FEV1) maximum mid-expiratory flow rate (MMFR).

Note:
- ❑ All static volumes can be measured by spirometer except residual volume, functional residual capacity and total lung capacity.
- ❑ All values have to be changed to STPD for comparison by using the "gas equation".
- ❑ **Functional residual capacity** is determined **by nitrogen wash-out method** or **helium dilution method**, and then residual volume and total lung capacity are calculated.

Static lung volumes (Table 2)

1. **Tidal volume:** It is the amount of air inspired or expired with each normal breath (tidal respiration).
2. **Inspiratory reserve volume:** It is the extra volume of air that can be inspired over and above the normal (resting, quiet) tidal volume (i.e. from the spontaneous end-inspiratory point), with maximum effort.
3. **Expiratory reserve volume:** It is the extra amount of air that can be expelled from lungs by forceful effort after normal expiration, i.e. over and above the normal tidal expiration.
4. **Residual volume:** It is the amount of air that remains behind in the lungs after a maximum voluntary expiration. The lungs cannot be emptied out completely of air even with maximum effort because as the pressure outside small air passages increases (i.e. the high intrathoracic pressure due to maximum expiratory effort) they are compressed and thus block the flow of air out of the lungs.

Static lung capacities (Table 3)

1. **Vital capacity: Consult Experiment 2.3.**

Table 2: Static lung volumes.

Static volumes	*Definition*	*Normal volume*	*Importance*	*Factors affecting*
Tidal volume (TV)	Resting volume	500 mL	Normal breathing rate calculation	Restrictive and obstructive disorders
Inspiratory reserve volume (IRV)	Volume inspired above the TV	2.5–3.2 L	Reserve for exercise	Restrictive and obstructive disorders
Expiratory reserve volume (ERV)	Volume expired after TV	1,000–1,200 mL		
Residual volume (RV)	Air in lungs after maximal expiration	1,200 mL	• Maintains gas exchange • Prevents collapse	• In emphysema, old age • In fibrosis

Table 3: Static lung capacities.

Static capacities	Definition	Normal value	Importance	Factors affecting
Inspiratory capacity	TV + IRV	2.5–3.7 L	Exercise reserve	Strength of muscles
Vital capacity	TV + IRV + ERV	4.8 L in males 3.2 L in females	Important index of pulmonary function	Strength, age, size, posture, diseases
Functional residual capacity	RV + ERV	2.3–2.5 L	Same as RV	Same as RV
Total lung capacity	VC + RV or IC + FRC	6 L	Reserve for gas exchange	Age, lung diseases

2. **Inspiratory capacity:** It is the maximum amount of air that a person can breathe in with maximum effort starting from the normal end-expiratory point. [IRV (2,500 mL) + TV (500 mL) = 3,000 mL].
3. **Functional residual capacity:** This is the amount of air remaining in the lungs at the end of a normal (quiet) expiration. It cannot be determined directly by spirometry. Normal value is 2.3–3.3 L (30–35 mL/kg body weight).
   Determination of functional residual capacity:
   i. Nitrogen washout method
   ii. Helium dilution method
4. **Total lung capacity:** It is the volume of air that is present in the lungs at the end of a deepest possible inspiration.

Dynamic lung volumes and capacities

1. **Minute ventilation/Pulmonary ventilation:** It is the volume of air inspired or expired per minute. It equals the tidal volume multiplied by respiratory rate [TV (500) × RR (12) = 6 L/min].
2. **Alveolar ventilation:** Out of a tidal volume of 500 mL, 150 mL air remains in the upper respiratory pass-ages up to respiratory bronchioles (anatomical dead space), while only 350 mL reaches the respiratory zone (respiratory bronchioles, alveolar ducts and alveoli) for exchange of gases. Thus, alveolar ventilation would be = (500 – 150 = 350) × 12 = 4.2 L/min.
3. **Maximum voluntary ventilation (Maximum ventilation volume):** It is the amount of air which can be moved into or out of the lungs with maximum effort during 1 minute. It was formerly called **maximum breathing capacity (MBC)**, the MVV amounts to 80–170 liters/min (average 120 L/min). The subject breathes quickly and deeply for 15 seconds, and MVV is calculated for 1 minute. (This means that pulmonary ventilation of 6–8 L/min can be increased by 15–20 times with maximum effort, though for short periods). MVV is profoundly reduced in patients with emphysema, airway obstruction and very poor respiratory muscle strength.
4. **Timed vital capacity/Forced vital capacity (FVC):** It is the largest volume of air a person can expel from the lungs with maximum effort after first filling the lungs fully by a deepest possible inspiration. It amounts to 3.5–5.5 liters.
   Components of TVC/FVC (Fig. 8): The volume of expired air can be timed by recording the FVC on a spirograph moving at a known speed. From the graph so obtained the FVC can be divided into the following components:
   i. **Forced expiratory volume during 1 second (FEV1):** Volume of air expired during the 1 second of FVC. It is the most commonly used screening test for airway diseases. FEV1 is actually a flow rate. FEV1% is the percentage of VC expired in 1 second. FEV1% = FEV1/FVC × 100 (Normally FEV1% = about 80% of FVC). The FEV1 recorded is a dynamic capacity. In a normal person, a single forced expiration takes about 3 seconds, and the tracing thus obtained is called an **"expiratory spirogram". Figures 9A to C** shows such a tracing where the fractions of FVC are: 80% in 1 second (FEV1), 95% in 2 seconds, and 98% in 3 seconds. The FEV1 is called the "first expiratory volume at 1 second (FEV1)" or "forced expiratory volume in 1 second".
   ii. **Forced expiratory volume in 2 seconds (FEV2):** It represents the volume of air expired in the first 2 sec of an FVC, FEV2% is about 90% of FVC under normal condition.
   iii. **Forced expiratory volume in 3 seconds (FEV3):** It represents the volume of air that expired in the first 3 seconds of an FVC, FEV3% is 98–100% of FVC under normal condition.

Physioclinical Significance of Timed Vital Capacity: It is useful in distinguishing between restrictive and obstructive lung disease. FEV1 and the ratio FEV1/FVC help in differentiating between two major patterns of abnormal ventilation—**obstructive** and **restrictive** lung diseases.

I. **Obstructive pattern:** Patients with obstructive lung disease (bronchial asthma) have relatively low

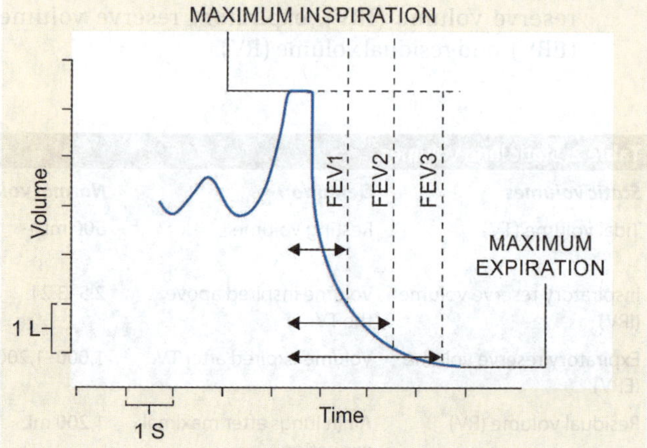

FIG. 8: Components of timed vital capacity.

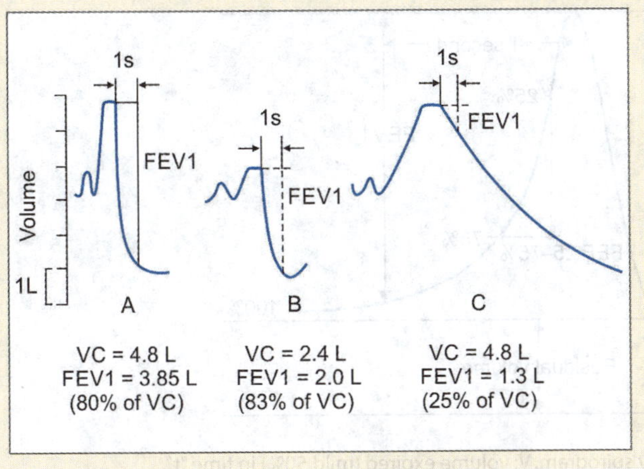

FIGS. 9A TO C: The expiratory spirogram: Forced expiratory volume in 1 second (FEV1) component of timed vital capacity. (A) Normal patient; (B) Patient with restrictive lung disease; (C) Patient with obstructive lung disease.

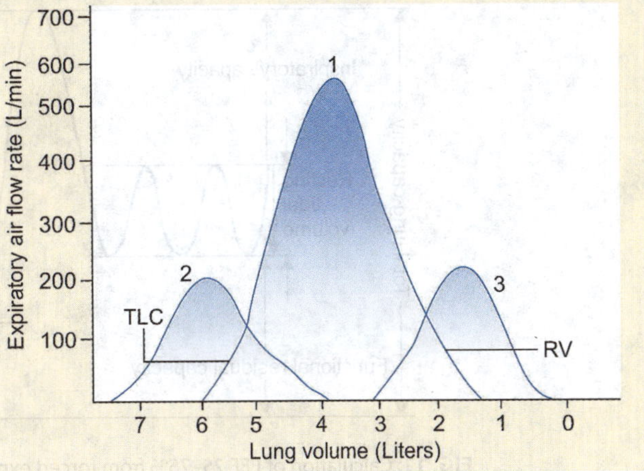

FIG. 10: Maximum expiratory flow volume curve. 1. Normal, 2. Chronic obstructive lung disease, 3. Restrictive lung disease.

expiratory flow rate throughout expiration as a result of high airway resistance therefore, their **FEV1% is abnormally low.** The main feature is a **decrease in PEFR, FEV1, FEV1/FVC, and MMEFR are all reduced (Figs. 9 and 10).** Over many years more and more air tends to remain in the lungs which increases TLC and RV **(Fig. 10).**

II. **Restrictive pattern:** Patients with restrictive lung disease (kyphoscoliosis, ankylosing spondylitis) have a reduced FVC but are able to achieve relatively high flow rates; therefore, their FEV1% exceeds 80%. The main feature is reduced lung volume (mainly TLC and RV), which may be due to *interstitial lung* disease *(ILD)* or *chest wall deformity* that reduces the air in the lungs. There is no obstruction to the outflow of air. **FEV1 is normal though FVC is low and FEV1/FVC may be normal or slightly increased as shown in Figure 9 and Table 4.**

Maximum expiratory flow-volume curve (MEFVC) (Fig. 10): It represents outflow of air from lungs during a forceful expiration after a deep inspiration. The curve starts at a TLC of about 6.0 L, quickly reaches a peak of 550 L/min, and then falls gradually to a residual volume of 1,100 mL. The decline in expiratory flow rate is due to compression of airways by the increasing intrathoracic pressure due to compression of chest by the forced expiration.

5. **Forced expiratory flow during 25–75% of expiration (FEF 25-75%):** It is the mean expiratory flow rate during the middle 50% of FVC. Normal value: 300 L/min. In addition to FVC and FEV1, the average expiratory flow rate during the middle 50% of FVC also called **"maximal mid-expiratory flow rate" (MMEFR; or FEF 25- 75%)** can also be calculated **(Fig. 11).** A horizontal line drawn from 25% (t) and a vertical line from the 75% mark (V) will denote FEF 25–75%. This indicates the patency of smaller airways.

Figure 11 also shows that in the middle 50% of FVC, 2.0 liters of air is expired in 0.5 second (t). This is also known as **mid-expiratory time (MET).** Thus, V/t = 2.0 L/0.5 sec = 4.0 liters per second. **Normal range = Males:** 1.5–4.5 L/sec. **Females:** 1.3–3.0 L/sec. This is increased in obstructive lung disorders.

6. **Forced expiratory flow during 200–1,200 mL of expiration (FEF200–1,200):** FEF200–1,200 refers to the mean expiratory flow rate between 200–1,200 mL segments of FVC. Normal value: 350 L/min. This indicates the patency of larger airways.
7. **Pulmonary reserve (PR) or breathing reserve:** PR refers to the maximum amount of the air above the pulmonary ventilation that can be inspired or expired in 1 minute. It equals maximum ventilation volume minus pulmonary ventilation (minute ventilation), i.e. PR = MVV – PV/min.

Pulmonary reserve is usually expressed as percentage of MVV and is known as percentage pulmonary reserve or ***dyspneic index (DI)***, i.e. DI = (MVV – PV)/MVV × 100.

- Normal values of DI or % PR range from 70% to 95% with an average of 75%.

Table 4: Restrictive pattern of lung diseases.

Interpretation	*FVC*	*FEV1*	*FEV1/FVC% (Tiffeneau index)*
Healthy person	Normal (>80%)	Normal (>80%)	Normal (>0.7)
Airway obstruction	Low/normal	Low	Low
Restrictive	Low	Low/normal	Normal/increased (>0.7)
Mixed	Low	Low	Low

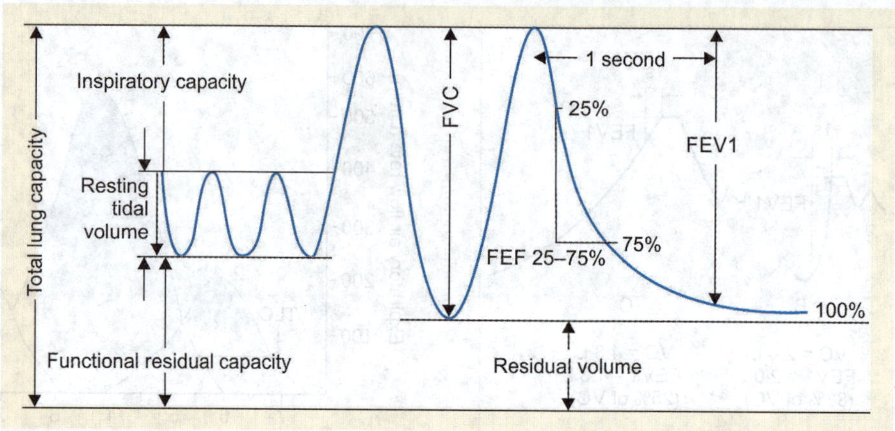

FIG. 11: Calculation of FEF 25–75% from forced expiratory spirogram. V: volume expired (mild 50%) in time "t".

- Dyspnea is usually present when the value of DI becomes less than 60%.

8. **Peak expiratory flow rate (PEFR):** It is the maximum or peak rate (or velocity), in liters per minute with which air is expelled with maximum force after a deep inspiration. **Normal range** = 350–600 liters per minute. **The Wright's peak flow meter** is a simple device for the measurement of the PEFR. A mini version is available which can be carried in one's pocket for bedside use **(Figs. 12A and B)**. The flow meter is a short cylinder made of plastic material. An indicator (pointer) moves in a slot alongside a scale with numbers on it which indicates liters/min. There is a handle provided near the mouthpiece. The end, opposite the mouthpiece, has holes in it for allowing air to exit from the apparatus.

Procedure

1. Ask the subject to hold the peak flow meter by its handle making sure that the fingers are clear of the scale and the slot, and are not obstructing the holes at the end of the apparatus.
2. Tell the subject to take a deep breath, place the mouthpiece firmly between the teeth and lips, and then to blow out with a short sharp blast. Note the reading on the scale. Bring the indicator back to zero by pressing the button located near the mouthpiece.
3. Take 6 readings at intervals of 1 minute, and select the maximum value for the report.

Precautions

1. Subject should be instructed to blow out rapidly, completely and forcefully into the mouthpiece.
2. There should be no leakage from the mouthpiece.

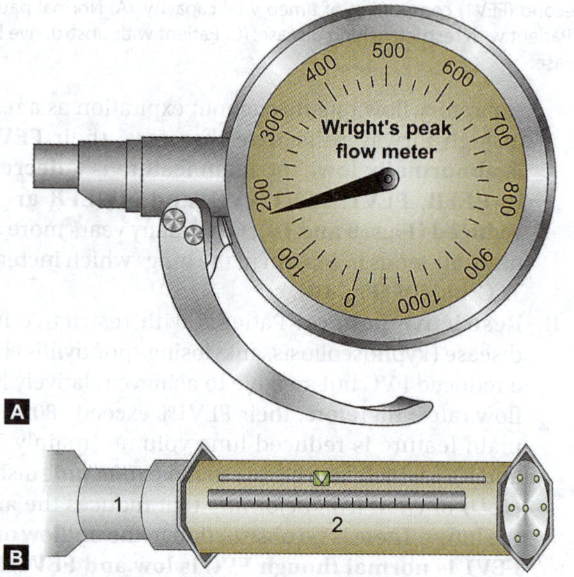

FIGS. 12A AND B: (A) Wright's peak flow meter. It directly measures expiratory flow rate; (B) Mini Wright's peak flow meter. 1. Mouth-piece, 2. Calibrated scale with marker.

Measurement of Dead Space

Dead space air is the portion of minute ventilation that does not take part in the exchange of gases. Normally, it is constituted by the air present in the conducting zone of respiratory passages *(anatomical dead space)*, but in some diseases may additionally also include poorly perfused alveoli *(physiological dead space)*. Anatomical dead space can be measured by the **single breath N_2 curve**.

Measurement of Compliance

- Compliance (C) expresses the distensibility (expansibility) of the lungs and chest wall. Compliance is defined as the change in lung volume (ΔV) per unit change in transpulmonary pressure (ΔP) where transpulmonary pressure is the difference in the pressure between the alveolar pressure and pleural pressure.

$$C = \Delta V/\Delta P$$

  a. Total respiratory compliance or combined compliance of lungs and chest wall, i.e. lungs inside the thoracic cavity. Normal value of total respiratory compliance is 0.13 L/cm H_2O.
  b. Pulmonary compliance, i.e. of lungs only (lungs outside the chest wall). Normal value of compliance for the lungs alone is 0.22 L/cm H_2O.

- **Measurement of total compliance:** Total respiratory compliance (combined compliance of chest wall and lungs) can be measured by the pressure—volume curve of the respiratory system. Pressure-volume curve of the respiratory system can be obtained in living subjects by using a spirometer.

Static versus Specific Lung Compliance

- **Static compliance:** The static compliance of any system is dependent on its size. Thus the lung compliance depends upon the amount of functional lung tissue.
- **Specific compliance:** It is the compliance of the lung at relaxation volume (the point at the end of a tidal expiration), i.e. the functional residual capacity. The compliance is corrected for lung volume which is referred to as specific compliance. It is expressed per liter of FRC. If the FRC is 2.2 L then specific compliance with both intact lungs will be: 0.22/2.2 = 0.1 L/cm H_2O.

Measurement of Airway Resistance

- Airway resistance is one of the fundamental features of the respiratory system. Total airway resistance (Raw) the driving pressure is the pressure difference between the mouth (P_{mouth}) and the alveoli (P_A).

$$Raw = \frac{P_{mouth} - P_A}{V}$$

Normal value in healthy adults = 1–3 cm of H_2O/L per second.

Flow-Volume Loop

- In contrast to the spirogram which displays airflow (in L), over time (in sec), the flow-volume loop displays airflow (in L/sec) as it relates to lung volume (in L) during maximal inspiration from complete exhalation (residual volume) and during maximum expiration from complete inhalation (TLC).
- The principal advantage of the flow-volume loop is that it can show whether airflow is appropriate for a particular lung volume.
- **A normal flow-volume loop:** A normal flow-volume loop begins on the X-axis (volume axis): At the start of the test both flow and volume are equal to zero. After the starting point the curve rapidly mounts to a peak: Peak (Expiratory) Flow. After the PEF the curve descends (= the flow decreases) as more air is expired. A normal, nonpathological F/V loop will descend in a straight or a convex line from top (PEF) to bottom (FVC) **(Fig. 13)**.

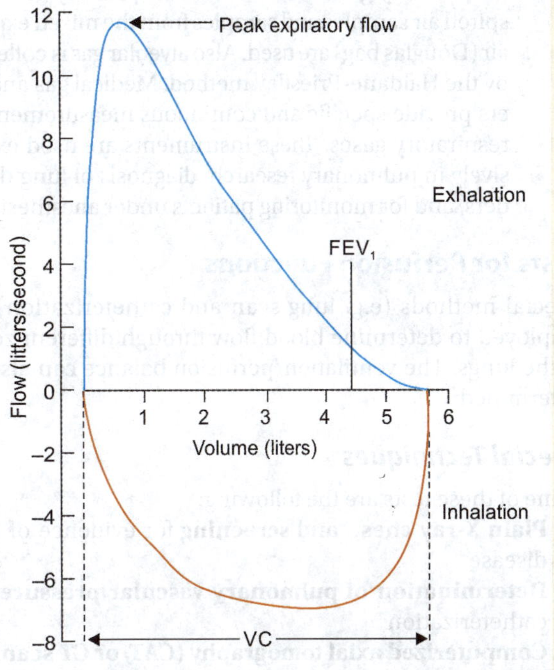

FIG. 13: Normal flow-volume loop.

Tests of Gas Exchange Functions

- **Tests of diffusion:** Pulmonary diffusion refers to the transfer of gases across the alveoli to the capillary blood across the respiratory membrane. Diffusion capacity is defined as the volume of any gas that diffuses across the alveolar-capillary membrane per minute per mm Hg difference of pressure across the membrane.
- **Diffusion capacity/Transfer factor for gases:** The diffusion of gases across the alveolar-capillary membrane depends not only on pressure gradients of O_2 and CO_2 across the membrane, but also its surface area and thickness, ventilation/perfusion balance, volume of blood in pulmonary capillaries, and the concentration of Hb in the blood. Therefore, the term **transfer factor (TF)** rather than diffusion capacity is used these days.
- **CO method for measuring TF for O_2:** Since it is technically difficult to measure the diffusing capacity of lungs (TF) for O_2 directly, CO is used instead. The diffusion capacity measured for CO at rest is about 17 mL/min/mm Hg.
- Since the diffusing coefficient for O_2 is 1.23 times that for CO, the diffusing capacity for O_2 is = 17 × 1.23 = 21 mL/min/mm Hg.
- **Estimation of arterial pO_2, pCO_2, pH:** For blood gas analysis, arterial blood sample is usually taken from the radial artery or femoral artery. The estimation of pO_2, pCO_2 and pH can be done within a minute or so using a very small sample of blood with the help of miniaturized glass electrodes.
- **Arterial pO_2** levels in young healthy adults vary from 85 mm Hg to 105 mm Hg with a mean of 95 mm Hg. The value may drop by up to 15% in healthy elderly patients due to an increase in ventilation-perfusion inequality.
- **Arterial pCO_2 and pH** levels in normal adult are about 40 mm Hg and 7.4 mm Hg, respectively and are basically determined by the volume of alveolar ventilation.
- *Methods of measuring blood and respiratory gases.*
  a. ***Blood gases:*** Miniature glass electrodes can quickly estimate the blood gases and pH on a very small arterial blood sample.

b. ***Respiratory gases:*** To measure respiratory gases inspired air samples and samples from the mixed expired air (Douglas bag) are used. Also alveolar gas is collected by the Haldane-Priestley method. Medical gas analyzers provide specific and continuous measurements of respiratory gases. These instruments are used extensively in pulmonary research, diagnosis of lung disorders, and for monitoring patients under anesthesia.

Tests for Perfusion Functions

Special methods (e.g. lung scan and catheterization) are employed to determine blood flow through different zones of the lungs. The ventilation/perfusion balance can also be determined.

Special Techniques

Some of these tests are the following:

1. **Plain X-ray chest, and screening** for evidence of lung disease
2. **Determination of pulmonary vascular pressures** by catheterization
3. **Computerized axial tomography (CAT, or CT scan)**
4. **Magnetic resonance imaging (MRI)**
5. **Bronchoscopy:** A fiberoptic (flexible) bronchoscope is introduced through the nose or mouth, through the larynx and trachea into the bronchial tree. A local anesthetic is sprayed at every step. This instrument allows the inside of trachea and lower bronchial passages to be directly visualized. A biopsy of a growth can also be taken.
6. **Lung scan:** This test is employed to determine any blockage in the blood flow from the heart into the lungs. A radioactive substance is injected into a vein and detected in the lungs by a scanning camera. In this way, cold spots (areas of decreased blood flow), and hot spots (areas of high flow) can be detected as the scanner converts this information into an image.
7. **Ventilation scan:** This test measures the flow of air into and out of the lungs. A radioactive gas is inhaled; once it is in the lungs, a scanning camera produces an image. Normally the gas is equally distributed in both lungs.
8. **Computerized multifunctional spirometers:** Computerized spirometers that can monitor lung volumes and capacities from breath to breath are employed in research laboratories and hospitals. They can graphically display the results, and show predicted values, and their interpretations, if so desired.

OBJECTIVE STRUCTURED PRACTICAL EXAMINATION

Aim: To record the normal spirogram using a recording spirometer and PEFR using Wright's peak flow meter.

Procedural steps: See text.

Checklist:

1. Check out the apparatus.
2. Seat the subject on a stool with the back facing the recording spirometer.
3. Ask him to relax and explain the procedure.
4. Record the spirogram following the instructions.

QUESTIONS

Q.1. What is meant by the terms lung volumes and capacities? How can they be measured and what are their normal values?

See text above.

Q.2. What is the purpose of testing lung functions?

See text above.

Q.3. Name the lung volumes and capacities that cannot be measured on a spirometer.

The lung volumes and capacities that cannot be measured on a spirometer include: total lung capacity (TLC), functional residual capacity (FRC), and residual volume (RV).

Q.4. What is the difference between minute ventilation and maximum voluntary ventilation?

See text above.

Q.5. What is timed vital capacity (FEV1) and what is its clinical importance?

See text above.

Q.6. What is peak (expiratory) flow rate and what is its significance?

- **The peak expiratory flow rate (PEFR):** The peak expiratory rate is the maximum flow rate, or peak flow rate of air, during a single forced expiration. This estimation is useful in distinguishing reversible (e.g. asthma) from irreversible (e.g. emphysema) diseases.
- The peak flow meter which measures PEFR is of special value in cases of asthma where the effectiveness of treatment with a bronchodilator can be quickly evaluated. For example, a PEFR of, say, 150 liters/min may improve to 300 liters/min within a short time of inhalation of the drug. But the meter is not useful for assessing the degree of disability of patients with lung fibrosis and other restrictive conditions because they may have normal expiratory flow rates. The measurement of the effect of training in athletes is yet another application of the Wright's peak flow meter.
- The major factor that limits expiratory flow rate during most of a maximal forced expiration is the narrowing of small airways. Thus, the flow rate is a function of lung volume rather than the effort exerted. This condition is called **"effort-independent flow"**.

Q.7. What is the physiological significance of functional residual capacity (FRC)?

- **Functional residual capacity (FRC),** the air that remains in the lungs at the end of a normal (quiet) expiration is important for the gas exchange function of the lungs. The FRC amounts to about 2,200 mL, half of which is residual volume which cannot be expired into the spirometer.
- Out of the 500 mL of tidal volume, 150 mL remains in the dead space, while only 350 mL reaches the depths of the lungs. There, it is added to the large amount of 2,000–2,500 mL of FRC. This causes dilution of the gases and a steady gas exchange throughout the respiratory cycle.

- The steady exchange prevents sudden changes in arterial PO_2 and PCO_2 which would make the control of breathing extremely difficult. The FRC is increased when lungs are overinflated with air as in old age, emphysema (due to loss of elasticity), asthma, etc.

Q.8. Name the precautions that must be observed during spirometric recording?

See text above.

Q.9. What is breathing reserve and what is its clinical importance?

See text above.

Q.10. What is the purpose of testing lung functions?

See text above.

Q.11. Demonstrate any two simple lung function tests.

The student may perform a *vital capacity estimation* and *respiratory endurance test* (or any other two function tests of his/her choice).

Q.12. How will you assess gas exchange functions of the lungs?

The gas exchange functions can be tested by analyzing respiratory and blood gases. **See text above.**

Q.13. What is the structure of alveolar-capillary membrane? What are the factors that affect the diffusion of gases through it?

This membrane, about 0.1–0.4 µm thick, consists of a thin layer of fluid, a layer of type I and type II cells and macrophages of alveolar wall, epithelial basement membrane, capillary basement membrane, endothelial cells of capillary, and a thin layer of fluid plasma. See text above for *factors affecting gas diffusion.*

Q.14. What is meant by the term ventilation? Name the forces that oppose the movement of air into the lungs during inspiration.

The term ventilation refers to the movement of air into and out of the lungs. The forces that oppose expansion of lungs (and air inflow) include:

i. Elastic recoil of thorax and lungs (elastic resistance).
ii. Nonelastic (viscous) resistance due to movement of tissues.
iii. Airway resistance due to friction between the air passages and the moving column of air. The contraction of inspiratory muscles must overcome all these forces before lungs can expand and pull air into their depths.

2.3: DETERMINATION OF VITAL CAPACITY AND EFFECT OF POSTURE ON VITAL CAPACITY

STUDENT OBJECTIVES

After completing this experiment, the student should be able to:

- Define vital capacity (VC) and name the muscles involved in carrying it out.
- Record the VC and explain the effect of posture on it.
- Describe the physiological and pathological factors that affect VC.

PY6.8: Demonstrate the correct technique to perform and interpret Spirometry.

VITAL CAPACITY

- The vital capacity (VC) is defined as the total volume of air that can be displaced from the lungs by maximal expiratory effort after maximal inspiration. It is the most commonly performed pulmonary function test.
- It is normally 60 to 70 mL/kg and in normal persons is determined primarily by the size of the thorax and lungs.
- Reduction of VC to 30 mL/kg is associated with weak cough, accumulation of oropharyngeal secretions, atelectasis, and hypoxemia.

Slow Vital Capacity

It is the volume of air expired (after maximum inspiration) during a slowly performed maximum expiratory effort without regard to time. It is used to evaluate the size of lungs. The VC can be decreased by either decrease in total lung capacity (TLC) as in restrictive disease or by increase in residual volume as seen in obstructive lung disease.

Forced Vital Capacity/Timed Vital Capacity/ Forced Expiratory Volume

It is the largest volume of air a person can expel from the lungs with maximum effort after first filling the lungs fully by a deepest possible inspiration. It amounts to 3.0–5.0 liters.

Note: Slow vital capacity is more than forced vital capacity in patients with airway obstruction.

Measurement of Vital Capacity

- The measurement of VC requires the subject to inhale as deeply as possible and then to exhale fully, taking as much time as required.
- The measurement can also be obtained by adding two of its components: the expiratory reserve volume (ERV), obtained by having the subject exhale maximally from the resting end-tidal level; and the inspiratory capacity (IC), obtained by having the subject inspire fully from the resting end-tidal level.
- The sum of these two measurements yields the "combined VC"; as long as the resting end-tidal lung volume is the same for the two component maneuvers, the combined VC and the VC are equal.
- Many sophisticated tests are available for assessing respiratory functions, VC is a simple and useful

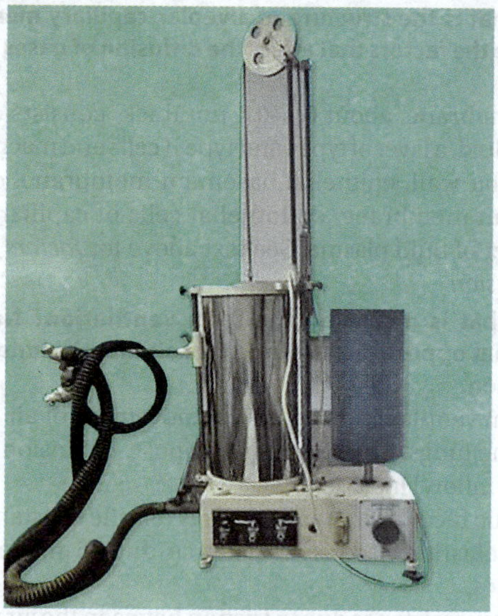

FIG. 14: Vitalograph.

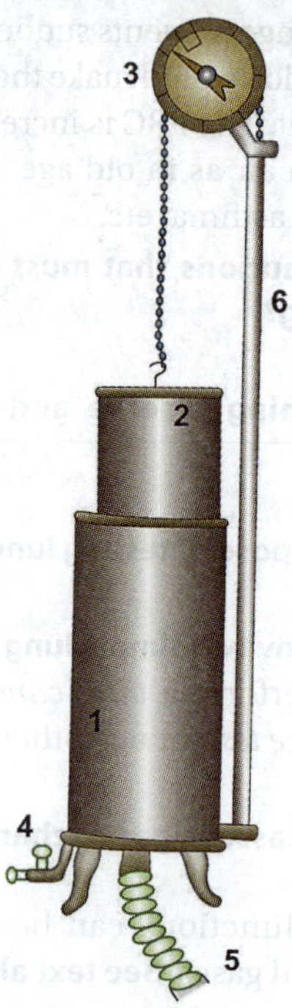

FIG. 15: Simple spirometer. 1. Outer container, 2. Gas float, 3. Calibrated pulley with spring-mounted indicator needle, 4. Tap for draining water, 5. Wide-bore inlet tube, and 6. Counterpoise system.

measurement for assessing the ventilatory functions of the lungs in health and disease. VC may be measured either on a simple spirometer or a recording spirometer (spiro = breathe; meter = measuring device).

- **Simple spirometer (student spirometer; also called a vitalograph):** It is a common low-cost instrument, either a metallic or a bellows type, used in colleges, hospitals, sports facilities, and gymnasia **(Fig. 14)**.
- **Recording spirometer:** It is a sophisticated, electrically-driven, recording system used in respiratory physiology laboratories, hospitals, etc. It provides a graphic record of various lung volumes and capacities.

Note: Wright's peak flow meter is a small portable instrument which can give information about the state of respiratory passages (it can be carried in one's pocket for bedside use by the physician).
In this experiment, the students will use a simple spirometer and the peak flow meter to measure some of the ventilatory functions of the lungs under normal conditions. The working of a recording spirometer will then be briefly described.

SPIROMETRY (VITALOMETRY)

Apparatus and Materials

Spirometer; potassium permanganate solution.

Spirometer [Vitalograph; "Student" (or Simple) Spirometer]

- It consists of a double-walled metal cylindrical chamber, having an outer container filled with water in which a light-metal gas bell of 6 liters capacity floats.
- The bell (or float) is attached on its upper surface to a chain which passes over a graduated frictionless pulley.
- The pulley bears a spring-mounted indicator needle that moves with the pulley and indicates the volume of air present in the bell.
- The gas bell is counterpoised by a weight (counterweight) attached to the other end of the chain **(Fig. 15)**. This weight allows a smooth up and down movement of the bell.
- The inlet tube, through which air moves into or out of the bell, is corrugated canvas-rubber tubing bearing a mouthpiece (this tube is attached to a metal pipe fitted at the bottom of the apparatus, the upper end of which lies above the level of water in the outer container).
- When air is blown into the inlet tube, it raises the bell, the water acting as an airtight seal.

Procedures

Note: One can record not only VC with this apparatus but also a few other lung volumes and capacities, though only approximately. Their accurate recording is done on a recording spirometer, as described later.

Important: Explain the procedure in detail to the patient and even give her a pilot rehearsal to ensure that the procedure has been fully understood. Also, the patient should be encouraged to exert full expiratory effort during the test. Record the *age, height and body weight* before starting the test.

1. **Measuring vital capacity by collecting expired air in the spirometer (standard method):**
   - Bring the bell to its lowest position by gently pushing it down. Adjust the pointer needle at zero, which indicates that the bell is completely empty.
   - Ask the patient to stand comfortably, facing the spirometer so that she/he can see the movement of

the bell. Tell her to breathe normally (quietly) for a minute or so.

- Now direct her to inspire as deeply and as fully as possible to fill the lungs. Then, while keeping the nostrils closed with a thumb and fingers, and the mouthpiece held firmly between the lips, tell him to expel all the air that he can with maximum effort into the spirometer.
- The bell moves up and the pointer on the pulley indicates the volume of expired air. The forced expiration should be deep and quick but without haste (normally, this procedure takes about 3 seconds).
- Take two more readings at intervals of 5 minutes in the standing position as before.
- ***Effect of posture:*** Ask the subject to sit comfortably on a stool and record the VC three times as before, at intervals of 2 minutes.
- Then ask her to lie down on the couch in supine position (face up) and record the VC three times (see Q/A 4 for the effect of posture on VC).

2. **Measuring vital capacity by breathing in from the full spirometer:** This method is a variation of the earlier method.
   - Raise and lower the bell a few times, finally raising it to its highest position so that it gets filled with fresh room air. Note the reading.
   - Tell the subject to breathe deeply a few times, then to expel air, with maximum effort, from the lungs into the atmosphere. This leaves only the residual volume (RV) in the lungs.
   - Now ask the subject to hold the mouthpiece firmly between the lips and then to breathe in maximally from the spirometer [thus breathing in expiratory reserve volume (ERV), tidal volume (TV), and inspiratory reserve volume (IRV) in that order, as shown in **Figure 16**]. Note the reading. The difference between the two readings is the VC.

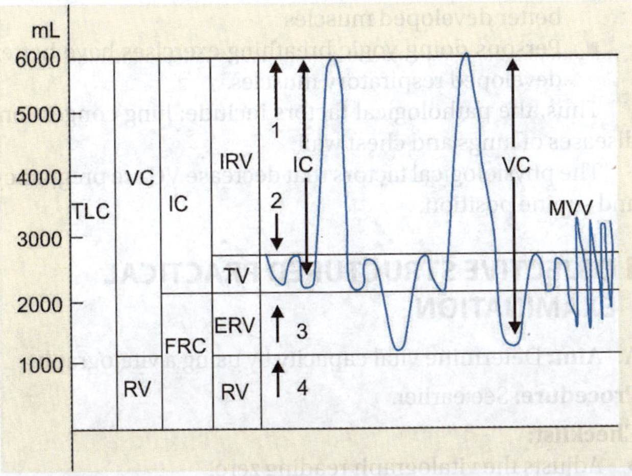

FIG. 16: Lung volumes and capacities. The volumes do not overlap; the capacities are made up of two or more volumes. Arrows: 1. Maximum inspiratory level, 2. Resting inspiratory level, 3. Resting expiratory level, and 4. Maximum expiratory level. Standard abbreviations used.
(ERV: expiratory reserve volume; FRC: functional residual capacity; IC: inspiratory capacity; IRV: inspiratory reserve volume; MVV: maximum voluntary ventilation; RV: residual volume; TV: tidal volume; TLC: total lung capacity; VC: vital capacity).

   - Compare this value with that obtained with the standard method, and explain the difference, if any.

3. **Two-stage vital capacity determination:**
   a. ***Stage I:*** Fill the spirometer with fresh room air, and note the reading. Ask the patient to breathe normally a few times. Then, starting from resting end-expiratory position, ask him to take maximum inspiration from the spirometer bell. Note the reading. The difference will give the inspiratory capacity (IC).
   b. ***Stage II:*** Bring the bell to its lowest position (zero level). Tell the patient to breathe normally a few times. And then, starting from resting end-expiratory position, to expel all the air from the lungs with maximum effort into the spirometer. This will give ERV.
   - The sum of the two, i.e. IC and ERV will determine VC.
   - Compare it with the value obtained with the standard method and explain the difference, if any.
4. **Measurement of inspiratory capacity:** This can be done in two ways:
   1. **By breathing from the spirometer:** Fill the bell with fresh air as before and note the reading. Carry out the procedure described earlier for the stage I employed for VC. This gives IC.
   2. **By breathing out into the spirometer:** Bring the bell down to zero level. Then tell the subject to take a deep breath and to expire forcefully into the spirometer up to the point of resting end-expiratory position. This will give IC, i.e. TV + IRV.
5. **Measurement of expiratory reserve volume:** Carry out the procedure described earlier for stage II for VC.
6. **Tidal volume:** Only an approximate idea can be obtained by breathing 2–3 times in and out of the spirometer and taking the readings. This step cannot be repeated for more than 2–3 times because this spirometer is a closed system and there is no provision for absorbing carbon dioxide (CO_2) from the expired air.

Observations and Results

All the readings should be taken in standing, supine, and sitting positions.

Record your observations as indicated here:

Name....... Age....... Sex....... Date of experiment.........
Weight....... kg........ Height……..cm
1. Rate of respiration………/min
2. Tidal volume…………/mL
Minute ventilation (at rest):………..liters/min

	Readings (mL) 1st	2nd	3rd	Maximum value
3. Vital capacity:				
a. Standard method				
b. Two-stage method	......	......	......	......
4. Inspiratory capacity:				
Breathing from the spirometer	......	......	......	......
Breathing out into spirometer				
5. Expiratory reserve volume	......	......	......	......
6. Effect of posture on VC:				
a. Standing	......	......	......	......
b. Sitting	......	......	......	......

c. Supine ......

Calculate the vital capacity:

Per kg body weight ......

Per cm height ......

Per m^2 BSA (vital index) ......

(Consult nomogram for body surface area calculation at the end of the book).

Physioclinical Significance

The VC is an effort-based measurement, therefore, it indicates the strength of the respiratory muscles.

See text above and refer to Q2.

QUESTIONS

Q.1. What is the normal vital capacity? Can it be predicted?

The normal VC varies between 3 and 5 liters, the value being 20% lower in females. In general, the VC (and other volumes and capacities) are larger in males, taller persons, and in younger adults. Thus, since the VC depends on age, sex, body build, occupation, etc. various formulae have been introduced to predict VC in an individual. Various disorders may then be diagnosed by comparing the actual (determined) values with the predicted normal values for one's age, sex, height, etc.

1. **Relation to height:**
   Males = Height in cm × 25
   Females = Height in cm × 20
   Athletes = Height in cm × 29
2. **Relation to body surface area (BSA):**
   This is called the vital index.
   Males = 2.5 L/m^2 BSA
   Females = 2.1 L/m^2 BSA
3. **Relation to age, sex, and height:**
   Males = [27.63 – (0.112 × Age)] × Height in cm
   Females = [27.78 – (0.101 × Age)] × Height in cm
4. **Relation to body weight:** For an average healthy person, the prediction formula is: VC (in mL) = W0.72/0.690, where W is the body weight in grams.

The VC is high in athletes, swimmers, divers, etc. but is low in persons who have sedentary habits.

Q.2. What is the clinical importance of determination of vital capacity?

The VC is frequently determined clinically as an index of lung function and provides useful information about abnormal ventilation due to airway obstruction, fibrosis of the lungs, mechanical interference with chest expansion and compression, strength of respiratory muscles, and so on. However, it cannot help in differentiating between obstructive and restrictive lung diseases, where timed VC is of greater help.

Q.3. What is a two-stage vital capacity?

See text above.

Q.4. Describe the effect of posture on vital capacity.

The VC is maximum in the standing position, less in the sitting position, and least in the supine position. This effect of posture is due to the following factors:

- In the sitting and supine positions, the muscles of respiration (both primary and accessory) cannot be employed as forcefully and effectively for the expansion and compression of lungs and chest.
- In the supine position, the abdominal viscera push the diaphragm up and interfere with its movements. The mobility of the chest is also reduced by the contact of the back with the bed.
- There is accumulation of more blood in the blood vessels of the lungs (especially veins) in the supine position. This decreases the total lung capacity, and hence the VC.

Q.5. Name the factors that affect vital capacity.

The main factors affecting VC are:

- Size of the lungs and chest wall
- Condition of the lungs and chest wall
- Magnitude of compressing forces, i.e. contraction of respiratory muscles.

Associated with these factors, the following factors affect VC:

1. **Age:** The net air capacity (size) is lower in young children. VC decreases in old age due to loss of elasticity of lungs and weaker compressing forces.
2. **Sex:** Males have larger chests, greater body surface area, and greater muscle power.
3. **Net air capacity of lungs:**
   - Volume of blood in the lungs, e.g. pulmonary congestion reduces air capacity
   - Condition of lungs, e.g. loss of elasticity, emphysema, and chronic interstitial lung disease
   - Destruction of lung tissue, e.g. carcinoma
   - Patency of lung passages, e.g. asthma reduces patency
   - Mechanical interference with expansion of lungs, e.g. pregnancy, deformities of spine
   - *Posture*: In supine position, the abdominal viscera push up against the diaphragm thus reducing the thoracic space.
4. **Magnitude of compressing forces:**
   - Swimmers, divers, and athletes have stronger and better developed muscles
   - Persons doing yogic breathing exercises have better developed respiratory muscles.

Thus, the pathological factors include: lung congestion, diseases of lungs and chest wall.

The physiological factors that decrease VC are pregnancy and supine position.

OBJECTIVE STRUCTURED PRACTICAL EXAMINATION

A. **Aim:** Determine vital capacity by using a vitalograph.

Procedure: See earlier.

Checklist:

- Adjusts the vitalograph reading zero.
- Asks the subject to sit comfortably facing away from the vitalograph.
- Gives instruction to the subject to put in maximum effort during the recording.
- Instructs the subject to repeat the procedure three times and record the best reading.

B. **Aim:** Effect of posture on vital capacity.

Procedure: See earlier.

Checklist:
- Adjusts the vitalograph reading zero.
- Instructs the subject to lie down supine on a couch.
- Gives instructions to the subject to exhale forcefully and maximally after a deep inspiration and record the reading.
- Asks the subject to repeat the procedure in sitting and standing position.
- Compares all the readings and report.

2.4: CARDIOPULMONARY RESUSCITATION

STUDENT OBJECTIVES

After completing this experiment, the student should be able to:
- Define cardiopulmonary resuscitation (CPR).
- Explain the aim of doing CPR.
- List the indications for CPR.
- Describe the procedure for mouth to mouth breathing.
- Describe the procedure for external cardiac massage.
- List the various steps of basic life support (BLS).
- List the various steps of advanced cardiac life support (ACLS).

INTRODUCTION

PY11.14: Demonstrate Basic Life Support in a simulated environment.

- **Cardiopulmonary resuscitation** is a first aid procedure performed to maintain blood circulation and oxygenation in a person who has suffered cardiac arrest. It involves repeated cycles of compression of the chest and artificial respiration, and must be started without losing a second. It is not the treatment, however.
- **Cardiopulmonary arrest (CP arrest)** is said to have occurred when there is a sudden stoppage of heart or breathing or both. It is an extreme emergency that threatens life. Consciousness is lost within 10–15 seconds of stoppage of oxygen supply to the brain and some brain damage occurs in 5–6 minutes. Circulatory arrest for more than 10–15 minutes causes permanent damage to the brain.

Important: Artificial respiration (AR) alone may be needed if breathing has stopped suddenly though the heart is still beating (as it happens in many cases). However, if breathing is not restarted within 3–4 minutes, the heart will also stop. In this case, both AR and external cardiac compression will be required (see general plan here).

Note: The survival rates of out-of-hospital CP arrest (say due to a heart attack on a roadside, or in a building) are, sadly, very low. The main reason is ignorance of the value of CPR in saving lives, but even in trained health personnel and bystanders, there is unwillingness to provide CPR for fear of catching acquired immunodeficiency syndrome (AIDS), hepatitis or tuberculosis through mouth-to-mouth respiration. Also, when professionals do CPR, it is often not done well.

It is for this reason, that medical/dental, and other life-sciences students must be seriously trained in this life-saving procedure.

AIM OF CARDIOPULMONARY RESUSCITATION

The aim of CPR is to "artificially" push oxygen-containing blood to the brain and other vital organs (when the heart and lungs fail to do this vital job), till the heart and lungs regain their normal function or the victim is shifted to the hospital.

GENERAL PLAN FOR CARDIOPULMONARY RESUSCITATION

Management of a case of cardiopulmonary arrest involves two phases:

Phase I: Emergency measures: Basic life support **(BLS)**

The management sequence of BLS

Initially the sequence of management in order of importance was **ABC**, i.e.

A—Airways

B—Breathing

C—Circulation.

According to the new guidelines of CPR, this order has been changed to—**CAB, i.e.**

Circulation: Re-establish circulation if there is insufficient heart beat, or if the heart has stopped.

Airway: Establish an airway, or maintain it if it is open.

Breathing: Provide artificial ventilation if breathing has stopped.

Note: These procedures must be performed in that order.

C-Circulate: Give external cardiac massage. One/two operators: (2:30). Alternate 30 cardiac compressions with two quick lung inflations. Continuous compressions at the rate of 100–120/min.

If unconscious, but breathing and pulse are present:

A-Airway: Tilt the head back with a hand under the neck to maintain an open airway.

If not breathing:

B-Breathe: Give mouth-to-mouth respiration (or mouth-to-nose). Inflate lungs 14–16 times/min to provide adequate oxygen supply. Maintain head tilt to avoid flaccid tongue from falling back into pharynx.

Feel the carotid pulse. If a pulse is present, continue lung inflations.

If pulse is absent (death-like appearance, fixed, dilated pupils).

Phase II: Definitive treatment: Advanced cardiac life support

This phase of treatment is carried out in the hospital, and includes:

D—Drugs (adrenalin, intravenous sodium bicarbonate for acidosis, etc.)

E—Electrocardiogram (ECG) monitoring

F—Fibrillation treatment with a defibrillator, lidocaine or procaine

G—Gauging and restoration of normal breathing and circulation
H—Hypothermia, and
I—Management of the patient in the intensive care unit (ICU) of the hospital.

CAUSES OF CARDIOPULMONARY ARREST

Acute Conditions

1. Massive, acute myocardial infarction (MI) leading to cardiac standstill (asystole) or fibrillation
2. Drowning
3. Hanging
4. Electric shock
5. Inhalation of poisonous gases (e.g. carbon monoxide)
6. Overdose or sensitivity to an anesthetic agent, poisoning with narcotics and drugs (accidental or suicidal) (e.g. barbiturates, opium, etc.), acids, and other chemicals
7. Head injuries
8. Obstruction of respiratory passages by inhalation of a foreign body (e.g. a fishbone)
9. Anaphylactic shock.

Chronic Conditions

1. Poliomyelitis
2. Diphtheria
3. Ascending paralysis
4. Obstruction of air passages by a tumor of pharynx, larynx, etc.

SIGNS AND SYMPTOMS OF CARDIOPULMONARY ARREST

1. The victim is unconscious, the lips, face, earlobes, fingers, and toes are blue, and there is a death-like appearance.
2. The skin is pale, cold, and moist, and the pupils are dilated and fixed, i.e. unresponsive to light (these features are due to sympathetic stimulation).
3. **Absent or weak arterial pulse:** The carotid artery must be palpated because the radial pulse may be too weak to be felt.
4. **Absence of heart sounds:** Put your ear on the chest of the victim and try to confirm presence or absence of heart sounds.
5. **Breathing is absent:** There is no movement of the chest or the alae nasi (nostrils). There is no air coming out of the nose or mouth.
6. **Blood pressure is not recordable.**

What to Do Immediately?

Confirm the diagnosis: Unconsciousness, absent carotid artery pulse. Note what time it is. One person should be incharge.

1. **Assess:**
   - **Thump the chest** (if there is no carotid pulse). This may stop fibrillation. Recheck pulse. If absent, start CPR.
   - Make sure you are in a safe place. Trying CPR on the road may risk your life as well.

   First establish unresponsiveness:
   - Determine the responsiveness of the victim by tapping him/her on the shoulder and asking "Are you all right?".
   - Check carotid pulse and breathing *to make sure that the heart and breathing have really stopped.* Because if the heart is still beating, there will be enough muscle tone so that external cardiac massage may cause fracture of the ribs.

Note: CPR is never demonstrated on a normal waking person for the same reason. Demonstration dummies are available for CPR training.

2. **Start CPR routine** after confirming CP arrest, and find out if a bystander can help.
3. **Ask a bystander to phone the hospital emergency** for an ambulance because you do not have time to do so yourself. If no one is available, continue CPR till the victim is revived.

What Not to Do?

1. Do not delay resuscitation; immediate intervention is required after establishing unresponsiveness.
2. The victim must not be made to sit or stand. No pillow should be placed under the head or neck, as this will bend the head and close the trachea.
3. The feet and legs should be raised by placing a pillow, etc. under the hips/legs. This will help promote venous return to the heart.
4. Nothing should be given by mouth to a semiconscious or unconscious individual for fear of aspiration of the fluid into the lungs.
5. There should be no crowding around the victim.

ARTIFICIAL RESPIRATION (PULMONARY RESUSCITATION)

Artificial respiration (AR; assisted ventilation) may be given by ***manual methods, mouth-to-mouth method*** (sometimes called ***"kiss of life"*** or ***"rescue breath"),*** or by ***mechanical methods.***

Note: Though mouth-to-mouth respiration has been found to be the best general first-aid procedure, which method to use in a given case will depend on the cause of CP arrest. For example, in a case of drowning or near drowning, face injuries, fracture of jaw, and chemical burns on lips and in the mouth, it may not be possible to give mouth-to-mouth respiration. In such cases, the International Red Cross recommends Holger Nielsen method.

Manual Methods

The old prone or supine position methods—*Schafer's* prone position, back pressure, *Sylvester's* supine position arm lift, and *Thomson's hip-lift chest pressure* methods are no longer employed since they rely on compressing the thorax to cause expiration, and then allowing lungs to expand passively. The

Holger Nielsen method described here is used when mouth-to-mouth respiration is not possible.

Holger Nielsen Method (Back-pressure Arm-lift Method)

1. Place the victim, face downward **(Figs. 17A to D)** on a hard surface, with the arms bent, and the head turned to one side and resting on the hands.
2. Kneel down on one knee at the victim's head, with the opposite foot placed near the elbow.
3. Place your hands, with fingers widespread, on the victim's back just below the scapulae. Now rock forward, with the arms held straight at the elbows, until your arms are vertical and pressing down on the back. This compresses the chest and produces expiration.
4. Slide your hands sideways and outward onto the victim's arms just above the elbows. Now rock backward, lifting the victim's elbows until some resistance is felt at her/his shoulders. This movement expands the thorax, decreasing the intrathoracic pressure and causing inspiration.
5. Repeat this cycle of compression and expansion (that lasts for about 3 seconds each) for about 12 times a minute.

Mouth-to-mouth Respiration (Rescue Breath; Exhaled-air Ventilation)

Mouth-to-mouth respiration **(Figs. 18A to C)** has proved to be superior to all the manual methods in all age groups. Comparative studies have proved it to be the only technique capable of producing satisfactory ventilation.

Advantages and Disadvantages of Mouth-to-mouth Respiration

The method is simple, safe, and easy to perform, even by a layman with minimum instruction. Above all, it does not require any apparatus. The only disadvantage is that the victim's flaccid (toneless) tongue tends to fall back into the pharynx and thus obstruct the airway. However, this can be avoided by extending the neck and turning the head slightly to one side.

Procedure

1. Place the victim on his/her back on firm ground, and loosen the clothing around the neck, chest, and waist.
2. Remove any mucus, food, saliva, or any foreign material (e.g. grass, dentures, etc.) from the mouth and nose with your fingers wrapped in a handkerchief.
3. Open the airway by tilting the head back. Kneel by the right side of the victim. Place your right hand under the neck and lift it, while keeping a pressure on the forehead with the heel of the other hand **(Figs. 18A to C)** (the extension of the neck lifts the flaccid tongue from the back of the throat). Using your right thumb and fingers, lift the chin, and angle of the jaw upward and forward. This simple procedure keeps the airway open.
4. Clamp the nostrils with your left thumb and fingers, take a deep breath, apply your mouth firmly on the victim's mouth (or nose if the pharynx cannot be cleared), and blow a liter of air into the victim's lungs, watching the expansion of the chest at the same time (remember, the expired air contains 15% oxygen).
5. Remove your mouth, turn your head to one side, and take another deep breath as the elastic recoil of the chest causes expiration. You may feel and hear the expiratory airflow from the victim's mouth and nose.

Note: If the airway is clear, only a moderate resistance will be felt when you exhale air into the victim's lungs.

6. **Repeat the cycle of** blowing out—turning the head—breathing in—about 14-16 times a minute, till spontaneous breathing returns or the victim is shifted to the hospital.

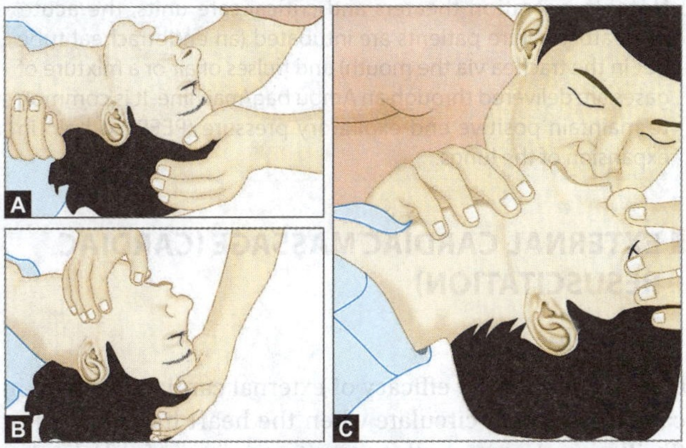

FIGS. 18A TO C: Mouth-to-mouth respiration. (A) Tilting the head back; (B) Lifting the chain and angle of law; (C) Clamping the nostrils and blowing air into the victim's lungs.

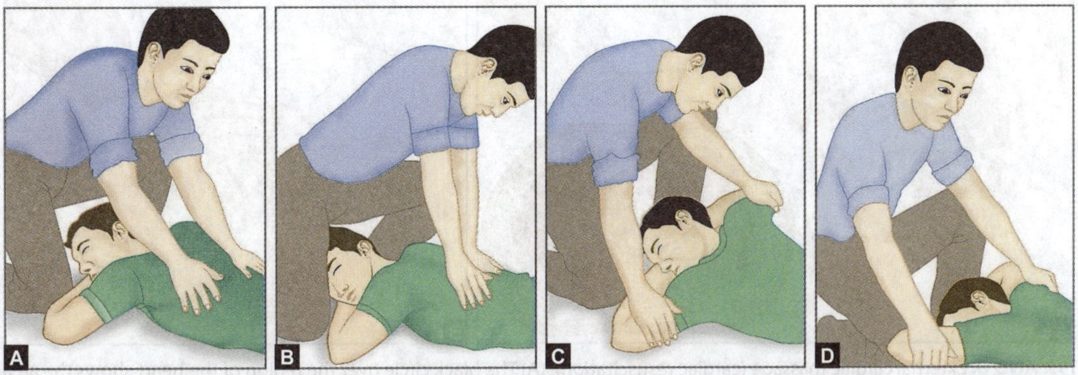

FIGS. 17A TO D: Holger Nielsen (back-pressure arm-lift, BPAL) method of artificial respiration. (A and B) Back pressure; (C and D) Arm lift.

7. **Important:** Feel the carotid pulse. If, after 6–8 lung inflations, there is no improvement in the color of the victim, suspect cardiac arrest, and start external cardiac massage as well.

Mechanical Respirators

Mechanical ventilation is employed when AR has to be given for long periods, e.g. during chronic respiratory failure. Air-tight metallic or plastic devices are placed around the chest and negative pressure is applied at intervals; this draws air into the lungs. The elastic recoil of the lungs and chest causes expiration.

Alternate positive and negative pressures are also employed.

1. **Drinker's tank respirator (also called the "iron lung"):** It is an iron chamber in which the patient is placed, with the head kept outside, an air-tight collar sealing the body inside. The pressure in the chamber is alternately raised (2–3 cm water) for expiration, and lowered (–10 cm to –14 cm H_2O) for inspiration, by means of a pump.
2. **Sahlin's jacket model, Bragg–Paul pulsator**, and their modifications employ inelastic chest jackets in which pressure can be increased and decreased at intervals.
3. **Eve's rocking method:** The victim is laid on a stretcher or a plank and the shoulders and ankles are fastened to it. A rhythmic rocking up and down like a see-saw causes the abdominal viscera to push up against the diaphragm (expiration) or pull it down (inspiration).

Note: In operation theaters and critical care units, the acute respiratory failure patients are intubated (an endotracheal tube put in the trachea via the mouth) and pulses of air or a mixture of gases are delivered through an Ambu bag/machine. It is common to maintain positive end-expiratory pressure (PEEP) to help in expansion of the lungs.

EXTERNAL CARDIAC MASSAGE (CARDIAC RESUSCITATION)

Rationale

One may doubt the efficacy of external cardiac massage in causing blood to circulate when the heart has stopped or fibrillating. However, there are two reasons for believing that cardiac output and coronary perfusion can be partially maintained by CPR:

1. When the heart stops suddenly, the pulmonary veins, left heart, and the arteries are full of oxygenated blood. Cardiac massage causes this blood to start flowing.
2. Since the heart is situated between two rigid structures—sternum in front, and vertebrae behind—pressure (compression) applied on the chest in front of it squeezes it, thus producing a mechanical systole. The right and left ventricular pressures exceed the pulmonary and aortic pressures, which cause a forward flow of blood. When the pressure is released, it causes diastolic filling of the ventricles due to the pressure gradient between the large peripheral veins and intrathoracic structures—especially the thin-walled right ventricle.

Procedure

1. Lay the victim on a firm surface. Kneel beside him and place the heel of your left hand (fingers extended and not touching the chest) on the junction of the upper two-thirds and lower one-third of the sternum. Place the heel of the other hand over the first, parallel to it **(Figs. 19A and B)**.
2. Keeping the elbows straight, bend forward, and depress the sternum toward the spine by 4–5 cm at a rate of 80–90/min. The movement should be at the shoulders so that the force can be transmitted through the hands to the chest.

Cardiopulmonary resuscitation by one/two persons—(30:2). Alternate 30 cardiac compressions with two quick lung inflations.

Note: If the CPR is being given correctly, you will quickly see an improvement in skin color of the victim; pupils will return to normal size, and neck pulsations will be visible, and heart sounds will be heard.

In Infants

Press the sternum with two fingers of a hand, or with a thumb, with the fingers supporting the back of the infant. Compress by 2–3 cm and maintain cardiac compressions at a rate of 100–110/min.

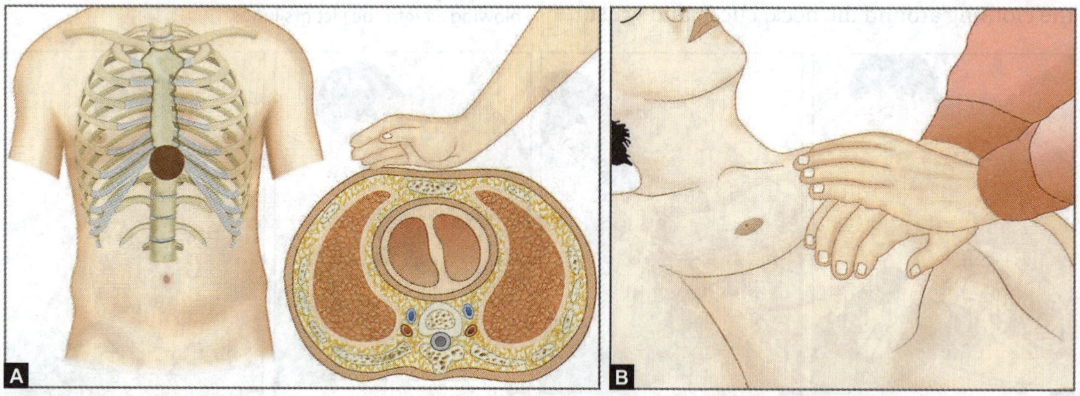

FIGS. 19A AND B: External cardiac massage (cardiac resuscitation). (A) The black circle over the region of the heart shows the area where compression should be applied; (B) The position of hands for chest compression. The victim must be placed on a firm surface.

INTERNAL OR OPEN CARDIAC MASSAGE

This procedure is employed in hospitals. The chest is opened in the left intercostal space in the midclavicular line; a hand is inserted into the thorax and the heart is compressed against the chest wall. There is a transdiaphragmatic approach as well.

CARDIOPULMONARY RESUSCITATION FOR ONESELF

What to do when one gets an attack of MI when alone. Coughing very vigorously and repeatedly can save life. A breath and a forceful cough, repeated every 3 seconds, without let up till help arrives or the heart is felt to be beating normally.

REASONS FOR FAILURE OF CARDIOPULMONARY RESUSCITATION

In every case you must try your best to get the heart and lungs functioning again. However, in some cases, all efforts at CPR may fail. It may be that:

- The injury to the heart is very severe, or
- Acid-base disturbances (lactic acidemia) and electrolyte imbalance do not allow the heart rate and rhythm to be restored.

VENTRICULAR FIBRILLATION

Ventricular fibrillation (VF) is the most common cause of cardiac arrest because a fibrillating (*trembling*) heart cannot act as an effective pump. It is most frequently caused by acute MI as a result of which an "ectopic" irritable focus starts to discharge action potentials (APs) in a fast and irregular manner. The heart responds to these APs and goes into fibrillation. If VF is not stopped within 2–3 minutes, it almost always leads to death. The specific treatment includes:

1. **Electroshock defibrillation (cardioversion):** While a weak AC current (as in accidental shock or in death penalty) causes VF and death, a strong, high voltage current applied to the chest via large, flat electrodes, can stop fibrillation. All APs stop and the heart remains quiescent for 4–5 seconds, after which it starts to beat at the normal rate and rhythm. The shock may have to be repeated a couple of times.
2. **Intravenous injection of 100 mL of 8% sodium bicarbonate** is used to neutralize lactic acidemia.
3. **Intravenous injection of 5–10 mL of 1% calcium chloride.**
4. **Intravenous or intracardiac injection of 0.5 mL of 1:1000 adrenaline** often revives the heart.

HEIMLICH MANEUVER (ABDOMINAL THRUST) FOR INHALATION OF FOREIGN BODY

This procedure can be life-saving when a person begins to choke on something he/she is eating (e.g. a fishbone) or in a child who puts something in his mouth and inadvertently "inhales" it, e.g. a coin, a marble, etc.

Important: Choking must not be confused with an attack of MI. A person who chokes on something cannot speak but only makes gestures, while a heart attack victim can (and, of course, choking is likely to occur while eating. Therefore, ask, *can you speak?*).

Procedure

1. Stand behind the person, place your clenched fist below his epigastrium (between the costal margin and the umbilicus), and grasp this fist with the other hand.
2. Now give a sudden upward and inward thrust. It is important the thrust be applied to the upper abdomen and not to the thorax.
3. The sudden thrust pushes the diaphragm up so that the forceful blast of air from the lungs carries the foreign body out of the respiratory passages. The maneuver may be repeated until the foreign object is expelled.

Important: In many cases of choking, the respiratory passage is not completely blocked (though there may be laryngeal spasm), so that if the person breathes quietly and without panic, enough air may reach the lungs to keep him alive until he is shifted to the hospital.

If you happen to choke on something, when alone, position yourself over the high back of a chair, or some other suitable furniture, and thrust your abdomen suddenly and forcefully against it. Repeat if necessary.

Emergency Procedure in Children

Bend the head of the victim forward and downward so that it is lower than the chest. Then, with the heel of a hand, give a few blows on the child's back between the scapulae till the offending object is expelled.

Note that the head must be kept lower than the chest, otherwise the foreign object is likely to be pushed further down into the lungs rather than upward.

QUESTIONS

Q.1. Name the indications for cardiopulmonary resuscitation.
Cardiopulmonary resuscitation is a first-aid measure and is indicated when there is a sudden stoppage of breathing or heart, or both.

Q.2. What are the causes and signs of cardiopulmonary arrest?
See text above.

Q.3. Name the advantages and disadvantages of mouth-to-mouth respiration.
See text above.

Q.4. How will you handle a case of drowning?

1. As soon as the victim is brought out of the water, check the carotid pulse and breathing. If both present but unconscious, press on the lower abdomen to expel water from the stomach, if any. Then place the victim in "recovery position", i.e. partial supine position, head turned to one side, left arm under left thigh, right arm above the head, and right leg bent.

2. If the pulse is present, but the victim is not breathing—start mouth-to-mouth breathing or Holger Nielsen method of AR.
3. If both pulse and breaching are absent—start CPR, till the victim recovers or is shifted to the hospital.

Q.5. How does defibrillation help in ventricular fibrillation?

A strong, high-voltage AC current applied to the chest can stop a fibrillating heart. However, within a few seconds, normal heart beat usually returns.

Q.6. What is the Heimlich maneuver?

It is an emergency procedure to clear the upper respiratory passages after a foreign body has been accidentally inhaled.

UNIT II: CARDIOVASCULAR SYSTEM

2.5: EXAMINATION OF THE ARTERIAL PULSE

STUDENT OBJECTIVES

After completing this experiment, the student should be able to:

- Define arterial pulse.
- Examine the radial pulse properly.
- Enumerate the common causes of increased, decreased and irregular pulse.
- Explain high and low volume pulse and water hammer pulse.
- Access the volume of the pulse.
- Know the various parameters under which the radial pulse is to be examined.
- State the importance of radial pulse examination.

INTRODUCTION

PY5.16: Record arterial pulse tracing using finger plethysmography in a volunteer or simulated environment.

- After each systole, the alternate expansion and recoil of the aorta sets up a pressure or pulse wave. This rhythmic pulsatile wave travels from segment to segment of the arterial tree and causes expansion and recoil of their walls which is felt as the **arterial pulse**.
- The arterial pulse has a velocity of about 6–10 m/sec and should not be confused with the flow of blood that has a velocity of 0.5 m/sec. A similar pulsatile phenomenon occurs in the pulmonary arterial tree, which, of course, cannot be felt.
- The examination of arterial pulse includes—inspection, palpation and auscultation of some important vessels, especially radial, brachial, carotid, temporal, retinal, femoral and popliteal arteries and their branches, especially the dorsalis pedis artery.
- ***Why is the radial artery chosen?***
  The routine examination of arterial pulse is done on radial artery because:
  - It is conveniently accessible as it is located in an exposed part of the body.
  - The artery lies over the hard surface of the lower end of the radius.

EXAMINATION OF RADIAL PULSE

- The radial artery is palpated with the tips of three fingers compressing the vessel against the head of radius bone **(Fig. 20)**. The subject's forearm should be slightly pronated and the wrist slightly flexed.
- The index finger (toward the heart) varies the pressure on the artery, the middle finger feels the pulse, while the distal finger prevents reflections of pulsations from the palmar arch of arteries. The following observations are made as follows:

Rate of Pulse

- The normal pulse rate at rest averages about 72 beats/min (60-90 beats/min). The rate is normally higher in children (90–110 beats/min) and slower in old age (55–65 beats/min). An increase in heart rate above 90 beats/min is called *tachycardia*. A decrease in heart rate below 60 beats/min is called *bradycardia*.
- The pulse rate normally increases during deep inspiration and decreases during deep expiration. When this happens during quiet breathing, it is called **sinus arrhythmia**, which is due to irradiation of impulses from the inspiratory center to the cardiac center. Quite trivial factors increase the pulse rate— climbing stairs, a brisk short walk, nervousness, etc. For this reason, the pulse rate should be counted two or three times at intervals of 10–15 minutes.
- The pulse rate should always be compared with the heart rate, as in some cases the pulse rate may be less than heart rate (pulse deficit).
- The pulse rate should be counted for a full 1 minute.

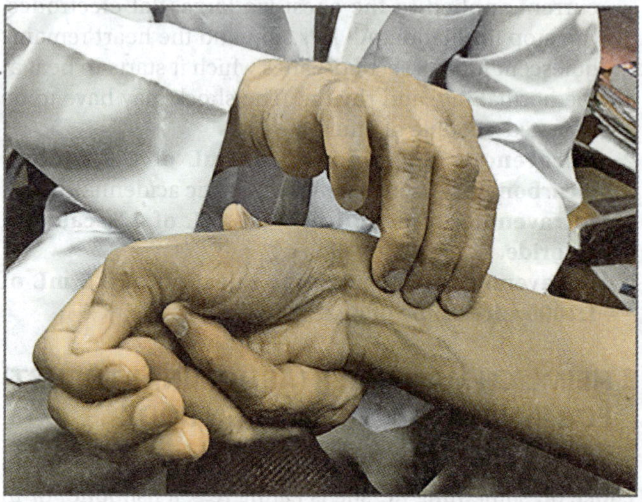

FIG. 20: Examination of radial pulse.

Rhythm

- The normal pulse waves follow at regular intervals, i.e. the rhythm is regular.
- The common irregularities in the pulse, which may be:
  - **Regularly irregular:** Irregularity of pulse occurring at regular intervals, e.g. in extrasystoles (premature ectopic beats)
  - **Irregularly irregular:** Irregularity of pulse seen at irregular intervals, e.g. atrial fibrillation.

Volume

- The "volume" of the pulse refers to the amplitude of the movement or expansion of the artery during the passage of the pulse wave.
- It is a rough guide to the pulse pressure. It can be:
  - **Low volume pulse** (thin, thready pulse) of low stroke volume seen in **shock**.
  - **High volume pulse** of hyperkinetic circulation seen in: Pregnancy, exercise, fever, anemia, thyrotoxicosis.

Condition of the Vessel Wall

- The index finger is used to obliterate the flow of blood and the ring finger should be used to empty the blood vessel. The middle finger is then used to palpate the vessel wall. The emptied vessel should then be rolled against the underlying bone.
- In young individuals, the "empty" artery is so compliant that it cannot be felt as a separate structure. However, the vessel becomes palpable in old age and is felt as a cord-like structure due to atherosclerosis and calcification. The surface may show irregularities and the vessel may be tortuous.
- Another way to note the condition of the vessel wall (when emptied out of blood) is to compress the brachial artery with a thumb and then palpate the radial artery by rolling it against the bone (a "full" radial artery is normally palpable in many thin individuals).

Radiofemoral Delay

- When the left femoral artery and the right radial artery are palpated simultaneously the two pulses normally beat together i.e. there is no delay between occurrence of the pulse in femoral and radial artery.
- Radiofemoral delay is seen in **coarctation of the aorta**.

Equality on the Two Sides

- The arterial pulse of one side is always compared with that of the other side for all of its features described above.
- Normally, there is no difference between the two.

Character or Form

- By character or form is the waveform and volume of the pulse, i.e. whether the individual pulse wave has a normal rise, maintenance or fall (its contours) as the pulse is being palpated.
- The character should be evaluated at the right carotid artery, i.e. the pulse closest to the heart, and least subjected to distortion and damping in the arterial tree.
- Since the contours of the pulse waves cannot usually be clearly felt by palpation, one has to record the pulse with an electronic transducer **(Dudgeon's sphygmograph** used to be employed in the past).

NORMAL PULSE WAVE

The normal pulse wave **(Figs. 21A to C)** shows the following components:

- **Percussion wave or the anacrotic limb:** This is the sharp upstroke. It is due to expansion of the artery due to ventricular systole and corresponds to the maximum ejection phase. The leisurely down stroke is called the catacrotic limb.
- **Tidal wave:** This pre dicrotic wave is due to elasticity of the aorta. It is sometimes recorded soon after the peak of the tracing.
- **Dicrotic notch and wave:** These are seen on the descending limb. The notch, the negative wave, is due to recoil of the elastic aorta that causes the blood column to momentarily sweep back toward the heart. The reverse flow closes the aortic valve and rebounds from it to cause the positive dicrotic wave. The systolic and diastolic phases of the ventricle can be indicated on the arterial pulse tracing. The maximum ejection phase lasts from the upstroke to the peak of the percussion wave, while the reduced ejection phase lasts from the peak to the dicrotic notch. Thus, the systole is from the upstroke to the dicrotic notch.

TYPES OF ABNORMAL ARTERIAL PULSE WAVES

- **Dicrotic pulse:** There are two palpable waves, one in systole, and the other in diastole. It is seen most commonly in low stroke volume.

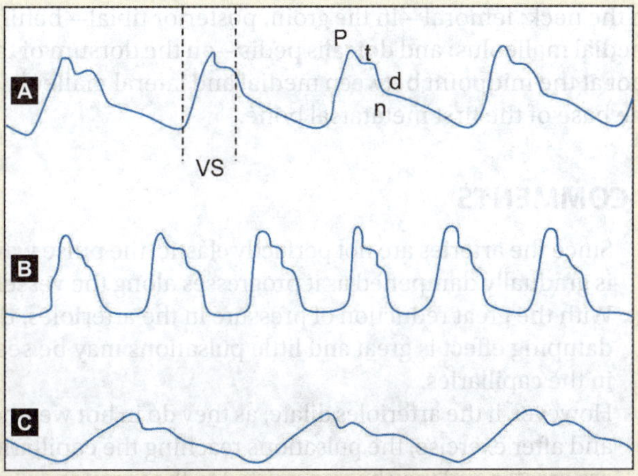

FIGS. 21A TO C: From the arterial pulse. (A) Normal pulse tracing; P: percussion wave; t: tidal wave; d: dicrotic notch; n: dicrotic wave, VS: period of ventricular systole (aortic valve open); (B) Water-hammer (Corrigan's) pulse-showing rapid upstroke and descent; (C) Pulse tracing in aortic stenosis-showing a gradual upstroke and slow descent.

- **Corrigan's, Water-hammer or collapsing pulse:** It is characterized by an abrupt rise, and a sudden fall of the pulse wave in early diastole. It is seen most commonly in aortic regurgitation in which the incompetent valve cannot close properly to prevent backflow of blood from the aorta back into the ventricle. The rapid upstroke is due to greatly increased and vigorous stroke volume while the collapsing is caused by two factors—the diastolic "run-off" of blood back into the left ventricle and the rapid "run-off" of blood toward the periphery due to low peripheral resistance resulting from arteriolar dilatation. This type of pulse is also found in patent ductus arteriosus, or a large arteriovenous fistula.
- **Pulsus parvus or slow-rising pulse:** It is a small (parvus = small), weak, pulse which rises slowly and has a late systolic phase. The weak upstroke is due to decreased stroke volume and a narrow pulse pressure. It is seen especially in aortic stenosis, left ventricular failure and hypovolemia.
- **Alternating pulse (pulsus alternans):** The pulse beats are regular but alternately large and small in amplitude, i.e. large and small systolic peaks. It is seen in left ventricular failure when the ventricle is severely diseased. The variation in strength should not be confused with an arrhythmia. The mechanism, however, is not known.
- **Pulsus paradoxus:** The term describes the marked decrease in pulse volume (and blood pressure) which occurs on deep inspiration. It is an accentuation of normal physiological fall in systolic pressure by 8–10 mm Hg. The paradox is that while the pulse may not be felt at the wrist, heart sounds may still be heard at the precordium. It occurs in patients with large pericardial effusion.
- **Thready pulse:** Thin, thready pulse is a feature of shock and due to decrease in stroke volume.

Examine all other arterial pulses: The examination of other pulses is important: brachial—at the elbow; carotids—in the neck; femoral—in the groin; posterior tibial—behind medial malleolus; and dorsalis pedis—on the dorsum of the foot at the midpoint between medial and lateral malleoli, at the base of the first metatarsal bone.

COMMENTS

- Since the arteries are not perfectly elastic, the pulse wave is gradually dampened as it progresses along the vessels. With the great reduction of pressure in the arterioles, the damping effect is great and little pulsations may be seen in the capillaries.
- However, if the arterioles dilate, as they do in hot weather and after exercise, the pulsations reaching the capillaries are greater and may be transmitted to the venules.
- Similarly, when the pulse pressure is greatly increased as in aortic regurgitation, the pulsations are seen in the capillaries. Properly applied pressure on a nail-bed, or on the mucosa of the lip (with a glass slide) will show alternate flushing of the blanched margin.

PRECAUTIONS

1. The pulse should be examined after the subject has rested and relaxed for at least 5 minutes.
2. The forearm of the subject should be semi-pronated and the wrist be slightly flexed.
3. The pulse rate should be counted for a minimum of 1 minute.
4. To detect radiofemoral delay the femoral artery should be examined simultaneously with the radial artery.
5. Pulses of both sides should be examined and compared.
6. While examining the radial pulse three fingers should be used. The index finger is used to obliterate the flow of blood, and the ring finger should be used to empty the blood vessel. The middle finger is then used to palpate the vessel wall.
7. All the peripheral pulses should be examined.

QUESTIONS

Q.1. Why is the radial artery chosen?
See text above

Q.2. List the various precautions taken during radial pulse examination.
See text above

Q.3. Why are three fingers used for radial pulse examination?
See text above

Q.4. How much is the normal pulse rate and what determines the pulse rate?
See text above

Q.5. Define sinus arrhythmia.
See text above

Q.6. What is tachycardia and what are its causes?
Tachycardia: An increase in heart rate above 90 beats/min is called tachycardia.

Physiological tachycardia is seen in:

1. **Emotional excitement, nervousness, and apprehension:** For example, at the time of an interview.
2. **Muscular exercise.**
3. **In the newborns:** The heart rate may be 120–150 beats/min; it gradually decreases during infancy and childhood.
4. **Sex:** The rate is comparatively higher in females; there may be tachycardia during pregnancy.
5. **Diurnal variations:** Higher rates are seen in the evening and may exceed 100 beats/min.

Pathological tachycardia is seen in:

1. **Fever due to any cause:** For every 1°C rise in temperature, the heart rate increases by about 10–14 beats/min. The raised temperature acts directly on the SA node and generates more action potentials per unit time.
2. **Thyrotoxicosis:** Increased metabolism of SA node generates more action potentials.
3. **Atrial flutter and fibrillation:** The pulse is fast and irregular.
4. **Paroxysmal atrial tachycardia:** Sudden onset and as sudden an offset are characteristic features.
5. **Circulatory shock:** The pulse is fast and weak (thready pulse).

Q.7. What is bradycardia and what are its causes?

Bradycardia: A decrease in heart rate below 60 beats/min is called bradycardia.

Physiological bradycardia is seen in:

1. **Athletes:** The resting heart rate may be 50-55 beats/min; it is due to increased vagal tone.
2. **Sleep and meditation:** The rate may be below 55 during deep meditation.
3. The rate may be below 60 beats/min under **basal conditions**, i.e. before a person gets out of bed after a good night's sleep.

Pathological bradycardia is seen in:

1. **Myxedema:** Hyposecretion of thyroid hormone is commonly associated with low pulse rates.
2. **Heart block:** The rate depends on the degree of heart block. In complete heart block, the ventricular rate may be 30-40 beats/min (idioventricular rhythm).
3. **General weakness and debility** following prolonged illness.
4. **Drugs:** Treatment with drugs such as digitalis and sympatholytics (e.g. propranolol).

Q.8. What is pulse deficit?

Normally the pulse rate and the ventricular rate (as determined by auscultation at the heart) are identical. However, in the case of extrasystoles (premature beats) and atrial fibrillation, some of the ventricular beats are too weak to be felt at the radial artery so that the heart rate is higher than the radial pulse rate—a condition called **pulse deficit or apex pulse deficit.**

Q.9. Examine the arterial pulse in the subject provided and comment on your findings.

See text above.

Q.10. List some different types of abnormal pulse.

See text above.

OBJECTIVELY STRUCTURED PRACTICAL EVALUATION

Aim: To examine the radial artery of the subject provided.

Procedural steps: See text above.

Checklist:

1. Stands on the subject's right side and explains the procedure. (Y/N)
2. Holds the subject's right hand in a semi-pronated and slightly flexed position. Then places her three middle fingers on the radial artery and compresses it slightly against the bone. (Y/N)
3. Notes the rhythm, volume, and character of the pulse. Counts the rate for 1 minute and notes the result. (Y/N)
4. Compresses the artery with the proximal finger and tries to roll the artery against the bone with the other two fingers. (Y/N)
5. Compares the equality of pulses in both arms. Counts the heart rate to see if there is any pulse deficit. (Y/N)

2.6: RECORDING OF SYSTEMIC ARTERIAL BLOOD PRESSURE

STUDENT OBJECTIVES

After completing this experiment, the student should be able to:

- Define blood pressure (BP) and its determinants.
- Define systolic, diastolic, pulse and mean arterial pressures (MAPs). Indicate their significance.
- Determine BP by palpatory, oscillometric, and auscultatory methods. Name the advantages and disadvantages of each method.
- Indicate the precautions that must be taken before and during recording of BP.
- Describe the Korotkoff sounds, and their physiological basis.
- Detect the appearance and muffling/disappearance of Korotkoff sounds while recording BP.
- Name the factors controlling BP.
- List the physiological variations in BP.
- Explain how BP is regulated on short-term and long-term basis.
- Define auscultatory gap and explain its significance.
- Describe the clinical conditions of hypertension and hypotension and their pathophysiology.
- Explain the importance of sinoaortic mechanism (baroreceptor reflex).

INTRODUCTION

PY5.12: Record blood pressure and pulse at rest and in different grades of exercise and postures in a volunteer or simulated environment.

- The term **blood pressure** (BP) refers to the force exerted by the blood as it presses against and attempts to stretch the walls of blood vessels.
- Although blood exerts this outward force throughout the CVS, the term BP, used unqualified, refers to systemic arterial BP (others are: venous, capillary pressure, etc).
- The BP is not steady (unchanging) throughout the cardiac cycle but fluctuating, i.e. it is pulsatile.
  - The maximum pressure is reached during the maximum ejection phase of systole and is called the **systolic blood pressure (SBP).**
  - The minimum pressure is reached during diastole and is called the **diastolic blood pressure (DBP).**
  - The **mean arterial pressure (MAP) or mean arterial blood pressure (MABP)** is the average of all the pressures measured during the cardiac cycle. Since the duration of systole is shorter than that of diastole, the MAP is slightly less than the average of systolic and DPs. MAP is calculated as: **MAP = DBP + 1/3 PP.**
  - **Pulse pressure (PP)** is the difference between systolic and DPs, the average PP being about 40 mm Hg.
- The cardiovascular system (CVS) is slightly overfilled with blood, i.e. its contents are more than its capacity. As a result, the blood exerts an outward force against the vessel walls as it flows through them.

NORMAL VALUES IN ADULTS

Systolic blood pressure (SBP)—100-140 mm Hg

Diastolic blood pressure (DBP)—60-90 mm Hg.

Measurement of BP is an important clinical procedure as it provides valuable information about the CVS under normal and disease conditions.

There are two methods for measurement of systemic arterial blood pressure:

Direct Method

- The direct method of recording BP in which an artery is punctured with a cannula connected to a manometer. It measures the end pressure which is the sum of **lateral pressure and pressure due to kinetic energy.**
- The direct method was first employed in man in 1856 by Favre, a French physician. He employed a Poiseuille manometer and recorded pressures in three patients prior to amputation—in the upper part of brachial artery in two patients and in femoral artery in one patient. In each case, pressure of about 120 mm Hg was recorded, which he thought was the mean aortic pressure.
- *Disadvantage:* This method is not safe and convenient in clinical practice as it is an invasive procedure and involves high risk of infections.

Note: These days, direct method is used in research work in animals, and during cardiac and arterial catheterization in man.

Indirect Method

Obviously, the direct method is not suitable as a routine clinical procedure. Indirect methods were, therefore, introduced; methods that are variations of a procedure called sphygmomanometry.

PRINCIPLE

The brachial artery is first compressed by inflating a rubber bag (connected to a manometer) placed around the arm to stop the blood flow through the occluded section of the artery. The pressure is then slowly released and the flow of blood through the obstructed segment of the artery is studied by:

- **Palpatory method:** Feeling the radial pulse.
- **Oscillatory method:** Observing the oscillations of the mercury column.
- **Auscultatory Method:** Listening to the sounds produced in the part of the artery just below the obstructed segment.

BP can also be measured in the femoral artery by indirect method.

APPARATUS

Stethoscope (Steth = Chest, Scope = To Inspect) (Fig. 22)

Though introduced in its present form by Laennec in 1819, it was not until 1905 that Korotkoff used it for recording the BP. The sounds produced in the chest and elsewhere in the body are heard with a stethoscope. The instrument has the following *three parts:*

1. **The chest piece:** The chest piece has two end pieces—(1) a *bell* and (2) a flat *diaphragm,* though some have only the diaphragm.

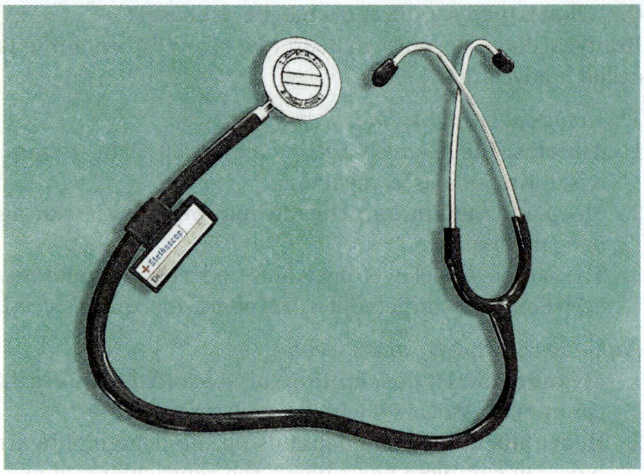

FIG. 22: Stethoscope.

2. **The rubber tubing:** In the commonly used stethoscope, a single soft-rubber pressure tube (inner diameter 3 mm) leads from the chest piece to a metal Y-shaped connector. The plastic diaphragm causes magnification of low-pitched sounds though it distorts them a little. The bell-shaped chest piece conducts sounds without distortion but with little magnification. Murmurs which precede, accompany or follow the heart sounds are better heard with the bell.
3. **The ear frame:** It consists of two curved metallic tubes joined together with a flat U-shaped spring which keeps them pulled together. The upper ends of the tubes are curved so that they correspond to the curve of the external auditory meatus, i.e. they are directed forward and downward. Two plastic knobs threaded over the ends of the tubes fit snugly in the ear. Two rubber tubes connect the Y-shaped connector to the metal tubes.

Sphygmomanometer (Commonly called the "Blood Pressure Apparatus") (Fig. 23)

The sphygmomanometer is the instrument routinely used for recording arterial BP in humans. The term "sphygmomanometer" is derived from three Greek roots with

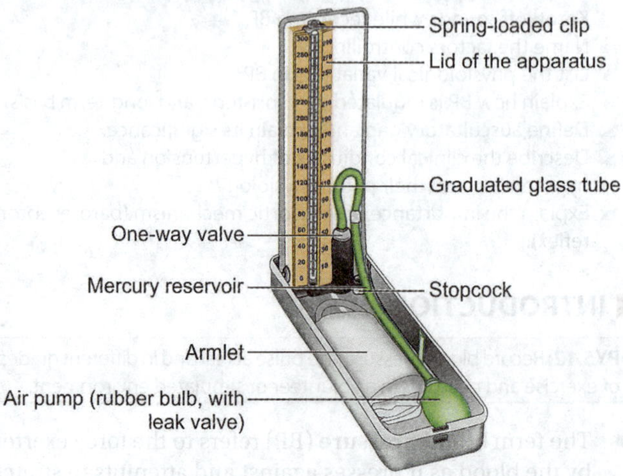

FIG. 23: Sphygmomanometer [the blood pressure (BP) apparatus].

Latin equivalents "sphygmo" means pulse, "manos" means thin, and "metron" refers to measure. In early procedures, when physicians used to feel the pulse during measurement of BP, they described its first appearance as "thin", hence the term. Different types of BP instruments are in use, but the one in common use is the mercury sphygmomanometer. It consists of the following parts:

- **Mercury manometer:** The manometer is fitted in the lid of the instrument. One arm of the manometer is the reservoir for mercury—a broad and short well that contains enough mercury to be driven up in the other limb—the graduated glass tube **(Fig. 24A)**.
- **Graduated tube:** The manometer glass tube is graduated in mm from 0 to 300, each division representing 2 mm, though actually slightly less than 2 mm. The reason for this is the greater diameter of the mercury reservoir than that of the glass tube. For example, when mercury is driven up the tube for, say, 20 mm Hg, the meniscus in the reservoir falls less so that the actual pressure on its mercury is slightly greater than 20 mm Hg.
  And, to compensate for this, the tube is calibrated with divisions that are slightly less than 2 mm apart.
  A stopcock between the two limbs, when closed, prevents the mercury from entering the glass tube. The one-way valve fitted at the top of the mercury well prevents spilling of mercury when the lid is closed, while allowing pressure to be transmitted from the rubber bag to the mercury reservoir. A spring-loaded clip at the top of the tube keeps it firmly pressed into a rubber washer at its lower end to prevent leakage of mercury.
- **The armlet (rubber bag; Riva-Rocci cuff):** The "cuff" as it is usually called, consist of an inflatable rubber bag, 24 cm × 12 cm, which is fitted with two rubber tubes—(1) one connecting it to the mercury reservoir and (2) the other to a rubber bulb (air pump). The bag is enclosed in a long strip of inelastic cloth with a long tapering free end. The cloth covering keeps the rubber bag in position around the arm when pressure is being measured. In some cuffs, two Velcro strips are provided in appropriate locations for the same purpose **(Fig. 24B)**.
  - The rubber bag is 12 cm wide which is enough to form a pressure cone that reaches the underlying artery even in a thick arm.
  - As a general rule, the **width** of the bag should be **20% more than the diameter** of the arm, though it should be wider in an obese person.
  - The **length** should cover two-thirds of the arm circumference.
  - The recommended width of the bag in different age groups is as under:
    - *Infants (below 1 year)*: 2.5 cm
    - *Below 4 years*: 5 cm
    - *Below 8 years*: 8 cm
    - *Adults*: 12 cm

Note: The problem of miscuffling (inappropriate size of the cuff) constitutes the most frequent error in the recording of BP. In order to prevent that, the **American Heart Association guidelines** specify that the proper cuff should have a bladder length (rubber bag) of 80% and a width of at least 40% of arm circumference. It is also to be remembered that BP measurement error is greater with an undersized cuff than it is with an oversized cuff.

- **Air pump (rubber bulb):** It is an oval-shaped rubber bulb of a size that conveniently fits into one's fist. It has a one-way valve at its free end, and a leak valve with a knurled screw, at the other where the rubber tube leading to the cuff is attached. The cuff can be inflated by turning the leak valve screw clockwise, and alternately compressing and releasing the bulb. Deflation of the bag is achieved by turning this screw anticlockwise.

Note: Since the criteria for classification of hypertension are based on BP reading taken in seated subjects in doctor's clinic. It is preferable to take BP measurements in sitting position. However, BP can also be measured in supine position if the patient is very sick or in standing position (to detect orthostatic hypertension). It is to be remembered that BP measures are not the same in seated and supine position.

- **Aneroid manometer:** In this manometer, in which metal bellows, mechanical links, and a calibrated dial replace the mercury manometer, is also in common use. However,

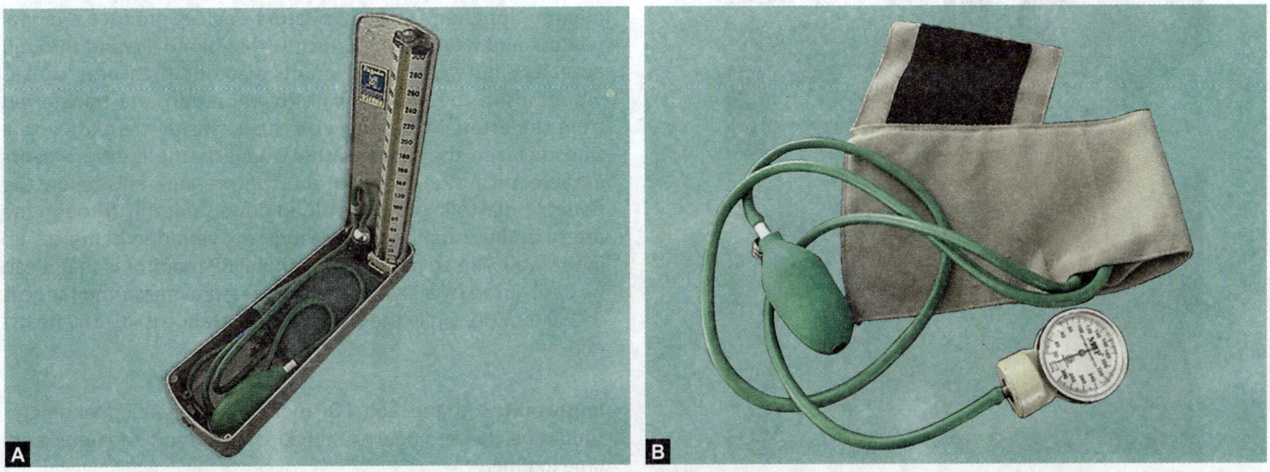

FIGS. 24A AND B: (A) Sphygmomanometer; and (B) Aneroid sphygmomanometer showing Riva-Rocci cuff.

it should be calibrated against a mercury manometer from time to time.

Note: Although mercury sphygmomanometer is the "gold standard" for taking BP measurements. However, because of the environmental issues other types of devices (e.g. aneroid sphygmomanometer/digital electronic pressure transducers) are increasingly being used.

PROCEDURE

Palpatory Method (Riva–Rocci, 1896)

1. Make the subject sit or lie supine and allow 5 minutes for mental and physical relaxation.
2. Open the lid of the apparatus. Release the lock on the mercury reservoir and check that the mercury is at the zero level. If it is above zero, subtract the difference from the final reading. If it is below zero, add the required amount of mercury to bring it to zero level.
3. Place the cuff around the exposed upper arm, with the center of the bag lying over the brachial artery, keeping its lower edge about 3 cm above the elbow. Wrap the cloth covering around the arm so as to cover the rubber bag completely, and to prevent it bulging out from under the wrapping on inflation. The cuff should neither be too tight nor very loose.
4. The upper arm on which the BP cuff is to be tied must be at the level of the heart (in the supine position, the arm resting on the bed will be nearly at the heart level **(Fig. 25)**. In the sitting position, the arm resting on the table of a suitable height will be at the correct level).
5. Palpate the radial artery at the wrist and feel its pulsations with the tips of your fingers. Keeping your fingers on the pulse, hold the air bulb in the palm of your other hand, and tighten the leak valve screw with your thumb and fingers.
6. Inflate the cuff slowly until the pulsations disappear; note the reading then raise the pressure of another 30–40 mm Hg.
7. Open the leak valve and control it so that the pressure gradually falls in steps of 2–3 mm Hg. Note the reading when the pulse just reappears. **The pressure at which the pulse is first felt is the SBP** (it corresponds to the time when, at the peak of each systole, small amounts of blood start to flow through the compressed segment of the brachial artery). Deflate the bag quickly to bring the mercury to the zero level.

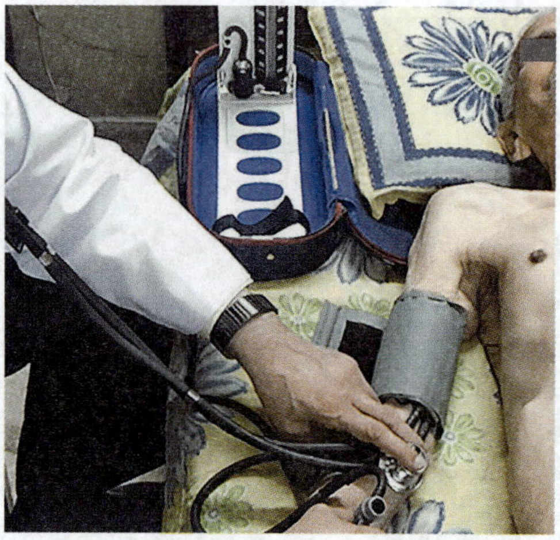

FIG. 25: Recording of blood pressure (BP) in supine position.

Note: It is easier to detect the reappearance of radial pulse than its disappearance. The first 2–3 beats being thin, may be missed so that the actual SP is 4–6 mm Hg higher than the recorded value.

8. Record the pressure in the other arm. Take three readings in each arm, deflating the cuff for a few minutes between each determination.

Advantages of Palpatory Method

This method avoids the pitfall of the auscultatory method in missing the auscultatory gap.

Disadvantages of Palpatory Method

- This method measures only the SBP, the DBP cannot be measured.
- This method lacks accuracy because the SBP measured by it is lower than the actual by 4–6 mm Hg. It assumes that the first escape of blood under the cuff will cause pulsations in the peripheral artery (radial in this case). But in reality definite pulsation may not occur until the cuff pressure has been reduced by 6–8 mm Hg.

Oscillatory Method

- Riva–Rocci, in 1896 (i.e. before Korotkoff sounds were described) measured SBP by the palpatory method while the DBP was recorded from the oscillations of the mercury column.
- As the cuff pressure is raised and then lowered, oscillations appear which become maximum and then disappear (*oscillations are best seen with an aneroid manometer).*
- The appearance of oscillations represent the SBP while their disappearance represents the DBP.

Note: Digital blood pressure monitor: It is a small, compact, battery-operated, palm-top unit with an LCD display screen and memory function. These oscillatory devices produce a digital readout and work on the principle that blood flowing through an artery between systolic and diastolic pressures causes vibrations in the arterial wall. The vibrations are transferred from the arterial wall, through the air inside the cuff, into a transducer in the monitor that converts the measurements into electrical signals. When the cuff pressure falls below the patient's diastolic pressure, blood flows smoothly through the artery in the usual pulses, without any vibration being set up in the wall. The advantage of a digital BP monitor is that it can be easily used by a layperson. The pressure measuring range is 0–280 mm Hg, while the heart rate (HR) range is 40–180 beats/min.

Important: Both the digital BP monitor and aneroid manometer should be checked against standard sphygmomanometer from time to time.

Auscultatory Method (Korotkoff, 1905)

Note: Before recording the BP by the auscultatory method, it should always be first recorded by the palpatory method so as to avoid missing the auscultatory gap.

Note: Ordinarily no sounds are heard when the chest piece of a stethoscope is applied over the brachial (or any other) artery. However, if the cuff pressure is raised above the expected SP and then gradually lowered, a series of sounds, called **Korotkoff sounds,** are heard over the artery just below the cuff.

1. Place the cuff over the upper arm as described earlier, and record the BP by the palpatory method.
2. Locate the bifurcation of brachial artery (it divides into radial and ulnar branches) in the cubital space just medial to the tendon of the biceps.
3. Place the chest piece of the stethoscope on this point and keep it in position.

Note: The chest piece should not rub against the cuff, rubber tubes, or the skin in this area because these disturbing noises will interfere with auscultation of sounds.

4. Inflate the cuff rapidly, by compressing and releasing the air pump alternately (sounds may be heard as the mercury column goes up). Raise the pressure to 40–50 mm Hg above the systolic level as determined by the palpatory method.
5. Lower the pressure gradually until a clear, sharp, and tapping sound is heard. Continue to lower the pressure and try to note a change in the character of the sounds. These Korotkoff sounds show the following phases:
   - **Phase I:** This phase starts with a clear, sharp tap when a jet of blood is able to cross the previously obstructed artery (sometimes this phase may start with a faint tap, especially when the SBP is very high). As the pressure is lowered, the sounds continue as sharp and clear taps. This phase lasts for 10–12 mm Hg fall in pressure **(Fig. 26).**

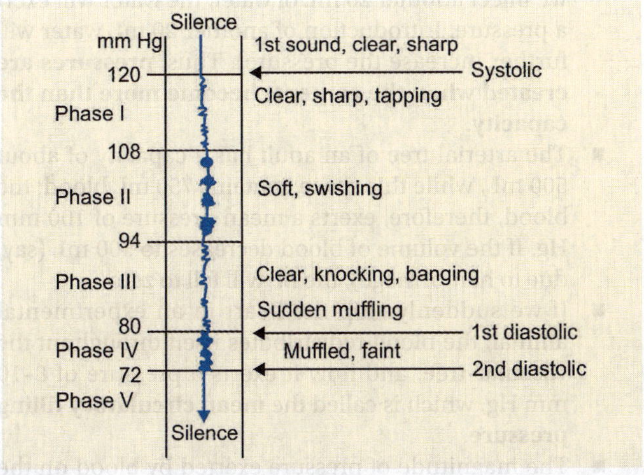

FIG. 26: Phases of Korotkoff sounds, showing the changes in their character during each phase as the mercury column is gradually lowered. Systolic pressure: first appearance of sounds. Diastolic pressure: sudden muffling of sounds.

Note: Criterion of systolic pressure: The level at which the first sound (clear, sharp or faint) is heard, is taken as the SBP.

   - **Phase II:** The sounds become murmurish and remain so during the next 10–15 mm Hg fall in pressure.
   - **Phase III:** It starts with clear, knocking or banging sounds that continue for the next 12–14 mm Hg pressure.
   - **Phase IV:** The transition from phase III to phase IV is usually very sudden. The sounds become muffled, dull, faint, and indistinct (as if coming from a distance) lasting for the next 4-5 mm Hg fall in pressure.

Important: Note the reading at muffling and another at disappearance of sounds, after which deflate the cuff quickly.

   - **Phase V:** This phase begins when the Korotkoff sounds disappear completely. If you reduce the pressure slowly, you will note that total silence continues right up to the zero level.
6. Take three readings with the auscultatory method and repeat three readings on the other arm.

COMMENTS, OBSERVATIONS AND RESULTS

1. It may be noted that the Korotkoff sounds are not heard equally well in all individuals.
2. Sometimes muffling of the sounds (first DBP) may not be distinguished though their disappearance is clear. In such cases, 5 mm are added to the level at which they disappeared (second DP). In cases like aortic regurgitation, the Korotkoff sounds may continue right down to the zero level. In others, the sounds may disappear only after 15–20 mm Hg after muffling. In these cases, placing the stethoscope over an artery and pressing its rim on the vessel may produce sharp tapping sounds called "pistol shot" sounds.
3. **Criterion of diastolic pressure:** *The criterion for DBP is the muffling of the sounds or their disappearance.*

Simultaneous recordings of BP with auscultatory method and intra-arterial recordings with pressure transducers have shown that the DBP correlates better with the disappearance of sounds (i.e. **phase V**). However, *in adults after exercise, patients with severe hypertension and in children, the DBP has better correlation with muffling (i.e.* ***phase IV****).* Therefore, the BP may also be expressed as: 120/80/76, the last figure indicating the disappearance of sounds (first and second diastolic) **(Fig. 26).**

Note: The BP readings are seldom identical in the two arms. It has been suggested that both arms be used, preferably the right arm and then the left arm.

Tabulate your results as shown here **(Table 5).**

For report, express your result as: **SBP/DBP mm Hg**

For report, express your result as:

- Right arm: Systolic/first diastolic/second diastolic; (e.g. 120/80/76).
- Left arm: Systolic/first diastolic/second diastolic; (e.g. 118/76/72).

Table 5: Record of systemic arterial BP.

A. Palpatory method (mm Hg)				
First reading				
Second reading				
Third reading				
B. Auscultatory method (mm Hg)				
	Systolic pressure	Diastolic pressure	Mean arterial pressure	Pulse pressure
First reading				
Second reading				
Third reading				
Average Reading				

PRECAUTIONS

1. The subject should be physically and mentally relaxed and free from tension and anxiety. He/she should be assured and rested for 5 minutes or so to avoid the condition of **"white coat hypertension"** (i.e. some people have higher BP readings in the clinician's office than during their normal daytime activity). It is good practice to compare the pressures in the two arms when recording BP for the first time. If the readings are above the upper normal limits, the measurement must be repeated under basal conditions, i.e. early in the morning before the subject gets up from the bed. A diagnosis of hypertension must never be made lightly and in haste.
2. The sphygmomanometer should be checked for zero error if any. Before applying the cuff the position of the mercury column should be checked. If it is lying above zero level, the same should be noted and this difference of mercury column should be subtracted from the final reading.
3. The arm, with the cuff wrapped around it, should be kept at the level of the heart to avoid the influence of gravity. The cuff tubing should lie anterolateral to the cubital fossa so that they do not rub against the chest piece of the stethoscope.
4. The cuff should not be too tight nor too loose.
5. The cuff should not be left inflated with high pressures for any length of time, because the discomfort and reflex spasm of the artery and its branches will give false high readings.
6. Do not apply pressure on the artery with the chest piece as this may produce partial obstruction of the artery and a fake low reading.
7. Check the pulse rate at the time of recording BP as the HR affects the BP.
8. The palpatory method must always be employed before the auscultatory method.
9. In suspected and known cases of hypertension, the pressure should always be raised well above 200 mm Hg, or above the level estimated by the palpatory method.
10. In obese subjects, a cuff that is wider than the standard should be used. Similarly, when measuring the pressures in the thigh, the cuff should be wider, because the thick layer of fat in the obese, or the large amounts of tissues in the thigh dissipates some of the cuff pressure, thus giving false high results (the BP may be recorded with the cuff on the forearm while palpating and auscultating the radial artery).

QUESTIONS

Q.1. Define blood pressure. Why does blood exert a pressure on the walls of the blood vessels? Is this pressure constant throughout the cardiac cycle? What are the units employed for blood pressure?

- The vascular system is "overfilled" with blood so that it is slightly stretched by the blood. As a result, the blood exerts an outward lateral force on the inside of the vessels. The term **blood pressure** (BP) refers to the force exerted by the blood as it presses against and attempts to stretch the walls of blood vessels. Although blood exerts a force (pressure) throughout the vascular system, the term BP, used unqualified, refers to systemic arterial pressure.
- **The cause of blood pressure–relation between contents and capacity:**
  - The relation between the contents and capacity of a distensible container determines whether or not the fluid will exert a pressure. So long as the contents are equal to or less than the capacity, no pressure is exerted, i.e. the pressure is zero, or atmospheric (all pressures in the body are described with reference to the atmospheric pressure which is taken as zero. Thus, a pressure of 120 mm Hg means a pressure of 760 + 120 mm Hg; a pressure of –5 mm Hg is equal to 760 – 5 = 755 mm Hg).
  - A pressure is exerted only when the volume of contents exceeds the capacity, i.e. when extra fluid is injected into the container (an example will clarify the point: we have a rubber ball of 200 mL capacity. When we inject 200 mL water into it, say, with a syringe, the pressure exerted will be zero or atmospheric. Now, if we inject another 20 mL of water, the water will exert a pressure. Introduction of another 20 mL water will further increase the pressure). Thus, **pressures are created when the contents become more than the capacity.**
  - The arterial tree of an adult has a capacity of about 500 mL, while this space contains 750 mL blood; the blood, therefore, exerts a mean pressure of 100 mm Hg. If the volume of blood decreases to 500 mL (say, due to hemorrhage), the BP will fall to zero.
  - If we suddenly stop the heart in an experimental animal, the blood redistributes itself throughout the vascular tree, and now it exerts a pressure of 8–10 mm Hg, which is called the **mean circulatory filling pressure.**
  - The magnitude of pressure exerted by blood on the vessel walls is determined by:
    - The degree of stiffness of the aorta and its large branches.

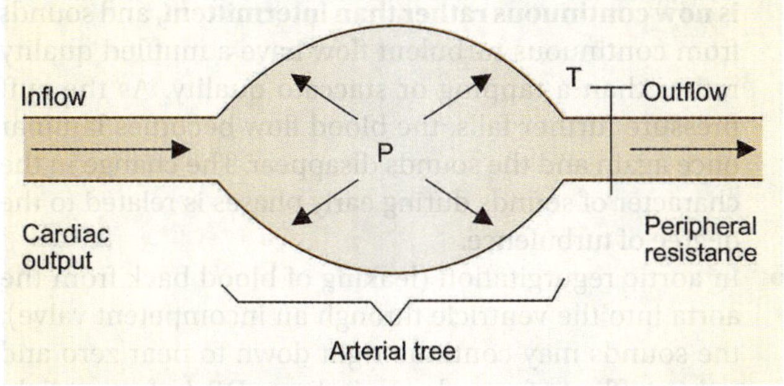

FIG. 27: Relation between inflow, outflow, and pressure (P) in the arterial tree. With each systolic input, the pressure rises to a maximum (during systole) and then falls to a minimum (during diastole). The arterioles act as taps (T) and control the outflow of blood from the arterial tree (the capacity of the arterial tree is about 500 mL but it contains about 750 mL blood; therefore, it exerts a pressure).

- ▸ The volume of blood which in turn is determined at any point of time by:
  - ✦ The inflow of blood into the arterial tree (controlled by cardiac output).
  - ✦ The outflow of blood from the arterial tree controlled by arteriolar tone (i.e. peripheral resistance) **(Fig. 27)**.
- **Arterial BP is pulsatile**: The BP does not remain constant at one level but rises and falls rhythmically with systole and diastole of the heart, i.e. it is pulsatile. It reaches a maximum during systole and falls to a minimum during diastole.
- Units employed for blood pressure:
  - Pressure is a force acting on a unit area (e.g. dynes/cm^2). The pressure exerted by blood is usually expressed in terms of the height of a column of fluid that the pressure will support.
  - The SI unit of pressure is the Pascal (Pa). This is the pressure exerted by 1 Newton force on an area of a square meter (1 Pa = 1 N/m^2); 1 mm Hg = 133.3 Pa = 0.1333 kPa).

Q.2. What is systolic blood pressure? How is it produced and what is its significance?

- With each systole of the left ventricle, 70–80 mL of blood is ejected into the aorta and its branches and the pressure sharply rises. These vessels, which are highly elastic, get stretched (expanded) and accommodate some of this stroke volume, while the rest runs off down the arterial tree.
- During diastole of the heart (when the ventricles are relaxing and getting filled with blood from the atria), the large elastic vessels recoil and the blood that was accommodated earlier, now moves down the arterial tree. Thus, these vessels act as **"secondary pumps"** which produce a pressure and blood flow during diastole of the heart.
- The periodic entry of blood into the arterial tree causes the pressure within to alternately rise to a maximum and fall to a minimum. **The maximum pressure is reached during the maximum ejection phase of systole and is called the SP. The minimum pressure is reached during diastole and is called the DP.**
- **Significance of systolic blood pressure:** The SBP indicates the force of contraction of the heart and thus it represents the work done by the heart in overcoming the resistance of the vessels. It is an important predictor of cardiovascular disease.

Note: It may be pointed out that during systole, the pressure rises to a maximum and then begins to fall as blood runs off down the arteries. The pressure would fall to zero but for the next systole when another stroke volume is ejected into the aorta and the pressure rises again. This rise and fall of BP is repeated over and over again.

Q.3. What is diastolic blood pressure and what is its criterion and significance?

- Diastolic blood pressure is the **minimum pressure** reached in the arteries during diastole of the heart, i.e. just before the next systole.
- Two factors, both outside the heart, combine to produce a pressure in the arteries during diastole:
  - Elasticity of aorta and large branches (i.e. recoil of aorta)
  - Peripheral resistance.
- If the aorta and large arteries were rigid, there would be no DBP; also the SBP would rise to a much higher level (thus, the elasticity buffers the SBP and does not allow it to rise very high). Similarly, there would be no DBP if there were no peripheral resistance, as most of the blood would run off into the periphery.
- **Criterion of diastolic blood pressure:** See text above.
- **Significance of diastolic blood pressure:** Clinically, greater importance is attached to the DBP because this much pressure is being exerted all the time during systole and diastole, while SBP is reached only momentarily during systole. Since a sustained high pressure causes damage to the vessel walls, diastolic hypertension is much more dangerous than systolic hypertension.

Q.4. What does mean arterial pressure mean and what is its significance?

- The mean arterial pressure (MAP) or mean arterial blood pressure (MABP) is the average of all the pressures measured during the cardiac cycle. Since the duration of systole is shorter than that of diastole, the MAP is slightly less than the average of systolic and DPs (the true MAP can be determined only by integrating the areas of the pressure curves). However, a reasonable approximation is: one-third of PP plus DP (e.g. SP = 120; DP = 80; so MABP is equal to 13 + 80 = 93 mm Hg). Another approximation is 40% SP + 60% DP (e.g. 40% of 120 = 48, and 60% of 80 = 48; thus 48 + 48 = 96 mm Hg).
- **Significance of mean arterial pressure:** The MAP of about 95 mm Hg provides the pressure head, or the driving force (vis-a-tergo) for the flow of blood through the arteries, capillaries and veins, etc. The MAP in medium-sized arteries (e.g. radial) is about 90 mm Hg. Thus, most viscera, muscles, and other tissues are perfused at a relatively high pressure. The mean pressure of about 85–80 mm Hg at the start of arterioles falls to about 32 mm Hg at their capillary ends (thus, maximum fall in pressure

occurs in the arterioles). The pressure then continues to fall progressively till it reaches zero in the right atrium. The pressure gradient of about 95 mm Hg is responsible for the circulation of blood and tissue perfusion.

Q.5. What is pulse pressure and what is its significance?

- Pulse pressure (PP) is the difference between systolic and diastolic pressure, the average PP being about 40 mm Hg.
- Other factors remaining unchanged, *the magnitude of PP indicates the stroke volume*. Thus, it provides information about the condition of CVS. For example, conditions such as atherosclerosis (hardening of blood vessels) and patent ductus arteriosus generally increase the PP. The normal ratio of SP to DP and to PP is about 3:2:1.

Q.6. Name the precautions that you will observe while recording blood pressure.

See text above.

Q.7. What are the advantages and disadvantages of the palpatory method of recording blood pressure?

See text above.

Q.8. What will be the effect of using a wrong-sized blood pressure cuff in different age groups or a standard cuff in a very obese person?

- If an over or undersized cuff is used, the reading will be higher than actual because more pressure would be required in the cuff to overcome tissue resistance and to form a cone of pressure.
- When a standard cuff is used in an obese individual, the reading will be higher than actual because of loss of pressure in overcoming tissue resistance.

Q.9. What are Korotkoff sounds and how are they produced?

- Normally, the blood flow through the arteries is laminar or streamline, and no sounds are heard when a stethoscope is placed on them.
- When the cuff pressure is raised above the expected SP, and then gradually lowered, a time comes, when at the peak of each systole, the intra-arterial pressure just exceeds the cuff (extra-arterial) pressure. But, in between these peaks, the artery is still constricted. Now, it is known that constriction of an artery increases the velocity of blood flow through the constricted part. Thus, when the small amounts of blood are jetted through the partially constricted artery, their velocity increases and then exceeds the critical velocity. This produces **intermittent turbulence** that in turn produces ***Korotkoff sounds*** (beyond the constriction) which have a staccato quality (tapping intermittent sounds).
- Also, the blood column in the distal part of the artery, i.e. below the cuff, is set into vibration by the jets of blood striking against it, which contributes to the sounds (the velocity of blood has to increase beyond a certain critical level before turbulence and hence sounds are produced. This velocity is sometimes normally exceeded in the ascending aorta at the peak of systolic ejection. Turbulence also occurs commonly in anemia because the viscosity of blood is low. This probably explains the systolic murmurs in these cases).
- When the cuff pressure is near the diastolic level, the artery is still partially constricted, but **the turbulent flow is now continuous rather than intermittent**, and sounds from continuous turbulent flow have a muffled quality rather than a tapping or staccato quality. As the cuff pressure further falls, the blood flow becomes laminar once again and the sounds disappear. The change in the character of sounds during early phases is related to the degree of turbulence.
- In aortic regurgitation (leaking of blood back from the aorta into the ventricle through an incompetent valve), the sounds may continue right down to near zero and only muffling of sounds can indicate DP. In fact, a slight pressure with a stethoscope alone (without the cuff on the upper arm) may produce sharp, clear and snapping sounds, called "pistol shot" sounds, in this condition.

Q.10. What is an auscultatory gap and what is its significance?

- In some patients of hypertension, there may be a gap in the Korotkoff sounds. As the mercury is lowered, a few faint sounds are heard which soon disappear only to reappear once again at a lower pressure.
- This brief interruption, which may range from 40 to 60 mm Hg, is called the **"auscultatory" or "silent" gap**. If the mercury column is raised to this gap, and then the pressure lowered, one may miss the first appearance of sounds, which indicate SP, and thus record a false low SP.
- To avoid this mistake, the BP should always be recorded by the palpatory method first. Then during the auscultatory method, the mercury column must be raised 30–40 mm Hg above the level found by the palpatory method.

Q.11. When recording blood pressure, why should the upper arm with the cuff wrapped around it, be kept at the level of the heart?

The force of gravity exerts an important effect on the BP readings. The degree of its effect varies with the vertical distance above and below the level of the heart. Consult next Experiment 2.7 on the effect of gravity on BP.

Q.12. What is the effect of muscular exercise on blood pressure?

Consult next Experiment 2.8 for the effect of exercise on BP.

Q.13. What is the oscillatory method of recording blood pressure?

See text above.

Q.14. How does the blood pressure recorded in the femoral artery differ from that recorded in brachial artery?

- A cannula inserted in an artery, with the artery tied off beyond this, records an end pressure (flow in the artery is interrupted and all the kinetic energy is converted into pressure energy). If a T-tube is inserted in an artery and pressure is measured in the sidearm of the tube, it records the side pressure, which is lower than the end pressure.
- The subclavian and the brachial arteries represent the side arms from the wall of the aorta. The pressure recorded in the brachial artery, thus, represents the side pressure or the lateral pressure in the aorta. On the other hand, the femoral arteries are the direct extensions of the aorta.
- When pressure is recorded from a femoral artery, the end pressure is represented in the recording. For this reason, even in the supine position, pressures recorded in the

lower limbs are somewhat higher than those in the upper limbs.

- A low pressure in the femoral artery with hypertension in the arms is the basic clue to the diagnosis of coarctation of aorta. With the normal person standing, the femoral pressure is higher than brachial pressure.

Q.15. What are the physiological variations in blood pressure?

Normally, variations in BP occur as mentioned here:

- **Age:** The average SP at birth is about 40 mm Hg, reaches 70 mm Hg at 2 weeks, and 80 mm Hg at 1 month. The SP/DP averages 90–100 mm Hg/60–70 mm Hg between 4 and 10 years and adult levels are reached by 18–20 years. Both SP and DP rise with age; at 60 years, the BP may be 160/90 mm Hg.
- **Sex:** The BP is generally lower in females by about 8–10 mm Hg. It remains so till the age of menopause, after which it remains slightly higher than the male average.
- **Body build and obesity:** Overweight individuals tend to have higher BP. Since resistance to blood flow through a blood vessel depends on its length, increased length of blood vessels is bound to increase the resistance and hence BP (each extra kg of adipose tissue is associated with the development of an additional 400 km of blood vessels).
- **Diurnal variations:** The BP is lowest under basal conditions, the peak being seen in the late afternoon, mainly in the systolic level. The SP shows a significant fall during sleep.
- **Digestion:** The SP shows a rise of 8–10 mm Hg after meals and lasts for about 1 hour. Diastolic is little affected, though it may decrease a little due to vasodilation in the viscera.
- **Emotional stress:** Hypertension is a natural response to pain, and stress in nonhypertensive individuals. The SP rises during anger, apprehension, excitement, etc. Some hypertensives, because of nervousness, have higher BP in the clinician's office than during their normal daytime activity—a condition which has been called **white coat hypertension**.
- **Posture:** See next Experiment 2.7.
- **Muscular exercise:** See next Experiment 2.8.

Sleep: The BP, both systolic and diastolic, tend to be low during the early restful stage of sleep, especially SP which may fall by 15–20 mm Hg due to general relaxation, decrease in sympathetic tone, etc. Meditation has the same effect.

Pregnancy: The increased blood volume (due to hemodilution) increases cardiac output which in turn raises systolic BP. However, the diastolic BP may decrease a little (due to dilatation of peripheral vessels) or remain unchanged. The peripheral resistance decreases due to the action of progesterone which relaxes the smooth muscle of blood vessels. As a result, the PP rises. After delivery, the BP returns to normal.

Q.16. How is arterial blood pressure maintained and controlled?

- **BP is the product of cardiac output and peripheral resistance.** It means that any BP reading is the result of the interaction of these two factors. Cardiac output controls the inflow of blood into the arterial tree, while peripheral resistance controls the outflow.
- There are five basic factors involved in establishing and maintaining systemic arterial BP. They include: (1) pumping action of the heart, (2) peripheral resistance, (3) elasticity of large blood vessels, (4) the volume of circulating blood, and (5) the viscosity of blood. Normally, the last three factors do not take part in the control of BP on a short-term basis. This leaves the first two factors, i.e. (1) cardiac output and (2) peripheral resistance **(Fig. 27)** for the regulation of BP.
  - **Pumping action of the heart:** The **rate** and **force of cardiac contraction** determines the cardiac output, i.e. the volume of blood ejected into the arteries by each ventricle separately. The HR and force of contraction are controlled by the cardiovascular centers in the medulla, ventricular end-diastolic volume, and myocardial contractility. **Cardiac output** increases in emotional upsets such as bouts of anger, mental stress (they release cortisol), and muscular exercise. **Cardiac output decreases in** severe hemorrhage, ischemia of heart, posture and intense pain during severe trauma.
  - **Peripheral resistance:** This refers to the resistance (opposition) that the blood encounters while passing through small vessels, especially arterioles (two-thirds of the peripheral resistance lies here). All the arterioles, except a few, are innervated by the sympathetic nervous system, which maintains them in a state of slight constriction (a phenomenon called vasomotor tone). Thus, these vessels can further constrict by increase in sympathetic activity or relax by decrease in sympathetic activity. Increase in peripheral resistance raises BP while decrease in resistance has the opposite effect. Peripheral resistance increases in activation of renin-angiotensin system, chemoreceptor reflex. Peripheral resistance decreases in severe hemorrhagic shock, emotional upsets such as sight of blood, fright, and anaphylactic shock.
  - **Elasticity of large arteries:** The elasticity of aorta and its major branches determines both systolic and DBP. With increasing age, these vessels become less elastic (arteriosclerosis). This results in an increase in SBP with a normal DBP (systolic hypertension) (but since peripheral vessels also harden, the DBP may also rise).
  - **Volume of circulating blood:** Increase in blood volume, as during salt and fluid retention, raises the BP, while loss of body fluids, such as due to severe diarrhea and vomiting, and hemorrhage result in a fall in BP (of course, changes in blood volume are not involved in short-term regulation of BP).
  - **Viscosity of blood:** The viscosity of blood partly determines resistance to blood flow through the small vessels. Polycythemia increases viscosity while anemia decreases it.

Q.17. How is blood pressure regulated on a short-term, intermediate-term and long-term basis?

- An adequate pressure of blood is required to perfuse vital organs and other tissues. On the other hand, a high BP can damage the blood vessels in vital organs and can cause serious complications. Under normal conditions, therefore, many different but interdependent negative feedback subsystems control BP by adjusting HR, stroke volume, peripheral resistance, and to some extent, blood volume.
- The BP regulatory mechanisms may be divided into: **short-term, intermediate-term and long-term processes. Short-term regulation is mainly neural while long-term regulation is hormonal.**
  - **Short-term regulation of blood pressure:** This mechanism is **life-saving,** and functions from moment-to-moment and minute-to-minute. (e.g. sudden standing from supine position may decrease the BP significantly and cause fainting; see next Experiment 2.7). It involves baroreceptors, chemoreceptors, and central nervous system (CNS) ischemic response.
    - ***Sinoaortic mechanism:*** Baroreceptors (stretch receptors) in the walls of heart, large arteries, and veins of the thorax monitor (sense) *the pressure within these structures. They are stimulated by distension* (stretching) of their walls by the pressure inside. They oppose sudden increase or decrease in BP. The *most well-known baroreceptors are present in carotid sinus and aortic arch.* The action potentials (APs) from these receptors affect the cardiovascular center in medulla. A sudden rise in BP sends APs from these receptors via IX and X nerves to the nucleus tractus solitarius (NTS). They are relayed to the medulla where they inhibit tonic discharge of vasoconstrictor nerves and excite vagal nerves to the heart. The result is vasodilatation, venodilatation, decrease in cardiac output, and bradycardia—and thus a fall in BP. A fall in BP has the opposite effect because it decreases the inhibitory APs from the baroreceptors so that the vasoconstrictor nerves are released from inhibition while cardiac vagal nerves are inhibited. The result is tachycardia, increase in carbon dioxide (CO_2), and vaso and venoconstriction.
    - ***Baroreceptors in atria and pulmonary veins:*** These are low pressure receptors so that they cannot detect changes in BP. However, they detect and respond to changes in blood volume (degree of fullness), and control the release of antidiuretic hormone (ADH), atrial natriuretic peptide (ANP), and renin-angiotensin-aldosterone system (RAAS).
    - ***Chemoreceptors:*** When the BP falls below a critical level, the blood flow to carotid and aortic bodies chemoreceptors decreases. The increased CO_2 and H^+ and decrease in O_2 stimulate these receptors and the BP is restored to some extent (these chemoreceptors play a much more important role in the regulation of respiration).
    - ***Central nervous system ischemic response:*** This response, in which the vasomotor center is stimulated (by increased CO_2 and decreased O_2), is the last ditch effort to raise the BP when it falls below 60 mm Hg. When the intracranial pressure increases, as by a brain tumor, the blood flow to the vasomotor center decreases as a result of compression of vessels. This stimulates the vasomotor center (accumulation of CO_2 also contributes to this) which increases the BP. Increased BP excites baroreceptor reflex that causes bradycardia. This response to increased intracranial pressure is called Cushing's reflex.
  - **Intermediate-term regulation of blood pressure:** This mechanism is **life-sustaining** and functions from day-to-day and from week-to-week. It involves movement of tissue fluid into circulation by ***capillary fluid shift*** and ***stress relaxation*** of vessels.
  - **Long-term regulation of blood pressure:** This mechanism is **life-stabilizing** and functions over months and years. It involves ***renal-body fluids volume system*** because the kidney is the major organ that regulates extracellular, and thus intracellular, fluid volume. The hormones involved include: renin-angiotensin-aldosterone, catecholamines, vasopressin (ADH), ANP, and nitric oxide (NO).

Note: The sinoaortic baroreceptors are not effective for intermediate and long-term regulation of BP because they become "reset" at a higher level in 1–2 days.

Q.18. What is hypertension and what are its causes and complications? Give its classification.

- Chronic elevation in BP beyond 140/90 is generally labeled as hypertension. The higher the BP, the greater the risk of complications. A diagnosis of hypertension requiring treatment is usually made on the basis of more than three high pressure readings on different days.
- A recognized classification of Joint National Committee (JNC) 7 is given below **(Table 6)**.

Etiological classification of hypertension

The disease is grouped into the following two main categories:

1. **Essential hypertension:** About 90–95% of hypertensives belong to this category in which the cause of the high pressure is not known—although obesity, high salt intake, alcohol ingestion, heredity, and mental make-up

Table 6: JNC 7 Classification of hypertension.

Category	*Systolic (mm Hg)*		*Diastolic (mm Hg)*
Normal	<120	and	<80
Pre-HTN	120–139	or	80–89
Hypertension			
Stage I	140–159	or	90–99
Stage II	≥160	or	≥100

(tense, irritable, and overambitious individuals; the type I personality) are believed to play a role.

2. **Secondary hypertension:** The remaining 5–10% of hypertensives belongs to this group, in which the cause of high BP is known. Secondary hypertension, which is curable, should always be considered in patients under the age of 30 years or those who develop hypertension after age of 55 years.
   a. **Renal diseases:** Parenchymal disease, polycystic kidney, and narrowing of renal artery.
   b. **Coarctation of aorta**
   c. **Endocrine diseases:** Pheochromocytoma (catecholamine-secreting tumor of adrenal medulla), hyperaldosteronism, Cushing syndrome, hyperthyroidism, oral contraceptives, and acromegaly.
   d. **Toxemias of pregnancy.**

Note: Malignant hypertension: In some patients, the BP, especially the DP, is accelerated and rises to very high levels within a short time (DP above 120 mm Hg is a medical emergency). If untreated, the patient may die within 1–2 years.

Complications of hypertension

Hypertension has been called a "silent killer". It may go unnoticed and undiagnosed for years when permanent damage has already occurred in vital organs (this shows the importance of regular medical checkups). The common causes of death are myocardial infarction (*heart attack*), hemorrhage or occlusion of a blood vessel in the brain (*brain attack*), and renal failure. Hemorrhages in the retina may cause blindness.

Q.19. What is hypotension and what are its effects?

Hypotension, or low BP, is hardly, if ever, considered a disease or a cause of alarm in otherwise healthy individuals. However, the BP may show low readings under certain conditions.

- ***Sudden fall in blood pressure:*** This may be due to myocardial infarction, acute loss of large amounts of blood, severe diarrhea and vomiting, and excessive intake of diuretics. The person may go into a state of shock.
- ***Postural hypotension:*** When the SBP falls by 20 mm Hg or more on sudden standing from supine position, it is called postural hypotension. It is usually due to autonomic insufficiency as a result of diabetic polyneuropathy, and during treatment with sympatholytic drugs in hypertension. Rising from bed after prolonged illness may also cause fall in BP.
- ***Chronic primary hypotension:*** It is seen in some elderly persons, but its cause is not known.

OBJECTIVE STRUCTURED PRACTICAL EXAMINATION-I

Aim: To record the BP of the subject provided by the palpatory method.

Procedural steps: See text above.

Checklist:

1. Check the zero reading of the manometer. Explain the procedure. Expose the arm up to the shoulder. (Y/N)
2. Wrap the cuff firmly around the upper arm, keeping its lower edge about 3 cm above the elbow, its middle lying over the brachial artery, and the tubes lying anterolaterally. (Y/N)
3. Keep the BP apparatus at the level of the heart. Open the stopcock between the two limbs of the mercury manometer. (Y/N)
4. Palpate the brachial artery and marks its position. Then holds the rubber bulb in her right hand, closes the leak-valve screw, and inflates the cuff slowly until the radial pulse disappears. (Y/N)
5. Release the pressure in the cuff slowly till the radial pulse reappears. Note the reading. (Y/N)

OBJECTIVE STRUCTURED PRACTICAL EXAMINATION-II

Aim: To record the BP of the subject provided by the auscultatory method.

Procedural steps: See text above.

Checklist:

1. Check the BP apparatus and stethoscope, and exposes the upper arm. (Y/N)
2. Record the BP by the palpatory method. (Y/N)
3. Correctly locates the lower end of the brachial artery. Then applies the ear pieces of the stethoscope to her ears and places its chest piece over the brachial artery. (Y/N)
4. Inflates the cuff rapidly and raises the mercury column to a high level. (Y/N)
5. Lower the pressure slowly in steps of 2–3 mm Hg till systolic and DPs are recorded, note the readings. (Y/N)

2.7: EFFECT OF POSTURE ON BLOOD PRESSURE AND HEART RATE

STUDENT OBJECTIVES

After completing this experiment, the student should be able to:

- Record blood pressure (BP) and heart rate (HR) changes after change in body posture.
- Explain the mechanism of BP and HR changes after change in posture.
- To describe physioclinical significance of the test.

INTRODUCTION

PY5.12: Record blood pressure and pulse at rest and in different grades of exercise and postures in a volunteer or simulated environment.

- In humans, circulating blood is subjected to gravity. Gravity affects the fluid distribution in man. It is due to gravity that postural changes result in fluid shifts. As the person change the position from lying to sitting and then to standing, the blood is redistributed to regions below heart toward the splanchnic, pelvic and leg vasculature (**Fig. 28**).

- This results in decreased venous return causing fall in BP; unchecked this can lead to loss of consciousness and ultimately death. Maintaining arterial pressure in a standing man is of vital importance for the perfusion of the brain.
- Considering the circulatory demands of the human brain, fast and efficient response to gravity-induced fluid shifts is crucial. There are physiological adaptations in the human cardiovascular system to counteract the effect of gravity on the circulatory system under postural changes, such as in standing, sitting and lying down position (**Flowchart 1**).

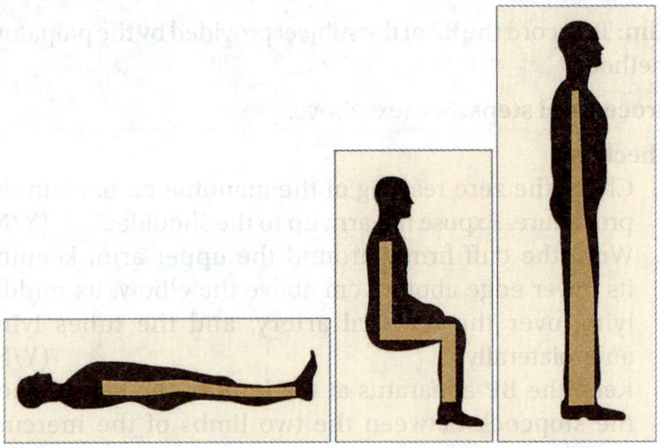

FIG. 28: Blood volume distribution on change in posture.

BLOOD PRESSURE AND HEART RATE RESPONSES AFTER CHANGE IN POSTURE

- The effect of changes in posture on BP and HR depends on whether these are recorded immediately after sitting or standing from supine position, or after prolonged standing.
- They also depend on whether a person stands with a support (e.g. against a wall), or is standing "free" and still.

FLOWCHART 1: Compensatory mechanism on immediate sitting/standing from supine position.

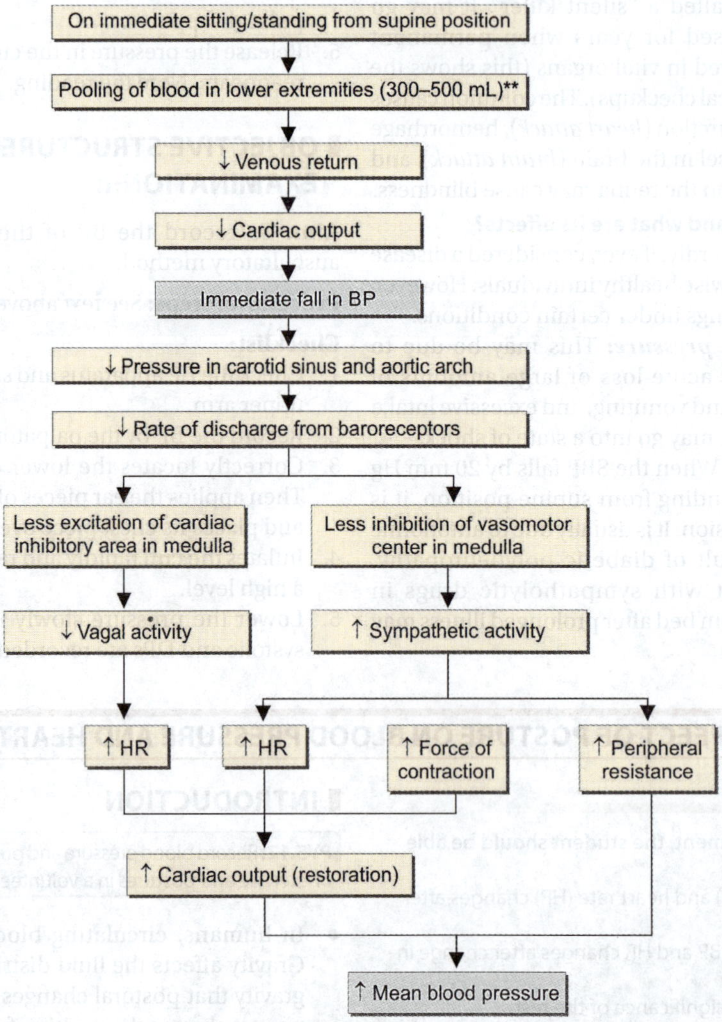

(BP: blood pressure; HR: heart rate)

**In standing position, BP changes are more marked as compared to that in sitting position, because of greater pooling (300–500 mL) of blood in lower extremities. HR increases in sitting and standing position as compared to that in supine position because of decreased vagal tone.

- Prolonged standing poses an additional problem because of increased capillary hydrostatic pressure which causes fluid to be filtered out into the tissues that leads to further decrease in venous return. The cardiac output (CO) and BP fall, may result in cerebral ischemia causing the person to fall down unconscious (*fainting).
- There is also increased catecholamine release and renin-angiotensin-aldosterone system (RAAS) activation to restore the BP during prolonged standing.

APPARATUS

Sphygmomanometer (or digital BP apparatus), stethoscope and stopwatch.

PROCEDURE

1. Allow the subject to rest and relax for a few minutes in the supine position. Record the HR (pulse rate) and BP by the palpatory method and auscultatory method (later on by auscultatory method alone). Disconnect the cuff from the BP apparatus.
2. Ask the subject to sit up and immediately record the BP and HR. Repeat the determinations after 1 minute, 2 minutes and 5 minutes.
3. Make the subject lie down again and rest for a few minutes. Then record the BP and HR. Now ask him to suddenly stand up, and record the BP and HR immediately. Repeat the determinations after 1 minute, 2 minutes and 5 minutes.
4. Record the observations in the workbook.

OBSERVATIONS

Compare heart rate, systolic blood pressure, diastolic blood pressure, pulse pressure and mean arterial pressure in lying, sitting and standing position. Enter the readings in **Table 7**.

PRECAUTIONS

1. The subject should relax for 5 minutes before recording BP and pulse rate in the supine position.
2. Record the BP in the arm, with the cuff wrapped around it, at the level of the heart.
3. Do not remove the cuff in between the estimations but leave it in position by disconnecting the connection between the cuff and the mercury reservoir (Aneroid BP apparatus is preferred nowadays).
4. Record the pulse rate and BP as soon as possible after a change in posture within 30 seconds (preferably within 10–15 seconds) because the changes in BP are rapid and short lasting.

PHYSIOCLINICAL SIGNIFICANCE

1. Effect of change in posture on BP and HR helps to assess the ***integrity of the autonomic nervous system (ANS)***.
2. The consequences of prolonged standing are commonly seen in sentries, soldiers, and ***traffic policemen***. They are, therefore, advised to tense their leg muscles and walk around from time to time (to promote venous return by the *muscle pump*). They also wear "wrappings" (tight strips of thick cloth) around their legs.
3. Through this practical, we can come to know if the person is having postural hypotension or not.
   a. In some individuals, within 3 minutes of sudden standing there is a significant fall in BP (fall in systolic pressure of more than 20 mm Hg or fall in diastolic pressure of more than 10 mm Hg), which results in fainting. This is called ***postural or orthostatic hypotension*** (orthostatic = upright posture of the body; hypo = less + tension = pressure).
   b. Symptoms are: lightheadedness, weakness, blurred vision and syncope.
   c. Seen in patients with—old age (because of decreased baroreceptor sensitivity).
      i. Dehydration, blood loss.
      ii. On antihypertensive medication.
      iii. Autonomic neuropathy (diabetes and syphilis).
      iv. Primary autonomic failure.

Table 7: Blood pressure and heart rate responses after change in posture.

Posture		*HR*	*SBP*	*DBP*	*PP*	*MAP*
Lying						
Sitting	Immediately	–	–	–	–	–
	After 1 minute	–	–	–	–	–
	After 2 minutes	–	–	–	–	–
	After 5 minutes	–	–	–	–	–
Standing	Immediately	–	–	–	–	–
	After 1 minute	–	–	–	–	–
	After 2 minutes	–	–	–	–	–
	After 5 minutes	–	–	–	–	–

(DBP: diastolic blood pressure; HR: heart rate; MAP: mean arterial pressure; PP: pulse pressure; SBP: systolic blood pressure)

***Fainting:** Homeostatic mechanism to restore venous return, CO, and cerebral blood flow in the horizontal position by automatic change of posture.

QUESTIONS

Q.1. With the help of a diagram, illustrate the changes in SBP, DBP, and heart rate on standing. Discuss briefly the physiological explanation of these changes.

See text above.

Q.2. Draw carotid baroreflex pathway.

See text above.

Q.3. Why should BP be recorded within 15–30 seconds of change of body posture?

See text above.

Q.4. What is vasovagal syncope?

- A sudden drop in heart rate and blood pressure leading to fainting, often in reaction to a stressful trigger. It is also called neurocardiogenic syncope.
- Common triggers include extreme emotional distress, prolonged periods of standing, fasting, dehydration, heat exposure or the sight of blood.
- Symptoms include paleness, nausea, sweating, a rapid heartbeat and fainting.
- Vasovagal syncope is usually harmless and requires no treatment. Trigger avoidance is advisable.

Q.5. What is Frank–Starling law?

The Frank–Starling Law states that the stroke volume of the ventricle will increase as the ventricular volume increases due to the myocyte stretch causing a more forceful systolic contraction. It implies that the increased filling pressure stretches the heart and increases its force of contraction.

OBJECTIVE STRUCTURED PRACTICAL EVALUATION

Aim: To record the effect of sudden standing from sitting position on the BP of the patient provided.

Procedural steps: See text above.

Checklist:

1. Explain the procedure to the patient and checks the BP apparatus and stethoscope.
2. Record the BP by the palpatory and auscultatory methods. Note the heart rate.
3. Without removing the cuff, asks the patient to stand up quickly without support.
4. Record the blood pressure within 30 seconds.
5. Note the heart rate.

2.8: EFFECT OF MUSCULAR EXERCISE ON BLOOD PRESSURE AND HEART RATE

STUDENT OBJECTIVES

After completing this experiment, the student should be able to:

- Determine heart rate (HR) and blood pressure (BP) changes after exercise.
- Describe physiological and clinical significance of exercise.
- Explain the difference between isotonic and isometric exercise.
- Assess the intensity of exercise.

INTRODUCTION

PY3.15: Demonstrate effect of mild, moderate and severe exercise and record changes in cardiorespiratory parameters.

PY5.12: Record blood pressure and pulse at rest and in different grades of exercise and postures in a volunteer or simulated environment.

The effect of muscular exercise on BP and HR depends on the following:

1. **Type of muscular exercise:** Whether the exercise is primarily isotonic or primarily isometric **(Table 8)**.
2. **Intensity of exercise:** Depending on the increase in HR, and relative load index (RLI), i.e. percentage of maximum oxygen utilization, there is WHO grading of exercise into light (mild), moderate, heavy, and severe **(Table 9)**.
3. **Whether the individual is trained or untrained:**
   i. Training of an individual results in lower basal HR (because of higher vagal tone and a lower sympathetic tone), lower submaximal HR with exercise, increased stroke volume and lower peripheral resistance than they had before training.
   ii. During exercise, the maximal HR of a trained individual is the same as that in an untrained person, but it is attained at a higher level of exercise.

Table 8: Types of muscular exercise.

Isotonic exercise	*Isometric exercise*
Exercise in which there is a change in muscle length	Exercise in which there is no change in muscle length
E.g. walking, jogging, and running	E.g. pushing against the wall
Systolic blood pressure (SBP) rises only moderately, whereas diastolic blood pressure (DBP) usually remains unchanged or falls (because of fall in total peripheral resistance due to vasodilation in exercising muscles)	Within a few seconds of the onset of exercise, SBP and DBP rise sharply
Cardiac output increases markedly due to increase in HR and stroke volume	Stroke volume changes relatively little
Blood flow to exercising muscle increases	Blood flow to steadily contracting muscle is decreased, as a result of compression of their blood vessel

APPARATUS

Sphygmomanometer, stethoscope, Harvard step, and hand grip dynamometer.

PROCEDURE

Various types of exercises of varying degrees and duration may be devised and their effects may be compared.

Table 9: World Health Organization (WHO) grading of exercise.

Grade	Level	Heart rate (beats/min)	O_2 consumption (l/min)	Relative load index (RLI) (% of max. O_2 consumption)	METS
I	Mild	<100	0.4–0.8	<25	<3
II	Moderate	100–125	0.8–1.6	25–50	3.1–4.5
III	Heavy	125–150	1.6–2.4	51–75	4.6–7
IV	Severe	>150	>2.4	>75	>7

VO_2 max is the maximum oxygen consumption.
Metabolic expenditure test (METS) is the oxygen consumption in multiples of basal oxygen consumption.
RLI (Relative load index) is the oxygen consumption as a percentage of VO_2 max.

Note: If during exercise the subject feels discomfort, fatigue and pain in the legs, breathlessness, giddiness and suffocation tell him/her to discontinue the exercise.

Effect of Isotonic Exercise

1. Make the subject comfortable and explain the procedures to be followed in this experiment.
2. Record the BP and the pulse rate of the given subject after 5 minutes of rest.
3. Ask the subject to perform any of these exercises: "running in place" (spot running) with the thighs brought up to the horizontal alternately, for 3–5 minutes (if a metronome is available, the speed of running can be varied); hopping on each foot for 3 minutes, raising the feet 12–15 inches off the ground; climbing up and down the stairs; jogging or Harvard step **(Fig. 29)** test.
4. Graded exercises can be given on a treadmill, if available.
5. Record the pulse rate and BP immediately, 2, 5 and 10 minutes after exercise.
6. Calculate pulse pressure, mean pressure, and compare the pre-and post-exercise values.

Effect of Isometric Exercise

1. Ask the subject to press the hand grip dynamometer to his maximum effort.
2. Note the force applied by looking at the movement of the needle over the circular scale. This is known as maximum voluntary contraction (MVC).
3. Repeat the test by applying force which is 30% of maximum voluntary contraction and sustain it for 1 minute.
4. Record the BP during and immediately after the exercise.

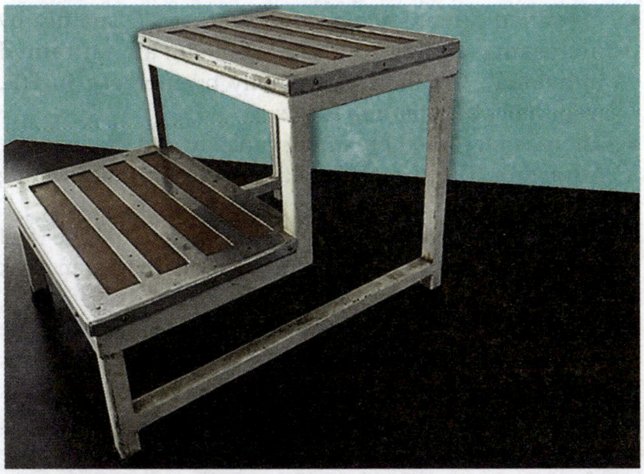

FIG. 29: Harvard step.

Important: If during exercise the subject feels discomfort, fatigue and pain in the legs, breathlessness, giddiness, suffocation, etc. tell him/her to discontinue the exercise.

OBSERVATIONS

Record your observation in tabular form **(Table 10)**.

Note: Blood pressure returns to normal within 5–7 minutes of termination of exercise whereas the HR takes a longer to return to normal.

PHYSIOCLINICAL SIGNIFICANCE

See Question 4 below.

PRECAUTIONS

1. The recording of HR and BP before and after exercise should be recorded in the same position.
2. The sphygmomanometer cuff should be disconnected from the tubing while exercising.
3. The BP and HR should be recorded as soon as following the exercise.

Table 10: Exercise observation table.

	PR	SBP	DBP	PP	MAP
Before exercise					
Immediately after exercise					
Two minutes after exercise					
Four minutes after exercise					
Six minutes after exercise					
Eight minutes after exercise					
Ten minutes after exercise					
HR returned to resting level after _____ minutes BP returned to resting level after _____ minutes					

(PR: pulse rate; SBP: systolic blood pressure; DBP: diastolic blood pressure; PP: pulse pressure; MAP: mean arterial pressure).

QUESTIONS

Q.1. Why is it important to record the HR (pulse rate) when studying the effect of muscular exercise on blood pressure?

The HR is noted because the effect of exercise on blood pressure varies with the intensity of exercise. So, heart rate gives us information about the intensity of exercise (**Refer Experiment 2.10** on "Additional chapters CVS").

Q.2. What are the different types of exercises?

1. **Aerobic and anaerobic exercise (depending upon O_2 usage):**
   - "Aerobics" are those exercises where one "huffs and puffs" to supply oxygen to the exercising muscles (these exercises are beneficial to the cardiovascular and respiratory systems).
   - **Aerobic exercises** include jogging, cycling, spot running, rebounding (running in place on a mini trampoline), swimming, skipping rope, etc. These exercises do not require excessive speed or muscular strength.
   - **Anaerobic exercises** are those where oxygen is not used for that duration, e.g. sprinting where one runs so fast that one does not take a breath. These exercises do not last long. This type of exercise helps in building muscle mass, strength and power. Weightlifting is another example of anaerobic exercise.
2. **Isotonic and isometric exercise (depending upon muscle length):**
   - **Isotonic exercises** are those where body movements are performed. The two types of isotonic contractions are **concentric isotonic** where a muscle shortens and produces movement (e.g. flexion of elbow) and **eccentric isotonic** where a muscle gradually lengthens while continuing to contract (e.g. gradually lowering a weight held in the hand such as in weight lifting).
   - In **isometric exercises,** much tension is generated without shortening of the muscle.

Q.3. What are the effects of muscular exercise on the cardiovascular system?

The cardiovascular responses depend on whether the muscle contractions are primarily isometric or isotonic, with the performance of work in the latter.

- **Effects of acute isometric exercise**
  - In **isometric exercise,** the heart rate rises due, largely to decreased vagal tone, and also due to psychic stimuli and sympathetic excitation.
  - Both SP and DP rise within a few seconds (the SP increases with the severity of exercise).
  - The blood flow through the contracting muscles is reduced due to compression of blood vessels.
- **Effects of acute isotonic exercise**
  - **Heart rate:** There is a quick rise in HR, the increase depending on the severity of exercise. The maximum HR achieved in young persons may be 180–200/min. In older persons it usually tops at 150–160/min.
  - **Cardiac output:** There is an increase in HR and cardiac output (CO), the latter may increase to 25 L/min or even more. This is due to generalized sympathetic excitation.
  - **Systolic blood pressure:** The increased rate and force of heart causes a prompt rise of SBP.
  - **Diastolic blood pressure:** The diastolic blood pressure may remain the same, increase a little, or even decrease somewhat, i.e. it is affected to a much less degree.
  - The above mentioned changes in BP, CO, and HR are mainly due to increased activity of noradrenergic sympathetic nerves. This results from psychic stimuli and afferent signals from the muscles, tendons, and joints. Venous return increases due to many factors.
  - **Muscle blood flow:** As a result of local metabolites in contracting muscles (increased CO_2, K^+, H^+, adenosine, increased osmolality, and decreased PO_2) and activity of sympathetic vasodilator nerve supply to the exercising muscles, there is vasodilatation. This increases the run-off of blood from the arterial system. At the same time, there is vasoconstriction **in the splanchnic** area. As a result of these changes, the DBP is affected little.
  - **Respiratory changes:** There is increased ventilation and thus increased oxygen supply and removal of CO_2 and heat. Increased pulmonary blood flow increases the perfusion of alveoli.
  - **Other changes:** These include raised metabolism, stimulation of glycogenolysis in liver and muscles, rise of body temperature, secretion of catecholamines from adrenal medulla, and glucocorticoids from adrenal cortex due to the stress of exercise.
  - After the exercise is over, the BP and HR gradually return to the pre-exercise levels over a variable period of time.

Q.4. What are the effects and benefits of regular exercise?

- The effects of regular exercise are well-known, as evidenced by the large number of gyms and health clubs. There is a marked improvement of cardiovascular function, especially endurance.
- The heart rate decreases due to increased vagal tone while stroke volume increases due to increased cardiac muscle mass (hypertrophy).
- A trained athlete achieves the target CO mainly by increasing cardiac output, while in an untrained individual, CO increases chiefly by increase in HR, respiratory benefits also follow.
- There is increased breathing capacity and maximal O_2 extraction. The size of skeletal muscles increases along with work capacity.
- Exercise also promotes better mental functions. The "feel good" effect and busting of stress of modern life can work as a powerful treatment of depression.
- **Long-term benefits:** Experts say that if one does moderate exercise, say, brisk walking for 30–40 minutes most days of the week, one can cut down the risks of heart attacks and strokes, hypertension, diabetes mellitus, arthritis, etc. This exercise regimen, combined with dietary and lifestyle changes raises the "good" high-density lipoprotein

(HDL) cholesterol, while lowering the "bad" low-density lipoprotein (LDL) cholesterol.

OBJECTIVE STRUCTURED PRACTICAL EXAMINATION

Aim: To record the effect of exercise on the BP of the subject provided.

Procedural steps: See earlier.

Checklist:

1. Explains the procedure to the subject and checks the BP apparatus and stethoscope. (Y/N)
2. Records the BP by the palpatory and auscultatory methods. Note the heart rate. (Y/N)
3. Without removing the cuff, asks the subject to do exercise. (Y/N)
4. Records the BP and HR following exercise at appropriate intervals. (Y/N)

2.9: ELECTROCARDIOGRAPHY

STUDENT OBJECTIVES

After completing this experiment, the student should be able to:

- Define electrocardiogram (ECG) and identify the various waves, segments, and intervals.
- Explain the basic working mechanism of the ECG equipment.
- Explain the physiological basis of ECG.
- Record and analyze the normal ECG.
- Determine the heart rate (HR) and mean QRS axis of the heart.
- Indicate the clinical uses of ECG.
- Interpret changes in various waves and intervals.

INTRODUCTION

PY5.13: Record and interpret normal ECG in a volunteer or simulated environment.

- **Electrocardiogram** (ECG, EKG) is a graphic representation of the electrical activity associated with heart beat. In fact, this electrical activity initiates the heartbeat. ECG does not represent the mechanical events of the heart.
- The heart is a mass of muscle tissue, and like other muscle tissues of the body, its activity is associated with action potentials. Thus, it acts as a small generator located in the body. During activity, the wave of depolarization spreads through the heart during each cardiac cycle.
- Since the body is a good *volume conductor*, this electrical activity spreads from the heart to the body surface from where, after suitable amplification, it can be graphically recorded as the ECG. Thus, the ECG recorded at the body surface represents the algebraic summation of activity of individual cardiac muscle cells.

APPARATUS

I. **The electrocardiogram machine (Fig. 30):** The **electrocardiograph** works on the household current AC-230 V, or on battery, and has a very sensitive galvanometer. The potentials picked up from the surface of the body are suitably amplified before flowing through the galvanometer. **The ECG machine can have a single channel/3 channel/6 channel or 12 channel recording facility.** The machine has the following *controls*:
   - **Mains switch:** The on/off switch controls the power supply. A filter cuts off unwanted 50 Hz interference.

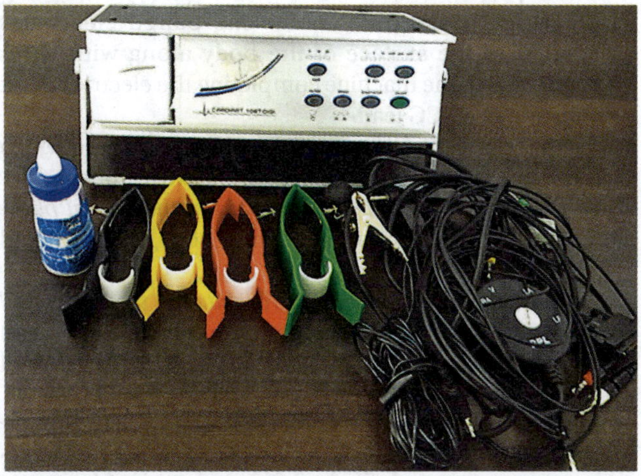

FIG. 30: Electrocardiogram (ECG) machine (single channel recording) and recording electrodes.

   - **Calibration/sensitivity switch:** A commonly used sensitivity is 1 mV/10 mm, so that a calibration signal of 1 mV causes a pen deflection of 10 mm.
   - **Centering:** The baseline control knob is used for bringing the pen to the center of the paper. This knob is not required in modern machines.
   - **Lead selector switch:** It permits selection of various unipolar or bipolar electrodes.

   In modern ECG machines, there is a mode switch. In auto mode, there is no need to adjust the machine for sensitivity, speed, and numbers of QRS complexes recorded per lead.

II. **Electrodes:** The electrodes for the limbs are flat metal plates which are kept in position by rubber straps or plastic clamps. The chest electrode is a metal cup which is kept in position by "suction" produced by a rubber bulb **(Fig. 30)**.

   The electrode jelly contains fine sand and glass particles. When it is rubbed on the skin it causes mild erythema, thereby reducing the skin resistance and enhancing the conduction of electric current. Cable lead wires connect the subject to the machine.

III. **Electrocardiogram paper:** The ECG paper is thermosensitive, wax coated/chemically treated standard graph paper which is divided into 1 × 1 mm squares. The horizontal axis represents time and the vertical axis denotes the voltage. Horizontally, each small square represents 0.04 second and on the vertical axis 10 mm denotes 1 mV. Since the machine is capped at the standard speed of 25 mm/s normally so the machine covers a distance of 1,500 mm horizontally in 1 minute. In normal ECG, the HR can be calculated by dividing 1,500 mm by RR interval in mm. When the RR interval is irregular, i.e. not uniform, the number of QRS complexes counted in 5 s are multiplied by 12 to determine the average HR.

IV. **Pen recording system:** This system is an electrically-heated stylus that inscribes on a chemically treated/wax coated paper.

V. **Electrocardiographic leads:** The paired electrodes applied to the surface of the body along with wires connected to the machine completing the electric circuit constitute an ECG lead.

In clinical practice, 12 conventional leads are used which are further divided physiologically into two groups:

1. *The frontal plane leads (oriented in the frontal plane of the body)*: They are standard leads I, II, and III and leads aVR, aVL, and aVF.
2. *The horizontal plane leads (oriented in the horizontal plane of the body)*: These are the precordial (chest) leads designated by the letter V. These are 6 precordial leads—leads V1-V6.

The leads can also be classified as unipolar/bipolar leads depending upon whether ECG is recorded using one exploring/active electrode (unipolar) or two exploring electrodes (bipolar). Standard limb leads I, II, and III are bipolar leads and precordial (chest) leads and augmented leads (aVR, aVL, and aVF) are unipolar leads. In bipolar leads, one electrode forms the positive pole and the other acts as a negative pole. In unipolar lead, the active electrode acts as the positive pole and the other electrode is kept at zero potential. During heart surgery experiments, leads can be directly applied to the exposed heart (direct leads).

CLASSIFICATION OF ELECTROGRAPHIC LEADS

The classification of ECG electrodes is described in **Flowchart 2.**

FLOWCHART 2: Classification of electrocardiogram leads.

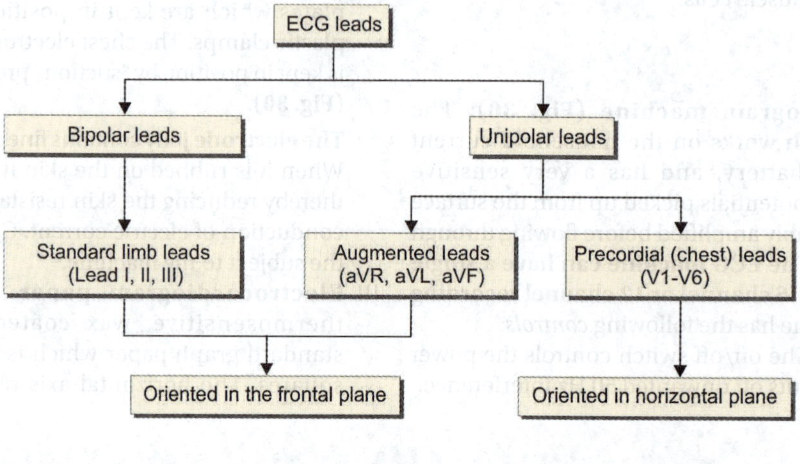

A. Bipolar Limb Leads/Standard Limb Leads or "Classical" Limb Leads I, II, and III

- These were the earliest leads to be used (Willem Einthoven of Leyden, 1860–1927). These leads measure the potential using two active electrodes placed on any two limbs and represent the algebraic sum of the potentials of two constituent active (electrodes) leads.
- The two shoulders and the left thigh where it joins the torso form the ***Einthoven triangle*** **(Fig. 31)** as described below.
- Since the potentials at these points are the same as at the wrists and left ankle, the limb electrodes can be attached at these locations, as they are more convenient to use. The right leg (RL) is used as a ground electrode to reduce electrical interference. There are three bipolar limb leads:
  1. **Lead I:** It records the potential at the left arm (LA) minus the potential at the right arm (RA), or LA-RA (LA positive).
  2. **Lead II:** It is the potential at the left leg (LL) minus the potential at RA, or LL-RA (LL positive).
  3. **Lead III:** This leads records the potential at the LL minus the potential at the LA, or LL-LA (LL positive).

Einthoven Triangle

As pointed out earlier **(Fig. 31)** the two shoulders and the LL (left foot) form the apices of an equilateral triangle—the

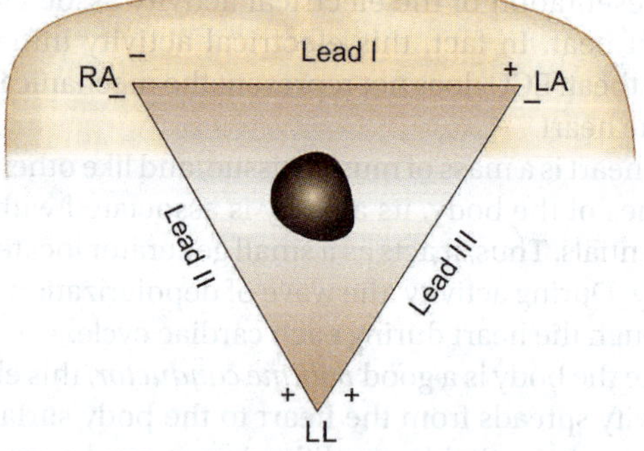

FIG. 31: The Einthoven's triangle.
(LA: left arm; LL: left leg (left foot); RA: right arm)

Einthoven triangle—that surrounds the heart. The heart is thus placed approximately in the center of a volume conductor. Lines that bisect each side of the triangle (i.e. at the zero axis of each side, where the potential is zero at all times), meet the center of the triangle at the heart.

Einthoven Law

The Einthoven law states that the sum of the potentials recorded in leads I and III will equal the potential in lead II:

$$I + III = II$$

In other words, if the potentials of any two of the three limb leads are known at any instant, the third can be obtained mathematically just by summing the first two.

B. Unipolar Leads

- These leads record the potential from a single region of the body (limbs or chest). One electrode, the indifferent electrode, is kept at zero potential by connecting the three limb leads to a common central terminal in the machine where the currents from the limbs neutralize each other.
- The other electrode can be ***on a limb*** or ***on the chest***. Thus, there are three such limb leads and a number of chest leads:
  1. **Unipolar limb leads:** Any of the limb electrodes can be used to record cardiac potentials in comparison to the indifferent electrode kept at zero potential. Thus, there are three limb leads, each denoted by the letter V (vector)—(1) VR, (2) VL, and (3) VF (left foot).
  2. **Augmented limb leads:** Since the recorded voltages are small, disconnecting one lead from the common terminal increases the potential difference by 50%. Thus, the augmented limb leads are:
     - **aVR** = Between RA and (LA + LL)
     - **aVL** = Between LA and (RA + LL) and
     - **aVF** = Between LL and (RA + LA).

     The disconnection of a lead is automatically done in the ECG machine.
  3. **Unipolar chest leads (also called unipolar precordial leads):** These leads record the potentials from the anterior surface of the heart, from the right side to the left side of the chest in relation to the indifferent electrode (RA + LA + LL).

     The standardized sites for the unipolar chest leads are as follows **(Fig. 32)**:
     - **V1** is in the fourth intercostal space (ICS), just to the right of the sternum.
     - **V2** is in the fourth ICS, just to the left of the sternum.
     - **V3** is halfway between V2 and V4.
     - **V4** is at the midclavicular line in the fifth ICS.
     - **V5** is in the anterior axillary line at the same level as V4 in the fifth ICS.
     - **V6** is in the midaxillary line in the fifth ICS.

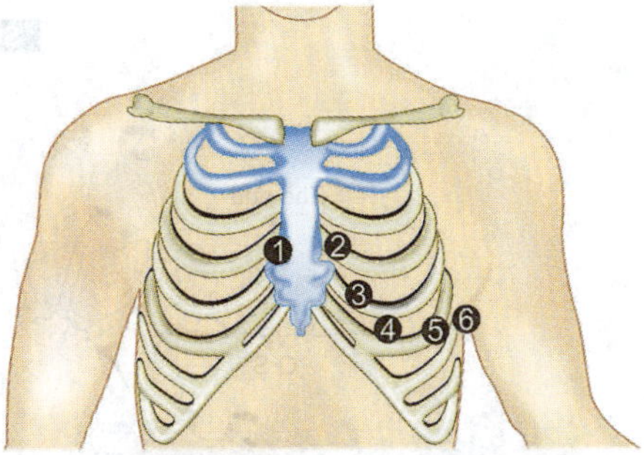

FIG. 32: Diagram to show the placing of unipolar precordial (chest) leads for recording electrocardiogram (ECG).

Note: The 12-lead ECG is used to gain information about the orientation of the heart, size of its chambers, and general direction of activation in the myocardium during any interval. It is also used to evaluate arrhythmias, conduction abnormalities, electrolytes disturbances, drug effects and location, extent and progress of myocardial ischemia, and infarction.

PHYSIOLOGICAL BASIS OF ELECTROCARDIOGRAM

- The wave of depolarization that spreads through the heart during each cardiac cycle has *vector properties* defined by its *direction and magnitude*.
- The net direction of the wave changes continuously during each cycle which causes changes in the deflections of the ECG.
- The size of the deflections is a function of muscle mass, while the direction of the waves depends on the direction of depolarization.
- The electrical field of the heart decreases algebraically with the distance from the center. With distances greater than 15 cm from the heart, this decrease in the intensity of the electric field is very small. Therefore, the electrodes when placed at a distance greater than 15 cm from the heart will record the same potential irrespective of the distance.
- If the wave of depolarization spreads toward the positive electrode of a lead, the deflection is positive (upward). If it spreads toward the negative electrode, the deflection is negative (downward).
- The ECG deflection produced by the atria (P wave) is smaller than that produced by the ventricular muscle (QRS) **(Fig. 33)**.
- The ventricular depolarization vector has two components:
  1. *Septal vector*: It represents septal depolarization and is directed transversely from left to right through the lower third of the interventricular septum.
  2. *Ventricular vector*: This represents the activation of the walls of left and right ventricles. It is directed from endocardium to epicardium and since the left ventricular muscle depolarization is dominant, the resultant direction is from right to left.

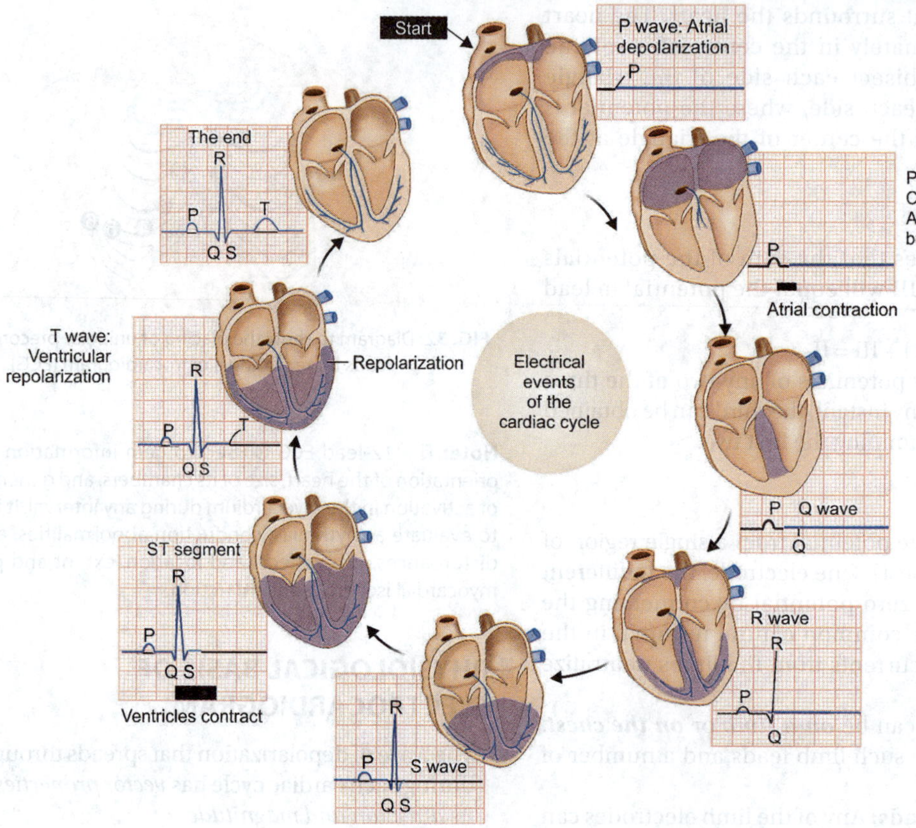

FIG. 33: Electrical events of cardiac cycle.

Cardiac Vector or Cardiac Axis

- In electrophysiology, a vector represents both the magnitude and direction of the potential generated by the current flow. A vector is represented by an arrow. The arrow is directed from negative to the positive direction. The length of the arrow represents the voltage of the potential. The average vector of all of the instantaneous vectors is called the mean vector. The direction of the mean vector is called the mean electrical axis.
- **Cardiac vector:** The magnitude and direction of the electromotive force generated in the heart represents the cardiac vector. The direction of the mean cardiac vector is called the mean cardiac axis.
- The QRS complex, which represents ventricular depolarization, is used for the determination of the electrical heart axis.
- The term, electrical heart axis, usually refers to the electrical axis in the frontal plane as measured by the limb leads.
- The mean frontal axis is the sum of all the ventricular depolarization forces. The average direction of the flow of current is called the electrical axis of the heart (the mean QRS axis) lies between -30° and +110° and averages around 59°.

Calculation of Mean Electrical Axis of the Heart (The Mean QRS Axis):

- This is generally calculated from leads I and III (any two of the limb leads can be used in reality).
- Net QRS amplitudes are calculated in millimeters in the two leads by subtracting any negative peak deflections (usually the negative peaks of the Q and S waves) from the R wave peak.
- The two values obtained are then plotted in the appropriate polarity direction along **the** respective lines (leads I and III here) in the hexaxial system **(Fig. 34)**.
- The two perpendiculars are drawn from those two points until they intersect.
- A line is then drawn from the center of the hexaxial system to the point where the two perpendiculars intersect with each other.
- This line represents the mean QRS vector in the heart at that moment in time **(Fig. 34A)**
- The mean QRS axis lies between -30° and +110°.
- Right axis deviation is said to be present if the calculated axis falls to the right of +110°. In right axis deviation, the QRS waves in these leads (leads I and III) point toward each other.
- Left axis deviation is when they point in opposite directions. In left axis deviation, the calculated axis falls to the left of -30°. If the QRS complex is primarily positive in these two leads, the axis is normal.
- Because the orientation of each lead to the depolarization is different, the direction and magnitude of deflections of ECG are different—still the sequence of deflections—P wave, QRS complex and T wave is identical.
- **The mean frontal axis** is the sum of all the ventricular depolarization forces. *The average direction of the flow*

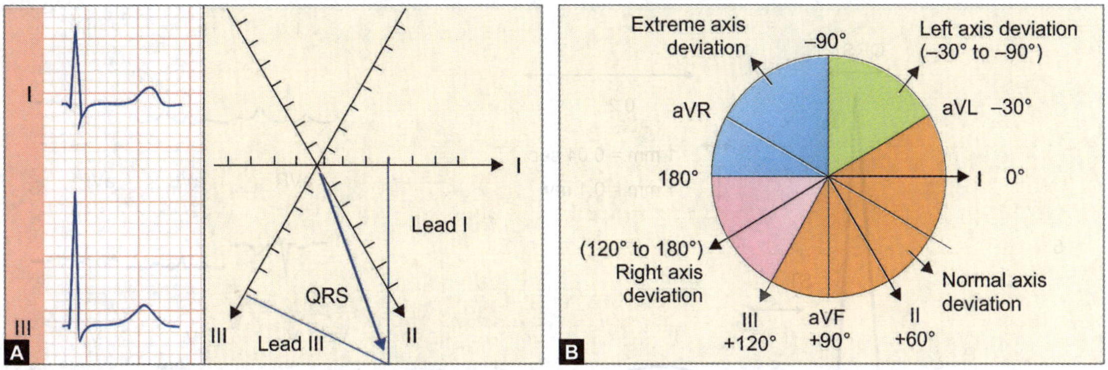

FIGS. 34A AND B: (A) Calculation of cardiac vector; (B) Hexaxial system (Cabrera system).

of current is called **the electrical axis of the heart** (the mean QRS axis) lies between -30° and +110°, though most believe it to be +50°.

- This is generally calculated from leads I and III (any two of the limb leads can be used in reality). Net QRS amplitudes are calculated in mm in the two leads by subtracting any negative peak deflections (usually the negative peaks of the Q and S waves) from the R wave peak. The two values obtained are then plotted in the appropriate polarity direction along the respective lines (leads I and III) in the hexaxial system. The two perpendiculars are drawn from those two points until they intersect. A line is then drawn from the center of the hexaxial system to the point where the two perpendiculars intersect with each other. This line represents the mean QRS vector in the heart at that moment in time **(Fig. 34)**
- **Right axis deviation** is said to be present if the calculated axis falls to the right of +110°. In the right axis deviation, the QRS waves in these leads point toward each other **(Fig. 34B)**.
- **Left axis deviation** is when they point in opposite directions. In left axis deviation, the calculated axis falls to the left of -30°. If the QRS complex is primarily positive in these two leads, the axis is normal **(Fig. 34B)**.
- Because the orientation of each lead to the depolarization is different, the direction and magnitude of deflections of ECG are different—still the sequence of deflections—P wave, QRS complex, and T wave is identical.

THE 12-LEAD ELECTROCARDIOGRAM COMPONENTS (FIGS. 35A AND B; TABLE 11)

The important features of the ECG components are shown in **Figures 35A and B.**

- **P wave:** Commonly called the "atrial complex", represents the start of depolarization at the sinoatrial (SA) node (the first part of the heart to be depolarized), and depolarization of atria. Normally, it is upward except in lead aVR where it is inverted. **Duration = 0.11 s; Amplitude** = usually

Table 11: Components of ECG.

Components of ECG	*Duration and amplitude*	*Cause*	*Remarks*
P wave	Duration: 0.08–0.10 sec Amplitude: Not greater than 2.5 mm (Lead II)	Atrial depolarization	Duration >0.10 sec—left atrial enlargement Amplitude >2.5 mm—right atrial enlargement
QRS complex	Duration: 0.08–0.10 sec	Ventricular depolarization	Duration >0.10 sec may represent a bundle branch block
T wave		Represents ventricular repolarization	
U wave		Slow repolarization of papillary muscles	
PR segment	Isoelectric	Extends from the end of P wave to the start of QRS complex	
PR interval	Isoelectric Duration: 0.12–0.20 sec Average: 0.18	Beginning of P wave to the start of QRS complex It includes the conduction delay in the AV node	It shortens as heart rate increases
QT interval	QT interval: 0.39 sec at a heart rate of 60/min Duration QTc: 0.35–0.43 sec	Onset of Q wave to end of T wave Represents ventricular depolarization + repolarization and corresponds to the duration of electrical systole	Shortens with tachycardia and lengthens with bradycardia so it must be corrected for the effect of the associated heart rate (QTc)
ST segment	Isoelectric	Extends from the J point to the onset of T wave	
ST interval		End of S wave to the end of T wave	

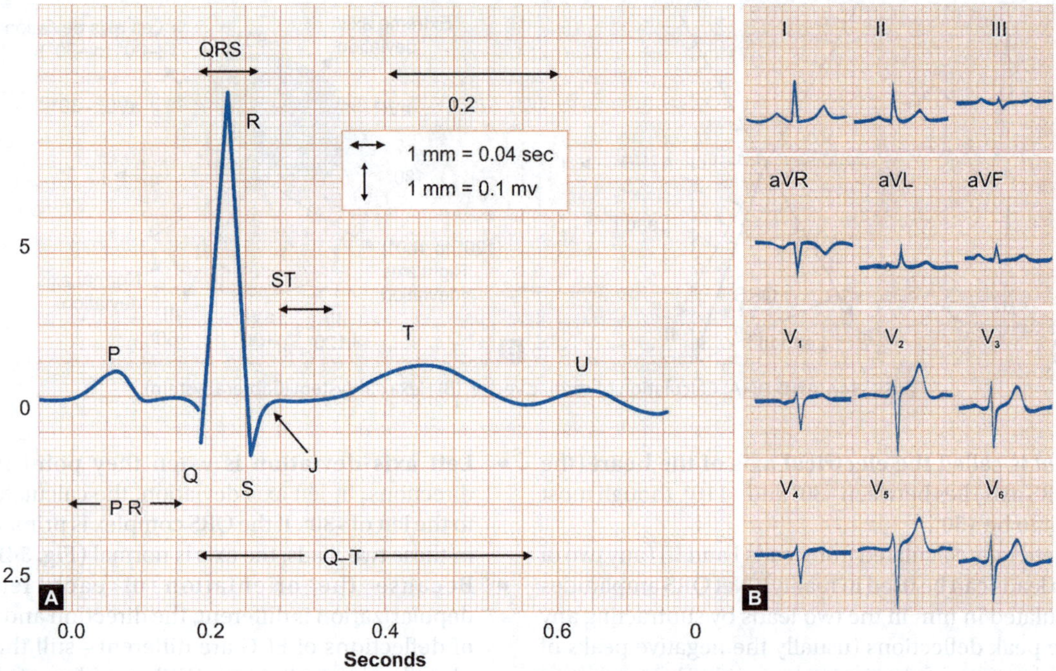

FIGS. 35A AND B: (A) The diagram of normal electrocardiogram (ECG) showing the various waves, segments, times, and voltages; and (B) The normal sequence of PQRS and T wave in an actual 12-channel ECG record; leads I, II, III, aVR, aVL, aVF, V1, V2, V3, V4, V5, and V6.

less than 2.5 mm. It is replaced by F (flutter or fibrillation waves) in atrial fibrillation.

- **PR segment:** It extends from the end of P wave to the start of QRS complex and is usually isoelectric. **PR** or **PQ interval if Q** wave is present. It is the interval between the beginning of the P wave to the start of the QRS complex. It is a measure of *atrioventricular (AV) conduction time*, i.e. the time taken by the excitatory wave to pass from the atria to the ventricles including the delay at the AV node. Thus, it indicates **the conduction time of the bundle of His** which connects the atria and the ventricles. The AV node is activated at the top of the P wave. **Normal duration = 0.12–0.2 second** depending on the HR. The PR interval is prolonged in various types of heart block.
- **Atrial repolarization:** It is associated with very small electrical changes **(atrial T wave)** that are not recorded in the conventional surface ECG because they are almost always obscured by the QRS waves.
- **QRS complex (ventricular complex):** The QRS complex represents ventricular depolarization. **Duration** = less than 0.08 second (maximum = 0.12 s), i.e. two small squares. **Amplitude** = 1.5–2 mV.
  - The **Q wave** is the first negative wave after the P wave and represents excitation of upper interventricular septum. It is often inconspicuous.
  - The **R wave** is the first prominent positive wave after the P wave. It represents excitation of the anteroseptum and major part of myocardium.
  - The **S wave**, the negative wave after R, represents activation of the posterior basal part of ventricles (these three waves represent three instantaneous vectors). If the entire QRS complex is negative, it is called **QS complex**.
- **T wave:** This wave is due to ventricular repolarization.
- **J point:** The J point occurs at the end of the QRS complex. At this point, the entire ventricular muscle is depolarized. Normally, the J point is on the isoelectric line but it is displaced up or down by the current of injury resulting from myocardial ischemia or infarction.
- **ST segment:** This segment extends from the J point to the onset of T wave. Normally it is isoelectric but may vary from +0.5 mm to +2.0 mm in chest leads. Elevation or depression of ST segment (due to current of injury), indicates myocardial damage [since the current of injury continues to flow during diastole of the heart (TP interval), it shifts the *zero* potential line (drawn through the J point) up or down, giving the impression of elevation or depression of the ST segment]. During the ST segment interval, the entire ventricular myocardium is depolarized.
- **U wave:** The U wave is seen just after the T wave in some individuals. It is due possibly to slow repolarization of the intraventricular contracting system (papillary muscles).
- **QT interval:** It is measured from the beginning of Q (or R wave) to the end of T wave. **Duration** = 0.40–0.43 second. It represents ventricular depolarization and repolarization. It corresponds to the duration of electrical systole.
- **ST interval:** It is measured from the end of S wave to the end of T wave. It represents the ventricular repolarization. **Duration** = 0.32 second.
- **TP segment:** It is measured from the end of the T wave to beginning of the next P wave. **Duration** = 0.2 second (depending inversely on HR).
- **PP interval:** It is the interval between beginning or peaks of two successive P waves.
- **RR interval:** This is the interval between the peaks of two successive R waves. It is measured for calculating HR (ventricular rate).

PROCEDURE

1. Ask the patient to lie down supine on the bed and be comfortable and relaxed.
2. Check that the ECG machine is properly earthed. Rub small amounts of electrolyte jelly on the fronts of wrists and just above the ankles.
3. Apply the limb electrodes firmly on these points and fix them in place with plastic clamps. Fix the lead wires, identified with the letters—RA, LA, LL, and RL electrodes. Connect the connector cable to the machine.
4. Switch on the machine and "center" the stylus (pen); run the paper and using the CAL (calibration), push the button 2–3 times and adjust the pen deflection to 10 mm.
5. Using the lead selector switch, record 4–6 ECG complexes in the standard order—leads I, II, III, aVR, aVL, and aVF—in this order **(Figs. 35A and B)**.
6. Stop the machine and apply the electrode jelly on the chest positions for V1-V6. Using the chest electrodes, record the ECG from these positions one after the other.
7. Tear off the paper from the machine and label the various leads. Note down the name of the person and date.

Note: Color coding of limb leads (red—RA, yellow—LA, black—RL, and green—LL). Color coding of chest leads (white/red—V1, white/yellow—V2, white/green—V3, white/brown—V4, white/black—V5, and white/violet—V6).

PRECAUTIONS

1. The patient must be completely relaxed and comfortably supported. Explain the procedure to him. This will alleviate his anxiety and help in smooth recording.
2. Electrocardiogram should be recorded in the supine position. Hair should be parted or shaved.
3. Electrocardiogram machines should be properly earthed.
4. Electrode jelly should be rubbed properly to ensure good conduction of current.
5. There should be good contact between the electrodes and the skin. Poor contact may result in instability of the baseline.
6. Ensure that RL is properly grounded.
7. Ask the subject to remove any magnetic or metallic articles which interfere at the time of recording.
8. Ensure that the ECG machine is properly calibrated (with respect to sensitivity, speed, and number of complexes recorded per lead) before recording the ECG.
9. Ensure the sequential recording of ECG machine with respect to sequence of leads. Recording should be done in a proper sequence. I, II, III, aVR, aVL, aVF, and V1-V6 in manual mode.

Note: In modern machines, there are three modes of recording, i.e. manual mode, auto mode and analysis mode. Under manual mode the operator can choose which lead group needs to be recorded and determine the record length. Under auto mode, the leads switch and calibrate automatically while recording. In analysis mode, the machine will sample the ECG for a prefixed time (1–3 minutes) and analyze all the waveforms of lead II for R-R analysis.

RECORDING OF ELECTROCARDIOGRAM ON STUDENT PHYSIOGRAPH

The student physiograph with ECG coupler can be used for recording ECG. Calibration of sensitivity, centering of pen, connecting subject to five-pin junction box through patient cable, and the latter to the coupler are required for recording ECG.

SYSTEMATIC ANALYSIS OF ELECTROCARDIOGRAM

1. **Heart rate:** It can be determined by any of the following two methods:
   a. By dividing 1,500 by the number of small squares between two successive R waves (1,500 small squares represent 1 min). For example, number of small squares between two R waves = 21
   Heart rate = 1,500/21 = 70 beats/min.
   b. By dividing 60 by the RR interval in seconds. For example, number of small squares between two R waves = 20
   RR interval = 20 ×0.4 = 0.80
   Heart rate = 60/0.80 = 75 beats/min.
2. **Rhythm:** In normal sinus rhythm, P waves precede each QRS complex. Atrial, junctional, and ventricular arrhythmias are detected by in-hospital and ambulatory ECG monitoring.
3. **Mean cardiac vector:** Evaluation of the frontal plane QRS axis provides the information.
4. **Morphology of various waves, intervals, and segments are** carefully studied.

CLINICAL APPLICATIONS OF ELECTROCARDIOGRAM

Electrocardiogram provides useful information in:

1. Diagnosis and prognostic information in ischemic heart disease [coronary artery disease (CAD)] such as angina, heart attack (acute CAD).
2. Detection of cardiac arrhythmias—both atrial and ventricular.
3. Different types of heart block. For example, in complete heart block, diseases of AV node or bundle of His which is the only pathway from atria to ventricles, there is complete dissociation between atria and ventricles. The HR may be 15–20 beats/min and serious emergencies may arise with prolonged periods of asystole. Due to cerebral cortical ischemia (Stokes-Adams syndrome), there is dizziness or "faints". It is in such cases that artificial pacemakers are implanted.
4. Hypertrophy of atria and ventricles.

5. Electrical activity resulting from general metabolic and electrolyte changes.

SPECIAL USES OF ELECTROCARDIOGRAM

1. **In-hospital electrocardiogram monitoring:** Cardiac arrest or severe arrhythmia patients who are shifted to the hospital need special care.
2. **Ambulatory electrocardiogram monitoring (Holter):** Patients with episodic palpitation and dizziness or unstable angina, are given a Holter monitor to wear for 24 h. Analysis of the recorded tape often identifies the cause of the condition.
3. **Exercise electrocardiogram:** The ECG recorded during exercise [treadmill test (TMT)], as per Bruce protocol in otherwise normal. Arrhythmias and ST segment changes are more likely to be detected during TMT.

SOME COMMON ABNORMALITIES OF ELECTROCARDIOGRAM

These include abnormalities of HR (tachycardia and bradycardia), new rhythm centers (e.g. extrasystoles), axis deviation, ischemic cardiac conditions, and various types of heart block.

OBSERVATION AND RESULT

Enter the observations in relation to heart rate, P wave, QRS complex, PR interval, QT interval, ST segment and mean QRS axis.

Heart rate	*Wave form*	*Duration*	*Amplitude*
P wave			
QRS complex			
PR interval			
QT interval			
ST segment			
Mean QRS axis			

QUESTIONS

Q.1. What is ECG and what is its basis?
See text above.

Q.2. What is meant by the term lead?
See text above.

Q.3. What do the lines on ECG paper indicate?
See text above.

Q.4. What are the different waves recorded in normal ECG and what do they represent?
See text above.

Q.5. Which wave represents atrial repolarization?
See text above.

Q.6. What is a complete heart block? Is this condition compatible with life?
See text above.

Q.7. What is the function of the electrode connected to the right leg?
See text above.

Q.8. How do you calculate the HR and mean QRS axis from an ECG record?
See text above.

Q.9. Where is the indifferent electrode in your recording setup?
See text above.

Q.10. Why 12 ECG leads are employed?

- The 12 ECG leads can be divided into two groups:
  - **Frontal plane leads:** The six limb leads I, II, III, aVR, aVL, and aVF, look at the heart in a vertical (frontal) plane. They record the electrical activity moving up and down and transversely (left and right) across the heart.
    - Lead aVR is oriented toward the cavities of the heart.
    - Leads I and aVL view the left ventricle.
    - Leads II, III, and aVF view the inferior surface of the heart.
  - **Horizontal plane leads:** The six unipolar precordial (chest) leads rearranged across the heart in horizontal plane. They view the electrical forces moving anteriorly and posteriorly. Since the heart is placed obliquely in the chest, leads V1 and V2 lie directly over the right ventricle, V3 and V4 lie over the interventricular septum, and V5 and V6 lie over the left ventricle.
- 12-Lead ECG provides a complete picture of heart activity and is a very important tool in making clinical decisions related to heart disorders. It uses 10 different electrodes placed over predetermined positions on the body to record 3-dimensional electrical activity of the heart.
- Thus, it can be seen that 12-Lead ECG recording is a unified method of signal acquisition that can be used to diagnose almost all the possible cardiac pathologies in bedside monitoring, ambulatory recording and as standard electrocardiography also.

Q.11. Why is the T wave of repolarization is positive?

- The T wave on the ECG represents repolarization of the ventricular myocardium.
- Unlike the situation in the single muscle cell or the atria where depolarization and repolarization travel in the same direction, depolarization and repolarization of the ventricular myocardium occur in opposite directions.
- Thus, depolarization starts from endocardium to epicardium and repolarization is reverse, occurring from epicardium to endocardium. This causes the QRS complex and T wave to be inscribed in the same direction (one of the reasons for this is that the endocardial areas have a longer period of contraction and are thus slow to repolarize).
- A vulnerable period occurs during the down slope of the T wave when the ventricle is partially repolarized and the cardiac muscle fibers are in a state of relative refractoriness. An ectopic stimulus in the ventricles due to myocardial damage may bring on extrasystoles or fibrillation.

2.10: ADDITIONAL CHAPTERS CVS

STUDENT OBJECTIVES

After completing this experiment, the student should be able to:

- Explain the grading of exercise.
- List the different cardiac efficiency tests.
- Explain the cardiac efficiency index and cardiac reserve.
- Explain the function of sino-aortic baroreceptor reflexes.
- Know about the normal venous pressure.
- Define the central venous pressure.
- Explain the mechanism of triple response.

PY3.16: Demonstrate Harvard Step test and describe the impact on induced physiologic parameters in a simulated environment.

CARDIAC EFFICIENCY TESTS (EXERCISE TOLERANCE TESTS)

- The response of the cardiovascular system to standardized exercise (**"exercise tolerance test"**, also called **"stress testing"**) is the single and the best test for assessing the efficiency of the heart.
- During exercise, there is a progressive increase in the heart rate (HR) and blood pressure (BP). However, after the exercise is over, these values return to the pre-exercise levels during the next few minutes.
- When compared to a trained person there is a greater increase in the HR and BP in an untrained individual during exercise, and that these values take a longer time to return to basal levels, forms the basis of exercise tolerance tests.
- The response to physical exercise depends on the cardiac reserve (i.e. efficiency of the heart), muscle power, training, motivation, and the state of nutrition. Therefore, the cardiac efficiency tests can also be used to test physical fitness in an individual.
- **Record the basal pulse rate,** then ask the subject to hop 20 times on each foot, raising the shoulders 6 inches at each step.If the heart is healthy, there should be little disturbance of breathing and the pulse rate should not increase by more than 10–20 beats per minute, and should return to pre-exercise level in about a minute.
  Record these timings in your workbook.
- **Harvard step test.**
  Protocol: Record the basal pulse rate. Then ask the subject to alternately step up and down, lifting each foot about 20 inches (16 inches in females) off the ground, at a rate of 30 double steps per minute for a period of 5 minutes [Alternately, ***the subject may step up and down a 50 cm bench (40 cm in females), at a frequency of 30 times/min for 5 minutes (300 secs)]***. Stop the test if the subject feels breathless and exhausted and is unable to continue the test.

  Count the pulse rate 1 minute after the end of the exercise. The pulse rate is inversely proportional to the degree of cardiac efficiency. To obtain an approximate idea of the cardiac efficiency index, count the pulse rate at the following intervals:
  - Between 1 and 1 1/2 minutes =............/min (a)
  - Between 2 and 2 1/2 minutes =.........../min (b)
  - Between 3 and 3 1/2 minutes =............/min (c)
  - Time after which the pulse rate returns to basal levels = ...minutes

  Cardiac Efficiency Index

  $$\frac{\text{Duration of exercise in seconds (300 sec)}}{a+b+c} \times 100$$

  In normal individuals, the cardiac efficiency index is nearly 100%, but is more in sports persons.

  Efficiency Index

  Over 90% efficiency is excellent.
  81–90% efficiency is good.
  55–80% efficiency is average.
  Below 55% efficiency is poor.
- **Master's step test:** The Master's step test, employed in the past, was a two-step wooden bench, each step being 9 inches high. The subject steps on and off the steps 12 times a minute and the pulse rate is noted. The time of recovery is about 5 minutes (the test also used to be repeated with stepping rates of 18 and 24 times a minute).

QUESTIONS

Q.1. How is physical exercise graded?

Grading of exercise: The WHO grading of muscular exercise, according to heart rate and relative load index (RLI; i.e. percentage of maximum O_2 utilization) is as follows **(Table 12)**.

Q.2. What is the purpose of the exercise tolerance tests?

Purpose of exercise tolerance tests: The exercise tolerance tests are the best tests for determining the efficiency of the

Table 12: World Health Organization (WHO) grading of muscular exercise.

Grade	*Level*	*Heart rate (beats/min)*	*O_2 consumption (L/min)*	*Relative load index (RLI) (% of maximum O_2 consumption)*	*METs*
I	Mild	<100	0.4–0.8	<25	<3
II	Moderate	100–125	0.8–1.6	25–50	3.1–4.5
III	Heavy	125–150	1.6–2.4	51–75	4.6–7
IV	Severe	>150	>2.4	>75	>7

VO_2 max is the maximum oxygen consumption.
Metabolic equivalent of task (METs) is the oxygen consumption in multiples of basal oxygen consumption.
RLI (relative load index) is the oxygen consumption as a percentage of VO_2 maximum.

heart as a pumping organ. These tests take the place of cardiac output (CO) measurements which cannot be made with ease in most clinical settings.

Q.3. What is meant by the term "cardiac reserve"?

Cardiac reserve: The cardiac reserve is the difference between the basal CO of an individual and the maximum CO that can be achieved in that person. It can also be expressed as cardiac reserve percent. For example, basal cardiac output = 5 liters/min; maximum achievable output = 25 liters/min. Thus, cardiac reserve percent = [(25 – 5) × 100]/25 = 80%.

Q.4. Name some other cardiac efficiency tests.

- **Treadmill test (TMT):** A very sophisticated "stress test" employed these days is the one using a treadmill or a bicycle ergometer. The individual is subjected to standardized incremental increase in external workload, according to a definite protocol (Bruce protocol), while the person's 12-lead ECG, arm blood pressure, and symptoms are continuously monitored by a physician present throughout the test.
- The performance is usually symptom-limited, and the test is discontinued as soon as there is evidence of chest discomfort, severe dyspnea, dizziness, fatigue, ST-segment depression of more than 2 mm, a fall in systolic pressure exceeding 15 mm Hg, or development of ventricular tachy-arrhythmia.
- The test is also done in cases of coronary artery disease to assess the degree of cardiac disability. The test can be enhanced by IV radioisotope (thallium 201) to assess regional myocardial perfusion by means of gamma camera. Radioisotope angiography using technetium 99 can also be employed to measure various parameters of ventricular performance.

Note: It may be noted that exercise testing can neither at present definitely exclude the presence of coronary artery disease, nor it is absolutely specific in predicting its presence.

DEMONSTRATION OF CAROTID SINUS REFLEX

Pressure sensitive sensory receptors are present in the walls of carotid sinuses. Since these are located close to the surface of the anterior neck, it is possible to stimulate these baroreceptors by exerting pressure on them or massaging them.

Procedure

- Ask the subject to lie down supine on the examination couch. Loosen his collar and lay the neck bare. Locate the anterior edge of sternomastoid muscle and feel the pulsations of the common carotid artery which lies deeper and medial to it. Locate the upper border of the thyroid cartilage, and feel the pulsations in the carotid sinus which is a small dilation of the internal carotid artery just above the bifurcation of the main trunk (the sinus lies just below the angle of the jaw).
- Palpate the radial artery with your left hand and with the thumb of your right hand press the carotid sinus against the vertebral bodies for 2 seconds only. The pulse can be felt at this site as well as in the radial artery.

Caution: Do not compress both carotids at the same time.

QUESTIONS

Q.1. What is the effect of compressing the carotid sinus?

Compressing the carotid sinus stimulates the stretch receptors (presso or baroreceptors) in its tunica adventitia. Impulses from these receptors pass along the sinus nerve, a branch of 9th cranial nerve to the medulla where the cardioinhibitory center (nucleus ambiguus, the motor nucleus of the vagus) is stimulated and the vasomotor center is inhibited (impulses also pass to the hypothalamus and cerebral cortex). The result is a reflex slowing of the heart, and decrease in peripheral resistance due to inhibition of the tonic discharge in the vasoconstrictor nerves supplying the arterioles.

Q.2. What is the function of sinoaortic baroreceptor reflexes?

Sinoaortic baroreceptor reflex is a powerful short-term mechanism for the regulation of BP. The inhibitory impulses along the sinus and aortic nerves (buffer nerves) can affect both CO and PR and can thus increase or decrease the BP as required.

Q.3. If the sinoaortic mechanism is so effective in regulating BP, why do people suffer from hypertension?

This mechanism is very effective on a short-term basis. However, if there are repeated episodes of increased BP (due to stress, anger, etc.), this mechanism is "reset" to maintain BP at a higher level and one gets into a state of hypertension.

Q.4. What is the practical significance of carotid sinus reflex?

Stretching or putting pressure on the carotid sinus such as by hyperextension of the head, carrying heavy shoulder loads, and wearing tight collars may decrease the HR and BP to cause **carotid sinus syncope**—when a person faints due to inappropriate stimulation of carotid baroreceptors.

Massage of carotid sinus is sometimes taken advantage of to slow the HR in cases of paroxysmal atrial tachycardia (PAT).

DEMONSTRATION OF VENOUS BLOOD FLOW

The flow of blood through the veins of the forearm and the presence of valves in these veins can be demonstrated by a simple experiment. William Harvey originally described it as one of the proofs for his theory of circulation.

Procedure

- Seat the subject on a stool with his arm resting on a table. Apply the BP cuff on his upper arm and inflate it to 30–40 mm Hg. The superficial veins of the forearm will become prominent.
- Place the tip of your right index finger (call it "R") over one of the veins, and mark the position of the valve (call it "V") above it, with a felt pen.
- Keeping the finger "R" in the same position, and using your left index finger, squeeze out the blood from this vein toward the elbow. Note that the segment of the vein

between points "R" and "V" remains collapsed and that there is no backflow of blood. However, the vein above the valve "V" is distended and the valve becomes prominent.

- Keeping the finger "R" in position, place the left index finger above the valve "V" and try to squeeze the blood downward toward the finger "R". It will be noticed that the blood cannot be forced backward across the valve "V" unless a pressure that would be enough to rupture the valve "V" is applied.

QUESTIONS

Q.1. What are the functions of the valves in the veins?

- The valves in the veins of the limbs (there are no valves in abdominothoracic veins) help in venous return especially during muscular exercise (the "muscle pump" for venous return).
- They also prevent the exudation of fluid out of the veins of the legs and feet (the pressure in these veins is very high due to the effect of gravity) by breaking the veins into short segments instead of there being a long continuous column of blood below the level of the heart.

Q.2. What is the function of the veins?

- Being thin-walled, the veins constitute the "capacitance" or storage vessels of the circulatory tree and contain about 70% of the blood.
- Although the amount of smooth muscle in the veins is small, considerable venoconstriction occurs by factors (e.g. sympathetic excitation) which cause vasoconstriction in arterioles.
- Local factors such as O_2 lack and CO_2 excess can also affect small veins. During hemorrhage, substantial amounts of blood can be translocated from the veins to the general circulation, thus helping in increasing the effective blood volume.

RECORDING OF VENOUS PRESSURE

- There is a pressure gradient from the arterial to the venous side in both systemic and pulmonary circuits.
- The gradient in the systemic circuit is about 95 mm Hg (MAP in aorta = 95 mm Hg; Right atrium = 0–4 mm Hg) and that in the pulmonary circuit is about 12–15 mm Hg (MAP in pulmonary artery = 15 mm Hg; Left atrium = 2–6 mm Hg).

There are three simple experiments to assess venous blood pressure.

Procedure

Experiment I

- Seat the subject on a stool, with his right arm hanging downward; the veins of the arm will become distended. While watching the veins on the back of the hand and the wrist, slowly and gently raise the subject's arm till these veins begin to empty out.
- Determine the vertical height between the wrist and the junction of third costal cartilage with the sternum (this point is the level of entry of superior vena cava into the right atrium). The distance measured in cm is the approximate measure of the right atrial pressure (in normal subjects, the hand will be a few cm above the heart when the veins empty out completely).
- Repeat the above procedure after asking the patient to close his nose and mouth and then perform a forced expiratory effort **(Valsalva maneuver)**. The venous pressure is now increased, i.e. the veins will remain engorged even when the hand is raised to the level of the head (the Valsalva maneuver increases the intrapleural pressure to + 20–30 mm Hg which interferes with the venous return. The normal intrapleural pressure remains negative, i.e. below the atmospheric, during quiet inspiration and expiration).
- Repeat the same procedure after asking the patient to close his nose and mouth and then to make a deep inspiratory effort **(Müller's maneuver)**. In this case, the intrapleural pressure becomes much more negative which facilitates venous return.

Experiment II

Apparatus: A flat glass cup with an outlet at the top (a small funnel will also serve the purpose); water manometer; air bulb of a BP apparatus; a glass T-tube; collodion, and rubber tubing will be required for this experiment.

Procedure:

- Connect the glass cup, air pump, and the water manometer to the T-tube.
- Seat the subject on a stool with his forearm resting on the table at the level of the heart. Apply the cup over a prominent vein on the forearm, and seal the cup with collodion.
- After the seal dries, gently increase the pressure in the cup till the vein just empties out. Read the manometer pressure at this point.
- Express the venous pressure in cm of water or mm Hg (1 mm Hg pressure = 13.6 mm H_2O). Repeat the Valsalva and Müller maneuvers to study their effects on venous pressure.

Experiment III

The venous pressure can also be directly recorded by inserting a wide-bore needle into a vein in the antecubital region, and connecting it to a manometer filled with normal saline containing an anticoagulant.

QUESTIONS

Q.1. What are the normal venous pressures?

- The pressure in the venules is 12–16 mm Hg. The peripheral venous pressure in the forearm (at the heart level) is 6–8 mm Hg and in the great veins near the heart is 3–4 mm Hg, but varies with respiration.
- The pressure in the dural sinuses (with the head upright) is subatmospheric (i.e. negative) because these venous channels are rigid and cannot collapse.

Q.2. When does the peripheral venous pressure increase?

- The peripheral venous pressure in the abdomen and limbs increases in cases of right heart failure (*congestive heart failure*).

- The failure of the right ventricle to effectively pump out all the blood that is returning to it causes back pressure in the systemic veins. Increased pressure in the portal veins causes exudation of fluid, a condition called *"ascites"*.
- In the limb veins, the back pressure increases the capillary hydrostatic pressure which leads to *edema*.

DEMONSTRATION OF TRIPLE RESPONSE

- The response of the skin to mechanical injury described first by Lewis in 1927 is called the **triple response** or the **Lewis' response.**
- With light injury, only the "white line" is seen, while with a stronger stimulus, all the three stages of the "triple response" can be seen.

White Line (White Reaction)

- Seat the subject on a stool with his forearm resting on the table. Draw a blunt-pointed object—a closed forceps, fingernail, a blunt pencil lightly on the skin of the ventral forearm. The response which appears in 8–10 seconds is a pale or white line in the track of the stimulus.
- The mechanical stimulus causes contraction of the precapillary sphincters, squeezes out blood from the capillaries and small venules leaving behind a white line.

Triple Response

After the white line disappears in about a minute, use a stronger stimulus with the forceps. The response will vary from person to person. A full-fledged triple response especially in sensitive skins consists of the following three stages:

1. **The red line (red reaction):** It appears in about 10 seconds, and is due to relaxation of the precapillary sphincters resulting from histamine, kinins, polypeptides, etc. that are released locally from injured cells. Passive capillary dilatation and increased blood flow cause the red line.
2. **The flare:** The flare which follows in a few minutes is an irregular, reddish, mottled area surrounding the red line. It is due to dilation of arterioles resulting from a local reflex called the **axon reflex.** In this case, impulses originating in the sensory nerve endings by the injury are relayed antidromically (i.e. opposite to the normal direction) down other branches of the sensory nerve fibers which supply the arterioles. This appears to be the only example of a physiological effect due to antidromic conduction in nerve fibers. The axon reflex is not a true reflex as it does not involve some part of the central nervous system.
3. **The wheal:** The flare is soon followed by local edema, (swelling) due to increased permeability of the capillaries and small venules, as a result of which fluid leaks out from these vessels. Histamine (released from local mast cells), kinins, substance P, and other polypeptides all contribute to increased permeability and edema. Injection of histamine in the skin produces flare and wheal via the H1 receptors. A common example of the triple response is the fingermarks left on the skin of the face following a hard slap.

UNIT III: SPECIAL SENSATIONS

2.11: PERIMETRY (CHARTING THE FIELD OF VISION)

STUDENT OBJECTIVES

After completing this experiment, the student should be able to:

- Define field of vision and physiological blind spot.
- Determine the field of vision in a subject and describe its extent in various meridians.
- Describe the printed perimeter chart.
- Name the factors that affect the field of vision.
- Trace the visual pathway and name the effects of lesions at different places.

INTRODUCTION

PY10.20: Demonstrate (i) Testing of visual acuity, color and field of vision, (ii) Hearing, (iii) Testing for smell, and (iv) Taste sensation in volunteer/simulated environment.

- The part of the external world visible to one eye when a person fixes his gaze on one point is called the **field of vision** for that eye.
- The visual field can be tested by confrontation method and perimetry.
- The process of charting the monocular field of vision is called **perimetry.** It is employed for the diagnosis of various lesions of the visual pathways.

VISUAL PATHWAY

- The optic nerve fibers (axons of ganglion cells of the retina) from the nasal (medial) half of each retina cross to the opposite side in the optic chiasma, while fibers from the temporal (lateral) half of each retina remain on the same side.
- For example, fibers in the right optic tract come from the temporal half of right retina and nasal half of left retina **(Fig. 36)**, thus serving the nasal (medial) half of field of vision in the right eye and temporal (lateral) field in the left eye (blindness resulting from lesions of the visual pathway are labeled in terms of defects in the visual fields).
- The optic tract fibers end in two ways: (1) Pretectum of midbrain to synapse on the **Edinger–Westphal nucleus** for light reflexes, and (2) Lateral geniculate body (LGB).

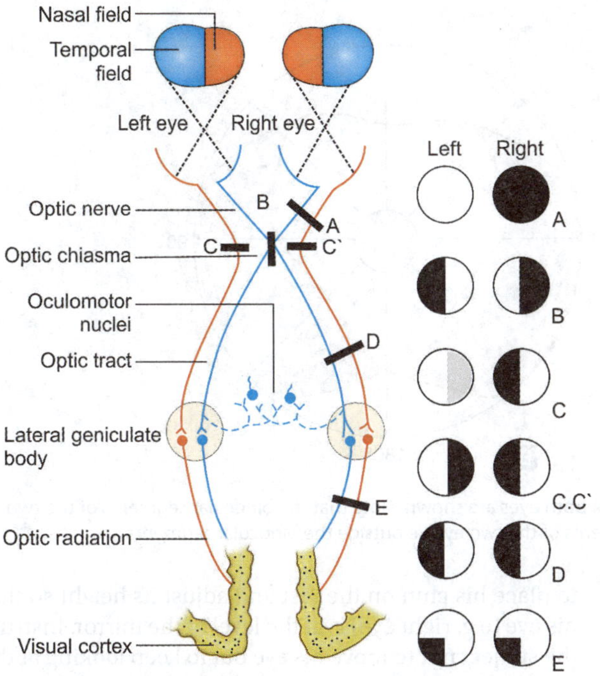

FIG. 36: Visual pathway. Lesions of the pathway at different locations produce defects in the fields of vision as shown on the right.

- Fresh relays from LGB pass back in the geniculocalcarine tract (optic radiations) which passes through the internal capsule where they lie behind the somatic sensory fibers to reach the *primary visual area (area 17 of Brodmann)* on the medial surface of the occipital lobe. Areas 18 and 19 on the lateral surface are the *visual association areas.*

PERIMETER

Priestley Smith **(Fig. 37)**, Lister perimeters, and student's perimeter (a simple *hand* perimeter) are commonly used instruments. These instruments accurately map the field of vision. The perimeter consists of the following parts:

1. **Stand:** A heavy stand on which a metal arc is fitted on a pivot provides stability to the apparatus. A large black disc

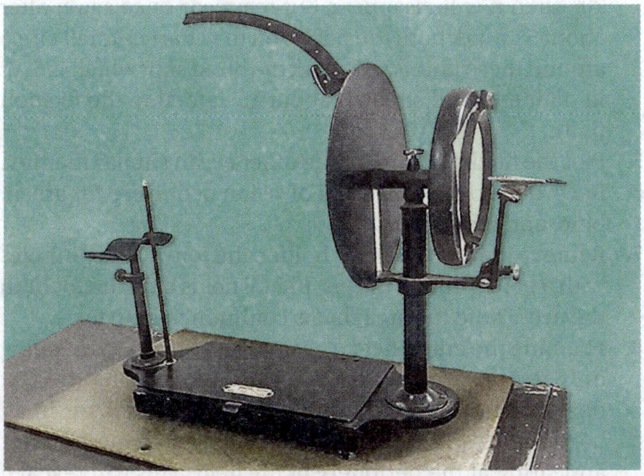
FIG. 37: Priestley Smith perimeter.

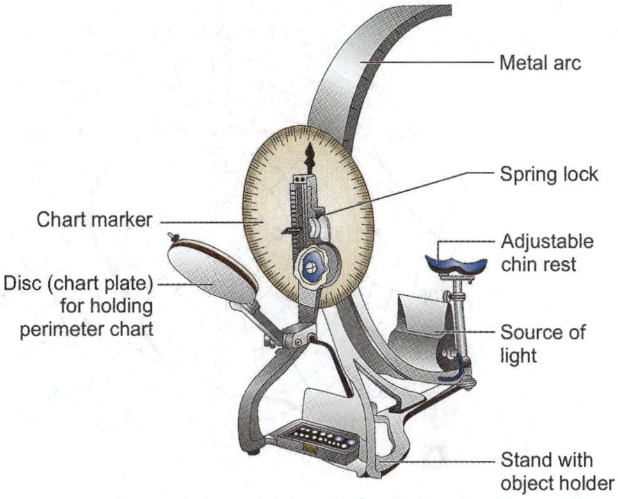

FIG. 38: Perimeter (Lister model).

with a frame for holding the perimeter chart is provided on the back **(Fig. 38)**.
2. **Metal arc:** A broad metal arc shaped like a half circle is mounted on the stand and can be rotated in any meridian around its central pivot. One half of the arc, the concavity of which is directed toward the subject, has a scale of 0–90° marked on its convex surface, while a source of light is fitted at the end of the other limb of the arc. A small plane mirror is fixed in the center of the arc. Test objects of various sizes and colors can be fitted in a carrier which moves in a groove in the graduated limb of the arc. When the test object is moved with a knob, a pin on the back of the apparatus moves correspondingly.
3. **Chin rest:** An adjustable chin rest is provided to keep the head steady. The chin of the subject rests on the right cup when the left eye is to be tested and the left cup is used when the right eye is tested.
4. **Scale and chart frame:** The chart frame or chart plate is meant to hold the chart paper in position. Priestley Smith model has a pricking point moving on the fixation chart along the scale. It marks the distance in degrees from central fixation point.
5. **Chart:** The perimeter chart **(Figs. 39A and B)** on which the field of vision is to be plotted is divided by circles from 0° to 90°, and by meridians at 15° intervals. Both the angles and the meridians are printed on the chart. The limits for the normal peripheral fields of vision for the two eyes, and the blind spots are printed on the chart for comparison with the plotted fields of vision. The term "peripheral field" refers to the peripheral or outer limits of the field.

Student Perimeter

In this model **(Fig. 40)**, the inclination of the arc is read from a plastic dial fitted behind the mirror. When an object which is moved along the inside of the arc becomes visible, the angle it subtends at the fixation point (i.e. the mirror) in a given meridian can be read from the scale engraved on the

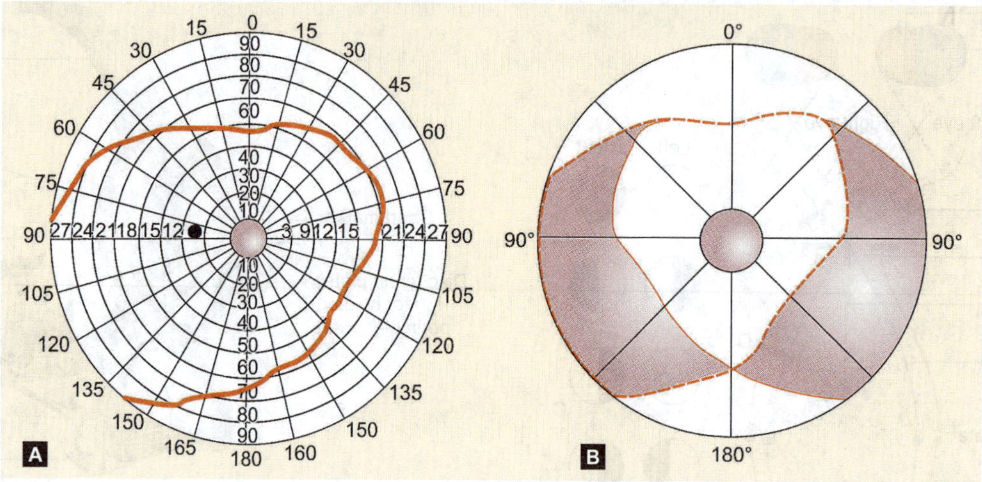

FIGS. 39A AND B: (A) The field of vision of left eye; (B) The fields of vision of both eyes are shown. Note that the binocular segments of the two eyes overlap and are seen by both eyes. The monocular segments of the two eye lie outside the binocular segments.

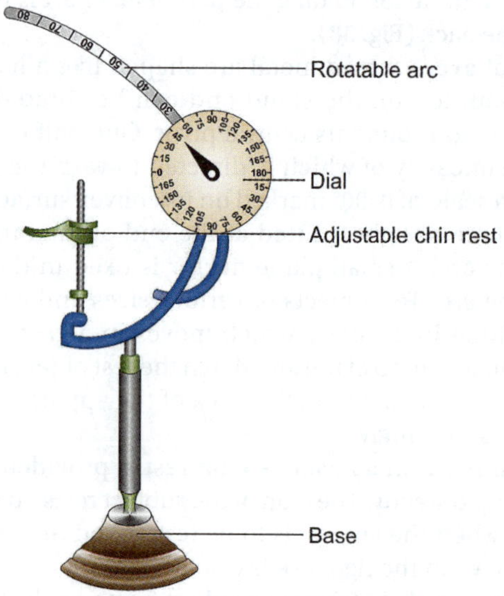

FIG. 40: The student perimeter.

outside of the arc. The readings—the meridian and the angle are then transferred to the corresponding points on the chart.

FACTORS AFFECTING VISUAL FIELD

1. **Visual acuity:** Obviously, the visual acuity should be sufficient to enable the subject to see the test object clearly.
2. **Size of object:** Though the visual field is better with a large object, a standard test object (5 mm in size) is used.
3. **Color of object:** The field is widest for white color, and smaller for blue, red, and green in that order.
4. **Brightness and contrast:** Adequate illumination affects the brightness and contrast of the object.

PROCEDURES

1. Place the perimeter on a table of suitable height and seat the subject in front of it. Fix a chart in the frame. Ask him to place his chin on the rest and adjust its height so that his eye (e.g. right eye) is at the level of the mirror. Instruct the subject not to move his eye but to keep looking at the mirror. Tell him to cover his left eye with a cupped hand.
2. Position the arc on zero meridian on the temporal side. Fix a 5 mm white object in the carrier and take it to the end of the arc; switch on the light. Ask the subject to say "yes" as soon as the object comes into view. Slowly move the object toward the mirror and as soon as the subject says "yes", strike the chart holder against the pin so that it punches a hole in the chart (the object will be visible beyond 90° on this side).
3. Rotate the arc downward (or upward) by 30°, take the object to the end of the arc, and move it toward the mirror. When it becomes visible, mark the angle on the chart paper as before. Repeat the procedure after moving the arc by 30° each time until the arc returns back to the starting position, i.e. through 360°.
4. To mark the blind spot, position the arc at 100° meridian (i.e. 10° below the horizontal) on the temporal side. Move the object from the periphery toward the center. The subject will continue to see the object up to about 20°, then it will disappear, but reappear once again after about 5°. Mark both the points on the chart; a small circle around these points will mark the blind spot which is 5–6° in diameter and situated about 15° lateral to the fixation point.
5. Plot the field of vision for the other eye in similar manner.
6. Record the peripheral field of vision of one eye for green, blue, and red objects.
7. Remove the chart from its holder and join all the pinholes with a pen to obtain the peripheral fields of vision for both the eyes. Note the area that is common to both eyes.
8. Examine the entire field of vision, in addition to mapping only the peripheral field of vision by bringing the test object right up to the fixation point at the mirror in all meridians, and noting if the object disappears after appearing at the periphery of the field. This will reveal if there is any scotoma in any part of the field.

PRECAUTIONS

1. The procedure should be explained to the subject, and instructed not to move the eye from the fixation point.
2. While testing for one eye, the other eye should be closed.
3. Adequate illumination should be provided.
4. If the subject wears glasses, these should be removed as they may restrict the field.
5. Healthy eye should be tested first.

QUESTIONS

Q.1. What is meant by field of vision? What is the extent of a normal field?

- The field of vision, visual field, or field of view is the cone of space with its apex at the eye which is seen by the subject, when that eye is kept fixed at one point. Of course, one can see much larger part of the outside world if the eye is moved.
- The whole of the view of a subject is subdivided into: (1) The right and left visual fields "seen" by the right and left eyes, respectively; (2) The binocular segment which is "seen" by both eyes; and (3) The right and left monocular segments outside of the binocular segment to the right and the left eyes **(Fig. 39B)**.
- The peripheral field of each eye extends up to about 100° on the temporal side, about 75° downward (it is limited by the cheek), 60° on the nasal side (limited by the nose), and about 60° upward where it is limited by the brow.
- The peripheral field is widest for the white color, and smaller for blue, red, and green colors in that order.

Q.2. Which parts of the retina are tested by perimetry?

Perimetry tests most parts of the retina except the macular region which contains the fovea centralis. The fovea contains only the cones and is the region of most acute vision. The acuity of vision is tested with Snellen chart for distant vision and Jaeger chart for near vision.

Q.3. Are all objects within the field of vision seen equally clearly?

- Objects whose images fall on the macula are seen in very minute details, and the colors are bright and distinct.
- Objects away from the point of fixation become less and less clear and colors are difficult to identify. Thus, only a small part of the field is seen in sharp focus. For example, when reading printed material only about 10 mm of each line is in sharp focus. At a distance of 6 meters, only a person's head and neck are in clear focus. We are normally unaware of this because the eyes are continuously moving over a scene and when they come to rest, much of what was seen in detail remains part of our perception.
- However, the peripheral part of the retina is very sensitive to movement—moving objects, flashes of light, etc. We can see a moving object much more easily through the "corner of the eye" than by directly gazing at it.

Q.4. What is physiological blind spot and what is its significance?

- The physiological blind spot refers to a zone of functional blindness all normally sighted people have in each eye, due to an absence of photoreceptors where the optic nerve passes through the surface of the retina.
- The *physiological blind spot* corresponds with the optic disc which is the region where the optic nerve leaves and the blood vessels enter the eye.
- The optic disc is 1.5 mm in diameter and is located 3 mm medial to and slightly above the posterior pole of the eye (the location of macula lutea).
- As there are no rods or cones in the optic disc, any image falling on it is not visible.
- Normally, we are not aware of the blind spot even if only one eye is used (see Experiment 2.13: Physiological Blind Spot).

Q.5. Describe the visual pathway.

See **Figure 36**.

Q.6. What is bitemporal hemianopia and what is its cause?

- Blindness in the temporal fields of vision of both eyes is called bitemporal hemianopia (or hemianopsia).
- A lesion of crossed fibers in the central part of optic chiasma, commonly due to a pituitary tumor causes this type of visual defect **(Fig. 36B)**.

Q.7. What is binasal hemianopia and what is its cause?

- Blindness in the nasal halves of fields of vision of both eyes is called binasal hemianopia. It occurs when the uncrossed optic nerve fibers in the lateral parts of optic chiasma are damaged.
- Usually, there is right or left nasal hemianopia as a result of a calcified internal carotid artery pressing on one or the other side of the chiasma **(Fig. 36C)**.

Q.8. What is homonymous hemianopia?

- Blindness in the temporal half of field of vision of one eye and the nasal field of the other eye is called *homonymous hemianopia.*
- A lesion of optic tract or optic radiation by tumors of parietal or temporal lobes produces this type of defect. A lesion on the right side will produce left homonymous hemianopia, and a lesion on the left side will produce right homonymous hemianopia (homonymous, because right half of field of one eye and right half of field of the other eye is affected.
- If the right half of field of one eye, and left half of field of the other eye is affected, it is called *heteronymous hemianopia,* e.g. binasal or bitemporal hemianopias). Partial damage to optic radiation will produce superior (lower part of radiation involved) or inferior (upper part affected) homonymous quadrantanopia **(Figs. 36D and E)**.

Q.9. What is stereoscopic vision?

The visual fields of the two eyes overlap, the portion common to both eyes having a diameter of 120°. The images of an object falling on the two maculae are slightly different from each other because of the separation of the two eyes. This is the basis of stereoscopic or binocular vision which is responsible for depth perception.

Q.10. What is a scotoma?

- Generally, the term scotoma (plural, scotomata) is applied to a small area of blindness (except the physiological blind spot) lying within a visual field.

- It is important clinically to detect the presence of scotomata and to map their location. Due to disease, a patch or patches of retina may get separated (retinal detachment) from the underlying choroid from where it gets its oxygen and other nutrients. The receptors in the affected parts degenerate and produce scotomata. Just as we are unaware of our own blind spots, similarly the patients are unaware of even quite large scotomata. Therefore, if detected early, the detached retina can be "welded" back into position with laser beams.

Q.11. Name any other method of determining the field of vision.

The confrontation test can provide a rough estimate of the peripheral field of vision.

2.12: MECHANICAL STIMULATION OF THE EYE

- Close the eyes and press on the outer corner of an eye with index finger. The pressure produces an impression of a dark circular spot surrounded by a bright circle in the field of vision directly opposite to the point of pressure. These visual sensations are called *pressure phosphenes* and are caused by "inadequate" retinal stimulation.
- This experiment supports the "Muller's law of specific nerve energy", which states that different types of stimuli applied to a sensory organ always produce the sensation peculiar to that receptor. In the case of retina, the natural stimulus of light requires minimum of energy to stimulate the rods and cones, while a mechanical stimulus requires many times the energy needed by the normal stimulus.

2.13: PHYSIOLOGICAL BLIND SPOT

PY10.20: Demonstrate (i) Testing of visual acuity, color and field of vision, (ii) Hearing, (iii) Testing for smell, and (iv) Taste sensation in volunteer/simulated environment.

- The physiological blind spot is a zone of functional blindness that all normally sighted people have in each eye.
- It is due to the absence of photoreceptors where the optic nerve passes through the surface of the retina.

PLOTTING THE BLIND SPOT

1. Seat the subject in front of a blackboard so that his eyes are 1 meter from it. If possible, fix the head to steady it.
2. Draw a small cross on the board, then ask the subject to cover his left eye with a cupped hand, and to gaze fixedly on the cross with his right eye.
3. Move a stick with a small white tip slowly on the board to the right of the cross until he can no longer see the white tip. Mark this spot with a chalk; this is the rough position of the blind spot.
4. Slowly bring the tip of the stick in vertical and oblique directions from the periphery toward the roughly positioned blind spot marking all the points when the white tip becomes visible. Join all these marks to obtain the outline of the projected image of the optic disc.
5. By using the method of similar triangles, the distances on the retina, i.e. the diameter of the optic disc, and its distance from the fovea can be calculated from the distances on the blackboard (i.e. the diameter of the projected image of the optic disc, and its distance from the cross). The point at which the rays intersect in the eye is the nodal point which can be assumed to lie 17 mm in front of retina. The distance of the nodal point from the board is 1 meter (the small distance from the nodal point to the cornea may be ignored).

$$\frac{\text{Size of object}}{\text{Size of image}} = \frac{\text{Distance of object from nodal point}}{\text{Distance of image from nodal point}}$$

MARIOTTE'S EXPERIMENT

- Draw a small cross on a blank sheet of your workbook, then draw a small spot about 10 cm to the right of the cross **(Fig. 41)**.
- Cover your left eye with your left hand and hold the figure in front of your right eye. Fix your gaze on the cross (the more nasally located of the two marks), then move the figures toward and away from you until, at a certain distance, the spot disappears. At this moment, the image of the spot is falling on the blind spot.
- Record the distance of the workbook from the eye.
- The presence of the blind spot in the left eye can be confirmed by fixing the left eye on the spot and moving the figures toward or away from the eye till the cross disappears.

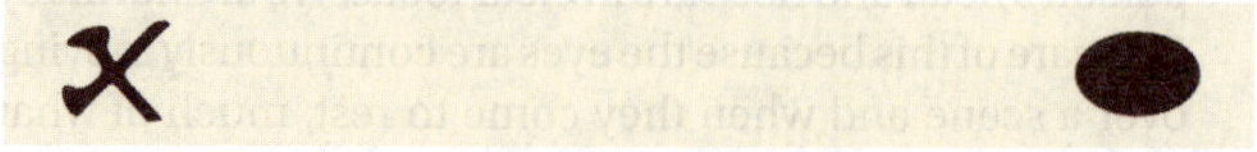

FIG. 41: Mariotte's experiment to demonstrate the physiological blind spot.

2.14: NEAR POINT AND NEAR RESPONSE

NEAR POINT

The nearest point at which an object can be seen clearly is called the near point.

Procedure

1. Seat the subject near a window in good light, and ask him to cover one eye with a cupped hand. Hold

a pencil in front of the other eye and slowly move it, preferably along a meter stick toward the eye until it can no longer be seen in *sharp* focus. Record the distance between the pencil and the eye to determine the near point.

2. Measure the near point for the other eye as well. If glasses are worn, measure the near point with and without glasses. Finally, measure the near point with both eyes open.

NEAR RESPONSE

The response showing convergence of eyes, constriction of pupil, and increase in the curvature of the lens when a distant object is brought near to the eye is called near response.

Procedure

- Seat the subject near a window and ask him to fix his eyes on a distant object. Then bring your finger in front of his eyes and ask him to focus his eyes on it. There is a convergence of eyes, constriction of pupil, and increase in the curvature of the lens.
- This three part response is called the near response or accommodation reflex.

RANGE OF ACCOMMODATION

The far point is the farthest point from the eye at which an object is seen clearly.

Procedure

1. Measure the far point in a manner similar to that used for the near point, remembering that if the subject is emmetropic (having normal vision), it will be infinitely far away (a distance of 6 meters from the eye is considered the practical far point because light rays coming from this distance are parallel).
2. If the patient wears glasses, record the near and the far points with and without glasses. Calculate the range of accommodation, i.e. the distance between the far and near points for each eye, separately.

QUESTIONS

Q.1. How does the eye accommodate for near vision?
Consult Experiment 2.19.

Q.2. What is meant by amplitude of accommodation?
Consult Experiment 2.19.

Q.3. What is presbyopia?
Consult Experiment 2.19.

2.15: SANSON IMAGES

- *Sanson images* are reflections, or images of reflections, of a light source from the various refracting surfaces of the eye.

PROCEDURES

A. Conduct the experiment in a dark room.

1. Seat the subject comfortably. Hold a burning candle to one side of his eye and observe the images of the candle flame from the other side.
   The following images are seen:
   - *On the anterior surface image #1 of the cornea*: The image is bright and upright.
   - *On the anterior surface of the lens (near the center of the pupil)*: The image #2 is upright, somewhat larger, and not so bright.
   - *On the posterior surface of the lens*: The image is smaller but inverted, and not so easily seen.
2. Ask the subject to look at the far wall of the room. While observing the images carefully, image #3 hold a finger in front of his eye and ask him to look at it.
   - **Result:** The image #2 (i.e. on the anterior surface of the lens) moves closer to the image #1; it also gets smaller and brighter. This shows that during accommodation for near vision, the *anterior surface* of the lens moves forward, i.e. this surface becomes more convex.

B. If a phakoscope is available, it should be employed to show that it is the anterior surface of the lens that becomes more convex during accommodation reflex.

C. See experiment 2.19: Visual Acuity for mechanism of accommodation.

2.16: DEMONSTRATION OF STEREOSCOPIC VISION

- ***Stereoscopic* vision** describes the ability of the visual brain to register a sense of three-dimensional shape and form from visual inputs. In current usage, stereoscopic vision often refers uniquely to the sense of depth derived from the two eyes.
- Simultaneous focusing of an object in both eyes enables us to perceive the depth and distance of that object. The overlapping of their images in the brain gives a three dimensional effect of the image.

PROCEDURE

1. Thread a needle first with both eyes open, and then repeat the experiment with one and then with the other eye. Note the time it takes in each case. Your hands should not touch each other otherwise the touch clues (such as relative position of the hands) will reduce the effect of closing one eye.
2. Hold a matchbox about 20–25 cm in front of your eyes. Draw its appearance as seen with only the right eye,

and then with the left eye. Compare the two sketches. The normal mechanism of vision fuses the two slightly different images into one to give an impression of solidity.

2.17: DOMINANCE OF THE EYE

- Ocular dominance, or dominant eye, is when one eye is used more than the other because of preference, have better vision in that eye, or can fixate on something better with this eye.
- Knowing which eye is dominant can be important for performing activities required to focus on a target.
- The dominant eye provides slightly more input to the visual cortex of the brain and relays information more accurately, such as the location of objects.
- Just as we habitually use one hand more than the other, we unconsciously have some other left-right preferences.
- The dominant eye is the one that a person normally employs to thread a needle or look into a camera.

PROCEDURE

Make a circle with your thumb and index finger, and holding it at arm's length, look through it with both eyes open at a small object across the room, say, a door handle. Close one eye and then the other; the eye that sees the object within the circle is your dominant eye.

2.18: SUBJECTIVE VISUAL SENSATIONS

- **Subjective visual sensations are those one originating within the eye and not occurring in response to an external stimulus.**
- **They appear as spots before the eyes due to cells and cell fragments in the vitreous body, aqueous and lens. They are called** *Muscae volitantes or floaters.*
- *Muscae volitantes or floaters* are a normal phenomenon especially as age advances. They are the shadows cast on the retina by cellular and other debris in the aqueous and vitreous humors. Images of the retinal blood vessels reflected from the posterior surface of the lens also contribute to the floaters.
- A sudden appearance of new floaters, if accompanied by bright flashes in the peripheral field of vision could indicate a retinal tear or detachment.

PROCEDURE

- Do this experiment on a clear day. Close one eye and look at the sky with the other and try to concentrate on what you see.
- You will observe small, circular, semitransparent, gray specks, or zigzag wispy filaments, or hair-like objects, or rows of cell-like structures that drift across the field of vision. These are called *muscae volitantes* or *floaters.*
- If you try to focus on them, they drift away or sink down, and if you jerk your eye up they rise up, but sink down or float away once again.

2.19: VISUAL ACUITY

STUDENT OBJECTIVES

After completing this experiment, the student should be able to:

- Give the definition of visual acuity (VA).
- Explain the importance of determining distant and near vision.
- How is distant and near vision tested and what are the factors that affect VA?
- Name the errors of refraction and how they are corrected?
- Define myopia and hypermetropia.
- Identify Snellen's and Jaeger's chart.

PY10.20: Demonstrate (i) Testing of visual acuity, color and field of vision, (ii) Hearing, (iii) Testing for smell, and (iv) Taste sensation in volunteer/simulated environment.

VISUAL ACUITY

- Visual acuity (VA) is the ability to see the details and contours of objects clearly. It is tested for both distant as well as near vision. This acuity of vision refers to the ability of the eye to recognize two point sources of light, or two parallel lines, as separate rather than one.
- It is expressed as minimum separable, i.e. the minimum distance between two points or lines when they can be recognized as two. If the distance is less than this, they will be seen as one. When perceived as two, they subtend an angle (the visual angle) of 1 minute (1') of arc at the nodal point (1° = 60 minutes).
- The nodal point lies at about the middle of the lens and is the optical center of the eye. Any ray passing through this point does not suffer refraction. This angle of 1 minute corresponds to a distance of 4.5 urns between the retinal images of the two points. Since the diameter of a foveal cone is about 1.5 μm, one unstimulated cone separates the two images. Some people can separate the two images even when the visual angle is only 25 seconds (retinal distance between images = 2 μm).

Factors Affecting Visual Acuity

The VA is a complex retinal and cortical mechanism that is affected by the following factors:

A. **Stimulus factors:** These include the following:
 1. **Illumination of the surface:** Bright illumination causes edge enhancement, i.e. the boundary between a bright field and a dark field is emphasized.
 2. **Size of the object** and its **distance** from the eye.
 3. **Color of the object:** Visual acuity is maximum for the white objects and is less for colored objects.
 4. **Wavelength of light:** The chromatic aberrations of the optical system tend to reduce the VA for mixed light sources, while monochromatic light increases VA. The VA is maximum for white light as compared to other colors.
 5. **Brightness contrast:** It depends on the luminescence of the dark and darker regions of the pattern.
 6. **Time of exposure:** A light flash of very short duration may not be perceived.

B. **Optical errors:** Obviously, the VA is reduced by any error of refraction because the images on the retina are blurred. In such cases, the VA will be raised by making the person look through a small aperture, which increases the depth of focus and reduces the amount of blurring caused by any error in focusing or by aberrations.

C. **Retinal factors (region of the retina stimulated):** The VA is maximal at the fovea centralis where cones are closely packed together. VA decreases away from this region.

TEST FOR DISTANT VISION

- **Snellen's Chart or Snellen's Types (Fig. 42):** The distant vision is clinically tested with this chart. It has a series of printed letters of varying sizes, black on a white background, and arranged in 8 lines. The top letter, the largest is visible to the naked eye at a distance of 60 meters, and the **subsequent letters at distances of 36, 24, 18, 12, 9, 6, and 5 meters, respectively. The distances for** each line are indicated above it (or below it in some charts). The letters are so designed that, from a specified distance, the letter as a whole subtends an angle of 5 minutes (5′) of arc at the nodal point. Further, the breadth of each line or stroke, and the breadth of gaps between two lines or two curves subtend an angle (visual angle) of 1 minute (1′) of an arc at the nodal point.

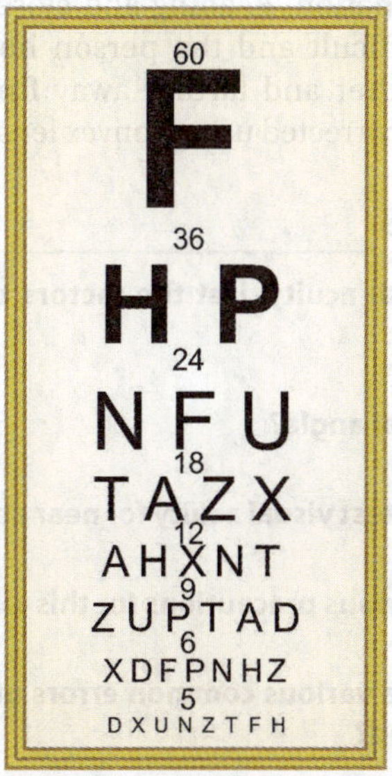

FIG. 42: Snellen's test types. Reduced in size from the standard chart seen at 6 meters.

- In the **Landolt ring chart**, the gap in the ring is positioned at random in the 8 lines. The width of the gap subtends an angle of 1 minute at the nodal point.
- In the **E Test chart**, the letter E is printed in 8 lines, the "legs" of the letters pointing in different directions. A person (or a child) who cannot read has to indicate the direction in which the legs of each letter are pointing.

Testing the Distant Visual Acuity

1. The subject is seated at a distance of 6 meters (20 feet) from a well-lighted chart and is asked to read the letters down the chart as far as she can read. Each eye is tested separately.
2. The VA is recorded according to the formula VA = d/D where d is the distance at which the letters are read, and D is the distance at which the letter should be read by a person with normal vision.
3. Thus, if only the top letter can be read, the VA is 6/60. If the subject can read only the first 4 lines, then the VA is 6/18, and so on. A normal person should be able to read at least the 7th line, i.e. have a VA of 6/6 (20/20 in terms of feet commonly pronounced *twenty-twenty* vision).
4. If the VA is less than 6/60, the subject is moved toward the chart until the subject can read the top letter. The VA is 2/60 the subject can read it at 2 meters. The VA less than 1/60 is recorded as "counting fingers" [CF; if she correctly counts fingers when held in front of her face; *hand movements* (HMs); *perception of light* (PL); or as *no perception of light* (no PL)].

TEST FOR NEAR VISION

- The subject is asked to read **Jaeger chart** held at the ordinary reading distance of 15 inches. This chart is made up of reading material of various sizes with the smallest size at the bottom **(Fig. 43)**.
- The subject reads the material down the chart and VA is recorded as the smallest type that can be read comfortably. The result used to be expressed as J1, J2, J3, J4, etc. J1—(the smallest size) indicates normal vision. These days a modification of the original Jaeger system is used and VA is expressed in terms of printers' point system—N36, N18, N8, N6, and N5 instead of J1, J2, etc.; N5 being the smallest type instead of J1.
- A **Landolt ring chart** for near vision is also available. Charts with pictures are used for children. In Sheridan-Gardiner test, Snellen's letters are matched with different types of objects.

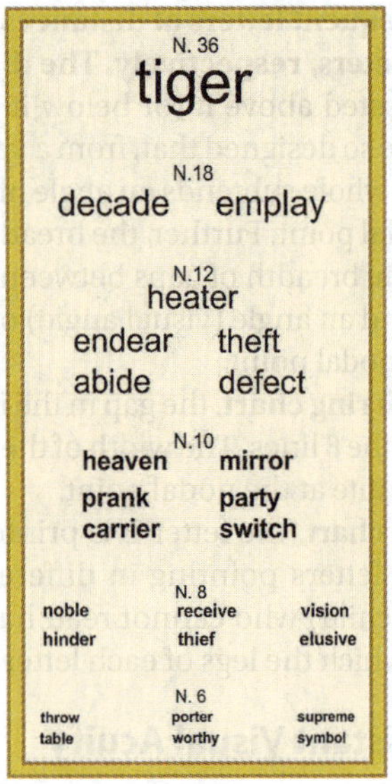

FIG. 43: Jaeger chart.

Accommodation for Near Vision

- The eye accommodates (adjusts) for near vision by increasing the refractive power of the lens, i.e. the lens becomes more convex mainly on the anterior surface.
- At rest, i.e. when the eye is looking at a distant object and the ciliary muscle is relaxed, the malleable and elastic lens is held under tension by its suspensory ligament and is pulled into a flattened shape. In this state, parallel rays of light coming from the distant object are brought to focus on the retina and the object is seen clearly.
- However, when the eye looks at a near object (closer than 6 meters), the divergent rays are brought to a focus "behind" the retina so that the image on the retina is blurred, i.e. out of focus. This *blurring of the image on the retina acts as a stimulus for the reflex contraction of ciliary muscle* which pulls the ciliary body forward and inward. As a result, the lens ligament becomes lax, the tension on the lens capsule decreases, and the lens due to its elasticity bulges forward. The increase in refractive power of the lens brings the image forward onto the retina and the image becomes clearly visible.
- When the gaze is shifted to a distant object, the ciliary muscle relaxes and the lens becomes less convex (the ciliary muscle is the most frequently used muscle in the body as we shift our gaze from distant to mid-distance and near objects, and then in the reverse order as we scan the environment).

Range of Accommodation

Far point: It is the farthest point from the eye at which an object is seen clearly. This point is infinity in the normal eye. A distance of 6 meters from the eye is considered as the practical far point because light rays from this distance are parallel.

Near point: It is the nearest distance from the eye at which an object can be seen clearly. It is 9–10 cm at age of 10 years.

Amplitude of Accommodation

- The difference in the refractive power of the lens in the two states of complete relaxation and maximal accommodation is called the amplitude of accommodation.
- The total refractive power of the eye is about 60 diopters (66 D in some cases). Of this 60 D, the cornea contributes 44 D, while the refractive power of the lens is 16 D in a young person. During maximal accommodation, the refractive power of the lens can add another 14 D to its refractive power. Thus, the amplitude of accommodation is 14 diopters (30 – 16 = 14 D).

COMMON ERRORS OF REFRACTION

- **Myopia (short-sightedness):** In this condition, parallel rays of light coming from a distant object are brought to a focus in front of the retina; the rays then diverge and form a blurred image on the retina. Thus, distant objects cannot be seen clearly. This error is corrected with concave lenses (the eyeball is longer than the *refractive power* of the eye).
- **Hypermetropia (long-sightedness):** This is the condition in which parallel rays of light from a distance are focused behind the retina (i.e. they are not *focused* on the retina but would have come to focus had the eyeball been longer). Thus, the near objects are not seen clearly. The condition is corrected with convex lenses.
- **Presbyopia:** The *near point* recedes throughout life, slowly at first, and then rapidly after age 40–45 years being 9 cm at age 10 years to about 80 cm by age 65 years. This is due to hardening of the lens that results in loss of accommodation. Reading and close work gradually becomes difficult and the person holds the reading material farther and farther away from the eye. The condition is corrected using convex lenses.

QUESTIONS

Q.1. Define visual acuity. List the factors that affect visual acuity.

See text above.

Q.2. What is visual angle?

See text above.

Q.3. How do you test visual acuity for near and distant vision?

See text above.

Q.4. State the various precautions for this experiment.

See text above.

Q.5. Describe the various common errors of refraction. How are they corrected?

See text above.

2.20: COLOR VISION

STUDENT OBJECTIVES

After completing this experiment, the student should be able to:

- Describe the receptors of color vision.
- Explain the mechanism of color vision.
- Perform Ishihara test on a patient.
- Name some other tests of color vision.
- Explain the practical importance of color vision.
- Define different types of color blindness.

PY10.20: Demonstrate (i) Testing of visual acuity, color and field of vision, (ii) Hearing, (iii) Testing for smell, and (iv) Taste sensation in volunteer/simulated environment.

INTRODUCTION

- **Colour vision is the ability to distinguish among various wavelengths of light waves and to perceive the differences as differences in *hue*.**
- **The human eye** is sensitive to all wavelengths of light from 400 nm to 700 nm which constitute the visible part of the electromagnetic spectrum.
- **The normal human eye can discriminate among hundreds of such bands of wavelengths as they are received by the color-sensing cells (cones) of the retina.**
- Colors-sensitive cones are concentrated in fovea and are sensitive to specific wavelengths of light.
- Hue refers to the origin of the colors one can see. Primary and Secondary colors (Yellow, Orange, Red, Violet, Blue, and Green) are considered hues; however, tertiary colors (mixed colors where neither color is dominant) would also be considered hues.

ATTRIBUTES OF COLORS

- Colors have three attributes: (1) **hue**, (2) **intensity**, and (3) **saturation** (degree of freedom from dilution with white). There are three **primary colors**—(1) *red*, (2) *green*, and (3) *blue*. For every color, there is a **complementary** color that when properly mixed with it produces a sensation of white.
- The sensation of white, any spectral color, and even extra-spectral color (e.g. purple) can be produced by mixing various proportions of primary colors (the paints used in painting are not pure colors but mixtures of different pigments).
- Black is the sensation caused by absence of light. It is probably a positive sensation because the blind eye does not "see black", it "sees nothing". Finally, the color perceived depends on the color of other objects in the visual field.
- Also, there are three types of cone pigments: (1) **erythrolabe** [red-sensitive or long-wave (723–647 nm) pigment], (2) **chlorolabe** [green-sensitive or middle-wave (575–492 nm) pigment], and (3) **cyanolabe** [blue-sensitive or short-wave (492–417 nm) pigment].

MECHANISMS OF COLOR VISION

Two mechanisms are involved:

1. **Retinal mechanism:** The **Young-Helmholtz theory** is based on the existence of three kinds of cones. The ganglion cells of retina add or subtract input from one type of cone to the output of another type. Further processing occurs in LGB and thalamus and then along specific pathways to the visual cortex.
2. **Cortical mechanism:** The fibers from lateral geniculate body (LGB) and thalamus project to clusters of cells (blobs) arranged in a mosaic in layer IV of the primary visual cortex (area 17) which along with visual association area (area 18) is involved in color perception.

TESTING OF COLOR VISION

I. **Ishihara charts:** These charts consist of lithographic color plates available in book form. The plates are so constructed that numbers and wavy lines made up of spots of confusing colors are printed against backgrounds of differently colored spots of identical size **(Fig. 44)**.

Procedure

1. Seat the subject in a room adequately lit by daylight. Direct sunlight or electric light may cause discrepancies in the result due to changes in the shades of the colors.
2. Ask the subject to read the numbers or trace the wavy lines on successive plates. The correct answers are given at the back of the book to exclude the possibility of examiner being color blind. For example, the person with normal color vision will read plate 3 in **Figure 44** as 5, while a person with defective color vision will reads it as 2. The results with other plates are given in **Table 13.**

II. **Eldridge-Green lantern:** In this electrical apparatus, different colored glass pieces (pure red, different intensities of red, yellow, green, and signal green) are fitted in a rotating disc.

These can be brought in front of a small illuminated area, the size of which can be varied. The effects of rain and fog can be added to the colors by bringing appropriate lenses in front of the colors. The subject sits 5–6 feet in front of the lantern set up in a dimly-lit room. He/she names the colors as they are brought in front of the aperture.

III. **Holmgren's wools (yarn matching test):** Small pieces of woolen threads of different colors and hues are placed in a heap on a table. The subject is given a test skein and is asked to pick out matching pieces. The subject only matches colors and does not name them.

CLINICAL SIGNIFICANCE

Color vision is tested as part of routine health check of persons entering government jobs or joining a professional course. It is particularly important in the following groups of people:

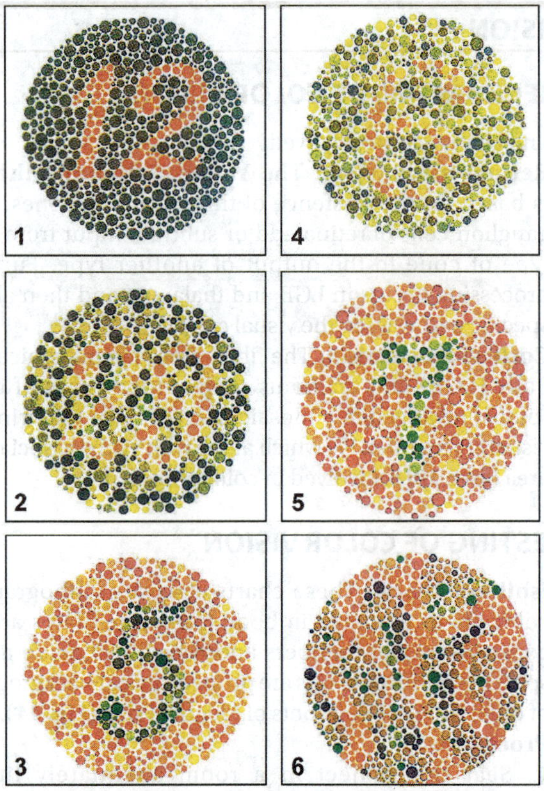

FIG. 44: Ishihara color plates.

Table 13: Results of Ishihara test.

Plate	Person with normal	Person with red-green deficiency	Person with total color blindness
1.	12	12	12
2.	29	70	X
3.	5	2	X
4.	6	X	X
5.	7	X	X
6.	X	5	X

The mark X shows that the plate cannot be read

1. Drivers of air, sea, and road transport vehicles, railway engine drivers, bus and truck drivers, pilots, etc.
2. Workers of textile industry where dyeing of cloth requires a high degree of color perception.
3. Paint and printing industries.
4. Interior decorators and visual artists.

DEFECTS OF COLOR VISION

- Abnormal color vision is present as an inherited defect. The prefix **deuter**—refers to green color, **trit**—refers to blue, and **prot**—refers to red color. The suffix—**anomaly** refers to color weakness while suffix—**anopia** refers to color blindness. **Monochromats** have only one cone system present, **dichromats** have two cone systems, and **trichromats** have all three cone systems but one may be weak.
- Physiological dichromatic vision is at the fovea centralis where only red and blue cones are present. The common defects of color vision in order of occurrence are: Deuteranomaly, deuteranopia, protanopia, and protanomaly. If either red or green or both cones are missing, the person cannot distinguish red from green. However, though the subject can see the other colors, they are not seen in the way a normal person does.

QUESTIONS

Q.1. Describe the theories of color vision.
See text above.

Q.2. How is color vision tested? What is the principle behind the chart used to test for color blindness?
See text above.

Q.3. What is color blindness? How is it classified?
See text above.

Q.4. What is the pathway for color vision?
See text above.

Q.5. Discuss the clinical significance of this practical.
See text above.

2.21: TUNING FORK TESTS OF HEARING

STUDENT OBJECTIVES

After completing this experiment, the student should be able to:
- Explain the importance of doing hearing tests in clinical physiology.
- Define sound, and name its characteristics that are perceived by the ear.
- Describe the principle underlying tuning-fork tests.
- Differentiate between air (ossicular) conduction and bone conduction.
- Trace the auditory pathway.
- Describe the principle of audiometry.
- Comment on cochlear implants.

PY10.20: Demonstrate (i) Testing of visual acuity, color and field of vision, (ii) Hearing, (iii) Testing for smell, and (iv) Taste sensation in volunteer/simulated environment.

INTRODUCTION

I. **Nature and characteristics of sound waves:**
   - Sound waves are alternating regions of high and low pressure traveling through some medium (e.g. air) in the same direction.
   - They are produced by some vibrating object and are perceived by us as the sound sensation.
   - The auditory analyzer perceives the following four properties of sound **(Fig. 45)**:
     1. ***Pitch:***
        - It is the psychological perception of the sound frequency; the higher the frequency, the higher the pitch.
        - The entire audible range extends from 16 Hz to 20, 000 Hz (1 hertz = 1 cycle/sec). The term **infrasound** refers to frequencies below 16 Hz,

while **ultrasound** refers to frequencies above 20,000 Hz.

- The human ear is most sensitive to frequencies between 500 Hz and 5,000 Hz. The average conversation voice frequency is 120 Hz in the males and 250 Hz in the females. The sounds from a distant plane range from 20 Hz to 100 Hz.
- Pitch discrimination is possible because different frequencies cause vibrations in different regions of the basilar membrane. Each segment of this membrane is thus "tuned" for a particular pitch—high-pitched sounds near the base of cochlea and low-pitched sounds near the apex.

Note: While the human ear cannot perceive (*hear*) ultrasounds, bats, dogs, and other animals can. Ultrasound is used extensively to study the internal organs of the body. The inaudible sounds are reflected from the organs and analyzed by a computer to provide a picture on the display screen.

2. ***Intensity (loudness):*** The intensity or loudness of a sound is the psychological term referring to the amplitude of the sound vibrations. The sound intensity is measured in units called decibels (Db; db) (see Q/A 1).
3. ***Timbre (quality or pattern):*** This property refers to the sensation perceived when we hear a mixture of related frequencies, i.e. harmonics or overtones (the same note played on different musical instruments is *perceived* or *sounds* differently).
4. ***Direction of sound:*** The ability to detect the position of the source of sound is called binaural effect.

II. **Mechanism of hearing:**

- The sound waves striking the tympanic membrane are magnified by the ossicles and set the basilar membrane to vibrate, which in turn, causes movement of the hair cells of the organ of Corti.
- The bending of the cilia of hair cells transducts mechanical vibrations into action potentials (APs) by releasing a neurotransmitter (probably glutamate) at the bases of hair cells where nerve endings of first-order sensory neurons synapse.
- The APs are carried up the auditory pathway to the primary auditory areas of the cerebral cortex (Brodmann areas 41 and 42). Since many fibers cross over from one auditory pathway to the opposite pathway in medulla, the primary auditory areas receive signals from both sides.

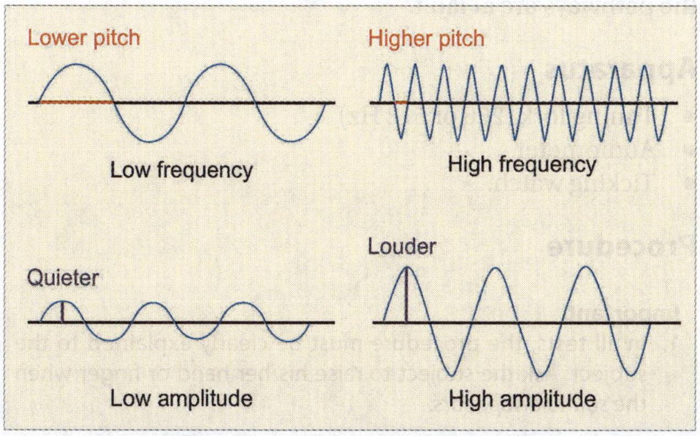

FIG. 45: Characteristics of sound waves.

III. **Auditory pathway:**

- The **pathway of hearing (Fig. 46)** from the cochlea to the auditory cortex consists of 4 to 6 neurons.
- The cell bodies of first-order neurons (bipolar) lie in the spiral ganglion. The peripheral processes end on the hair cells of the organ of Corti, while the central processes which form the auditory nerve enter the upper medulla to synapse on the dorsal and ventral cochlear nuclei.
- The second-order neurons from these nuclei take different routes through the nearby olivary nuclei and the trapezoid bodies of both sides (some fibers end here), cross to the opposite side, and turn upward to form the lateral lemniscus.
- The lemniscal fibers synapse on the neurons in the inferior colliculi and medial geniculate bodies from where fresh relays (third-order neurons) spread upward as auditory radiation to terminate in the primary auditory cortex (Brodmann areas 41 and 42).

IV. **Tests of hearing:**

1. *Whisper test:* See clinical testing of 8th nerve for these tests.
2. *Watch test:* See clinical testing of 8th nerve for these tests.
3. *Tuning fork tests:* These are the most commonly used tests in clinical practice.
4. Recording of brainstem auditory evoked potentials (BAEPs; see experiment 2.27: Electroneurodiagnostic Tests).
5. *Audiometry.*

TUNING FORK TESTS

Before one can understand the principles on which the tuning-fork tests are based, one must understand what is meant by **air conduction** and **bone conduction** of sound.

Air (Ossicular) Conduction

- Normally, most of the energy of incident sound waves is transmitted via the outer ear, tympanic membrane, and middle ear ossicles to the cochlea where it stimulates the sensory hair cells of the organ of Corti.
- This mode of conduction of sound is called **ossicular conduction**, though it is commonly and **misleadingly called air conduction. True air conduction**, i.e. vibrations of tympanic membrane, vibrations of air in the middle ear round window of cochlea (that is, where vibrations of the ossicles are not involved) does not play any role in normal hearing.

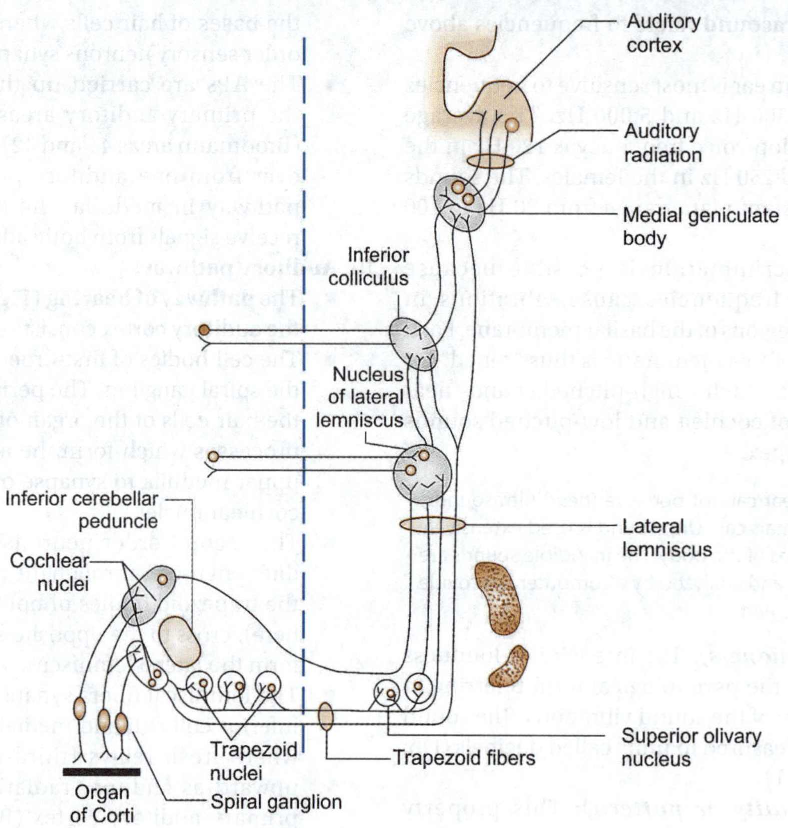

FIG. 46: The auditory pathway.

Bone Conduction

- Since cochlea is enclosed in a bony cavity (bony cochlea), vibrations of the skull bones themselves can be transmitted to the organ of Corti—a type of sound conduction called bone conduction (BC).
- In this case, sound from a vibrating tuning fork directly placed anywhere on the skull can be heard in both ears by bone conduction.
- However, even loud sounds in the environment do not possess enough energy to cause vibrations of the skull bones and thus stimulate the organ of Corti; they usually take the air and ossicular route.

Principles of Tuning Fork Tests

- Tuning forks which emit pure tones allow comparison of air conducted (AC) hearing and bone conducted (BC) hearing in an individual.
- In ***AC hearing***, sound from a vibrating tuning fork held in front of the external ear passes via the external auditory meatus, tympanic membrane, and middle ear ossicles to the organ of Corti.
- In ***BC hearing***, vibrations from a tuning fork directly placed on the skull are conducted to the organ of Corti and perceived as sound.
- **Normally, AC hearing is better than BC hearing (written as AC > BC, or Rinne positive).**

Conduction (or Conductive) Deafness

Pathology in the outer ear (e.g. wax), or damage to the tympanic membrane (e.g. perforation), or pathology in the middle ear (e.g. loss of mobility or destruction of ossicles), reduces AC hearing without affecting bone conduction (BC hearing), a condition called **conductive deafness.**

Nerve Deafness

Damage to the hair cells in the organ of Corti or auditory pathways will reduce both AC and BC hearing, a condition called **nerve deafness** or **perceptive deafness.** In other words, if BC is normal, the inner ear (cochlea) and auditory pathways must be normal, but if BC is reduced the cochlea or the pathways are at fault.

Apparatus

- Tuning fork (256 or 512 Hz)
- Audiometer
- Ticking watch.

Procedure

Important

1. In all tests, the procedure must be clearly explained to the subject. Ask the subject to raise his/her hand or finger when the *sound disappears.*

2. The sense of hearing should first be tested with the whisper test, and then with a tuning fork.
3. The student is advised to perform all these tests on herself and on her partner.

I. **Rinne test (Figs. 47A and B)**

This test compares the subject's AC hearing with his BC hearing in each ear separately.

1. Hold the stem of the tuning fork with the thumb and finger and set it into vibration by striking one of its prongs on the heel of your hand (the other prong will also start to vibrate).
2. Place its base on the mastoid process (the bony prominence behind the ear). The subject will hear a sound. Ask him to raise his hand when the sound stops. Note the time for which the sound is heard.
3. When the sound stops, bring the prongs in front of the ear the sound will become audible once again. Note the time for which it lasts (e.g. for another 10 seconds; total = 45 seconds).

   Results

   In normal individuals: For example, sound heard on mastoid process = 35 seconds.

   Sound heard in front of ear = 35 + 10 = 45 seconds.

   Thus, AC > DC (Rinne positive).

   In conduction deafness: BC sound remains normal at 35 seconds, but AC sound not heard after BC sound stops. Thus, AC < BC (Rinne negative).

   In nerve deafness: Hearing will be impaired in both BC and AC sounds.

   For example, BC becomes 15 seconds, AC becomes 20 seconds.

   Thus, AC > BC, if nerve deafness is partial.
4. Test the other ear and record the timings for BC and AC sounds.

II. **Weber's test (Fig. 48)**

This test compares the bone conduction of the subject in his two ears.

1. Set the tuning fork into vibration and place its base in the midline on the top of the subject's head or on his forehead. Ask the subject if he hears the sound equally well in both the ears, or louder on one side.

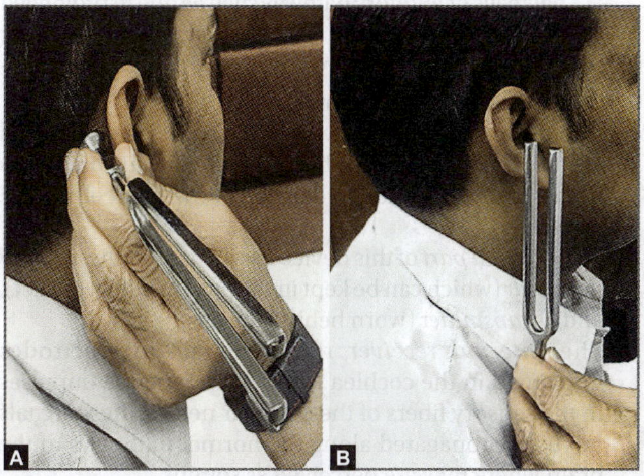

FIGS. 47A AND B: Rinne test.

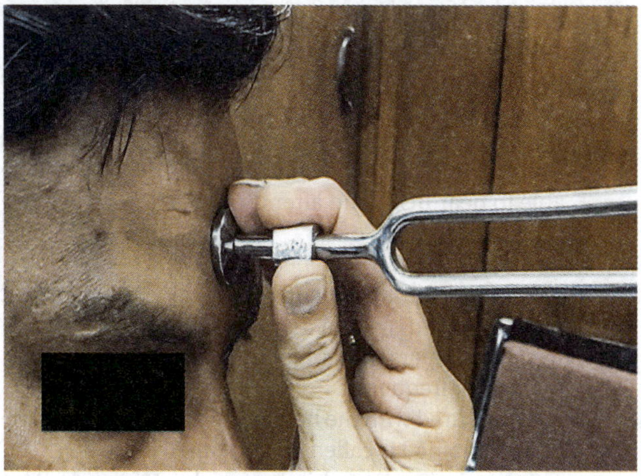

FIG. 48: Weber's test.

   In a normal subject: Bone conducted sounds are heard equally well on the two sides.

   In conduction deafness: Sound is louder/better heard in deaf or deafer ear because of masking effect of environmental noise is absent on diseased side.

   In nerve deafness: The sound is louder/better heard on the healthy side, i.e. the patient lateralizes the sound to healthy side.
2. Conduction deafness can be artificially created if you close one ear (say left) of the subject with your finger. Set the tuning fork into vibration once again and place it on his head or forehead.

   In a normal person: Sound is better heard in the closed ear due to bone conduction. Closing his ear produces a situation of conduction deafness, and demonstrates the masking effect of environmental noise.

III. **Schwabach's test**

This test compares the subject's bone conduction with the examiner's bone conduction. It is assumed that the examiner's hearing is normal.

Note: The Weber's and Schwabach's tests demonstrate the important masking effect of environmental noise on the auditory threshold.

IV. **Absolute bone conduction (ABC) test: This test is performed to identify sensorineural hearing loss.**

- Principle: This is a modified Schwabach's test where the bone conduction level of patient is compared to that of the clinician. It includes occlusion of the External Auditory Canal by pressing the tragus to reduce the ambient sound in the surrounding, which is not done in Schwabach's test.
- Pre-requisite: Clinician should have normal bone conduction level or at least he should know his bone conduction level.

Procedure

1. Set the tuning fork into vibration as before and place its base on the subject's mastoid process. Ask him to indicate by raising his hand when the sound stops.
2. After the subject stops hearing the sound, place the fork on your own mastoid process.

In a normal person: BC sound in the subject is nearly equal to your own.

In conduction deafness: The subject's bone conduction is better than your bone conduction.

In nerve deafness: BC sound in the subject is reduced as compared to your own (this means that you will be able to hear BC sound after the subject stops hearing this sound).

V. **Audiometry:**

- Audiometry (*audre* means to hear) is an accurate, painless, and noninvasive test for hearing that measures a person's ability to hear different sounds, pitches, or frequency.
- It is measured with the help of an audiometer and the graph obtained is called an audiometer.
- The test is conducted in a soundproof room. Pure tones of different frequencies and different intensities are presented to the ear from an oscillator connected by an amplifier to the earphones.
- Threshold intensity is the lowest decibel at which the subject hears the tone.
- Audiometric threshold as a function of frequency discrimination is plotted on a graph. This is called an audiogram.

VI. Brainstem **auditory evoked potential:** See experiment 2.27.

QUESTIONS

Q.1. What are the features of sound that are perceived by the hearing mechanism? What is the unit of intensity of sound?

- The auditory analyzer perceives the pitch, intensity or loudness, timbre or quality of sound, and the direction of the source of sound.
- The **intensity or loudness of sound** is expressed in decibels (db). The standard sound reference (faintest audible sound) corresponds to zero (0) db at a pressure level of 0.0002 dyne/cm^2. This is the minimum sound intensity that can be perceived by a normal person. Thus, a zero db sound is not inaudible, but just audible. Ordinary conversation at 6–8 feet is held at 50–60 db. The sound pressure that can damage cochlear receptors is more than 10^{14} times, i.e. more than a trillion times the auditory threshold (the db scale is logarithmic). This pressure approximately equals about 140 db. Loud stereo music with headphones on, or prolonged exposure to other loud noises causes selective loss of hearing.

Q.2. What is meant by the terms ultrasonic, infrasonic, and supersonic?

- The audible range for humans extends from 16 Hz to 20,000 Hz.
- *Infrasound* refers to frequencies below 16 Hz and *ultrasound* refers to frequencies above 20,000 Hz (see earlier).
- The speed of sound at sea level is about 770 miles per hour (about 1,250 km/hr). The term *supersonic* refers to an object (e.g. an aeroplane) that travels at a speed faster than that of sound (The term *mach 1* is used for planes flying at the speed of sound; twice this speed is *mach 2* and so on. Nowadays, planes can fly at over *mach 5–6*).

Q.3. What are the limitations of the tuning fork tests? What are audiometry and BAEPs?

- The tuning fork tests often provide valuable information, but cannot give quantitative estimates about the acuity of hearing. Furthermore, bone-conducted vibrations reach all parts of the skull irrespective of where the fork is placed on the head. Thus, when testing bone conduction in one ear, the patient will also be hearing sound in the other ear, which is likely to confuse him.
- **Audiometry:** An audiometer is an apparatus in which selected pure tones of 125–800 Hz can be fed into each ear separately through headphones. The threshold is determined at each frequency and is then plotted as a percentage of normal hearing. Audiometry is thus the only reliable method to determine the nature and degree of deafness in a patient.
- **Brainstem auditory evoked potentials (BAEPs):** The BAEPs recorded from the scalp after applying a suitable auditory stimulus are employed to localize the site of lesion in the central auditory pathways (consult experiment 2.27: Electroneurodiagnostic Tests).

Q.4. What is masking and what is deafness?

- **Masking:** It literally means "covering" (like a face mask). The auditory system cannot separate the different components of total sound stimulation. Auditory masking is the effect by which a faint but audible sound becomes inaudible in the presence of another louder audible sound. For example, if someone listens to a soft and a loud sound at the same time, he or she may not hear the soft sound.
- **Deafness:** This refers to the inability of a person to hear either partially or totally. It is of two types:
  1. ***Conduction deafness*** in which there may be wax or a foreign body in the external auditory meatus, thickening or damage to tympanic membrane due to infection (otitis media), and osteosclerosis (stapes gets fixed in oval window) interfere with hearing; and
  2. ***Nerve deafness*** in which there is damage to cochlear hair cells or auditory pathway such as due to prolonged exposure to industrial sounds, or very loud music, or damage to 8th nerve by drugs.

Q.5. What are cochlear implants?

- A cochlear implant is a device which converts sounds into electrical signals that can be interpreted by the brain. It is useful in deafness due to damage to the hair cells of the cochlea.
- The *external part* of this device has a *microphone, a sound processor* (which can be kept in the patient's shirt pocket), and a *transmitter* (worn behind the ear).
- The *internal receiver* relays signals to electrodes implanted in the cochlea where they generate impulses in the sensory fibers of the cochlear nerve. These signals are then propagated along the normal pathways to the brain where they are perceived as sounds.

Q.6. What is audiometry?

See text above.

OBJECTIVE STRUCTURED PRACTICAL EXAMINATIONS

Task: To demonstrate Rinne test on the subject provided.

Procedural steps: See text above.

Checklist:

1. Explain the test procedure and gives suitable instructions. (Y/N)
2. Select either 216 Hz or 250 Hz tuning fork and strikes one of the prongs on the heel of her hand. (Y/N)
3. Close the external auditory meatus of the subject's other ear with her finger. (Y/N)
4. Place the base of the tuning fork on the patient's mastoid process; when he raises his finger to indicate that the sound can no longer be heard. (Y/N)
5. Quickly transfer the vibrating tuning fork close to the patient's ear. Note if he/she can hear the sound once again. Note down whether air or bone conduction is better. (Y/N)

2.22: LOCALIZATION OF SOUNDS

PY10.20: Demonstrate (i) Testing of visual acuity, color and field of vision, (ii) Hearing, (iii) Testing for smell, and (iv) Taste sensation in volunteer/simulated environment.

- Sound localization refers to the ability to identify the direction of a sound source. There are two different aspects to sound localization.
  1. **Absolute localization, or localization acuity:** It refers to the ability to judge the *absolute position* of a sound source in three-dimensional space.
  2. **Relative localization:** It refers to the ability to *detect a shift* in the absolute position of the sound source.
- Use of both the ears to perceive the sound is defined as Binaural hearing. Binaural hearing makes it possible to identify the location of sound far more effectively. The ability to judge the position of the source of sound with both ears is called the **binaural effect.** Two factors are involved in this process:
  1. The difference in the loudness of the sounds at the two ears.
  2. The difference in the interval of sound at the two ears, i.e. the phase difference or interval between equal phases of sound waves entering the two ears.
- The human ear can gauge the direction of a sound's origin on a 0.00003 second difference in its interval at the two ears.
- When we want to localize a sound coming from a distance, we turn our head until the sound is equally loud in the two ears.
- The direction in which we are facing is the direction of the sound's origin.

PROCEDURE

- Seat the subject in a quiet room, and ask him to close his eyes.
- Use a forceps to produce clicking noises behind, in front, and to each side of his head, one after the other, and ask him to locate the direction of sound in each case.
- Enter the results in your workbook indicating the ability to localize the sound as excellent, good, fair, and poor.

2.23: MASKING OF SOUND

PY10.20: Demonstrate (i) Testing of visual acuity, color and field of vision, (ii) Hearing, (iii) Testing for smell, and (iv) Taste sensation in volunteer/simulated environment.

- **Auditory or Sound Masking** *is the process by which the threshold of hearing for one sound is raised by the presence of another sound.* This is when a signal, the sound that is desired to be heard, is made inaudible by a masker, noise or unwanted sound that is present throughout the signal.
- For example, if someone listens to a soft and a loud sound at the same time, he or she may not hear the soft sound. The soft sound is masked by the loud sound. The loud sound has a greater masking effect if the soft sound lies within the same frequency range, but masking also occurs when the soft sound is outside the frequency range of the loud sound.
- We raise our voices when traveling in a noisy bus or train. When the noise suddenly stops, we become aware of the loudness of our voice.
- The masking effect of noise is employed to detect malingering.

PROCEDURE

- Ask the subject to read from a book. After a few seconds, make a rattling noise near his ear by using a tin box containing some metal objects.
- The subject automatically increases the intensity of his voice. *Obviously, this would not occur in a deaf individual.*
- A person malingering deafness, on the other hand will raise his voice.

2.24: SENSATION OF TASTE

PY10.20: Demonstrate (i) Testing of visual acuity, color and field of vision, (ii) Hearing, (iii) Testing for smell, and (iv) Taste sensation in volunteer/simulated environment.

- Sensations of taste are commonly called chemical sensations because they are stimulated by chemicals (tastants for taste and odorants for smell) dissolved in oral and nasal mucus.
- These sensations help in avoiding ingestion of harmful foods and chemicals.
- Though the sensations of taste (gustation; gust = taste) and smell are closely related, they are anatomically distinct.

RECEPTORS FOR TASTE

- Different types of cells are present in 40–80 µm ovoid structures called taste buds (about 10,000 in humans). **The sensory receptor cells have vesicles and microvilli that project into the taste pore.**
- Their bases have synaptic connections with afferent nerve fibers of 7th, 9th, and 10th cranial nerves.
- The taste buds are present in fungiform and vallate papillae, but are absent in filiform papillae.
- The sensory cells are replenished from supporting cells.

BASIC TASTE MODALITIES

There are four basic tastes: (1) ***sweet,*** (2) ***salt,*** (3) ***bitter,*** and (4) ***sour.*** The fifth taste sensation—***umami,*** has recently been added by the Japanese to the list. It is excited by glutamate (especially monosodium glutamate, MSG); its taste is described as "meaty" or "savory". MSG is naturally present in many foods and is added to many Asian foods to enhance taste.

Taste Perception

- Taste perception occurs when water-soluble chemicals in the mouth contact the epithelial cells of the taste buds.
- The belief that there is a specific localization of basic tastes on the tongue—sweet at the tip, salt on the dorsum, sour along the edges, and bitter at the back—appears to be no longer valid.
- It is believed that all taste sensations are experienced from all areas of the oral cavity and that it is the pattern of stimulation of taste receptors that produces a particular taste. With some foods (e.g. *hot* sauces), there is an element of pain. Touch, temperature, and texture also contribute to taste.
- Flavor is a combination of different tastes and smells.

TASTE PATHWAY (FIG. 49)

- Three cranial nerves contain the axons of first-order gustatory neurons that innervate the sensory cells in taste buds—(1) 7th nerve from anterior two-third of tongue, (2) 9th nerve from posterior third of tongue, and (3) 10th nerve from part of pharynx and epiglottis.
- These first order afferent fibers relay in the nucleus of tractus solitarius (NTS).
- Second-order neurons originating from the nucleus of tractus solitarius travel up in the ipsilateral medial lemniscus to end in the nucleus lateralis posterolateralis of the thalamus.
- From thalamus, they are relayed to the taste area I in the postcentral gyrus.
- Other fibers from thalamus end in taste area II in the insula and to limbic system and hypothalamus.
- In addition the sensations of touch, pain, and temperature are carried from the oral cavity by the 5th cranial nerve.

Abnormalities of taste: Taste disorders fall under three broad descriptors: **hypogeusia** is a diminished sense of taste, **ageusia** is the complete loss of taste, and **dysgeusia** is an alteration or distortion in the perception of taste.

Note: The sweet taste is better experienced near the tip of the tongue, salt on the sides and top, bitter in the posterior part, and sour sensation in between these areas.

TESTING THE TASTE SENSATION

Materials Required

The following materials will be required:

- Strong solutions of sucrose (10%), sodium chloride (15%) and weak solutions of acetic acid (1%), and quinine sulfate (0.1%) all kept in drop bottles.
- A hand lens.
- Small cotton swabs or toothpicks; gauze.
- Four cards with sweet, salt, sour, and bitter printed on them.

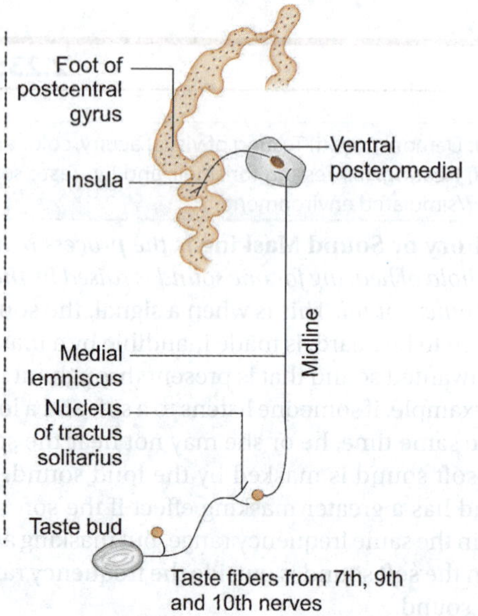

FIG. 49: The pathway for taste.

Procedure

Instruct the subject that he is to point to a card to indicate the taste felt by him.

1. Seat the subject near your work table. Ask him/her to protrude his tongue. Using the hand lens, examine and identify the areas which have large concentrations of papillae and taste buds. Locate the fungiform and circumvallate papillae.
2. Ask the subject to rinse his mouth; then dry it with gauze. Moisten a swab with a few drops of sugar solution, apply it to the tip of the tongue, and ask him/her to indicate without withdrawing the tongue, the taste experienced by him/her.
3. Have him rinse his mouth; dry the tongue with gauze, and repeat the procedure with the salt solution.
4. Repeat this procedure with all the four substances, one by one, on the sides, near the tip, the anterior two-third, and the posterior one-third of the dorsum of the tongue, and taking care that the test solution does not spread across the midline. The tip of the tongue may be held with gauze while testing.
5. Record the results, and grade the intensity of taste sensation as: Intense (++++), moderate (+++), mild (++), slight (+), or absent (0).

QUESTIONS

Q.1. What is the pathway for taste sensation?
See text above.

Q.2. What are the various abnormalities in relation to taste sensation?
See text above.

2.25: SENSATION OF SMELL

PY10.20: Demonstrate (i) Testing of visual acuity, color and field of vision, (ii) Hearing, (iii) Testing for smell, and (iv) Taste sensation in volunteer/simulated environment.

- Sense of smell is poorly developed (and least understood) in man as compared to lower animals such as dogs, etc. who are called macrosomatic.
- In these animals, smell is very highly developed. It has survival value in searching for food and animals; it is also involved in other instinctual behaviors such as mating.
- Humans have relatively simple noses with a weakly developed sense of smell (microsmatic).

OLFACTORY MUCOUS MEMBRANE

- The olfactory mucous membrane (area 5 cm^2) is the part of the nasal mucosa, and is located in the roof of the nasal cavity near the septum. It is here where there are sensory olfactory receptors for sense of smell.
- The 10–20 million sensory receptor cells are actually bipolar neurons originally derived from the central nervous system (this is the only place where the nervous system lies closest to the outside world).
- They are scattered among the supporting and basal cells.
- The dendritic ends of the cells are expanded to form olfactory rods that contain cilia and vesicles. Unlike other neurons these sensory cells are constantly replaced.
- Unlike primary colors or primary tastes, there are no definitely known primary odors, though 7 such odors are described—(1) peppermint, (2) camphoraceous, (3) floral, (4) ethereal, (5) musky, (6) pungent, and (7) putrid.
- **Olfactory adaptation:** Also called *olfactory fatigue*; the olfactory sensation decreases with continued exposure to an odorant. It occurs within seconds or minutes depending on the nature of the odorant.

PATHWAY FOR SMELL (FIG. 50)

- The axons from the sensory cells pierce the cribriform plate of ethmoid bone and enter the olfactory bulb.
- Here they synapse on the dendrites of mitral cells to form glomeruli.
- The axons of mitral cells which are the main output neurons in the bulb form the olfactory tract.
- As it enters the brain, it divides into two parts.
  1. One part (the primitive part) passes to the lateral olfactory cortex (piriform cortex, uncus, and entorhinal cortex) and part of the amygdala and hence to hippocampus. This circuit connects with the

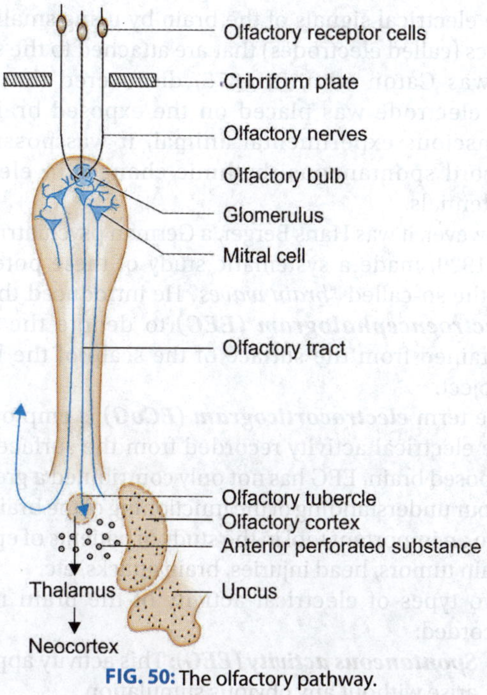

FIG. 50: The olfactory pathway.

lateral "feeding" area of hypothalamus and is involved in initiating eating behavior.

2. The other, the newer pathway, passes via olfactory tubercle and possibly thalamus to the neocortex—the lateral portion of the orbitofrontal cortex. It helps in conscious analysis of odor.

- **Abnormalities of the sense of smell: Anosmia** refers to complete absence of smell. **Parosmia** refers to alterations of smell sensation. **Hyposmia** is a decreased sense of smell.

PROCEDURE

1. Ask the subject to close his eyes, and occlude one of his nostrils. Then have him smell and distinguish the odors of each of the test substances, one by one, in each nostril, separately.
2. Ask him/her to occlude one nostril, and have him smell the oil of cloves until the odor can no longer be detected.
3. Immediately after this, ask the subject to try to distinguish with the adapted nostril between turpentine and alcohol.
4. Describe the result in the practical workbook.

QUESTIONS

Q.1. Describe the pathway for sensation of smell?

See text above.

Q.2. What are the various abnormalities associated with sense of smell?

See text above.

UNIT IV: NERVOUS SYSTEM

2.26: ELECTROENCEPHALOGRAPHY

STUDENT OBJECTIVES

After completing this experiment, the student should be able to:

- Define EEG and indicate the sources of these potentials.
- List the various waves that are seen in a normal recording.
- Describe the significance of alpha rhythm.
- Explain alpha block
- Indicate the significance of EEG.

PY10.12: Identify normal EEG forms.

INTRODUCTION

- An EEG, or electroencephalogram, is a test that records the electrical signals of the brain by using small metal discs (called electrodes) that are attached to the scalp.
- It was Caton who, in 1875, discovered that when an electrode was placed on the exposed brain of a conscious experimental animal, it was possible to record spontaneous rhythmic changes in electrical potentials.
- However, it was Hans Berger, a German psychiatrist, who in 1929, made a systematic study of these potentials, or the so-called *"brain waves"*. He introduced the term ***electroencephalogram (EEG)*** to denote the record obtained from the surface of the scalp of the human subject.
- The term ***electrocorticogram (ECoG)*** is employed for the electrical activity recorded from the surface of the exposed brain. EEG has not only contributed a great deal to our understanding of the functioning of the brain but is also an important tool in the study of patients of epilepsy, brain tumors, head injuries, brain attacks, etc.
- Two types of electrical activity of the brain may be recorded:
  1. ***Spontaneous activity (EEG):*** This activity appears to arise without any obvious stimulation.
  2. ***Evoked potentials:*** These are the electrical potentials that are caused (and recorded) by the stimulation of sensory receptors or sensory nerve fibers.

PRINCIPLE

- Gold-plated discs or shallow cups are placed on multiple analogous areas on the two sides of the scalp and simultaneous recordings are made from these areas for analysis and interpretation.
- The electrodes placed on the scalp record the electrical activity of the cerebral cortex.
- This electrical activity is because of the current flow in fluctuating dipoles on the dendrites of the cortical cells and cell bodies.

FEATURES OF EEG WAVES

- Normally, all the recurring oscillations in potentials (EEG waves, or brain waves) recorded from different areas of the scalp are more or less identical in waveform (shape), though their amplitude may wax and wane slightly.
- The dominant rhythm of the waves is 8-13/sec and an amplitude of about 50 μV which is called the alpha rhythm.
- Depending on their frequency and amplitude which are inversely related, the following rhythms are described (**Table 14**).

Table 14: Rhythms of the electroencephalogram waves.

Rhythm	*Frequency/sec*	*Voltage (μV)*
Delta	1–3.5	100–200
Theta	4–7	50–100
Alpha	8–13	30–70
Beta	14–25	10–20
Gamma	20–30	2–8

Alpha Rhythm (Berger Rhythm, 8–13/sec)

- The alpha rhythm is the dominant rhythm of a normal EEG, especially from the parieto-occipital region.
- It is found in almost all normal, waking, and relaxed adults with the eyes closed. It represents a resting state of cerebral activity, i.e. it is the rhythm of inattention.
- The alpha rhythm is called ***synchronized EEG;*** the synchronization is due to:
  1. The synchronizing effect of neighboring, densely packed, parallel-arranged fibers (dendrites) in the cerebral cortex.
  2. Rhythmic discharges from thalamus, and possibly other subcortical structures.

Changes in Alpha Rhythm

- ***Alpha rhythm is decreased in:*** Hypoglycemia, low body temperature, high arterial PCO_2, low levels of glucocorticoids, anesthesia, and sleep.
- ***Alpha rhythm is increased in:*** Hyperglycemia, rise in body temperature, low arterial PCO_2, and hyperventilation.

Note: Alpha rhythm, the rhythm of "inattention", is usually associated with a relaxed state of mind and a feeling of well-being. It can be promoted by "biofeedback" that is employed in the management of stress.

Desynchronization: Desynchronization, or *arousal response* refers to the replacement of a rhythmic EEG pattern by irregular, low-voltage activity. The ascending reticular activating system (ARAS) is responsible for this desynchronization that follows any type of sensory stimulation, e.g. cutaneous, visual effort at mental arithmetic, etc.

Delta Rhythm (1–3.5/sec)

- A rhythm slower than alpha rhythm, i.e. theta or delta rhythm does not usually occur in a normal waking individual (except in infants). However, the alpha rhythm is replaced by delta rhythm *in normal subjects during sleep.*
- The presence of delta rhythm during the waking state in adults may indicate the presence of organic brain disease.

Beta Rhythm (14–25/sec)

It is seen in infants instead of alpha rhythm.

Theta Rhythm (4–7/sec)

- It may be seen in children where it is blocked by visual stimulation.
- The frequency of alpha rhythm is decreased by low blood glucose and low temperature.

PHYSIOLOGICAL BASIS OF ELECTROENCEPHALOGRAM WAVES

- The neural basis of the EEG waves (they are not action potentials) is not fully known. However, their rhythmicity indicates that fluctuations in potentials are occurring in a number of neurons. The activity recorded is mainly that of similarly oriented and densely packed dendrites in the superficial layers of the cortex.
- These dendrites and the deeper-lying cell bodies function as fluctuating dipoles in response to the ascending inhibitory and excitatory signals from subcortical structures, especially from the thalamus.
- These oscillating potentials spread to the scalp from where they are recorded as the EEG waves.

INSTRUMENTATION

Electroencephalogram records may be *unipolar* or *bipolar.* A unipolar tracing records the potential difference between a *sensitive scalp electrode* and a theoretically *indifferent* or *reference electrode* placed at a distance away from the sensitive (or exploring) electrode. A bipolar recording shows the fluctuations in potential between two sensitive electrodes placed on the scalp or on the exposed brain.

1. ***Electroencephalogram machine:*** A variety of **electroencephalography** having different numbers of recording channels (up to 32) are available. The number of channels is important because simultaneous recordings can be made from wide areas of the scalp (the number of electrodes is fixed). In the present experiment, a 20-channel inkwriting oscillograph (Medicaid NG 8917) was used. The potentials picked up by the electrodes are suitably modified and amplified before being fed to the recording unit. The machine has the following controls:
   a. **Mains supply:** The ON/OFF power switch controls 220 volts AC, 50 Hz current supply. A 50 Hz filter excludes interference from the strong sources of AC current near the recording site. A wooden couch is used for the patient (earlier, a grounded wire-cage was employed for the patient).
   b. **Filters:** Special filters are provided to select desired frequencies and to modify the output of the amplifiers.
   c. **Sensitivity control:** A commonly used sensitivity is 7 μV/mm so that a calibration signal of 50 μV causes a pen deflection of about 7 mm.
   d. **Input selector switch:** Various combinations of electrode placements (montages)—unipolar, bipolar, and unipolar plus bipolar can be selected by this control. Three montages—A, B, and C are provided in this machine.
   e. **Photic stimulation:** A stroboscopic lamp can give light flashes of desired frequency (usually 25/sec) and duration of stimulation (usually 5 sec).
   f. **Hyperventilation time clock:** A time clock displays the duration of voluntary overbreathing (usually 3–4 minutes) during the EEG recording.
2. ***Electrodes:*** The surface electrodes are shallow silver cups about 10 mm in diameter, and have a central hole. Lead wires connect them to the electrode board. They are applied to the scalp with an electrode jelly which holds them in place and provides good mechanical and electrical contact with the skin. Cotton balls are placed over the electrodes to delay the drying of the conductive paste.

Electrode paste: It is a bentonite paste prepared by thoroughly mixing 100 g of bentonite powder with 100 mL of normal saline and adding glycerin slowly.

3. ***Electrode or input board:*** It connects the electrodes on the subject's head to the input selector switches of the machine. A diagram of the scalp showing various electrode positions is printed on the board. There is a provision for checking any loose connections. There is a provision in the machine for minimizing skin to electrode impedance (resistance). The EEG records brain waves using equipment called amplifiers and by looking at the information from the electrodes in different combinations. These combinations of electrodes are called **'montages'**.
   - In *bipolar montages*, consecutive pairs of electrodes are linked by connecting the electrode input 2 of one channel to input 1 of the subsequent channel, so that adjacent channels have one electrode in common. The bipolar chains of electrodes may be connected going from front to back (longitudinal) or from left to right (transverse).
   - Another type of montage is the *referential montage*. In this type, various electrodes are connected to input 1 of each amplifier and a reference electrode is connected to input 2 of each amplifier. Ideally, inactive electrodes (ones that are uninvolved in the electrical field being studied) are chosen as references.
4. ***Electrode placement:*** The standard set of electrodes for adults consists of 22 electrodes including one ground electrode. The international *"10-20" (ten-twenty) system* of electrode placement **(Fig. 51)** uses the distances between three bony landmarks of the skull—nasion (bridge of nose), inion (occipital protuberance on the back of the head), and preauricular point to generate a system of lines which run along and across the head and intersect at intervals of 10% or 20% of their total length. The electrodes are named with a letter and a subscript. The letter denotes the underlying region—frontopolar (Fp), frontal (F), central (C), parietal (P), occipital (O), and auricular (A). The subscript is either the letter z indicating zero or midline placement, or a number indicating lateral placement, odd numbers on the left and even numbers on the right side of the head. Thus, *Cz* is placed at 50% of the nasion-inion distance in the midsagittal plane, while *C3* and *C4* are 20% of this distance to the left and right of *Cz*.
5. ***Electroencephalogram paper:*** The paper transport system pulls the paper from a folded stack in a storage bin and moves it under the writing pens at the standard speed of 3 cm/sec (it can be increased or decreased). The paper has printed vertical lines at 3 cm intervals as shown in **Figure 51**.
6. ***Pen recording system:*** There are 21 recording pens, the lowermost being for the time tracing. The pens are 120 mm in length to minimize arc distortion. The contact tension of the pens on the paper can be adjusted, if required, with cradle springs. A pen lift knob can lift the pens from the paper.

Procedure

Records are taken simultaneously from multiple analogous areas of the scalp for at least 20-minute period.

1. No special preparation of the patient is required except that the scalp should not be oily. Ask the subject to lie down on the couch comfortably and relax.
2. Apply the reference electrodes on the earlobes and ground electrode above the bridge of the nose. Place the sensitive electrodes on the scalp as per the "20-20" system. Connect them to the electrode board and check for any loose connections.
3. Sensitivity calibration. Calibrate the machine so that an input of 50 μV gives a pen deflection of 7 mm.
4. Ask the subject to close his eyes and make a test recording. Normally, alpha rhythm is recorded as shown in **Figure 51**.

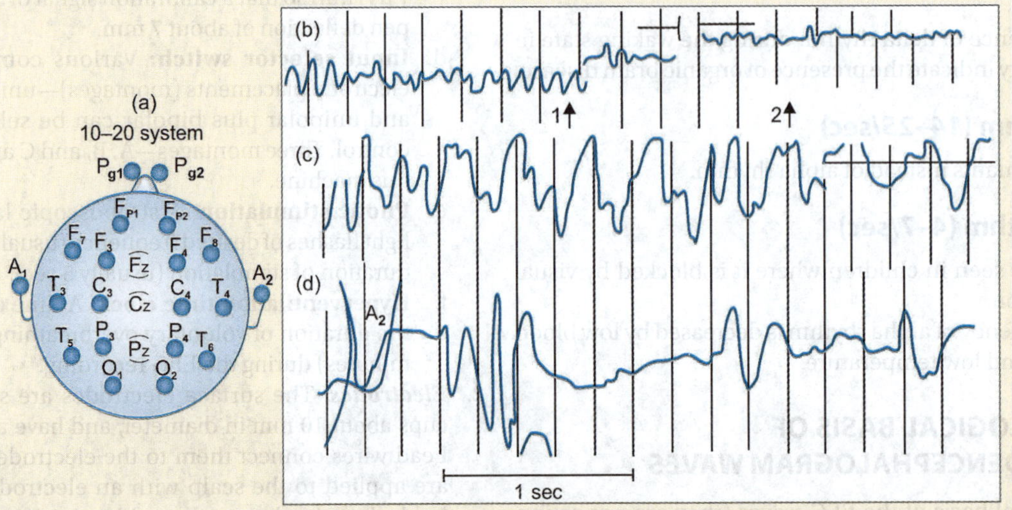

FIG. 51: Electroencephalogram. (a) The international "10–20" (ten–twenty) system of electrode placement. (b) Normal record showing alpha rhythm; and the effect of opening the eyes (arrow 1, alpha block) and closing the eyes once again (arrow 2) when the alpha rhythm is restored. (c) Delta rhythm; low-frequency high amplitude waves in a patient of focal epilepsy (channel O_2-A_2 right side). (d) Grand mal epilepsy, spike-wave pattern.

5. **Effect of opening the eyes:** Ask the subject to open his eyes. Note that the alpha rhythm is immediately replaced by desynchronization, i.e. by fast, irregular activity. Ask the subject to close his eyes, the alpha rhythm reappears.
6. **Photic stimulation:** As the record is running, deliver light flashes at a rate of 25/sec for 5 seconds, first with eyes closed, then with eyes open.
   Normally, there may be no change, but in abnormal cases (e.g. epilepsy), delta rhythm may appear. In some cases, even an attack of epilepsy may be precipitated (A flickering television is known to result in an attack of epilepsy).
7. **Effect of hyperventilation:** Ask the subject to breathe deeply and quickly for 3 minutes. Normally, the frequency of alpha waves decreases by low PCO_2 and the record may show theta or even delta rhythm. In epilepsy, an attack may be precipitated along with abnormal patterns.

Interpretation of Electroencephalogram

- If the electrical activity at the active electrodes is positive when compared to the activity at the reference electrode, the deflection will be downward.
- The interpretation of EEG depends on the frequency, amplitude, and distribution of the wave activity in various leads. Each record is then graded according to different systems.

CLINICAL APPLICATIONS OF ELECTROENCEPHALOGRAM

The EEG has its limitations in that a normal record may be obtained in spite of strong clinical evidence of organic disease. Also, an abnormal record may not always indicate an organic disease. Still, EEG is useful in the following disorders:

1. **Epilepsy:** In epilepsy, an excessive discharge from some part of the cerebrum is commonly associated with abnormalities of consciousness. In grand mal epilepsy, there are generalized tonic-clonic convulsions of the muscles followed by unconsciousness. The EEG shows high-voltage, high-frequency synchronous waves during tonic stage and slower and larger waves during clonic stage. In petit mal epilepsy, there are brief (lasting a few seconds) episodes of loss of contact with surroundings and the patient has a vacant look. The EEG shows a "spike and dome" pattern. In psychomotor or temporal lobe epilepsy, there are behavioral changes (they indicate involvement of the limbic system). The EEG may show low-frequency rectangular waves.
2. **Brain tumors and abscess:** Abnormal EEG recorded from a region overlying a tumor or abscess can help in the localization of these lesions.
3. **Head injuries and vascular lesions:** Serial EEG recordings can help in following the course of head injuries, e.g. an expanding hematoma.
4. **Encephalitis, meningitis, and congenital defects of the brain.**
5. **Electroencephalogram, organic and functional disorders:** Electroencephalogram may prove useful in differentiating between organic and functional disorders, i.e. nonorganic psychiatric disorders. However, its role in functional disorders is doubtful.

QUESTIONS

Q.1. How is EEG recorded? Describe the key features of the different EEG waves.
See text above.

Q.2. What is an alpha block?
See text above.

Q.3. Describe sleep spindles. In which phase are they seen?
See text above.

Q.4. What do you mean by "desynchronization"?
See text above.

Q.5. What are the clinical applications of EEG?
See text above.

2.27: ELECTRONEURODIAGNOSTIC TESTS

INTRODUCTION

- Electroneurodiagnostic tests are the investigations done by using the various devices to aid in the evaluation and examination of the nervous system. These devices receive and record the electrical impulses produced by the brain or other parts of the nervous system.
- The introduction of cathode ray oscilloscope (CRO), amplifiers, various types of stimulating and recording electrodes, single fiber preparations, and the use of computers in medical investigations have tremendously increased our knowledge of the functioning of the nervous system. It has also significantly improved diagnostic methods in clinical neurology.
- These techniques involve stimulating, recording, displaying, measuring, and interpreting action potentials (APs) and other electrical changes occurring in:
  - ***Peripheral nerves (nerve conduction studies; NCSs)***
  - ***Muscles (electromyography; EMG)***
  - ***Central nervous system (CNS): (EEG and evoked potentials).***

TERMINOLOGY

1. **Voltage:** This term represents the difference of potential between two points. It is measured in millivolts (mV) or microvolts (μV).
2. **Current:** It is measured in milliamperes.
3. **Time:** It is measured in milliseconds (ms, or msec) and microseconds (μsec).

EQUIPMENT

1. **Cathode ray oscilloscope:** A beam of electrons emitted by a cathode is focused on a fluorescent screen as a bright luminous spot, and is made to sweep from left to right in a

horizontal plane. The amplified potentials from the tissue under study are applied to plates above and below the beam to move it in a vertical plane above and/or below the baseline. The movement of the spot traces out the activity as a function of time. The display can be photographed or recorded directly on an ink-writing oscillograph.

2. **Amplifiers:** A variable degree of amplification is required in most applications because biological signals are very small because of intrinsic impedance (resistance) of the recording electrodes. Also the impedance of the electrode—skin contact point tends to reduce the amplitude of potential changes. Amplification also minimizes distortion of waveforms and improves noise rejection. The sensitivity of the amplifier can be adjusted as required.
3. **Filter:** It is a device that removes unwanted frequencies (high or low) from a signal and allows only desired frequencies to pass through.
4. **Averager:** This extracts small signals that are buried or hidden in large noise. For example, evoked potentials buried in electroencephalography (EEG) noise, sensory nerve APs hidden in EMG noise.
5. **Stimulators:** Stimulators are required in most applications in neurophysiology. They are of two general types:
   i. ***Electronic/electrical stimulators:*** They can provide variable constant current or constant voltage, single pulse or repeated stimuli.
   ii. ***Magnetic stimulators:*** These are employed for noninvasive stimulation of motor cerebral cortex, spinal cord, and peripheral nerves. Low-intensity stimulation causes current flow mainly in superficial soft tissues. With stronger stimuli, more current enters tissues at the cathode which may be painful in some persons.
6. **Stimulus artifact:** When a stimulus is applied, there is a brief, irregular deflection of the baseline, this is called a stimulus artifact and is due to leakage of current from the stimulating to the recording electrodes. It is employed for measuring the latent period (latency).
7. **Electrodes**

   Recording electrodes (REs): Three electrodes are employed for recording potential changes: (1) **active**, (2) **reference,** and (3) **ground**. The AP is measured between active and reference electrodes. The ground electrode serves as a "zero" voltage reference point.

   Electrodes are made of metal—platinum, silver, gold, stainless steel, chromium, nickel, etc. Silver and gold electrodes have the advantage of stable electrode polarizing potentials that give noise-free recordings [when a metal electrode reacts with an electrolyte such as sweat, or electrode paste, or extracellular fluid (ECF), an electrochemical reaction occurs that results in electrode polarizing potentials of 100–500 mV].

   The recording electrodes are of two general types:

   i. ***Surface electrodes:*** They are in the shape of discs, cups or rings, and are used for recording activity from the body surface. They are "attached" (applied) in place with electrode paste or jelly that is gently rubbed on the skin to reduce the resistance at electrode-skin contact point.
   ii. ***Concentric needle electrode:*** The concentric (or coaxial) needle electrode (usually 24 gauge) is a *bipolar electrode,* one pole of which is formed by the shaft, and the other by a teflon-coated wire threaded through the shaft. The electrode records activity at its tip, the recording area being 150–500 μm², thus sampling a restricted area in a muscle.

   The monopolar needle electrode is solid steel, 22–24 gauge needle, and coated with varnish or Teflon except at its tip. The reference electrode is placed on the skin.

   Stimulating electrodes (SEs): Stimuli can be applied through cup, disc, or ring electrodes.

PRECAUTIONS

1. The mains supply must be checked to confirm adequate voltage.
2. Proper earthing of the equipment must be ensured. The subject should also be properly grounded.
3. The procedure should be explained to the subject.
4. Loose wire and cable connections as well as the electrode placement may cause distorted APs.

Note: Although both median and ulnar nerves are mixed nerves, motor nerve conduction is discussed in median nerve in this experiment, while sensory nerve conduction will be taken up in the ulnar nerve in the next experiment.

NERVE CONDUCTION STUDIES

Nerve conduction studies are carried out in both motor and sensory nerves. The nerves commonly tested are:

- *In the upper limbs*: Median, ulnar, radial, and brachial plexus.
- *In lower limbs*: Sciatic, femoral, common peroneal, tibial, and sural nerves.

Clinical Significance

- Testing of conduction velocities in both motor and sensory nerves provides early and accurate diagnosis; there may be an increase in the latency or even complete block of nerve impulses.
- Nerve conduction tests are useful in: nerve injuries during accidents, fractures of bones, fracture dislocations of joints, local pressure on nerves by tumors or by ligaments, arthritis, neuropathies in diabetes mellitus, demyelination (multiple sclerosis), vitamin B deficiency, leprosy, and so on.

Nerves and Nerve Fibers

- The nerves (nerve trunks) dissected by the students during anatomical studies contain thousands of individual nerve fibers packed in bundles. The individual nerve fibers are the protoplasmic extensions of the neurons, their lengths varying from a few mm to over a meter. In the core of a fiber is the axis cylinder—the continuation of cell cytoplasm. The nerve cell membrane extends over the axis cylinder as the axolemma that is the site of all ionic fluxes and electrical processes.

- ***Medullated (myelinated) and non medullated (unmyelinated) nerve fibers:*** Fibers larger than 1 µm in diameter have a covering of lipoproteins called myelin (medullary) sheath. This insulating sheath is interrupted at regular constrictions, about 1 mm apart, called the *nodes of Ranvier*. In peripheral nerves, the myelin sheath is covered with glia-like cells called the cells of Schwann, there being one such cell to each internode (in the CNS, the cells of Schwann are absent and the myelin sheath is laid down by oligodendroglia).
- Nerve fibers, usually less than 1 µm lack myelin sheath, the axolemma being directly exposed to ECF throughout its length.

Nerve Fiber Type and Function

Table 15 shows a classification of nerve fibers, their type, location and function, diameter, and conduction velocity (after Erlanger and Gasser).

Motor Nerve Conduction

Principle

- When a current is passed through two electrodes placed on the skin, some of it penetrates deep into the tissues. If it is strong enough and in the neighborhood of a nerve, then it will stimulate enough fibers to produce a recordable muscle response.
- Nerve conduction velocity determination requires stimulation of a nerve at two places along its length.
- The velocity in m/sec can be calculated from the difference in the latent periods of the two responses and the length of the nerve segment between the two points stimulated (refer to experiment 4.6 on Velocity of Nerve Impulses in Frog's Nerve Muscle Preparation).

Table 15: Nerve fiber type and function.

Fiber type		*Location/Function*	*Diameter (µm)*	*Conduction velocity (m/sec)*
A	α	Somatic motor, proprioceptor	12–20	70–120
	β	Touch, pressure, and motor	5–12	30–70
	γ	Motor to muscle spindle	3–6	15–30
	δ	Pain, touch, and cold	2–5	12–30
B		Preganglionic autonomic	1–3	3–15
C	Dorsal root	Pain, temperature, and some mechanoreception reflex responses	0.4–1.3	0.5–2
	Sympathetic	Postganglionic sympathetic	0.3–1.3	0.7–2.3

A and B fibers are myelinated, while C fibers are unmyelinated.

Median nerve (C-6, 7, 8; T-1): It is a mixed nerve and arises from the brachial plexus. Its motor branches supply most of the flexor-pronator muscles of the forearm. It enters the hand through the carpal tunnel to supply the thenar muscles. It is sensory to the lateral palm and lateral two and one half fingers, and their distal ends. It has no innervation in the upper arm.

Apparatus

- Cathode ray oscilloscope
- Preamplifier
- Electronic stimulator
- Stimulating and recording electrodes
- Electrode jelly
- Spirit swabs.

Procedure

1. Ask the subject to sit on a chair near a table and explain the procedure to him.
2. Clean the skin over the thenar muscle pad and the areas over the median nerve at the elbow and the wrist. Rub electrode jelly over these areas (**Fig. 52**).
3. Apply the cup recording (active) electrode (A) over the motor point of abductor pollicis brevis, and the reference electrode (R) about 3 cm away from it. Place the ground electrode (G) between recording and stimulating electrodes (S-1). Connect the recording electrodes to the CRO through the preamplifier.
4. Apply the stimulating electrodes on the wrist 3 cm above the distal wrist skin crease (S-1) and apply a supramaximal stimulus. Note the response of the thenar muscles. Now shift the electrodes to the elbow and apply a stimulus (S-2). Note that at both the sites of stimulation (S-1 and S-2), the *cathode* is the stimulating electrode and it is placed distal to the anode.
5. **Observations and results:** In both cases, there is a stimulus artifact at the beginning of the sweep, followed by a latent period, and a biphasic AP with initial negativity, this is called ***a biphasic muscle potential*** or ***compound muscle action potential (CMAP).***

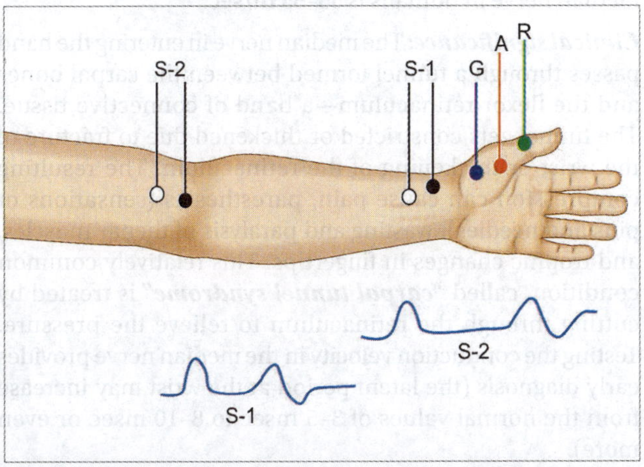

FIG. 52: Measurement of motor nerve conduction velocity in median nerve. S-1: stimulation at wrist; S-2: stimulation at elbow; A: recording (active) electrode; R: reference electrode; and G: ground electrode.

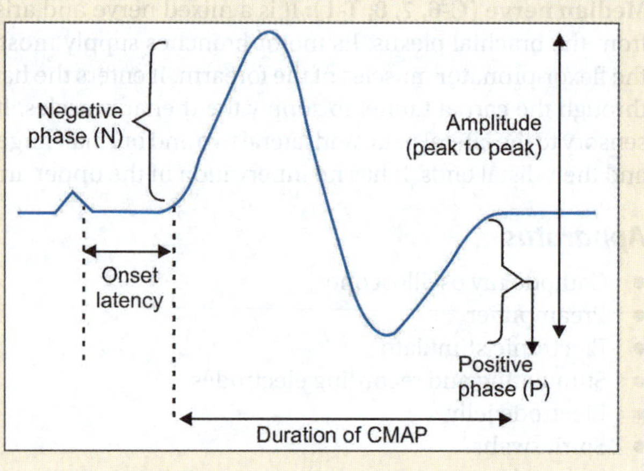

FIG. 53: Compound muscle action potential (CMAP).

Compound muscle action potential: It includes the onset latency, duration, and the amplitude of the biphasic AP, as shown in **Figure 53**.

Onset latency: It is the time from the stimulus artifact to the start of the first negative deflection. It is a measure of speed of conduction in fastest nerve fibers and includes neuromuscular transmission time, spread of AP over the muscle fibers, and the process of excitation-contraction coupling.

Amplitude of compound muscle action potential: It is measured from baseline to the negative peak (base to peak) or between negative to positive peaks (peak to *peak).*

Duration of compound muscle action potential: It is measured from onset to the negative or positive peaks, or the final return of the waveform to the baseline.

Calculation of velocity: For example: Latent period at S-1 = 5 msec
Latent period at S-2 = 9.5 msec
Length of nerve between the two stimulated points = 26 cm
Distance traveled in 4.5 msec = 26 cm
Distance traveled in 1 second = 58 meters.

Normal values: The normal velocity in the motor fibers of the median nerve in humans is 55–65 m/sec.

Clinical significance: The median nerve in entering the hand passes through a tunnel formed between the carpal bones and the flexor retinaculum—a band of connective tissue. The tunnel gets constricted or thickened due to fracture of the wrist or thickening of the retinaculum. The resulting compression can cause pain, paresthesias (sensations of pins and needles), wasting and paralysis of thenar muscles, and trophic changes in fingertips. This relatively common condition, called ***"carpal tunnel syndrome"*** is treated by cutting through the retinaculum to relieve the pressure. Testing the conduction velocity in the median nerve provides early diagnosis (the latent period at the wrist may increase from the normal values of 3–5 msec to 8–10 msec or even more).

Note: Working for long periods at the keyboard of a computer may also cause this type of syndrome.

Sensory Nerve Conduction

Ulnar Nerve

The ulnar nerve, like the median nerve, is also a mixed nerve. It arises from C-7 to T-1 segments of the spinal cord, passes behind the medial epicondyle of the humerus, and then down the ulnar side of the forearm. It gives ***motor*** branches to muscles in the forearm, and in the hand to the hypothenar and other muscles. Its ***sensory*** branches supply the skin of the medial half of the hand and of the little and ring fingers. ***Principle of sensory nerve stimulation:*** In the body, sensory nerve fibers conduct nerve impulses (APs) only in one direction, i.e. from the sensory receptors toward the CNS (orthodromic conduction). But when they are stimulated artificially, say, through the skin, they can conduct APs in the opposite direction as well, i.e. toward the sensory receptors (antidromic conduction).

Equipment

- Cathode ray oscilloscope with storage facility
- Electronic stimulator
- Stimulating silver ring electrodes
- Recording silver cup electrodes
- Electrolyte paste
- Spirit swabs.

Procedure

1. Clean the areas of the little finger and where electrodes are to be applied and rub electrode jelly over these points.
2. *Stimulating electrodes:* Place silver ring electrodes, one on the middle phalanx (active electrode) and the other on the terminal phalanx.
3. *Recording electrodes:* Apply two silver cup recording electrodes about 2–3 cm apart, proximal to wrist skin crease. Apply the ground electrode between the SE and the RE on the palm. Connect all these to the CRO through the preamplifier.
4. *Adjust the settings:* Filter = low cut: 5–10 Hz; high cut: 2–3 kHz; gain = 1–5 mV/div; sweep speed = 1–2 msec/div, or as desired.
5. Apply a supramaximal stimulus and note the response. Record a time tracing and note the distance between the SE and the RE.
6. For antidromic conduction, simply reverse the connections of SE and RE.

Observations and Results

Figure 54 shows a sensory nerve action potential (SNAP). It has a stimulus artifact, onset latency, amplitude, and duration.

Calculate the velocity of sensory nerve conduction velocity as follows:
Velocity = Length of nerve in mm/latency in msec
Normal value: 50–65 m/sec.

Comments: The orthodromic and antidromic conduction velocities provide similar information in clinical practice. The duration of SNAP gives information about the number of slow-conducting fibers, while amplitude reveals the density of nerve fibers. Both are affected in nerve injuries, neuropathies, vitamin efficiencies, leprosy, etc.

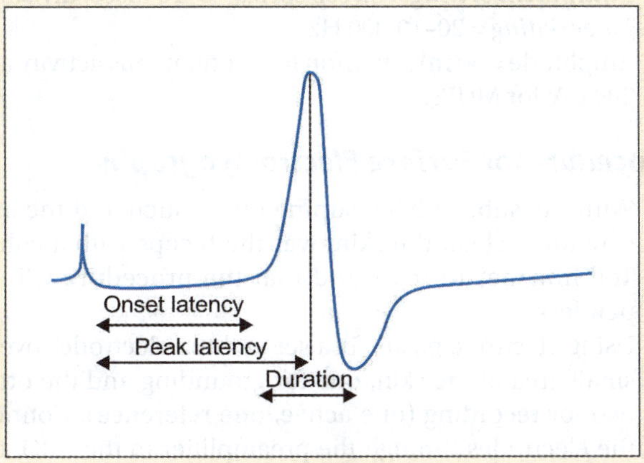

FIG. 54: Latency, amplitude and duration of sensory nerve action potential.

Note: Sensory nerve conduction velocity can also be determined in median nerve by placing stimulating ring electrodes on the index finger and recording electrodes at the base of the thumb. This will record orthodromic conduction velocity. Antidromic velocity can be recorded by reversing the locations of the electrodes.

QUESTIONS

Q.1. Name the equipment employed in electroneuro-diagnostic techniques.
See text above.

Q.2. What is the basis of working of a cathode ray oscilloscope?
See text above.

Q.3. What are electrodes employed for in these studies?
See text above.

Q.4. What is a waveform and what are its components?
See text above.

Q.5. Name some properties of nerve fibers.
Nerve fibers are excitable; they show RMP; they can conduct the excitatory state (AP); they show all-or-none response, i.e. either there is a full-fledged AP or no AP at all. They also exert a trophic influence on the structures innervated by them.

ELECTROMYOGRAPHY

Introduction

- Electromyography (EMG) is a recording of the electrical activity occurring in a muscle during voluntary contraction.
- It is the sum of APs of many muscle fibers. This change of potential sets up a current field that can be recorded either with needle electrodes or by surface electrodes.
- Although the EMG does not provide a specific clinical diagnosis, it can help in arriving at a diagnosis when its results are interpreted along with the results of other tests and clinical features of the patient.
- EMG is useful in the detection of lower motor neuron diseases, and disorders of neuromuscular transmission from certain muscle disorders such as muscular dystrophy.
- A skeletal muscle consists of a number of anatomically separate, parallely-arranged, cylindrical, multinucleated fibers (cells), 10–100 µm in diameter, and of varying lengths from a few mm to many cm. **They have no activity of their own, but contract only in response to nerve impulses arriving along their motor nerve supply from the CNS.**
- In normal muscles, the muscle fibers do not contract individually but as part of a motor unit consisting of a variable number of innervated muscle fibers. Thus, the motor unit is the functional unit of muscle activity.
- ***Motor unit:*** A motor unit consists of one anterior gray column motor neuron of the spinal cord (or the equivalent motor cranial neuron in the brainstem), its axon and all its branches as it enters a muscle, and all the muscle fibers innervated by these branches. The number of muscle fibers in a motor unit varies from a few (external ocular muscles) to many hundreds (muscles of the back, thighs, etc.).

Note: While a normal muscle fiber shows a RMP, and an AP when activated for contraction, a denervated muscle fiber shows unstable potential and spontaneous twitching.

Motor Unit Potential

The motor unit potential (MUP) is the potential change produced by the excitation of muscle fibers of a motor unit. Since these fibers discharge synchronously (at the same time) near the needle electrode, the MUP has higher amplitude and a longer duration than the AP produced by a single muscle fiber.

Characteristics of Motor Unit Potential

A MUP is characterized by its firing frequency, duration, amplitude, phases, and rate of rise.

- ***Frequency:*** With mild contraction, the MUP shows a frequency of 5–15 Hz. With stronger contractions, there is recruitment of additional motor units (and so of MUPs) that depends on the size principle—the smaller motor units being recruited first, then larger and larger units are brought into action.
- ***Duration:*** The duration of a MUP is measured from the initial take-off of the potential to the point of return to the baseline **(Fig. 55)**. It varies from 5 msec to 10 msec, being shorter in children and longer in adults. The duration of MUP is a measure of conduction velocity, length of muscle fibers, membrane excitability, and synchronization of response of muscle fibers.
- Short-duration MUPs are found in myopathies, myasthenia gravis, and early stage of reinnervation after nerve injuries.
- Long-duration MUPs are seen in lower motor neuron lesions and myopathies.
- ***Amplitude:*** It is measured from peak to peak and the normal value is 0.5–2.0 mV. It depends on the size, density and type of muscle fibers, synchrony of firing, nearness of needle to muscle fibers, age of the subject, and temperature of the muscle.

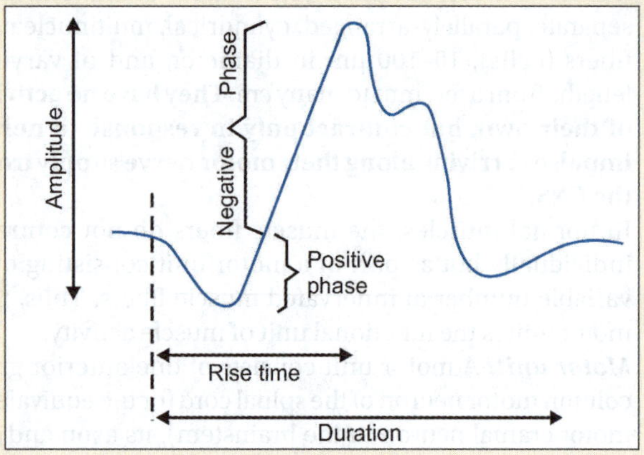

FIG. 55: Normal motor unit potential (MUP) recorded by needle electromyography (EMG).

- ***Phases:*** The MUP recorded by needle electrodes shows a triphasic potential, i.e. positive-negative-positive sequence, as shown in **Figure 55**. A phase is the part of a MUP between the departure and return of the potential to the baseline. A MUP with more than four phases is called polyphasic. Some potentials show directional changes without reaching baseline—these are called *turns*. Polyphasic potentials and turns are more commonly seen in myopathies when regeneration is occurring.
- ***Rise time:*** The rise time of a MUP is the duration from the initial positive to the next negative peak. The usual rise time is up to 500 msec and indicates the distance of the needle from the muscle fibers. A greater rise time indicates increased resistance of the intervening tissues.

Factors Affecting Motor Unit Potential

Technical factors: These include: Type of needle electrode and its location (superficial, deep, or near endplate of muscle fiber; the amplitude is smaller when it is superficial), preamplifier and amplifier, and method of recording, etc.

Physiological factors: These are: Age—the amplitude and duration increases while firing rate decreases as age advances. Sex and the temperature of muscle also affect MUPs.

Methodology

A resting muscle is electrically silent, i.e. it does not show any electrical potential. When it contracts, however, such changes can be recorded.

Instrumentation

1. *Cathode ray oscilloscope:*
   - Polygraph (paper recorder)
   - Preamplifier
   - Audio Amplifier with speaker.
2. Electrode paste, 70% alcohol, and cotton and gauze swabs.
3. *Recording electrodes:*
   - Surface electrodes
   - Needle electrode.
4. ***Equipment settings:*** *Sweep speed* = 5–10 msec/division; *Filter setting* = 20–10,000 Hz
   Amplitude = 50 mV/division for spontaneous activity and 200 mV for MUPs.

Procedure for Surface Electromyography

1. With the subject lying supine on a couch and the arm extended, clean the skin over the biceps with alcohol. Tell him/her to relax and that the procedure will be painless.
2. Using electrode paste, fix a set of three electrodes over a small area of the skin, one for grounding and the other two for recording (one active, one reference). Connect the electrodes through the preamplifier to the CRO, the recorder, and the audio amplifier. Observe if there is any electrical activity.
3. Ask the subject to flex the arm, and then pronate and supinate the forearm, first gently, then with greater force. Note the potentials.

Procedure for Needle Electromyography

1. Clean the skin with alcohol and let dry, and fix the ground electrode on the skin. Tell the subject that an injection needle will be inserted into the muscle.
2. Insert the concentric needle gently into the muscle, and advance it by steps to several depths.
3. *Make the following observations at each depth:* Activity evoked by insertion, activity produced by moving the needle, activity of relaxed (resting) muscle with the needle undisturbed, and activity during weak and then during stronger and stronger voluntary contractions.

Observations and Results

Note the following activities and draw diagrams in your notebooks.

1. ***Insertion activity:*** There is a brief burst of electrical activity of 0.5–1.0 msec due to mechanical damage by the needle, appearing as positive or negative bursts of high-frequency spikes.
2. ***Spontaneous activity:*** There is no spontaneous electrical activity except that when the needle electrode is near the endplate region when miniature endplate potentials (MEPPs) may be recorded. They are monophasic negative waves of up to 100 mV and of 1–2 msec durations.
   Abnormal spontaneous activities include: Fibrillation, fasciculation, and cramp potentials, and complex repetitive discharges (CRDs).
3. ***Voluntary contractions:*** With weak contractions, MUPs of 5–15 Hz are recorded. With stronger contractions, potentials of 0.3–2 mV and 5–15 msec are recorded. With still stronger contractions, the potentials run into each other and the resulting confused tracing is called interference pattern.

Audio signals: As audio signals, the MUPs produce knocking or thumping sounds on the loudspeaker.

QUESTIONS

Q.1. Define the term EMG. What is its relevance in clinical physiology and medical diagnosis?
See text above.

Q.2. Why are resting muscles electrically silent?
The resting muscle fibers only show a steady RMP across their cell membranes, negativity on the inside and positivity on the outside. So, when the recording electrode lies near them, no potential difference is recorded and they are electrically silent. They show APs only when they are reactivated by signals arriving along their motor nerves. This electrical activity is then followed by the mechanical activity of contraction.

Q.3. How is force of contraction graded?
The varying force of reflex or voluntary contraction of skeletal muscles depends on:

1. Number of motor units activated.
2. Frequency of nerve impulses.
3. Synchronization of nerve impulses.
4. Initial length of muscle fibers.

Q.4. How can recruitment of motor units be demonstrated experimentally without needle electrodes?
This can be done by placing recording electrodes on the skin over thenar region and then asking the subject to move the thumb slowly at first and then with greater force. MUPs of different amplitude and shape will be recorded.

EVOKED POTENTIALS

Introduction

- As mentioned earlier, electrical potentials can be produced (evoked) in the cerebral cortex by the stimulation of sensory receptors or sensory nerves.
- But since these cortical potential changes are small and buried in the background of spontaneous electrical activity (EEG), their details can only be studied and evaluated by repeated stimulation and averaging the responses obtained after each stimulation by a computer.
- The commonly tested evoked potentials are:
  1. Brainstem auditory evoked potentials (BAEPs)
  2. Visual evoked potentials (VEPs)
  3. Somatosensory evoked potentials (SEPs)
  4. Motor evoked potentials (MEPs).

Note: The BAEPs will be taken up to illustrate the technique of evoked potentials, while others will only be briefly mentioned.

Brainstem Auditory Evoked Potentials

- The BAEPs represent an objective test for hearing. They are a series of potentials generated by sequential activation of different parts of the auditory pathway.
- These APs cannot only be recorded from along this pathway but also from the body surface, especially from the scalp.

Auditory pathway: Experiment 2.21, **Figure 46.**

Apparatus

- Cathode ray oscilloscope
- Preamplifier
- Electroencephalography electrodes
- Electrode paste
- Alcohol or ether swabs
- Headphones.

Procedure

1. The test is carried out preferably in a soundproof room. Ask the subject to sit in a chair, with his back to the apparatus, and relax.
2. Clean the skin where electrodes are to be applied. Place the recording (active) electrodes on both earlobes, or on the mastoid processes. Place the reference electrode at the vertex (Cz position), and the ground electrode on top of the forehead.
3. Connect the REs to the amplifier. Use amplification of 200,000–500,000; set low filter at 100 Hz and high filter at 3,000 Hz.
4. Apply brief click stimuli of 70 db intensity above the subjects threshold, at a rate of 10/sec, and of 0.1 msec duration (the stimuli are usually square wave pulses; the pulse wave can move the diaphragm of the earphone either toward or away from the ear, i.e. condensation or rarefaction stimuli).
5. The sound clicks stimulate not only the ipsilateral ear but also travel to the opposite ear by bone and air conduction to stimulate that ear at an intensity of 40–50 db lower than the ipsilateral ear.
6. Observe the effect of intensity of stimulation on the BAEPs.

Observations and Results

The auditory nerve and BAEPs are "volume conducted" to the surface recording electrodes. At the vertex and earlobes, they form vertex positive and vertex negative potentials. A sequence of five or more distinct waveforms (vertex positive peaks) labeled I-V **(Fig. 56)** are recorded within 10 msec of

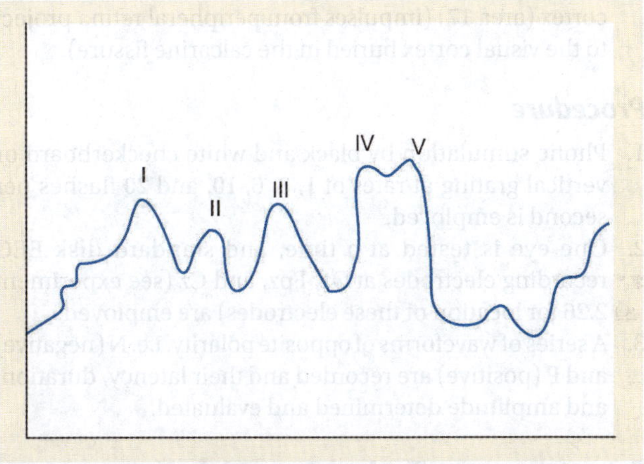

FIG. 56: Brainstem auditory evoked potentials in normal individuals. Interpeak latencies are measured from the top of one peak to the other. Refer to text for the origin of different waveforms.

the application of stimulation. If the recording is continued, a few more positive and negative waves are recorded. The origin of the waveforms is:

Wave I: From the peripheral part of the auditory nerve.

Wave II: From cochlear nuclei.

Wave III: From superior olivary nucleus.

Wave IV: From lateral lemniscus.

Wave V: From inferior colliculi.

Wave VI: From the medial geniculate body.

Wave VII: From auditory *radiation.*

Measurement of brainstem auditory evoked potential waveforms: The features noted are—absolute latency, amplitude, interpeak latencies, inter-ear-interpeak differences, and amplitude ratio of V/I.

Factors affecting brainstem auditory evoked potentials: These include—age, sex, height, temperature, drugs (alcohol and barbiturates prolong the latency of wave V), and hearing loss.

Clinical Significance

1. The auditory responses provide an objective assessment in infants and young children suspected of being deaf.
2. The BAEPs aid in assessing the degree of hearing loss.
3. The latencies of waveforms provide information in patients of vestibular nerve and brainstem tumors, demyelination, and in distinction of various kinds of coma and drug-induced and traumatic disease processes.

Visual Evoked Potentials

- The VEPs are the potential changes recorded from the scalp in response to visual stimuli. They represent the resultant responses of cortical and subcortical structures to photostimulation.
- Normal VEPs indicate the intactness of the entire visual pathway [see experiment 2.11: Perimetry (Charting the Field of Vision)]. They can detect abnormality, if any, but cannot exactly locate the site of lesion.
- The VEPs primarily represent the activity originating in the central 3–6° of visual field that is relayed to the visual cortex (area 17) (impulses from peripheral retina project to the visual cortex buried in the calcarine fissure).

Procedure

1. Photic stimulation by black and white checkerboard or vertical grating at rates of 1, 3, 6, 10, and 20 flashes per second is employed.
2. One eye is tested at a time, and standard disk EEG recording electrodes at Oz, Fpz, and Cz (see experiment 2.26 for location of these electrodes) are employed.
3. A series of waveforms of opposite polarity, i.e. N (negative) and P (positive) are recorded and their latency, duration, and amplitude determined and evaluated.

Somatosensory Evoked Potentials

- In humans, event-related, "far-field SEPs" are simultaneously recorded from several electrodes placed over the popliteal fossa, lumbar and thoracic vertebrae (spinal evoked potentials), and over the parietal region of the opposite side.
- The SEPs are generated mainly by the large diameter (12–20 μm) fibers in response to repeated stimuli applied to them anywhere along their course in peripheral nerves, or in ascending tracts in CNS [large fibers carry mainly proprioceptive impulses, while small diameter fibers (0.5 mm) carry pain and temperature].
- Though SEPs can be obtained by stimulation of any large peripheral nerve; in clinical practice they are generally recorded from **median nerve** (median SEPs) and the **posterior tibial nerve** (tibial SEPs). The method can prove useful in the evaluation of spinal defects such as multiple sclerosis, spinal injuries, etc.

Motor Evoked Potentials

- Sensory evoked potentials (auditory, visual, and somatosensory) are recorded from the scalp or from sensory pathways after sensory stimulation. The MEPs, on the other hand, are recorded from **target muscles as EMG** following stimulation of motor cortex or spinal cord.
- The stimuli used may be electrical or magnetic. Since electrical transcranial stimuli can be painful, magnetic stimuli are applied over the vertex, and cervical and lumbar regions. The target muscles include deltoid, biceps, thenar muscles, tibialis anterior, and abductor hallucis brevis.
- A very important precaution is to ensure that the subject is not using a cardiac pacemaker, a cochlear implant, or has a history of epilepsy.

THE HOFFMANN'S REFLEX (H-REFLEX)

Introduction

- Tendon jerks or deep reflexes (tested clinically) are reflex contractions of skeletal muscles in response to stimulation of their stretch receptors located in their muscle spindles. The stimulus is the **sudden stretch of their muscle spindles** that sends impulses via IA (Aα) afferents to the spinal cord where they stimulate the AHC that supply the muscle.
- The H-reflex is the electrical equivalent of a tendon jerk. It confirms the integrity of the reflex pathway.

Apparatus

- Cathode ray oscilloscope
- Electronic stimulator
- Stimulating and recording electrodes
- Swabs moist with alcohol or ether.

Procedure

1. Apply the stimulating electrodes on the skin over the tibial nerve behind the knee, and recording electrodes on the skin overlying soleus muscle in the calf region.
2. Apply a minimum strength of stimulus. Since the threshold of stimulation of Ia sensory fibers is much lower as compared to motor fiber, the H-wave (H-reflex) will

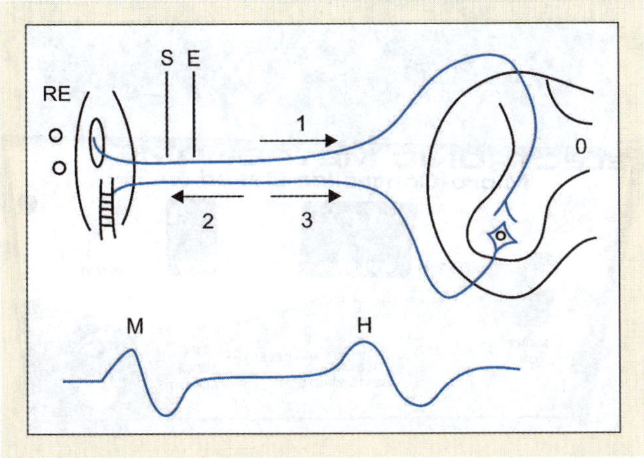

FIG. 57: Recording of H-reflex. SE: stimulating electrodes on skin over tibial nerve; RE: recording electrodes on skin over the muscle; M: M-wave due to direct (orthodromic) stimulation of muscle; and H-wave: due to H-reflex.

be recorded, as shown in **Figure 57**. It has a long latency because the Ia signals are conducted orthodromically (arrow 1) to monosynaptically stimulate AHC that innervate the soleus.

3. Increase the strength of stimulus to stimulate both sensory and motor fibers. Note that two responses are recorded from the muscle. The first waveform is the ***"M-wave"*** resulting from direct stimulation of motor fibers (arrow 2), while the second response is the ***"H-wave"*** due to H-reflex resulting from excitation of Ia sensory fibers.
4. Increase the strength of stimulus still further, and note that the H-wave gradually decreases and then disappears, leaving only the M-wave. The APs in motor nerves, in addition to normal orthodromic conduction toward the muscle, are also conducted antidromically (arrow 3) to cause depolarization of AHC so that when Ia signals arrive they find the motor neurons refractory—thus canceling their reflex response.

Note: Two clinical signs are associated with Hoffmann's name:
1. **Hoffmann's sign:** Flicking the distal phalanx of the index finger causes clawing movement of fingers and thumb. This response in the upper limb is equivalent to the Babinski response in the sole of the foot in upper motor neuron (UMN) lesions.
2. **Hoffmann's sign of tetany:** Electrical or mechanical stimulation of a sensory nerve produces muscle spasm (the ulnar nerve is usually selected for this test in parathyroid tetany).

QUESTIONS

Q.1. Describe the different waveforms in the recording of BAEP. What is the physiological basis of BAEP?

See text above.

Q.2. Name the factors affecting BAEP. What is the clinical significance of BAEP?

See text above.

Q.3. Describe the different waveforms of VEP. What is the physioclinical significance of VEP?

See text above.

2.28: STUDY OF HUMAN FATIGUE

STUDENT OBJECTIVES

After completing this experiment, the student should be able to:
- Define ergography.
- Explain the physioclinical significance of this experiment.
- Calculate the work done using Mosso's ergograph.
- Enlist the factors affecting fatigue and work done.
- Explain the effects of venous, arterial occlusion, and motivation on work done.
- Explain the difference seen in onset of fatigue using Mosso's ergograph and hand grip dynamometer.
- Measure the endurance time using a hand grip dynamometer.

INTRODUCTION

- Fatigue is defined as a temporary and reversible loss of the physiological property of contraction of skeletal muscles. There is also a subjective feeling of tiredness so that the onset of fatigue can be somewhat delayed by motivation. With rest, however, fatigue is completely reversible.
- Mosso's ergography is done to record the voluntary contractions of the skeletal muscles of a human being on a kymograph. The **erg** is the unit of work and **ergograph** is the apparatus used for recording voluntary contractions of skeletal muscle in humans.
- The Mosso's ergograph is employed not only to assess the performance of hand and forearm muscles but also to study the phenomenon of fatigue and the factors that affect fatigue.
- Human fatigue can be studied by using:
  1. ***Mosso's ergograph***
  2. ***Hand-grip dynamometer.***

MOSSO'S ERGOGRAPH

- It consists of a flat wooden board with two pairs of clamps and curved plates to fix, hold, and steady the forearm of the subject **(Figs. 58 and 59)**.
- There is a pair of metal tubes into which index and ring fingers are inserted. The middle finger remains free to be connected to a thick cord and hook.
- A sliding plate that can move to and fro carries a lever system to record muscle exertions on a kymograph cylinder.
- A sling fits over the middle finger, and a strong cord bearing a hook on which different weights can be hung (in some cases, the sliding plate can carry a chart paper on which a pencil or ballpoint pen can record the contractions).

Metronome: It is a clockwork device that functions as a "variable interrupter" to deliver "tick tock" sounds at a preselected frequency of up to 200/minute. There is a thin metal rod bearing a scale on which a sliding clip can set the

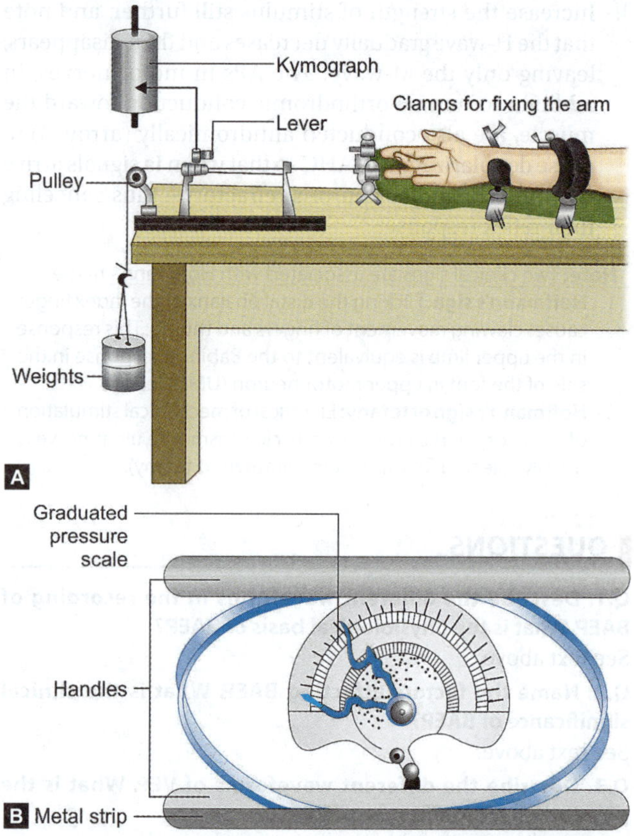

FIGS. 58A AND B: (A) Mosso's ergograph; (B) Dynamometer.

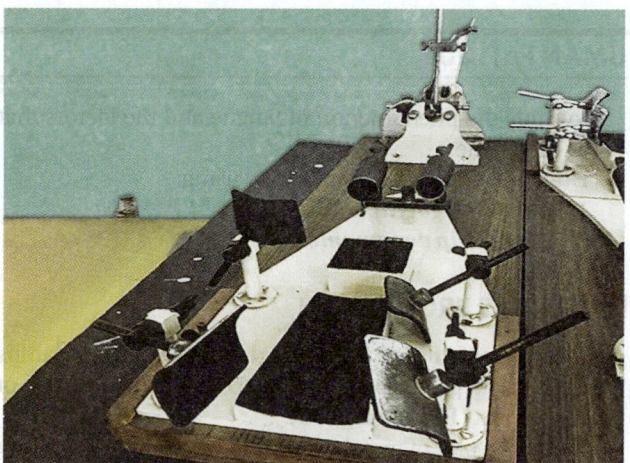

FIG. 59: Mosso's ergograph.

desired frequency (the metronome is commonly used to provide *beats* during training in piano playing) **(Fig. 60)**.

Procedure

1. Place the ergograph on a table such that the weight will hang down over its edge. Explain the procedure to the subject and seat her/him beside the table.
2. Fix the forearm on the ergograph, and insert the index and ring fingers in the finger holders. With the middle finger extended and the string with the cord attached to it, adjust the position of the forearm and fingers so that

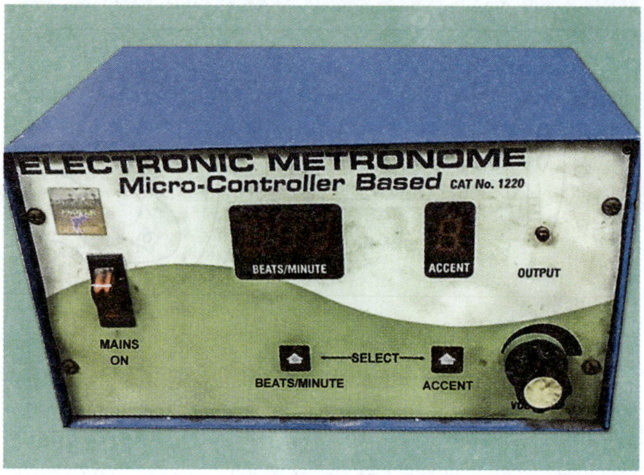

FIG. 60: Metronome.

the subject is comfortable. Apply a weight of 1–2 kg on the hook.

3. Ask the subject to flex the middle finger and check that the system works freely.
4. Adjust the beat of the metronome at 30/minute, i.e. one beat every 2 seconds, and set it oscillating. Ask the subject to contract the flexor muscles maximally and rhythmically, following each beat of the metronome, and to continue (without moving the shoulders) until fatigue is so great that the weight can no longer be lifted.
5. ***Motivation:*** Give a rest for 15 minutes and then repeat the whole procedure, telling the subject that she/he will do much better this time.
6. ***Effect of venous occlusion:*** After another rest period, apply the blood pressure (BP) cuff on the upper arm and **raise the pressure to 40 mm Hg to stop venous return.** Repeat the whole procedure. Fatigue sets in earlier because of accumulation of waste products in the exercising muscles.
7. ***Effect of arterial occlusion:*** After another period of rest, **raise the BP to about 160–170 mm Hg to stop arterial blood flow [the pressure increased should be above the systolic blood pressure (SBP)].** Tell the subject to repeat the muscle contractions. Fatigue sets in much earlier now because there is not only an accumulation of waste products but also a deficiency of oxygen and other nutrients.

Calculation of work done: Calculate the work done in each case as shown in **Figure 61**:

Work done (in kg meters) = Weight lifted × Distance

The distance through which the weight is lifted is the sum of all the heights of contractions, converted to meters.

$$\text{Total distance moved (D)} = \frac{\text{Area of triangle } (1/2 \times b \times h) + \text{Area of rectangle } (a \times h) \times \text{Number of contractions}}{\text{Total length of base } (a + b)}$$

Factors that Affect Onset of Fatigue

The degree, duration, and type of work done are the important factors that in general affect the onset of fatigue.

1. The weight to be lifted.

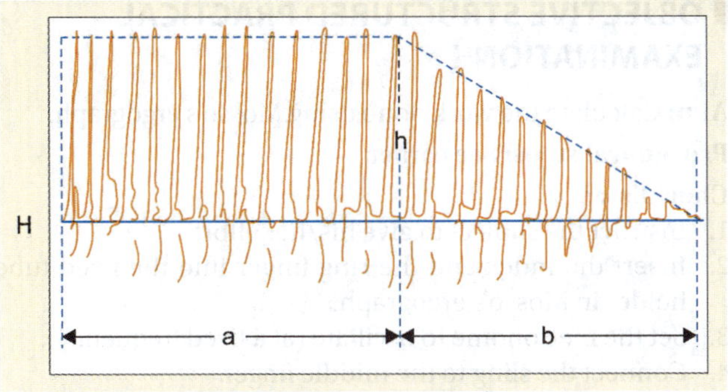

FIG. 61: Calculation work done.

2. Frequency of contractions.
3. Motivation.
4. Blood supply to contracting muscles.
5. Training.
6. Obesity.
7. Environmental factors such as temperature, humidity, and pollution affect the onset of fatigue.

HAND-GRIP DYNAMOMETER

- The hand-grip dynamometer is used for isometric exercise. It consists of two hollow metal tubes called handles which are connected together through a flexible (springy) metal strip **(Figs. 62A and B)**.
- The whole apparatus can be held in the palm of the hand and when compressed (squeezed), the metallic strip offers great resistance to compression. A graduated pressure scale is provided between the two handles for directly recording the compressing force.

Procedure

1. Show the use of the instrument to the subject before testing. Ask the subject to stand, with arms at the sides, and elbows slightly bent.
2. Ask him/her to hold it in her dominant hand to get a full grip of it.
3. Then ask him/her to close her eyes and to squeeze only once. Note the tension developed.
4. Tell him/her to make two more trials with a pause of about a minute between them to avoid fatigue. Take the mean of these readings; this is called **Tmax (maximal isometric tension)**.
5. Determine the **endurance time** for 60–80% of Tmax. This is the time of the onset of fatigue after starting the exercise on the dynamometer.
6. After a rest of 2–3 minutes, measure the endurance time for 60–80% of Tmax first after occlusion of veins and then after occlusion of arteries with a BP cuff on the upper arm.

Results

The Tmax varies widely between 30 and 50 kg. It depends on many factors such as sex, age, muscle strength, hand dominance, time of the day, nutrition, fatigue, and pain. There is a slight difference between the two hands.

Physioclinical Significance

Venous occlusion decreases the work done due to accumulation of metabolites in the muscle. Arterial occlusion further decreases the work done and brings in an early onset of fatigue as it prevents the supply of nutrients to the muscle. The performance of a person can be increased by encouragement and motivation.

QUESTIONS

Q.1. Define the term fatigue. What are the factors that affect the onset of fatigue?

See text above.

Q.2. How does motivation improve muscular performance?

Encouragement improves performance for a short time. This shows that the cerebral cortex is involved in fatigue in humans. In sports physiology, motivation plays an important role in enhancing performance.

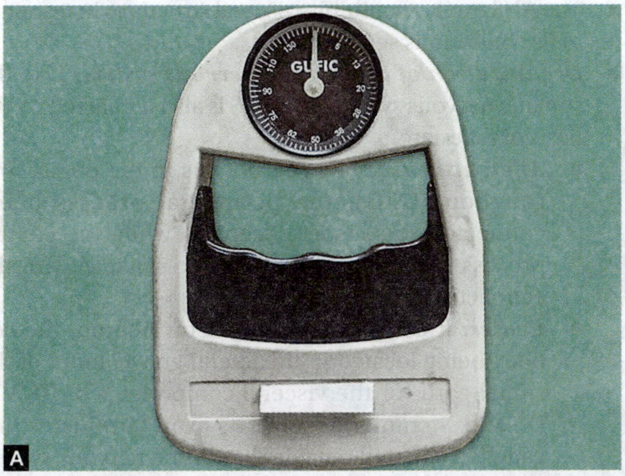

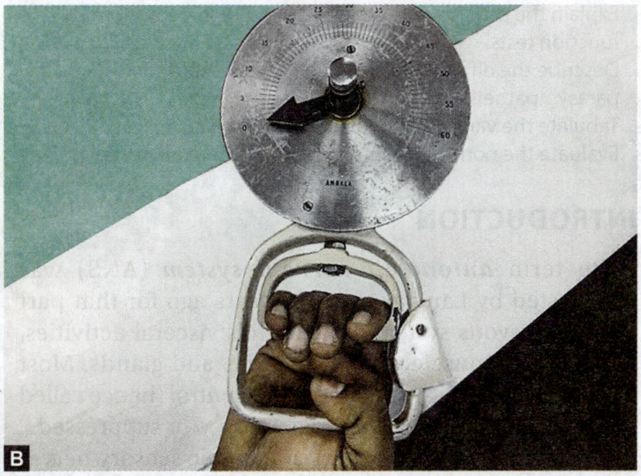

FIGS. 62A AND B: Hand-grip dynamometer.

Q.3. What is the site of fatigue in humans?

The first site of fatigue in humans is the central nervous system (CNS). This is proved by the fact that encouraging the person enhances the performance and delays the onset of fatigue. The next site of fatigue is the muscle followed by the neuromuscular junction.

Q.4. How will you demonstrate the site of fatigue in an intact muscle?

After the flexors of the fingers are fatigued, they will still contract on peripheral nerve stimulation. This will show that fatigue is a "central" phenomenon involving synapses.

Q.5. How does fatigue in this experiment compare with fatigue in frog's nerve-muscle preparation?

In frog's preparation (see experiment 4.10: Genesis of Fatigue), there is no blood supply. Hence, fatigue sets in early. Also, the seat of fatigue is the neuromuscular junction. In the present experiment, the seat of fatigue appears to be a central phenomenon.

Q.6. Name a clinical condition where venous or arterial occlusion can impair muscular performance.

In thrombosis of leg veins due to thrombophlebitis, the venous return is decreased so that fatigue sets in early. Arterial occlusion occurs in Buerger's disease (said to be due to chronic smoking); there is pain while walking. The narrowed vessels cannot keep pace with increased demands of muscles for oxygen. In coronary artery disease, ischemic muscle pain has a similar mechanism.

Q.7. How will the results be affected if the rate of work done is increased by setting the metronome faster? Give reasons.

See earlier.

Q.8. How is the work done affected following venous and arterial occlusions? Give reasons.

See earlier.

OBJECTIVE STRUCTURED PRACTICAL EXAMINATION-I

Aim: Calculate the work done using Mosso's ergograph.

Procedural steps: See earlier.

Checklist:

1. Instruct the subject to give his/her effort.
2. Insert the index and the ring finger into the fixed tube holder in Mosso's ergograph.
3. Set the metronome to oscillate (at a fixed frequency).
4. Connect the sling to the middle finger.
5. Ask the subject to lift the load by maximal contraction of the flexors of the middle finger.
6. Ask the subject to continue to lift the load till onset of fatigue.
7. Repeat the entire procedure with arterial and venous occlusions.

OBJECTIVE STRUCTURED PRACTICAL EXAMINATION-II

Aim: To measure your own endurance time for 60–80% of your Tmax by using the provided hand-grip dynamometer.

Procedural steps: See text above.

Checklist:

1. Check the instrument and hold it in her dominant hand to get a feel of it. (Y/N)
2. Close her eyes and then squeezes the handle with her maximum effort. Take a reading. (Y/N)
3. Wait for about a minute and then take the second reading of maximum tension. (Y/N)
4. Take the mean of the two readings (Tmax). (Y/N)
5. Measure her endurance time for 60–80% of her Tmax. (Y/N)

2.29: AUTONOMIC FUNCTION TESTS

STUDENT OBJECTIVES

After completing this experiment, the student should be able to:

- Explain the physioclinical significance of doing autonomic function tests.
- Describe the differences between sympathetic and parasympathetic function tests.
- Tabulate the various autonomic function tests.
- Evaluate the normal values of autonomic function tests.

INTRODUCTION

- The term ***autonomic nervous system*** (ANS) was suggested by Langley over 100 years ago for that part of the nervous system that controls visceral activities, i.e. cardiac muscle, smooth muscle, and glands. Most visceral activities are not under our control (hence called autonomic) and cannot be easily altered or suppressed.
- The main input to ANS is via autonomic sensory nerves from interoceptors (stretch receptors, chemoreceptors, etc.) in blood vessels and viscera that monitor the internal environment. Mostly, these signals are not consciously perceived.
- The ANS excites or inhibits visceral structures in response to its continuous sensory input.
- ***Organization of autonomic nervous system:*** Like the somatic nervous system, the ANS is also organized on the basis of reflex arc.
    - ***Afferent neuron:*** Its cell body is in the dorsal root ganglion (DRG), the peripheral process being connected to sensory receptors while the central process enters the spinal cord to synapse with the connector neuron.
    - ***Center:*** It consists of a connector neuron, the cell body being located in the lateral gray column of the spinal cord (or the visceral components of III, VII, IX, and X cranial nerves). Its axon terminates in a ganglion situated outside the central nervous system (CNS) [paravertebral ganglia in sympathetic system

(SS) and near or in the viscera in parasympathetic system (PSS)].

- ***Efferent pathway:*** While somatic efferent pathway consists of a single motor neuron (AHC), the visceral efferent pathway has two neurons—(1) preganglionic neurons and (2) postganglionic neurons.

- ***Divisions of autonomic nervous system:*** Depending on the anatomical location of connector or preganglionic neurons, the ANS is divided into **craniosacral (parasympathetic)** and **thoracolumbar (sympathetic)** components **(Fig. 63).**
- The preganglionic fibers in both systems are myelinated and **cholinergic**, while the postganglionic fibers are unmyelinated cholinergic is parasympathetic division and **noradrenergic** in sympathetic division, except those supplying sweat glands and blood vessels in skeletal muscles, which are **cholinergic**.
- The PSS conserves and stores energy and is **anabolic** while the SS is **catabolic** and prepares the body for emergency situations.
- The effects of PSS are localized and short-lived, the effects of SS are prolonged and widespread.

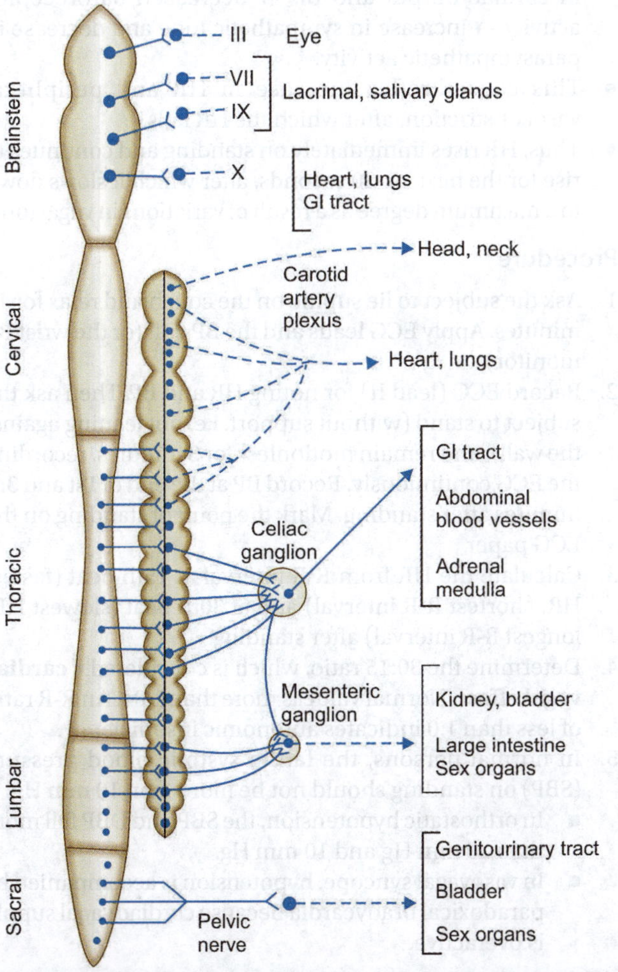

FIG. 63: Diagram to show the efferent pathways of the autonomic nervous system. The preganglionic neurons are shown as solid lines, postganglionic neurons as dashed lines.

CLASSIFICATIONS OF AUTONOMIC FUNCTION TESTS

- Assessment of sympathetic functions.
- Assessment of parasympathetic functions.

Apparatus

- Electrocardiogram (ECG) machine
- Blood pressure apparatus
- Multichannel polygraph
- Cathode ray oscilloscope (CRO)
- Electrodes
- Electronic stimulator
- Electromyography (EMG) machine and preamplifier.

Tests for Sympathetic Functions

QT-QS2 Ratio

This test is an index of sympathetic excitation of the heart.

Procedure

1. Ask the subject to lie down supine on the couch and relax. Attach ECG leads and place the contact microphone on the carotid artery to record heart sounds [phonocardiogram (PCG)].
2. Record lead II of ECG and PCG simultaneously at a paper speed of 50 mm/sec.
3. Measure QT interval from the beginning of the QRS complex to the end of T wave. Measure QS2 from the beginning of QRS to the first major vibration of the aortic component of second heart sound in PCG. Determine the QT/QS2 ratio.

Comments: QS2 is the total electromechanical systolic interval. A high value indicates greater sympathetic tone, while a low value represents low sympathetic tone.

Sympathetic Skin Response

Rationale

- The sweat glands distributed over the entire body are innervated by sympathetic postganglionic cholinergic fibers (except in palms and soles which are innervated by noradrenergic sympathetic fibers).
- The stratum corneum of the skin, which is punctured by the ducts of sweat glands, offers maximum resistance to the passage of current through the skin.
- However, when the sweat glands are activated, the ducts get filled with sweat (which is an electrolyte), so that an electric current can easily pass through the skin due to a fall in skin resistance.
- Change in skin potential in response to stimuli causing sympathetic activation is called **sympathetic skin response.** It is also called **galvanic skin response** (GSR).

Procedure

An EMG machine and a CRO are generally adequate to record the response to application of current. However, a polygraph may be used.

1. *Set the preamplifier to GSR and EMG machine*: Frequency response = 0.1–1,000 Hz, gain = 0.5 mV/ div, and set the sweep to record 5 seconds after the stimulus.
2. After cleaning the skin and applying small amounts of paste, place the active electrode (disk type) on the palm (or sole of foot), reference electrode on the dorsum of the hand (or foot), with the ground electrode between the two.
3. Apply a constant current of 5 μA, and note the response and calculate its latency and amplitude. Estimate the skin resistance in millivolts from the recording pen deflection (the deflection resulting from 1 mV to the amplifier is equal to a resistance change to 10 kOhm).
4. Give a stimulus in the form of startling sound (say, a sudden handclap near the head of the subject) and record the response, i.e. the SSR potentials, their latency, and amplitude (the stimulus will activate the SS).

Note: The SSR may be mono, di, or triphasic and the potentials may be 1.1–1.5 mV in amplitude and about 1.5 seconds in latency in the hands and 0.7–0.9 mV and 2.0–2.5 seconds in the feet. Abnormal SSR is usually seen in progressive autonomic dysfunction.

Cold Pressure Response

Rationale

Physical or mental stress causes stimulation of SS. Plunging a hand in cold water act as a pain stimulus and causes rise in BP (since this test is somewhat unpleasant, it is done at the end of ANS testing).

Procedure

1. Explain the test to the subject and seat him/her in a chair; record the baseline BP.
2. Ask the subject to immerse one hand in cold water at 4–5°C for 2 minutes. Record the BP from the other arm at 30 seconds intervals.
3. Note the maximum increase in systolic and diastolic pressures (DPs) and compare with the pretest readings. The systolic pressure (SP) may increase by 20 mm Hg, while the DP rises by 10 mm Hg.

Results

Reduced sympathetic activity is indicated by a smaller rise of BP. In some normal persons, there may be no significant rise in BP.

Handgrip Test (Isometric Exercise)

Sustained handgrip causes a rise in HR and BP. An ECG machine, a sphygmomanometer, and a hand-grip spring dynamometer will be required for this test.

Procedure

1. Apply the BP cuff on the non exercising arm, and lead II of ECG for recording HR. Record the resting BP and HR at 30 seconds intervals for 4 minutes. Then ask the subject to hold the dynamometer in the dominant hand and take a full grip on it.
2. Ask the subject to exert maximum force and note the maximum tension developed. Repeat three times at intervals of 2 minutes. Take the highest reading and note it as ***maximum isometric tension (T max)***.
3. Now ask the subject to maintain a tension of 30% of T max for 5 minutes. During this procedure, record the BP and ECG at 30 seconds intervals.
4. Note the diastolic blood pressure (DBP) at the point just before the release of handgrip.
5. Note the mean resting value of DBP readings during the last 3 minutes before starting the exercise.

Results

The rise in DBP in normal subjects is more than 15 mm Hg but less than 10 mm Hg in sympathetic insufficiency.

Tests for Parasympathetic Functions

Standing Test (30:15 RR Ratio)

Rationale

- Upon sudden standing from supine, there is pooling of blood in the lower parts of the body. This is followed by a sequence of events: fall of venous return → decrease in cardiac output and BP → decreased baroreceptor activity → increase in sympathetic tone and decrease in parasympathetic activity.
- This causes reflex increase in HR and peripheral vasoconstriction, after which the HR falls.
- Thus, HR rises immediately on standing and continues to rise for the next 15–20 seconds, after which it slows down to a maximum degree as a result of variations in vagal tone.

Procedure

1. Ask the subject to lie supine on the couch and relax for 15 minutes. Apply ECG leads and the BP cuff (or the wrist BP monitor).
2. Record ECG (lead II) for noting HR and BP. Then ask the subject to stand (without support, i.e. not leaning against the wall), and remain motionless for 3 minutes, recording the ECG continuously. Record BP at the end of 1st and 3rd minutes after standing. Mark the point of standing on the ECG paper.
3. Calculate the HR from R-R interval at 15th beat (fastest HR; shortest R-R interval) and at 30th beat (slowest HR; longest R-R interval) after standing.
4. Determine the 30:15 ratio, which is considered a **cardiac vagal effect**. Normal value is more than 1.04. An R-R ratio of less than 1.0 indicates autonomic insufficiency.
5. In normal persons, the fall in systolic blood pressure (SBP) on standing should not be more than 10 mm Hg.
   - In orthostatic hypotension, the SBP and DBP fall more than 20 mm Hg and 10 mm Hg.
   - In vasovagal syncope, hypotension is accompanied by paradoxical bradycardia because cardiac vagal supply is overactive.

Note: Similar responses can be better studied by passively tilting the subject on a tilt table from supine position to an inclination of 80° (head up) for a period of 3–4 minutes.

Standing to Lying Ratio (S/L Ratio)

Rationale

- When a normal person lies down from a standing position, there is at first a rise in HR which is followed by a slowing of the heart.
- This rise and fall of HR is due to changes in vagal tone.

Procedure

1. Explain the procedure to the subject. Connect ECG leads for recording lead II. Ask the subject to stand quietly for 2 minutes and then to lie down supine without any support.
2. Record ECG for 20 beats before and for 60 beats after lying down. Note the point of change of position on the ECG paper.
3. Repeat three times at intervals of 5 minutes.
4. **Calculation of S/L ratio:** Take the average R-R interval during five beats before lying down and shortest R-R interval during 10 beats after lying down. The maximum ratio of the three trials is reported. Any abnormally low ratio indicates parasympathetic insufficiency.

Valsalva Ratio

- Valsalva maneuver (effort) is forced expiration against a closed glottis.
- This straining, associated with changes in HR and BP, is a simple test for baroreceptor activity (**Fig. 64**).

Procedure

1. Seat the subject on a stool and explain the procedure. Connect ECG leads and BP cuff on him/her, and close the nostrils with a nose clip.
2. Disconnect the cuff from another BP apparatus and ask the subject to take a deep breath, blow into the manometer, and maintain the pressure of 40 mm Hg for 15 seconds (recall the 40 mm Hg test for lung functions).
3. Record ECG (lead II) for 1 minute before the straining, for 15 seconds during straining, and for 45 seconds after the release of strain. It may also be calculated as the ratio of longest R-R interval after the strain to the shortest R-R during the strain.

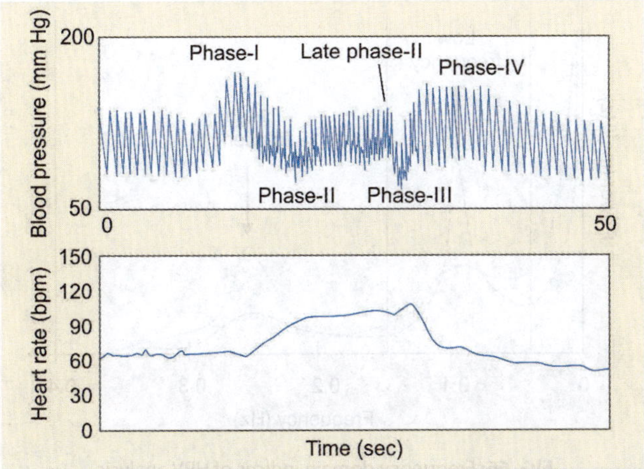

FIG. 64: HR and BP during Valsalva maneuver.

Observations

The Valsalva maneuver has four phases:

1. **Phase I:** It is the onset of strain. In this phase, there occurs a transient decrease in BP. Mechanical compression of the great vessels and increased intrathoracic pressure contributes to this rise. There is not much change in HR.
2. **Phase II:** During straining, there is decrease in venous return, fall in cardiac output and BP, and inhibition of baroreceptors, followed by tachycardia and vasoconstriction. The HR increases throughout straining due to vagal inhibition initially and sympathetic activation later.
3. **Phase III:** At the release of strain, there is a transient fall of BP without significant change in HR.
4. **Phase IV:** After further release of strain, the BP slowly rises with decrease of HR. These, in turn, stimulate baroreceptors causing bradycardia and drop in BP to normal levels.

The maximum Valsalva ratio of three trials is taken as the index of autonomic activity. A ratio of greater than 1.45 is normal, 1.20–1.45 is borderline, and less than 1.20 indicates autonomic disturbance.

Clinical Significance

Failure of HR to increase during straining suggests sympathetic insufficiency, while failure of HR to slow down after the effort suggests a parasympathetic insufficiency.

Tachycardia Ratio

- This ratio is related to Valsalva ratio and is defined as the ratio of shortest R-R interval during Valsalva effort to the longest R-R interval before the effort.
- It is believed to be a better index of vagal activity.

Deep Breathing Test

- The HR increases during inspiration (due to decreased cardiac vagal activity) and decreases during expiration (due to increased vagal activity).
- This is a normal phenomenon and is called ***sinus arrhythmia***.

Procedure

There are two methods to show the effect of breathing on HR. In one method, a single deep breath is taken and its effect noted. In the other method, the subject breathes deeply for 1 minute.

1. Explain the procedure to the subject, and ask him to lie down supine and relax, with the head raised to 30°.
2. Attach the ECG leads for recording lead II. Then ask the subject to breathe deeply and slowly at a rate of 6 breaths/min, with 5 seconds for inspiration and 5 seconds for expiration. Record ECG before and during deep breathing.
3. Determine the maximum and minimum HR with each respiratory cycle and note the average HR in inspiration and in expiration.
4. Calculate the expiration to inspiration ratio (E:I ratio). This is the mean of maximum R-R intervals during expiration

(slow HR) to the mean of minimum R-R intervals during deep inspiration (fast HR).

5. In normal persons, the fall in HR should be more than 15 beats/min. In vagal insufficiency, the HR slows less than 10 beats/min.

Other Tests

The smooth muscle of the iris and ciliary body are supplied by both SS and PSS nerve fibers. Sympathetic activity causes pupillary dilation while parasympathetic activity causes pupillary constriction, accommodation, lacrimation, and salivation.

Test for Pupillary Function

- Sympathetic activity causes pupillary dilatation while parasympathetic activity causes pupillary constriction, accommodation, lacrimation, and salivation.
- Local application of pharmacologic agonists is helpful in establishing pupillary denervation—resulting in denervation hypersensitivity.
- ***Denervation hypersensitivity:*** This is the phenomenon in which an effector tissue (muscle, in this case) becomes hypersensitive to a neurotransmitter 2–3 weeks after denervation of that tissue.

Procedure

- Put a drop or two of 0.125% pilocarpine drops in the eye of the subject. Normally, this causes minimal pupillary constriction. In parasympathetic denervation, there is a strong constriction of the pupil.
- In a similar way, 2–3 drops of 0.1% solution of epinephrine put three times in the eye at 1 minute intervals causes minimal dilatation of the pupil. But in sympathetic denervation, there is strong pupillary dilatation (checked at 15, 30, and 45 minutes).

Test for Lacrimation (Schirmer's Test)

- Take a strip of filter paper, 25 mm long and 5 mm wide, and place its one end between the lower eyelid and sclera, allowing its other end to hang down over the cheek.
- Measure the length of its wetting after 5 minutes. In normal persons, the filter paper wets by about 15 mm while less than 10 mm suggests parasympathetic insufficiency.

HEART RATE VARIABILITY

- Heart variability is defined as the cardiac beat-beat variation and represents the variation in cardiac cycle length during respiratory cycles at rest. The physiological phenomenon of variation in the time interval between heart beats is known as **HRV**. It describes oscillation in consecutive cardiac cycles.
- Heart rate variability (HRV) is a highly sensitive noninvasive indicator of autonomic functions. It is mainly important for assessment of sympathovagal balance. This is mainly used for prediction of cardiovascular dysfunction.
- The methodology is based upon the calculation of successive R-R intervals. These can then be plotted as frequency histogram (**time domain**) or undergo power spectral analysis to yield information in the **frequency domain**.

Heart Rate Variability Analysis

The variations in HR can be evaluated by the following two HRV indices:

1. Time domain analysis
2. Frequency domain analysis.

Time Domain Analysis (Fig. 65)

- This is one of the simplest methods to access the HRV. In this, the HR at any point in time or the intervals between successive complexes are determined.
- A continuous ECG record is taken and a normal to normal (N-N interval, i.e. all intervals between adjacent QRS complexes) are determined. The term N-N is used in place of R-R as the processed beats are normal beats.

Frequency Domain Analysis (Fig. 66)

- The HRV is comprised of various frequencies. Frequency domain analyses this by viewing different frequency components of the waveform. The main frequency components that represent autonomic activity are:
  - **High frequency (HF)—0.15–0.4 Hz**
  - **Low frequency (LF)—0.04–0.15 Hz**
  - **Very low frequency (VLF)—0.0–0.04 Hz**

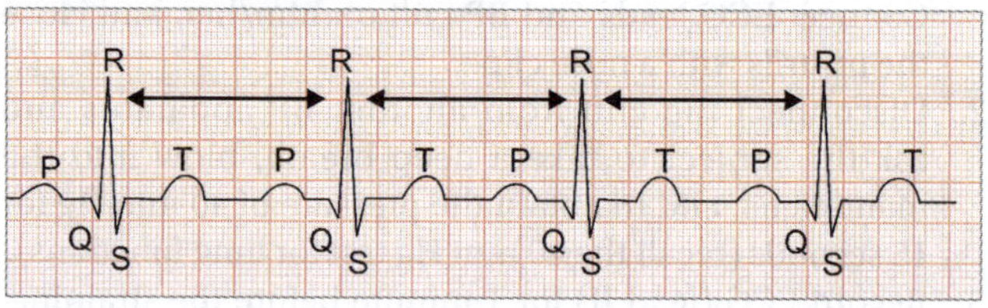

FIG. 65: Time domain analysis of heart rate variability (HRV) using R-R interval.

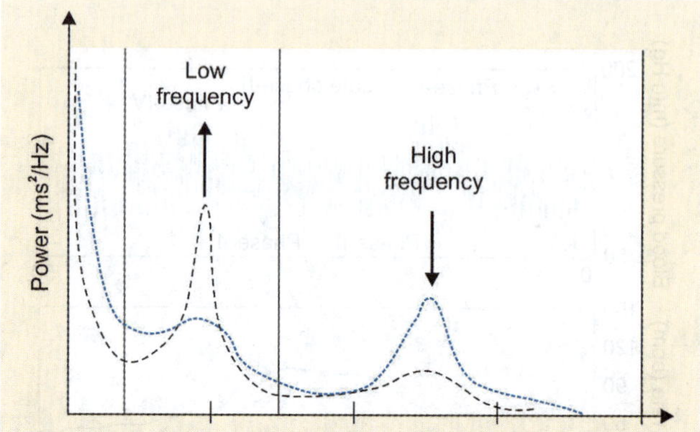

FIG. 66: Frequency domain indices of HRV analysis.

- The LF and HF components are relative indices of cardiac sympathetic and vagal activity, respectively.
- High frequency component is because of vagal tone during respiratory cycle.
- Low frequency component results from self-oscillation in the sympathetic component of the baroreceptor reflex loop as a result of negative feedback.
- All other HR changes such as associated with thermoregulation and humoral mechanisms are accounted by VLF components.

Heart Rate Variability Recording

- Two types of HRV recordings are done: Short-term (5 minutes) recording and Long-term (day-night) HRV recording.
- For research and clinical investigations, short-term HRV recording is preferred, although long-term HRV recording is more reliable.
- After 5 minutes of supine rest, lead II ECG recording is obtained from the subject at a rate of 1,000 samples/sec using computer software (data acquisition system).
- This data is further processed with the help of another software to get HRV analysis.

Physiological Significance

1. Heart rate variability analysis assesses the efficiency of vagal control precisely. During inspiration, vagal tone is inhibited thereby leading to increase in HR. The HR shows fluctuations with a frequency similar to the respiratory cycle. The vagal tone is inhibited during inspiration because of the irradiation of impulses from the respiratory to the cardiovascular center.
2. It also provides information about sympathovagal balance.
3. Heart rate variability alterations have also been seen during yoga and traditional exercise.
4. Heart rate variability is used as a prognostic tool after myocardial infarction and cardiac transplantation.
5. Decreased HRV is seen in many cardiovascular diseases.
6. There is a good correlation between decreased HRV and risk for sudden cardiac death in patients of heart disease.

QUESTIONS

Q.1. What are the divisions of autonomic nervous system?
See text above.

Q.2. Describe the functions of parasympathetic and sympathetic divisions of the ANS.
See text above.

Q.3. Name the various conventional autonomic function tests.
See text above.

Q.4. Discuss the physiological basis of clinical tests in assessing autonomic dysfunction.
See text above.

Q.5. Which is the most sensitive autonomic function tests?
See text above.

Q.6. Give the common causes of autonomic dysfunction.
In progressive autonomic dysfunction both preganglionic and postganglionic neurons undergo degeneration. This leads to **orthostatic or postural hypotension** (inability to maintain BP in the erect posture), constipation, sexual dysfunction, incontinence of urine, disturbances of sweating, etc.

Common causes of autonomic neuropathy are diabetic neuropathy, alcoholic neuropathy, and uremic neuropathy.

Q.7. What is HRV? What is its physioclinical significance?
See text above.

Q.8. What do the time domain and frequency domain indices of HRV represent?
See text above.

UNIT V: REPRODUCTIVE SYSTEM

2.30: SEMEN ANALYSIS

STUDENT OBJECTIVES

After completing this experiment, the student should be able to:

- Describe the relevance of semen analysis in physiology and clinical practice.
- Indicate the composition of semen.
- Perform the sperm count and assess the fertility problem of the patient.
- List the precautions observed during sperm counting.

PY9.9: Interpret a normal semen analysis report including (a) sperm count, (b) sperm morphology, and (c) sperm motility, as per WHO guidelines and discuss the results.

INTRODUCTION

A semen analysis, also called a sperm count, measures the quantity and quality of a man's semen and sperm.

- Semen (also known as spermatic fluid) is studied for sterility. It is a routine test to determine if the sterility is due to a defect in the semen.
- Study of semen is also done to confirm the completeness of vasectomy, a procedure commonly adopted for controlling birth.

Characteristics of Normal Semen and Comments

A sample of semen collected after 2–3 days of sexual abstinence has the following features:

Volume

Normal volume is 2.5–5 mL. It decreases in functional disorders, or inflammation of the male genital tract.

Physical Characteristics

White, opalescent, mucoid, and sticky.

pH

About 7.2–7.7. The alkaline pH brings the vaginal pH of 3.5–4.5 to about 6–6.5, the pH at which sperms show maximum motility.

Morphology

Normal sperms are actively motile. They are one of the smallest cells (5–6 µm). In contrast to an ovum, which is the largest cell of the body (about 120 µm). They have a head, neck, body, and tail.

Abnormalities in shape include: Bifid or absent heads, bifurcated tails, etc. If present in more than 70% of sperms, it indicates some pathology.

Motility

More than 80% sperms show a good forward motility due to "flail-like" movements of their tails. More than 70% of sperms in a specimen should show active motility within 3 hours of collection of specimen. Less than 40% motile sperms indicate sterility.

Count

Normal count is 60–120 million/mL, with an average of 100 million/mL. Counts between 20 million/mL and 40 million/mL indicate borderline infertility. Counts below 20 million/mL indicate sterility.

Clotting and Liquefaction

Normal semen clots within 5 minutes of ejaculation. There is no thrombin or prothrombin, the clotting is due to the conversion of fibrinogen into fibrin. However, the exact mechanism is not known. It undergoes secondary liquefaction due to the presence and activation of plasmin and other proteolytic enzymes, such as prostate-specific antigen (PSA), pepsinogen, hyaluronidase, and amylase.

Fructose

Normal semen contains fructose. It is used by sperms for production of adenosine triphosphate (ATP) via Krebs cycle.

Also present are: Calcium, citric acid, clotting proteins different from those of blood clotting, hyaluronidase, acid phosphatase, and prostaglandins.

PRINCIPLE OF SPERM COUNTING

Semen is collected from the subject, diluted 20 times in a white blood cell (WBC) pipette and the sperms are counted in a Neubauer chamber.

Apparatus and Materials

1. *Microscope*:
   - Improved Neubauer chamber
   - White blood cell pipette
   - Coverslips
   - Slides
   - Plasticine.
2. *Diluting fluid*: 5% sodium bicarbonate in 1.0% phenol solution.

Procedure

1. Collect a fresh sample of semen (after 2 days of abstinence) in a petri dish or a small beaker.
2. Wait for 25–30 minutes for secondary liquefaction. Observe if the liquefaction is uniform. Measure its volume.
3. ***Assessing sperm motility:*** Place a drop of semen on a coverslip and invert it on the rim of a small circle of plasticine previously made on a slide. Examine under low and high power, and watch the motility of sperms. Try to assess the percentage of motile to nonmotile sperms. Also note their morphology.
4. ***Counting the sperms:*** Gently shake the sample to assure uniformity.
   - Draw semen to 0.5 mark in the WBC pipette, then draw the diluting fluid to the mark 11. Mix the contents of the bulb for 2–3 minutes.
   - Discard the first few drops, then charge the counting chamber, and count the sperms under high power in the four WBC squares, as was done for total leukocyte count (TLC).
5. ***Calculation:***

   Number of sperms in 64 squares (volume = $4/10$ mm^3) = N

   Then number of sperms in 1 mm^3 of undiluted semen = $N \times 10/4 \times 20$

   To get sperm count in 1 mL = $N \times 50 \times 1{,}000$ Normal count = 60–120 million/mL

   Report: Morphology ....

   Count: .... million/mL.

QUESTIONS

Q.1. What is semen? Where are sperms formed?

- Semen is a mixture of spermatozoa and a liquid consisting of the secretions of seminiferous tubules, seminal vesicles, prostate, and bulbourethral glands. The liquid part provides nourishment and a transport system.
- About 60 million sperms are manufactured daily in about 1,000 seminiferous tubules in each testis, each tubule being 50–60 cm long. Leydig cells of testis secrete testosterone, the male sex hormone that promotes spermatogenesis, in addition to primary and secondary "male" sex characteristics.

Q.2. What are the indications for sperm analysis?

Semen is examined for four main purposes:

1. To determine whether a male is fertile or not.
2. In the investigation of genetic disorders like cryptorchidism and Klinefelter syndrome.
3. To diagnose inflammatory or neoplastic diseases of the genital tract.
4. To confirm the completeness of vasectomy.

Q.3. What is the composition of semen? Name some features of the sperms.

See text above.

Q.4. Why is abstinence advised for 2-3 days before collecting a sample of semen?

Since the volume and sperm count of semen decrease rapidly with frequent ejaculations, it might give a misleading low-count result if this precaution is not taken.

Q.5. What is the significance of clotting and liquefaction of semen?

These two features of semen—(1) clotting and (2) secondary liquefaction—appear to play a biological role. The initial coagulation helps to retain semen in the vagina, while the subsequent liquefaction aids the sperms to swim up the female genital tract.

Q.6. When is a male considered infertile?

The male infertility (or sterility) is the inability of a person to fertilize a secondary oocyte. It may be due to a low sperm count (<20 million/mL), or a high percentage of nonmotile or abnormal sperms.

Infertility should not be confused with impotence (erectile dysfunction), i.e. inability to perform the sexual act.

Q.7. For how long can sperms remain capable of fertilization in the female genital tract?

The maximum duration of fertilization capacity of normal sperms varies between 24 hours and 48 hours.

Q.8. Define the terms oligospermia, azoospermia, and necrospermia.

Oligospermia refers to a count less than 20 million/mL, azoospermia means total absence of sperms, and necrospermia refers to dead (nonliving) sperms in the semen.

Q.9. When only one sperm is required for the fertilization of ovum, Why has nature provided such a huge number of sperms?

The large and extravagant excess of sperms appears to be a reminder of (and a *fallback* on) life's origin in the sea. Some fish simply spray their sperms into water on the off chance that a drifting egg will be fertilized.

Q.10. What is vasectomy and why is it done? For how long sperms may appear in the semen after bilateral vasectomy?

- Vasectomy is the chief method for *the sterilization of males* by a simple surgical operation. Incisions are given on each side of scrotum, vas deferens is located, and a piece is removed from each.
- Sexual desire and performance are not affected since testosterone secretion continues normally. Sperm production also continues but they cannot reach outside. In time, they degenerate and are removed by macrophages.
- For the first 2 months after vasectomy, viable sperms may be released from their storage in ampullae of seminal vesicles.

Note: Though "recanalization" of the ducts is possible, the chances of regaining fertility are very slim.

2.31: PREGNANCY DIAGNOSTIC TESTS

STUDENT OBJECTIVES

After completing this experiment, the student should be able to:

- Name the different pregnancy diagnostic tests.
- Explain the principle of biological and immunological tests.
- Compare the advantages and disadvantages of the various pregnancy diagnostic tests.
- Discuss the role of various hormones in maintenance of pregnancy.
- Discuss the clinical significance of these tests.

PY9.10: Discuss the physiological basis of various pregnancy tests.

INTRODUCTION

- Most of the laboratory tests for pregnancy are based on the detection of the **presence of human chorionic gonadotropin (HCG) in the woman's urine.**
- Some tests are so sensitive that the earliest diagnosis of pregnancy can be made within a few days of the conception, i.e. even before the next missed period.
- These tests can be grouped into *biological, immunological,* and *radiological.*

BIOLOGICAL DIAGNOSTIC TESTS

These tests, which involve injection of urine into various animals, are time consuming and costly. They are, however, 99% accurate.

1. ***Aschheim–Zondek mouse test:*** Urine is injected subcutaneously into immature mice. Appearance of blood-filled ovulated follicles on 5th day confirms pregnancy.
2. ***Friedman rabbit test:*** Intravenous injection of urine into virgin female rabbits causes ovulation in 18 hours.
3. ***Galli–Mainini frog test:*** Injection of urine into the dorsal lymph sac of male frogs or toads causes shedding of sperms in about 3 hours.
4. ***Hogben test:*** Adult female toads are used in this test. Injection of urine into the lymph space causes ovulation within 18 hours.

IMMUNOLOGICAL TESTS

Principle

- The HCG secreted by syncytiotrophoblast cells of placenta is antigenic, and antibodies against this hormone can be produced by injecting it into rabbits.
- These antibodies are available commercially and are employed to detect the presence of HCG in the subject's urine or serum by precipitation, hemagglutination, or complement fixation, etc.

Procedure

- ***Collection of urine:*** The sensitivity level of HCG in urine is 1.5–3.5 IU/mL in the slide test and 0.2–1.2 IU/mL in the test tube test. This concentration is reached by the 10th day of fertilization (i.e. even before the missed period).

- The subject is advised to restrict water intake for 12–14 hours, and urine is collected in a clean container in the morning. The specific gravity of urine should be at least 1.015 and it should be free from protein and blood.

Latex Agglutination Inhibition (LAI) Test (Gravindex Test)

- ***Basis of test:*** Small globules of latex (rubber) particles coated with pure HCG, and antiserum to HCG, are available commercially in "kit" form.
- A sample of urine is treated with antiserum on a glass slide placed against a black background. If the urine contains HCG (i.e. if the woman is pregnant), then the antibodies in the antiserum are all "used up". Then if the coated latex particles are added, they do not get agglutinated.
- Urine (HCG present) + Antiserum + Latex particles = No agglutination.
- Therefore, **"no agglutination"** means a positive result, i.e. the woman is pregnant. If the urine sample does not contain HCG, then the antibodies in the antiserum are "remain free". Then if latex particles are added, antigen-antibody reaction occurs and the particles get agglutinated.
- Urine (HCG absent) + Antiserum + Latex particles = Agglutination.
- Therefore, **"agglutination"** means a negative result, i.e. the woman is not pregnant.

Hemagglutination Inhibition (HAI) Test

- In this test, sheep's red blood cells (RBCs) coated with HCG are employed in place of latex particles. The test is done in a test tube and observations are made after 2 hours.
- The principle is the same as LAI.

One-step Immunoassay Test

- This test is based on the combination of monoclonal antibody-dye conjugate with polyclonal solid phase antibodies for the qualitative detection of HCG in the urine.
- A sample of urine is applied to the test zone of the card or strip, and if it contains HCG, a pink-purple colored band develops.
- A control is provided to check the potency of the test reagents. A number of test kits under different proprietary names are available.

Radioimmunoassay (RIA)

- Human chorionic gonadotropin radiolabeled with iodine (iodine135) is treated with fixed amounts of antibodies and urine/serum sample.
- The method is much more sensitive and can detect as little as 0.003 IU/mL of beta subunit and 0.001 IU/mL of alpha subunit of HCG in the specimen.

Enzyme-linked Immunosorbent Assay (ELISA)

- Enzyme-linked immunosorbent assay has been widely used to detect a variety of antigens and antibodies.
- The principle of the test is the same as that of RIA except that an enzyme is used in place of a radioactive substance.
- The enzyme acts on the substrate to produce blue color which is a positive test for pregnancy.

ULTRASONOGRAPHY

- Pulses of ultrasonic waves at high frequency are generated from a piezoelectric crystal transducer that also acts as a receiver to detect waves reflected back from various parts of the uterus. The echoes (reflected waves) are displayed on the ultrasound screen.
- It is the most reliable method for detecting pregnancy. The gestational ring is evident as early as 5th week of pregnancy, cardiac pulsations by 10th week, and fetal movements by 11th week.
- The method is particularly useful in detecting fetal viability and position, site of placenta, multiple pregnancy, and fetal-maternal abnormalities, etc. The method, however, is being used for the determination of sex of the fetus. If the fetus is a female, many parents get the fetus aborted by unscrupulous doctors.

QUESTIONS

Q.1. What is the principle underlying biological tests for pregnancy?

See text above.

Q.2. What is the physiological basis of immunological tests for pregnancy?

See text above.

Q.3. Why are immunological tests preferred over biological tests?

Immunological tests are used routinely in all hospitals and clinics. Compared to biological tests, they are less costly, simpler and easy to carry out, take very little time for reporting, and can confirm pregnancy within 10 days of conception.

Q.4. What are the conditions in which false-positive and false-negative results may be obtained?

False-positive results: These may be obtained due to excessive protein or blood in the urine sample, or at menopause, or at the time of ovulation due to increased secretion of luteinizing hormone (LH). Such a result can also be seen in benign or malignant tumors of the placenta. Drugs such as thiazide diuretics and steroids may affect early pregnancy tests.

False-negative results: Such results may be seen when the concentration of HCG in urine/serum is very low (though the woman is pregnant), or testing too soon, or due to an ectopic pregnancy.

Q.5. What is the chief advantage of ultrasound method?

See earlier.

Q.6. What is the utility of pregnancy tests?

1. Use in diagnosing pregnancy.
2. The tests are also employed in detecting hydatidiform mole (a benign tumor of placenta), and chorioepithelioma (carcinoma of placenta). Repeated tests in these conditions show a high and rising concentration of HCG

(the urine diluted 1 in 500 may give a positive test) while in normal pregnancy, the HCG titer falls by 12th week.
3. They are employed in assessing and planning the course of action in cases of repeated abortions.

Q.7. Name the hormones released from the placenta during pregnancy. What are their chief functions?

1. **Human chorionic gonadotropin:** The most important function of HCG is to prevent degeneration of corpus luteum (which occurs about 2 weeks after ovulation) and maintain its viability. This allows it to continue to secrete estrogens and progesterone—an activity required to prevent menstruation and for continued attachment of embryo and fetus to the uterine endometrium.
   Human chorionic gonadotropin is now used for maintenance of pregnancy in women with history of repeated abortions. It is also used for stimulating the release of ova that can be collected and later employed for in vitro fertilization (for the so-called *test tube babies*).
2. **Human chorionic somatomammotropin (HCS); also called "human placental lactogen", (HPL):** The rate of secretion of HCS reaches maximum levels after 32 weeks and remains high after that. It prepares mammary glands for lactation, increases protein synthesis in the fetus and its growth, and causes retention of nitrogen, calcium, and potassium.
3. **Estrogens:** These are secreted by corpus luteum in early stages of pregnancy but placenta becomes the major site of estrogen secretion. Important effects are enlargement of uterus and breasts, protein anabolic effects including building of strong bones, and relaxation of pelvic ligaments for facilitating birth at term.
4. **Progesterone:** It is secreted by corpus luteum during early pregnancy and maintains pregnancy. From 4 months to 9 months, placental progesterone increases. It relaxes uterine muscle by decreasing spontaneous movements and helps in continuation of pregnancy and promotes growth of alveoli in breasts.
5. **Relaxin:** Secreted from placenta, it relaxes the uterus and helps in continuation of pregnancy. In later pregnancy, it relaxes pubic symphysis and dilates uterine cervix to facilitate delivery.
6. **Corticotropin-releasing hormone (CRH):** This hormone (normally secreted by anterior pituitary), has recently been shown to be part of the "clock" that establishes the timing of delivery. Its secretion begins at about 12 weeks and greatly increases toward the end of pregnancy. It also increases the secretion of cortisol that is required for the maturation of lungs and secretion of lung surfactant in the fetus.

Q.8. What is amenorrhea and what are its causes?

- **Amenorrhea** is defined as the absence of menstruation during the reproductive years of a woman's life. Physiological states of amenorrhea are seen, most commonly during pregnancy and lactation (breastfeeding). It can be classified as primary and secondary amenorrhea.
- *Primary amenorrhea is defined as a failure to reach menarche.* The most common causes of primary amenorrhea relate to hormone levels, although anatomical problems also can cause amenorrhea. The causes of amenorrhea are diverse.
- *Secondary amenorrhea* is the absence of regular menstrual periods for at least 3 months or the absence of irregular menstrual periods for 6 months or more. Pregnancy is the most common cause of secondary amenorrhea, although hormonal disturbances also can cause secondary amenorrhea.
- Secondary amenorrhea can be caused by various conditions that affect the menstrual cycle, including pregnancy, anovulation, estrogen deficiencies, and reproductive tract obstructions. In addition, certain lifestyles may increase the risk of secondary amenorrhea.
- In vigorous and competitive women athletes, amenorrhea results from reduced gonadotropin-releasing hormones (GnRHs) from the hypothalamus, and thus, LH and follicle-stimulating hormone (FSH) from the anterior pituitary. The result is a failure of development of ova and stoppage of ovulation. Low body weight, and low body fat (and low levels of leptin secretion by adipose cells) may be a contributing factor.
- Short periods of amenorrhea may be harmless, but long-lasting disruption of reproductive function may cause loss of bone density that is a part of the "female athlete triad" of osteoporosis, disordered eating, and amenorrhea.

2.32: BIRTH CONTROL METHODS

PY9.6: Enumerate the contraceptive methods for male and female. Discuss their advantages and disadvantages.

INTRODUCTION

- Birth control (contraception) is any method, medicine, or device used to prevent pregnancy.
- **Contraceptives** are temporary or permanent measures employed to prevent pregnancy in spite of sexual intercourse.
- With the explosion of population in our country, various methods of planning a small family have been in vogue for the last many decades. However, there is no single, ideal method of preventing pregnancy.
- The only method of preventing pregnancy with 100% surety is total abstinence, i.e. avoidance of sexual intercourse.
- Birth control methods are employed not only for limiting the number of children but also for the spacing of pregnancies because repeated pregnancies pose danger not only to the health of the mother, but also to that of the offspring.
- The requirements of different couples vary, so that one or more of the following methods may be recommended.

METHODS BASED ON PHYSIOLOGICAL PRINCIPLE

1. ***Rhythm method ("safe period"; periodic abstinence):***
   - Normally, only one viable ovum is released per menstrual cycle and it remains viable for about 24 hours, while the sperms, after entering the **uterus, survive** for about 48 hours.
   - Thus, there is a minimum period of 3 days during which intercourse must be avoided to prevent pregnancy.
   - For this method to be effective, the time of ovulation must be known. In most women who have regular periods, ovulation usually occurs ***14 days before the onset of the next menstruation*** (not the 14th day from the 1st day of a cycle).
   - For example, if the cycle starts on the 1st day of a month and lasts 30 days, the time of ovulation would be the 16th of that month. Pregnancy is unlikely to occur if coitus is avoided 4 days before and 4 days after the expected day of ovulation.

Note: The rhythm method, though physiological, is the most unreliable method because pregnancy has been reported to occur from coitus on every day of the cycle.

2. ***Withdrawal method***: Withdrawal of penis just before ejaculation (orgasm or climax) though practiced is not reliable, the failure rate of this method (coitus interruptus) being about 20%.

BARRIER METHODS (CONDOM AND DIAPHRAGM)

- Since it is very cheap and effective, the condom (a rubber sheath worn over the penis during coitus), is the most widely used method by the males.
- An added advantage is the protection it gives to the male against sexually transmitted diseases (STDs) like acquired immunodeficiency syndrome (AIDS), hepatitis, syphilis, and gonorrhea.
- A similar barrier, the rubber diaphragm, is fitted over the cervix by the female.
- In addition to these mechanical barriers, a spermicidal jelly is used by many couples at the same time.

USE OF SPERMICIDAL AGENTS

Use of creams, jellies, foams, suppositories, etc. in the female before coitus, and vaginal douches after intercourse may be combined with barriers.

INTERRUPTION OF THE NORMAL PATHS OF SPERMS OR OVUM (SURGICAL STERILIZATION)

- Interrupting the normal paths of sperm or ovum by vasectomy in males and tubectomy in females, appear to be the ideal methods suitable for our poor and illiterate population.
- However, restoration of the patency of these tubes, if required later on, has few chances of success.

INTRAUTERINE DEVICES

- Intrauterine devices (IUDs) or intrauterine contraceptive devices (IUCDs) are foreign bodies (plastic or metal) that are placed in the uterus and left there. "Copper T" and "loop D" (stainless steel) are the common devices used. They possibly make the endometrium unsuitable for implantation of fertilized egg by causing "aseptic inflammation" and/or by increasing uterine motility.
- IUDs have long-term use (6–10 years), can be removed when desired, and are as effective as tubectomy (the copper in *copper T* may also be spermicidal).

ORAL CONTRACEPTIVES (HORMONAL METHODS)

- It has been known for long that various doses of synthetic estrogens and progesterone given during the first half of menstrual cycle inhibit release of FSH and LH by negative feedback. This, in turn, reduces the levels of the normal ovarian estrogens and progesterone, the midcycle LH surge does not occur, and ovulation is not triggered.
- Even if ovulation does occur, changes in cervical mucus and in the endometrium prove hostile for sperms and implantation.
- The pills are started early in the cycle, continued beyond the expected day of ovulation, and then stopped to allow menstruation to occur.
- The *contraceptive "pills"* are 100% effective and are used by millions worldwide. The hormonal methods include:
  - ***The classical pill***: It contains orally active progesterone like substance—gestagen, and a small dose of estrogen.
  - In addition to inhibiting ovulation, these pills also render the cervical mucus hostile to sperm penetration. They may also induce endometrial changes which prevent implantation of the fertilized egg.
  - ***The sequential pill:*** It has a high dose of estrogen for 15 days followed by estrogen plus gestagen for 5 days. This pill inhibits ovulation by suppressing both LH and FSH.
  - ***Luteal supplementation pill***: These pills contain low doses of gestagen throughout the entire cycle. It controls fertility without inhibiting ovulation. The hormone may be acting on the cervical mucus, or on the endometrium, or perhaps by reducing the motility of the fallopian tubes.
  - ***The "morning-after pill" (emergency contraception, EC):*** These pills have high doses of estrogens and progestin. They inhibit FSH and LH, and stop the secretion of ovarian estrogens and progesterone. The sudden fall of these hormones causes shedding of uterine endometrium, thus blocking implantation. When two pills are taken within 72 hours of unprotected coitus, and another two tablets after

another 12 hours, chances of pregnancy are greatly reduced.

Other Hormonal Methods

- Subcutaneous implantation of hormone-containing capsules (they slowly release the drug into the circulation and are effective for about 5 years).
- Intramuscular injection of progestin (e.g. Depo-Provera) every 3 months.
- Once-a-month intramuscular injection of estrogen and progesterone, skin patches containing these hormones, once a week for 3 weeks of the cycle.

QUESTIONS

Q.1. How can the time of ovulation be determined?

1. The anterior pituitary hormone FSH is responsible for the early maturation of the ovarian follicle, while LH is responsible for its final maturation.
2. A burst of LH secretion at the midcycle causes the release of the ovum and the initial formation of corpus luteum. It is important to know the time of ovulation for the rhythm method to be effective in preventing pregnancy.

The following methods are employed to determine the time of ovulation:

1. **Change in the basal body temperature:** A fairly reliable and convenient indicator of the time of ovulation is a rise in the basal body temperature at the time of ovulation. Using a thermometer with wide graduations, and before getting out of bed in the morning, the oral temperature is recorded every day and charted on a temperature chart. The temperature continues to fall during the first half of the cycle, and then it starts to rise from the time of ovulation till the onset of the next cycle, the difference being 0.5–1.0°C. The cause of temperature rise is probably the increase in progesterone secretion, since this hormone is thermogenic.
2. **Examination of cervical secretions:**
   a. 'Fern like' pattern of cervical secretions when a specimen is allowed to dry on a glass slide and is viewed under a low-power microscope just before ovulation due to crystallization of sodium chloride on mucus fibers.
   b. *Spinnbarkeit test* refers to the "stringy and stretchy" quality of cervical mucus at the time or just prior to ovulation under the influence of oestrogen.
3. **Mittelschmerz:** Some people may have pain in their lower abdomen during ovulation. This is called mittelschmerz pain. It may last a few minutes.

Q.2. What is meant by medical termination of pregnancy (MTP)?

- MTP, which stands for Medical Termination of Pregnancy, is a procedure of terminating pregnancy using medicines. In the early stages of pregnancy (7-9 weeks), it can be terminated with the help of medicine, otherwise, the surgical process is needed.
- If the length of pregnancy is not exceeded 20 weeks then, medical termination of pregnancy is legal in India.
- Legally, only the consent of a major pregnant woman is needed in terminating the pregnancy and no other person's consent needs to be obtained.

Q.3. How can safe period be determined when the menstrual periods are irregular?

If the periods are irregular, the safe period can be calculated as indicated by the following examples:

Woman A:

- Menstrual cycles are regular, the duration of a cycle is 29 days.
- *Menstrual cycle:* 29 days.
- *Ovulation:* 15th day of the cycle (14 days before the onset of the next cycle).
- *Safe period:* Extends up to 11th day and continues from 19th day onward to the end of the cycle.

Woman B:

- Menstrual cycles are *irregular*, the duration of cycles varies between 26 days and 33 days to calculate the safe period in women with irregular menstrual cycles during the preovulatory phase, 18 is subtracted from the shortest recorded cycle.
- During the luteal phase, 11 is subtracted from the longest recorded cycle.
- Safe period: 26 - 18 = 8 and 33 - 11 = 22. Therefore, in this woman, the safe period extends up to the 8th day of any cycle and continues from day 22 onward till the end of the cycle (the first day of the menstrual cycle is the day when the menstrual bleeding starts).

Clinical Examination

SECTION 3

- 3.1: History Taking and General Physical Examination
- 3.2: Clinical Examination of the Respiratory System
- 3.3: Clinical Examination of the Cardiovascular System
- 3.4: Clinical Examination of the Gastrointestinal Tract and Abdomen
- 3.5: Clinical Examination of the Nervous System

Introduction

- While making a diagnosis the first step is observation of the patient which includes history taking, physical examination and other investigations.
- The second step is interpretation of the obtained knowledge.
- General physical examination is an important part of clinical examination of the patient. It should be performed before proceeding to the systemic examination.

3.1: HISTORY TAKING AND GENERAL PHYSICAL EXAMINATION

STUDENT OBJECTIVES

After completing this practical, the student should be able to:

- Communicate with the patients properly and empathically.
- Take a detailed, relevant and proper history.
- Evaluate the signs pertaining to systemic examination.
- Perform general physical examination.
- Evaluate the systemic examination under inspection, palpation, percussion and auscultation wherever applicable.

PY11.13: Obtain history and perform general examination in the volunteer/simulated environment.

CLINICAL EXAMINATION

- The word "patient" is derived from the Latin "patiens" meaning sufferance or forbearance.
- The clinical examination in the outdoor clinic begins the moment the patient is seen by the doctor. It is important to make the patient relaxed and comfortable.
- There are two basic steps in clinical examination of a patient/subject:

I. **History taking:** It includes general and special interrogation.

II. **Physical examination:** It is an orderly examination for evaluation of the patient's body and its functions. It includes noninvasive methods, along with measurement of vital signs. It has two components:

1. **General physical examination**
2. **Systemic physical examination.**

HISTORY TAKING

History taking is perhaps the most important and skilled part of clinical examination. The patient is asked for a description of what has happened. The history taking includes:

a. Age and address
b. Marital status
c. **Social and occupational history:** History of smoking, alcohol, recreational drugs, accommodation and living arrangements, marital status, baseline functioning, occupation, pets and hobbies
d. History of previous illness, accidents, operation etc. should be recorded.
e. **Family history:** State of health of parents and siblings. Any cause of death in the family.

f. **Presenting complaints:** Allow the patient to tell his chief presenting complaints in his/her own words. These are the primary reasons for seeking medical help. Note them in chronological order. All symptoms may not be of equal diagnostic importance.

g. **History of present illness:** Its mode of origin and when it began. Did it start slowly or suddenly? The order in which the symptoms appeared and how they have progressed. Ask for any treatment received. Enquire about any loss of weight, appetite, and strength (Note reliability of information).
Ask! "When were you free of any illness?"

h. Treatment history

History taking, though considered easy and tedious by a new medical student, is perhaps the most important and skilled part of clinical examination.

PHYSICAL EXAMINATION

1. **General physical examination**
2. **Systemic physical examination.**

Prerequisites for a Satisfactory Physical Examination

1. Establish a good rapport (sympathy) with the patient. He/she will be relaxed and reassured.
2. The room should be comfortable, with adequate natural daylight as artificial light may mask the changes in skin color.
3. If the patient is a female, the husband, female relative or a female nurse must be present.
4. The patient should be asked to expose the area which is to be examined.
5. The doctor, if right handed, must always stand on the right side of the patient.

General Physical Examination

General physical examination (GPE) necessitates a general examination of the patient from head to toe in order to have vital information. This should include:

"PICKLE"—Pallor, Icterus, Cyanosis, Clubbing, Lymphadenopathy, and Edema

I. **Pallor:** It is the paleness of skin which is usually detected by retracting the lower eyelids and examining the lower palpebral conjunctiva **(Fig. 1)**. It is seen in conditions where the blood flow to the capillaries is diminished or when the hemoglobin content in the blood is decreased. The degree of pallor is expressed as Plus 1–Plus 3.
   - Pallor 0: No anemia
   - Pallor +: Mild anemia
   - Pallor ++: Moderate anemia
   - Pallor +++: Severe anemia.

II. **Jaundice/Icterus:** It is the yellowish discoloration of sclera, skin and mucous membrane of the body due to presence of excess bilirubin in the blood **(Fig. 2)**. While examining for icterus/jaundice the preferred site is sclera which is rich in collagen fibers. They have high affinity

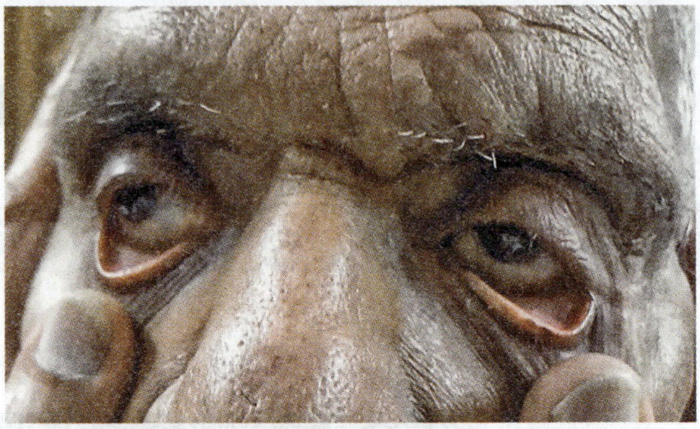

FIG. 1: Looking for pallor.

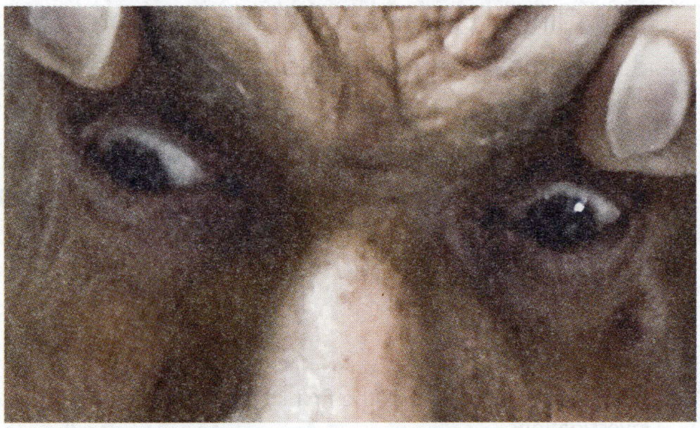

FIG. 2: Looking for icterus.

for bilirubin leading to yellow discoloration of sclera in jaundice. Normal serum bilirubin concentration—0.2 to 0.8 mg/100 mL of blood. When serum bilirubin levels exceed 2 mg% jaundice is said to appear clinically.

III. **Cyanosis:** It is the bluish discoloration of the skin and mucous membranes that occurs when the absolute concentration of deoxygenated/reduced hemoglobin is more than 5 g%. It is of two types:
   i. ***Central cyanosis*:** It is seen at the lips and tongue. Anemic or hypovolemic patients rarely have central cyanosis because severe hypoxia is required to produce the necessary concentration of deoxygenated hemoglobin. Patients with polycythemia can become cyanosed at normal arterial oxygen saturation.
   ii. ***Peripheral cyanosis*:** It is seen in the hands, feet or ears, usually when they are cold. It is also found with central cyanosis, but is most often seen with poor peripheral circulation due to shock, heart failure, peripheral vascular disease, Raynaud's phenomenon and venous obstruction, e.g. deep vein thrombosis.

IV. **Clubbing:** It is the bulbous enlargement of the soft parts of the terminal phalanges, the tissues at the base of the nail are thickened and the angle between the base of the nail and the adjacent skin of the finger is lost **(Fig. 3)**. Thus, the nail becomes convex both transversely and longitudinally. Clubbing can be detected by any of the following signs:
   i. **Fluctuation test:** Holding the base of the nail from both sides and gently press the tip of the nail to elicit fluctuation which increases in clubbing.

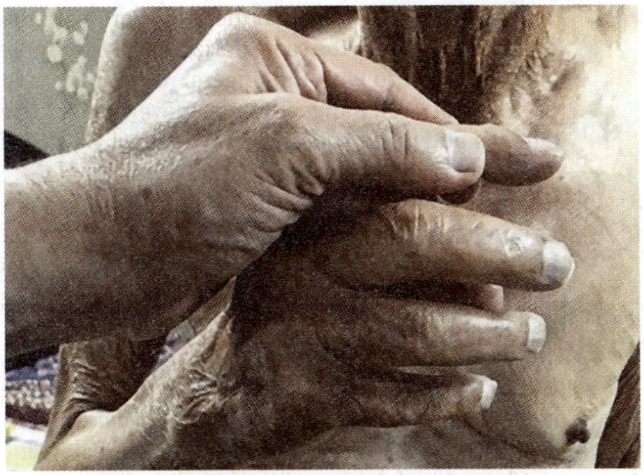

FIG. 3: Looking for clubbing.

ii. **Curving of the nails:** The nail becomes convex both transversely and longitudinally due to the hypertrophy of the nail bed tissue.

iii. **Schamroth's sign:** The two fingers are held together with their nails facing each other a space is seen at the nail fold, which is lost in clubbing.

iv. **Base angle:** Normally the angle between the base of nail and the adjacent portion of the dorsum of the terminal phalanx is an obtuse angle of about 160°. However in clubbing this angle gets obliterated and increases.

Causes of clubbing—cyanotic heart disease, bronchiectasis, bronchial carcinoma, inflammatory bowel disease and infective endocarditis.

Degree of clubbing:

- *1st degree*: Increased fluctuation of the nail bed.
- *2nd degree*: Curving of nail bed along with increased fluctuation of nail bed.
- *3rd degree*: Increased fluctuation, increased curving and obliteration of base angle of nail.
- *4th degree*: All of the above plus subperiosteal thickening of the wrist and ankle bones along with the presence of definite transverse ridge at the root of the nails.

V. **Lymphadenopathy:** Lymph nodes may be palpable in normal people, especially in the submandibular, axilla and groin. Areas on both the sides should be examined. Lymph nodes in the neck are examined by standing behind the subject keeping the head slightly flexed. The different groups of lymph nodes are examined. Distinguish between normal and pathological nodes. Pathological lymphadenopathy may be local or generalized, and is of diagnostic and prognostic significance in the staging of lymphoproliferative diseases and other malignancies. The lymph nodes are palpated to check for their size, shape, consistency, mobility and tenderness. The most common cause of lymphadenopathy in India is tuberculosis. Few other causes are: Connective tissue disorder (e.g. systemic lupus erythematosis and sarcoidosis), endocrine disorders (e.g. Addison's disease) and drug induced (e.g. phenytoin, carbamazepine).

Size

Normal nodes in adults are seldom greater than 0.5 cm in diameter.

Consistency

Normal nodes feel soft. In Hodgkin's disease they are characteristically "rubbery", in tuberculosis they may be "matted", and in metastatic cancer they feel hard.

Tenderness

Acute viral or bacterial infection, including infectious mononucleosis, dental sepsis and tonsillitis, causes tender, variably enlarged lymph nodes.

Fixation

Lymph nodes fixed to deep structures or skin suggests malignancy.

VI. **Edema:** It is the swelling of skin and subcutaneous tissues due to accumulation of free fluid in excess in the interstitial tissue spaces. It is diagnosed by usually pressing the skin against the bone in the dependent parts of the body. It can be of two types:

i. **Pitting edema:** Congestive heart failure, cirrhosis of liver, nephrotic syndrome (facial edema)

ii. **Non-pitting edema:** Filariasis

- ***General appearance:*** Does the patient look healthy, unwell, or ill? Apparent age, weight and height, body build, body mass index, and nutrition. Note if breathing is comfortable.

  $$BMI = Weight (kg)/[Height (m)]^2$$

- ***Posture in bed and gait:*** In congestive heart failure there is orthopnea (i.e. the patient is more comfortable sitting rather than lying down). Some diseases are obvious by the gait, e.g. drunken *(zig-zag)* gait of cerebellar ataxia, and the rigid gait of Parkinsonism.
- ***Face and speech:*** Note the expression, symmetry, and color of the face. Does he/she speak or is silent? Is the speech hysterical? Eyeballs, facial palsy, exophthalmos, nose, and lips.
- ***Skin:*** Look for the color, texture, eruptions, petechiae, and scars. There is pallor in anemia (color of oral mucosa and creases of palm give a better idea of paleness); yellowish in jaundice and hypercarotenemia; and bluish in cyanosis (due to presence of at least 5.0 g of reduced Hb in the skin capillaries).
- ***Neck:*** Look for enlarged lymph glands; thyroid; pulsations of vessels, venous distension; position of trachea.
- ***Chest:*** Shape; deformities, curvature of spine at the back. Note rate of breathing (Normal = 12–16 breaths/min).

  Odor of breath; breath may be sweet and sickly in diabetes and ketosis; ammoniacal in uremia; halitosis (bad breath) in poor dental and oral hygiene.
- ***Abdomen:*** Contour, skin, scars, pulsations.
- ***Hands:*** Look for attitude, tremors, skin, nails, clubbing of fingers, trophic changes.
- ***Extremities:*** Arms, legs, hands, feet, scars, wounds, deformities, edema, prominent leg veins.

- ***Vitals***:
  - ***Pulse rate***: Count for 1 minute. Note if there is tachycardia or bradycardia (Normal range = 60–90 beats/min).
  - ***Temperature***: Keep the thermometer under the tongue for 2 minutes (Normal range = 97.2°–98.8°F). Oral cavity temperature approximated the core body temperature. (In children, the axillary or groin temperature is less by about 1.0°F).
    - Core temperature refers to the measurement of temperature of body cavities.
    - Hyperpyrexia is said to occur when the core temperature exceeds 107°F.
    - Hypothermia is said to occur when the core temperature goes down below 95°F.
  - ***Respiratory rate***: The respiration is counted for full 1 minute by observing the subjects abdominal movements (Normal range = 12–16 respirations/min)
  - ***Blood pressure***: Record the blood pressure after a short period of rest (Experiment 2.6).

The average SBP (systolic blood pressure) in a healthy adult is 100–140 mm Hg, the average diastolic blood pressure (DBP) is 60–90 mm Hg. In elderly both the values, i.e. SBP and DBP reach or even exceed the higher figure. In children both SBP and DBP approximate to be lower figure. The difference between SBP and DBP is called pulse pressure. Normal pulse pressure is 30–60 mm Hg.

Outline of general physical examination:

General examination	*General appearance*
• General appearance • Hands and arms • Skin • Face • Eyes • Mouth • Neck • Edema • Lymph nodes • Vital signs – Temperature – Pulse – Respiration rate – Blood pressure	• General state of health: Healthy/ill/comfortable/distressed • Body built and nutritional status – Height – Weight – BMI – Obese/lean – Tall/short – Muscular/asthenic/cachexic • State of awareness or level of consciousness • Facial feature/expression/mood/attitude • Speech (tone/voice) • Position/posture and gait • Personal hygiene • Breath/odor

Systemic Physical Examination

1. **Inspection** is a very essential faculty in medical practice that has to be cultivated rigorously, is the hallmark of inspection. It should be carried out in good light, the part of the body should be fully exposed, and looked at from different angles. Note if there are any changes in the body that deviate from the normal.
2. **Palpation** (-palp = gentle touching)
   - It means touching and feeling a part of the body with the flat surfaces of your palm and fingers. The principle is to mold your hand to the body surface.
   - Place your right hand flat on the body part, with the forearm and wrist in the same horizontal plane. Apply a gentle pressure with the fingers, moving them at the metacarpophalangeal joints. Never "poke" the patient's body with your fingers. The ulnar border of your hand may also be used for palpation.
3. **Percussion** (percur- = beat through)
   - Percussion means giving a sharp tap or impact on the surface of the body, usually with the fingers. Its purpose is to set up vibrations in the underlying tissues, and listen to the echo.
   - The tip of the bent middle finger of the right hand strikes, two or three times, the middle phalanx of the middle finger (pleximeter finger) of the left hand placed firmly in contact with the skin. Two things are noted:
     - Character of the sound produced
     - The characteristic feeling imparted to the pleximeter finger.
4. **Auscultation** (auscult- = listening). It refers to listening to body sounds to assess the functioning of certain organs. A stethoscope is used to amplify the sounds. For example, listening to heart sounds and breath sounds.

COMMONLY USED TERMS

1. **Symptoms:** These are subjective disturbances in the body function resulting from disease, which a patient experiences and which cause him to feel he is not well. These subjective changes that are not visible to an observer are called symptoms.
2. **Physical signs:** These are objective marks of diseases that a trained person can see and measure using his senses, generally unaided, though the aid of a stethoscope is usually allowed under this definition (e.g. fever, high BP, and paralysis).
3. **Syndrome:** Constellation of symptoms which occur together and characterize a particular abnormality or condition.
4. **Disorder:** The term refers to any abnormality of structure or function.
5. **Disease:** It is a more specific term for an illness characterized by specific recognizable set of symptoms and signs. Thus, it is any specific change from the state of health. A disease may be a local one, affecting a part or limited region of the body. Or it may be a systemic disease affecting either the entire body or several parts of it.
6. **Diagnosis** (Dia- = through; -gnosis = knowing). It is the science and skill of distinguishing one disorder or disease from another. The patient's history of illness and physical examination (and sometimes various tests), and their correct interpretation builds up a picture of the patient's illness. Sometimes the diagnosis is only "provisional", which is usually confirmed after laboratory and/or special investigations.
7. **Prognosis:** After considering all aspects of a patient's illness, the doctor may be able to give an opinion about the possible future course of the disease, i.e. the degree of cure possible (or otherwise). This comment on the future course of the disease is called prognosis.

8. **Vital signs:** This term refers to the four signs which can be seen, measured, and recorded in a living person. They include: **pulse, blood pressure, respiratory rate,** and **body temperature**. The former three are controlled by the "vital centers" located in the medulla, while the body temperature is controlled by the hypothalamus.

The vital signs must always be checked during general physical examination.

QUESTIONS

Q.1. What is the importance of general physical examination?
Q.2. How do you detect jaundice clinically?
Q.3. What are the causes of yellowish discoloration of skin and mucous membrane?
Q.4. Define cyanosis. What are the different types of cyanosis? Discuss its physiological basis.
Q.5. What is clubbing? How is it detected?
Q.6. What are the causes of clubbing?
Q.7. What are vital signs?
Q.8. Define edema. What are the different types of edema?
Q.9. What is lymphadenopathy?

Refer text for answers to Q.1 to Q.9

3.2: CLINICAL EXAMINATION OF THE RESPIRATORY SYSTEM

STUDENT OBJECTIVES

After completing this practical, the student should be able to:
- Carry out a systematic examination of the respiratory system.
- Name the important signs and symptoms of respiratory diseases.
- List the abnormal forms of the chest.
- Perform percussion correctly.
- Describe the differences between vesicular and bronchial breath sounds.
- Describe the importance of vocal fremitus and resonance.

PY6.9: Demonstrate the correct clinical examination of the respiratory system in a normal volunteer or simulated environment.

IMPORTANT SIGNS AND SYMPTOMS OF RESPIRATORY DISEASE

1. **Breathlessness (dyspnea):** It is an unpleasant awareness of the necessity for greater respiratory effort and it may be present on effort or at rest.
2. **Cough:** It may be dry or productive of sputum.
3. **Expectoration (sputum):** Its amount, color, watery or frothy; it may contain pus or blood.
4. **Hemoptysis:** It means coughing out of blood in the sputum. It should never be dismissed lightly without proper evaluation because the blood may come from the gums or nose, or even from the stomach (hematemesis).
5. **Wheezing:** The patient must be asked if any sounds come from the lungs during breathing.
6. **Pain:** Apart from pain from the muscles and skeleton of the chest, pain due to lung disease comes usually from the pleura.
7. **Other symptoms include:** Fever, cyanosis, and clubbing of fingers. Some of these are also encountered in nonrespiratory diseases.

Note: Always take family history, occupational history and smoking history.

- **Important landmarks:** Vertical lines dawn on the front and back of the thorax constitute some of the important landmarks.
- These are: midsternal line; midclavicular lines; anterior axillary, midaxillary, and posterior axillary lines; mid spinal and midscapular lines **(Fig. 4)**.

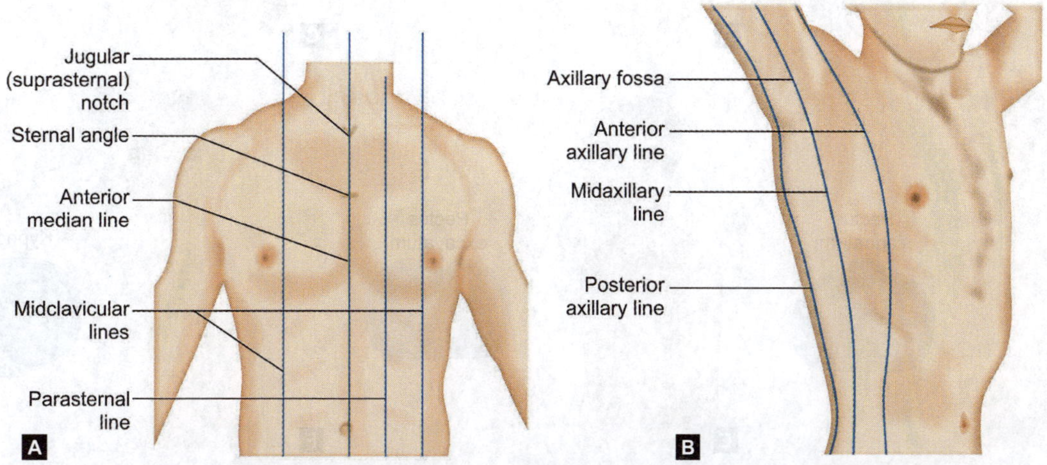

FIGS. 4A AND B: Important landmarks (vertical lines) of the respiratory system.

EXAMINATION OF THE RESPIRATORY SYSTEM

This is to be done as under the following headings:

- **General physical examination:** Any systemic examination is preceded by general physical examination. Already discussed in the previous chapter.
- **Systemic examination:** This is to be done under the following headings:
  - **Inspection**
  - **Palpation**
  - **Percussion**
  - **Auscultation**

INSPECTION

The subject is examined in good light, stripped to the waist, and preferably in a sitting position. Observe carefully the positions of trachea and apex beat, and note whether engorged veins are present over the chest. The chest should be inspected from all sides, especially from behind and over the shoulders.

Form of the Chest

- The normal chest is bilaterally symmetrical and there are no large bulges or hollows.
- It is elliptical in shape, the normal ratio of transverse to anteroposterior diameter **(Hutchinson's index)** being 7:5, (the chest becomes barrel shaped in emphysema). A depression runs down the sternum, and is most marked at its lower end.
- ***Abnormal forms of chest*** include—alar and flat chests due to poor posture, rachitic chest in rickets, pigeon breast chest; and barrel- shaped chest in emphysema **(Fig. 5)**.

Respiratory Movements

1. Rate:

- The rate should be counted surreptitiously, while keeping the fingers on the radial pulse, because a nervous patient may breathe rapidly and irregularly. The rate, depth, rhythm, and type (manner) of breathing should be noted.
- The normal rate of respiration is 14–20 breaths/min, one inspiration and one expiration making up one cycle. It is faster in children and in old age.
- The rate bears a definite ratio to pulse rate of about 1:4, which is usually constant in the same person. The rate and depth usually increase or decrease together.
- They are regulated by the respiratory center via reflexes arising in the thorax and the great vessels.

2. Depth:

- The rate and depth usually increase or decrease together. They are regulated by the respiratory center via reflexes arising in the thorax and the great vessels.
- Look whether the respiration is shallow or deep. In bronchial asthma, the respiration is shallow and it is deep when there is brain damage or uremia.

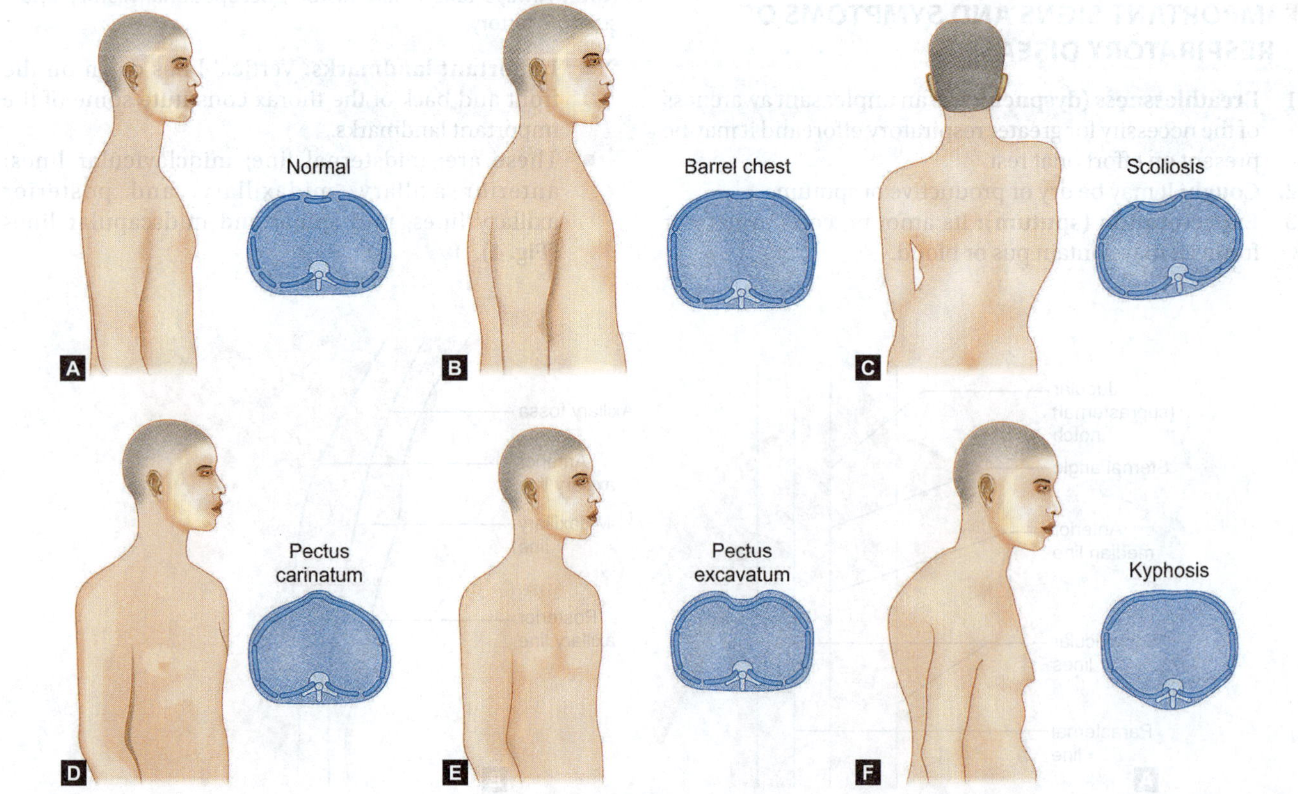

FIGS. 5A TO F: Shapes of chest.

3. **Rhythm:**
   - Normal respiration is regular.
   - Irregular breathing may be seen during brain damage, after voluntary hyperventilation or in left ventricular failure. It may also occur in obstructive airway disease.
4. **Type (manner) of breathing:**
   - The respiration can be predominantly thoracic or abdominal.
   - In women the respiration is thoracoabdominal while in males it is abdominothoracic.
5. **Expansion of chest:**
   - Both sides move equally, symmetrically and simultaneously.
   - Asymmetric expansion of the lungs may be seen when the underlying lung is diseased.
   - Fibrosis, consolidation, collapse or pleural effusion can all decrease chest expansion on the affected side though other physical signs will also be present.

> **Note:** Inspiration is an active process and involves elevation of the thorax and forward movement of the abdomen. Expiration is passive and is associated with depression of ribs and abdominal wall. (The main muscle of inspiration is the diaphragm, supplied by phrenic nerves).

Position of Trachea and Apex Beat

Inspection may not show the position of trachea, though cardiac pulsation may be visible; the lowermost and outermost point on which would be the apex beat. It will be confirmed by palpation.

PALPATION

- For successful palpation the hands must be warm and used as gently as possible. The chest is palpated in the upper, middle, and lower regions, on the front and the back.
- The movements of the upper zones of the lungs are compared by placing the hands over the two apices from behind, and the thumbs are approximated in the midline on the back. The movement of the thumbs away from the midline, as the subject breathes deeply, indicates equal or unequal expansion.
- The middle and lower regions are palpated by placing the hands on either side of the chest, with fingers stretched out and the thumbs just touching in the midline. The excursion of each thumb away from the midline indicates the degree of expansion of the lungs.
- Palpation also detects subcutaneous emphysema (air in the tissues) which results from fracture of ribs and gives a characteristic spongy feeling.
- Before palpating the chest, it is essential to confirm the:
  a. ***Position of trachea:*** Feel the rings of trachea in the suprasternal notch with the tip of your index finger, and try to judge the space between it and the insertion of sternomastoid muscle on either side of it. Normally, the trachea is in the midline or slightly to one side. However, in diseases, it may be pulled to the affected side (fibrosis, lung collapse), or pushed away from the affected side (pneumothorax, pleural effusion).
  b. ***Position of apex beat:*** (See next experiment for locating its position). Displacement of trachea and apex beat indicates shifting of the mediastinum.
  c. ***Presence of lymph glands:*** Note the presence or absence of lymph glands in the axillary and supraclavicular regions, because these may be the only evidence of carcinoma of the lungs.
  d. ***Expansion of chest:***
     - The expansion of the chest when measured with a tape placed around the chest just below the level of the nipples is 4–8 cm after a deep breath.
     - Chest expansion is tested by placing the fingertips of either hand at the patient sides in such a way that the tips of the two thumbs meet in the midline.
     - The patient is then asked to inspire deeply. The increase in distance between the thumbs indicates the extent of chest expansion (**Figs. 6A and B**).
  e. ***Palpate the chest for vocal fremitus***
     - ***Vocal fremitus:*** The detection of vibrations transmitted to the hands from the larynx through bronchi, lungs and chest wall during the act of phonation is called vocal fremitus.

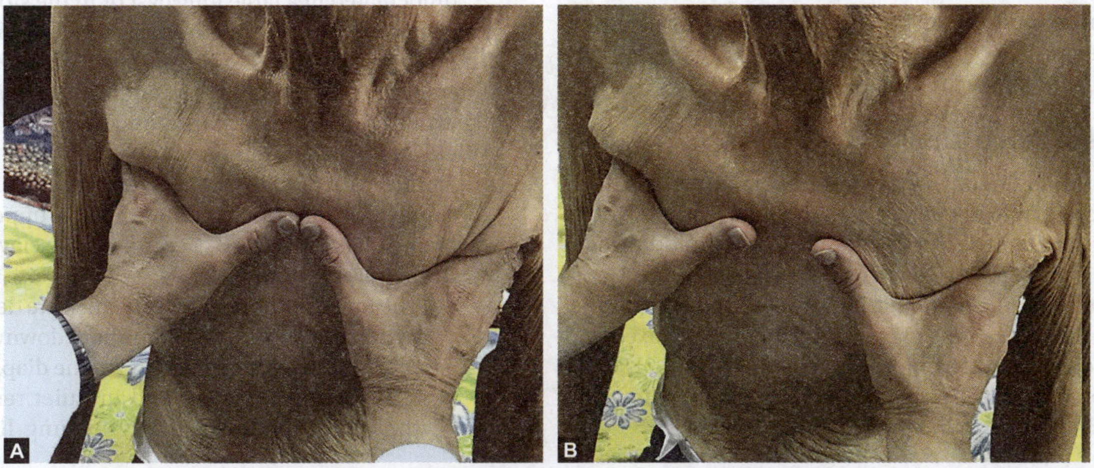

FIGS. 6A AND B: Chest expansion.

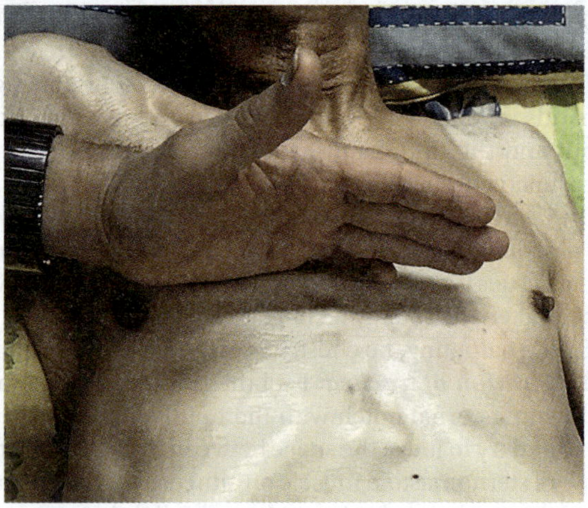

FIG. 7: Vocal fremitus.

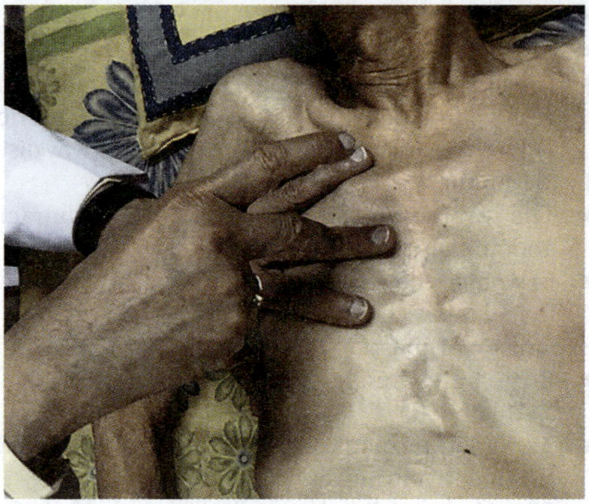

FIG. 8: Percussion.

- The palm, or the ulnar border of the hand which is more sensitive, is placed on the intercostal spaces while the patient is asked to say "ninetynine", "one-two-three", or "ek-do-teen", once or twice.
- The vibrations felt by the hand are compared on identical points, from above downward, on the front, axillary region, and on the back of the chest.
- Vocal fremitus may be ***diminished*** if the voice is feeble, or when a bronchus is blocked by a new growth which interferes with the passage of vibrations, or when the vibrations are dampened by fluid or air in the pleural cavity.
- It is ***increased*** when the vibrations are better conducted, as through solid lung (consolidation due to pneumonia) **(Fig. 7)**.

f. ***Tenderness:*** Palpate all the regions of the chest wall to elicit tenderness if any. It may be seen in injury or inflammatory conditions of the chest wall.

PERCUSSION

- Percussion is the procedure employed for setting up artificial vibrations in a tissue by means of a sharp tap, usually delivered with the fingers **(Fig. 8)**. Percussion is done for determining:
  a. The condition of the underlying tissues—lungs, pleura.
  b. The borders of the lungs.

Method of Percussion

- The middle finger (pleximeter finger) of the left hand is placed firmly in contact with the skin. The back of its middle phalanx is struck with the tip of the middle finger of the right hand, two or three times.
- The striking finger should lie, almost over and parallel to the pleximeter finger as it falls, should be relaxed and should not be lifted more than 2 or 3 inches. It must also be lifted clear immediately after the blow to avoid damping of the resulting vibrations.
- The movement of the hand should be at the wrist and not at the elbow or shoulder.
- If the percussed organ or tissue lies superficially, the percussion should be light, but heavier if the tissue lies deeper.

The following two things are to be noted while percussing:

1. **The character of the sound produced.** It differs in quality and quantity over different tissues.
   - Air containing organs, such as lungs, produce a note (sound) called **resonance.**
   - The opposite of resonance, i.e. lack of note, called **dullness**, is found over solid viscera like heart and liver, or when the lung becomes solidified as in pneumonia, growth, or fibrosis.
   - An increase in resonance (**hyperresonance**) though difficult to detect may be produced when there is air in the pleural cavity, i.e. pneumothorax.
   - An extreme form of **dullness** is called **stony dullness,** in which a feeling of resistance is felt by the tapping finger along with a dull note; such dullness is found by percussing over the thigh, and is encountered in pleural effusion.
   - The percussion note changes to **tympani** when air fills the pleural cavity, or when air is contained unloculated in a large lung cyst or in the stomach.
2. **The characteristic feeling imparted to the pleximeter finger.** The student should practice percussing over different parts of his/her body, and over various objects like wooden and steel furniture, and so on.
3. **Apical and basal percussion:**
   - **Apical percussion:** It is carried out in the supraclavicular fossae to determine the upper borders of the lungs which lie 3–4 cm above the clavicles.
   - **Basal percussion:**
     - The lower limits of lung resonance are determined by percussion the chest from above downward, with the pleximeter finger parallel to the diaphragm.
     - With light percussion and in quiet respiration, the lower border of the right lung lies in the

midclavicular line at the 6th rib, in the midaxillary line at the 8th rib, and in the scapular line at the 10th rib.

- Posteriorly, on both sides, and anteriorly on the right side, the percussion note changes from resonance to dullness, while anteriorly on the left side, the percussion note changes from resonance to tympani.

4. **Precautions:** The following precautions are to be taken while doing percussion:
   a. When the boundaries of organs are to be defined, percussion is done from resonance to dullness and from more resonant to less resonant areas.
   b. The direction of percussion should be at right angles to the edge of the organ.

AUSCULTATION

Auscultation of Lungs and Trachea

- Before using the stethoscope for auscultation of the lungs, **one should listen carefully to the patient's breathing.** The breathing of a normal resting subject cannot be heard at a distance of more than a few inches from the face.
- Audible breathing at rest can be an important sign of airway disease (narrowing, secretions) and in some other conditions. For example, the breathing sounds may be: ***stertorous*** (snoring like; in coma due to any cause); ***gasping, grunting and sighing*** (exercise, pain, fear, grief); ***wheezing*** (usually louder during expiration, as in asthma); ***hissing*** (Kussmaul's breathing, as in acidosis of diabetes and uremia); and ***stridor.***

Important: Quiet environment and a properly-fitting stethoscope are essential. Crackling noises due to hairs on the chest, rubbing of chest-piece on the skin or against clothes, and shivering and heart sounds are to be ignored. Sitting position is ideal; when auscultating at the back, the patient is asked to lean forward, flex the head, and cross the arms in front.

- Auscultation is done all over the lungs—front, axillary regions and back—and sounds at corresponding points on the two sides are compared. Since breath sounds during quiet breathing are insufficient for study, the patient is asked *to breathe deeply through open mouth* (it is best to show this to the patient). The following points are noted:
   a. **The type or character of breath sounds**—whether *vesicular* or *bronchial.*
   b. **Intensity of breath sounds**—whether diminished or absent.
   c. **Added or adventitious sounds**—crepitations, rhonchi, pleural rub, etc.
   d. **Character of vocal resonance.**

Vesicular Breath Sounds

i. The vesicular breath sounds are produced by passage of air in the medium and large bronchi; they get

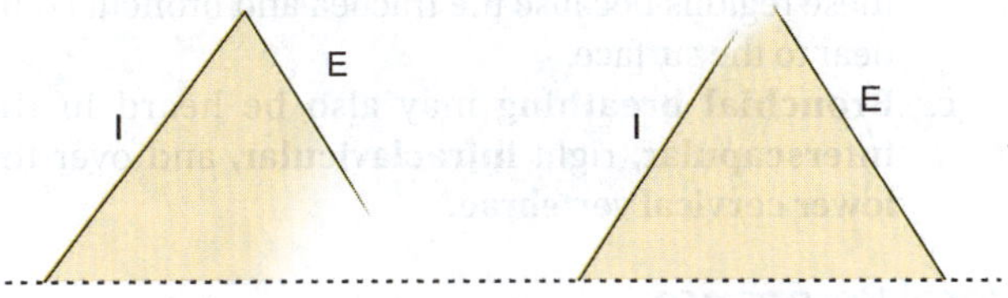

FIG. 9: The two main types of breath sounds. (I: inspiration, E: expiration)

filtered and **attenuated** while passing through millions of air filled alveoli before reaching the chest wall. These sounds are heard both during inspiration and expiration.

ii. The inspiratory sound is low pitched and rustling in character, and is always longer than the expiratory sound.
iii. The expiratory sound, which is softer and shorter, follows without a pause and is heard during the early part of expiration (it may commonly be inaudible) as shown in **Figure 9**.
iv. Normally, breathing over most areas of the chest is vesicular, and most typically so in the axillary and infrascapular regions.

Bronchial Breath Sounds

i. Bronchial breath sounds originate probably in the same medium and large bronchi, and replace vesicular sounds when the lung tissue between them and the chest wall becomes airless as a result of consolidation (as in pneumonia), tuberculosis, carcinoma and fibrosis. There is no filtration and attenuation of sounds because they pass directly from bronchi through diseased lung tissue instead of passing through air-filled alveoli.
ii. The bronchial breath sounds are loud, clear, hollow or blowing in character and of high frequencies.
iii. The inspiratory sound becomes inaudible just before the end of inspiration while the expiratory sound is heard throughout expiration. Thus, the bronchial breath sounds are loud and clear, the inspiratory and expiratory sounds being of about the same duration, and separated by a distinct pause.

Note

Tracheal breath sounds: The bronchial type of breathing resembles that heard over the trachea although tracheal sound is much harsher and louder. In fact, auscultation over the trachea can give the student an idea about bronchial breathing.

In children, the breath sounds normally are harsher than in adults, and are described as **puerile breathing,** and a similar type of breathing is produced by exercise.

iv. Bronchial breath sounds can normally be heard over the following areas:
   a. **Trachea and larynx:** The sounds are harsher and louder than those heard over diseased lungs.
   b. **Interscapular region and the apex of right lung:** There is more of bronchial element than vesicular in

these regions because the trachea and bronchi come near to the surface.

c. **Bronchial breathing** may also be heard in the **interscapular,** right **infraclavicular,** and over the **lower cervical vertebrae.**

Vocal Resonance

- Vocal resonance refers to the sounds heard over the chest during the act of phonation. The vibrations set up by the vocal cords are transmitted along the airways and through the lung tissues to the chest wall.
- The subject is asked to repeat "ninety-nine", or "ek-do-teen" in a normal, clear and uniform voice; and the sounds heard are compared on the identical regions on the two sides.

Intensity of Vocal Resonance

- The normal intensity of vocal resonance gives the impression of being produced near the chest piece of the stethoscope.
- When the intensity is increased, and the sounds appear to come from near the earpiece of the stethoscope, they are called ***bronchophony.*** It is heard over consolidation of lung tissue in pneumonia, over tuberculosis, or other resonating cavity or over lung apex when the upper lobe is collapsed and trachea is pulled to that side.
- When the words are clear and appear to be spoken (whispered) right into the ears, and the words can be clearly identified, the condition is called ***whispering pectoriloquy.***
- Vocal resonance may be decreased or even abolished when there is fluid in the pleural cavity, pneumothorax, or emphysema.

Adventitious or "Added" Sounds

The sounds which do not form an essential part of the usual breath sounds are called adventitious (extra) or "added" sounds. They are generally of three types:

1. ***Rhonchi (or wheezes):*** These are ***"dry sounds"*** and are produced by the passage of air through narrowed or partially blocked respiratory passages.
2. ***Crepitations (or "moist sounds"):*** They are discontinuous "bubbling" or "crackling" sounds produced by the passage of air through fluid in the small airways and/or alveoli. Crepitations may be "fine" or "coarse". (If you rub your hair between your thumb and a finger near your ear, the sound produced resembles fine crepitations).
3. ***Pleural rub (or "friction sound"):*** It is a "creaking" or "rubbing" sound produced by friction between the two layers of inflamed and roughened pleura. It is mainly produced during that part of respiration when the rough surfaces rub against each other, i.e. during deep inspiration. The pleural rub disappears when there is accumulation of fluid in the pleural cavity.

QUESTIONS

Q.1. Inspect the chest for its form and respiratory movements in the subject provided.

Q.2. Palpate the chest for position of trachea and respiratory movements in the subject provided.

Q.3. Palpate the chest for vocal fremitus.

Q.4. Percuss the lungs of the subject provided.

Q.5. Auscultate the lungs and trachea of the subject provided.

Q.6. Auscultate the areas where bronchial breath sounds can normally be heard.

Q.7. Auscultate the lungs for vocal resonance in the subject provided.

Q.8. What are adventitious or "added" sounds?

Refer text for answers to Q.1 to Q.8

OBJECTIVE STRUCTURED PRACTICAL EXAMINATION-I

Aim: To assess expansion of the chest.

Procedural steps: See text above.

Checklist:

1. Gives proper instructions to the subject. Expose the chest. (Y/N)
2. Places both hands on either side of the chest, with fingers stretched out on either side and thumbs just touching in the midline. (Y/N)
3. Asks the subject to take two or three deep breaths. (Y/N)
4. Observes the expansion of the chest by noting the movement of each thumb away from the midline. (Y/N)
5. Repeats the maneuver once again. (Y/N)

OBJECTIVE STRUCTURED PRACTICAL EXAMINATION-II

Aim: To test the vocal resonance in the subject provided.

Procedural steps: See text above.

Checklist:

1. Explains the procedure to the subject. (Y/N)
2. Applies the stethoscope to her ears and checks the diaphragm. (Y/N)
3. Places the diaphragm on the infrascapular region on the back. (Y/N)
4. Asks the subject to say 1, 2, 3 or 99 in a normal clear voice and listens to the sound. (Y/N)
5. Places the stethoscope on the other side of the chest and repeats the process. (Y/N)

3.3: CLINICAL EXAMINATION OF THE CARDIOVASCULAR SYSTEM

STUDENT OBJECTIVES

After completing this practical, the student should be able to:

- Name the important signs and symptoms of cardiovascular disease.
- List the headings under which the systematic examination of the cardiovascular system is to be carried out.
- Locate the apex beat and listen to the heart sounds.
- Locate the different cardiac areas.
- Differentiate between 1st and 2nd heart sounds.
- Explain the physiological basis of heart sounds and murmurs.

PY5.15: Demonstrate the correct clinical examination of the cardiovascular system in a normal volunteer or simulated environment.

IMPORTANT SIGNS AND SYMPTOMS OF CARDIOVASCULAR DISEASE

The important signs and symptoms of CVS disease include:

1. **Chest pain:** Chest pain is commonly a result of myocardial ischemia and may present as angina of effort, unstable angina, or myocardial infarction. Pericarditis and aortic aneurism are the other causes.
2. **Dyspnea:** It is an abnormal awareness of breathing occurring at rest or on low level of exertion.
   It is a major symptom of left heart failure. In **orthopnea,** the patient is more comfortable sitting than lying down.
3. **Palpitation:** Awareness of heart beat is common during exercise or heightened emotions. Under other circumstances, unpleasant awareness of heart beat may indicate abnormal rhythm. Extrasystoles, though common, rarely mean important heart disease. These are usually felt as "missed" or "dropped" beats. Rapid irregular palpitation is typical of atrial fibrillation.
4. **Tachycardia** and/or other arrhythmias, headache, dizziness, syncope, fatigue, postural hypotension, cyanosis, and vasovagal syncope are the other symptoms.
5. **Edema:** Subcutaneous edema that "pits" on pressure against a bone (pitting edema) is the chief feature of congestive heart failure. It is caused by salt and water retention which increase plasma volume and hence capillary hydrostatic pressure and filtration of excess fluid into the interstitial spaces.

Note: Cardiovascular disease may also be detected during a routine medical examination though the patient may be otherwise symptom free. Essential hypertension is such a disease and has, therefore, been called a "silent killer".

Anatomical Landmarks

Precordium: It refers to the anterior aspect of the chest wall overlying the heart. The positions of the valves and the different borders of the heart are delineated on the precordium **(Fig. 14)** for the clinical examination of cardiovascular system (CVS).

EXAMINATION OF THE CARDIOVASCULAR SYSTEM

This is to be done as mentioned below:

1. **General physical examination:** See practical 3.1
2. **Systemic examination:**
   a. **Examination of the arterial pulse:** This has been covered under practical 2.5.
   b. **Examination of venous pulse**
   c. **Examination of the precordium:** This is done under the following headings:
      - **Inspection**
      - **Palpation**
      - **Percussion** (Not very important in examination of the cardiovascular system. This is used to define the cardiac borders)
      - **Auscultation**

Examination of the Venous Pulse

Pulsations in the Neck

- Both arterial and venous pulsations may be seen in the neck, especially in thin persons. However, venous pulsations can be easily occluded by pressure with a finger above the clavicle.
- Arterial pulsations can be palpated and are stronger, increase with heart rate on mild exertion, and cannot be easily occluded.
- Jugular venous pulse differs from carotid arterial pulse in the following aspects **(Table 1)**. Jugular venous pulse (JVP) characteristics can also be remembered by the pneumonic **"POLICE"**, i.e.:
  Palpation—not palpable
  Occlusion—easily occluded
  Location—Between the heads of SCMs (Sternocleido-mastoid)
  Inspiration—Height of JVP drops with inspiration
  Contour—Biphasic waveform
  Erection/Position—Height decreases on sitting.

Table 1: Differences between carotid arterial pulse and jugular venous pulse.

Carotid arterial pulse	*Jugular venous pulse*
Palpable	Impalpable
Independent of respiration	Height of pulsation varies with respiration
Cannot be easily occluded	Can be easily occluded
Independent of abdominal pressure	Height increases with abdominal pressure
Independent of position of patient	Varies with position of patient
Rapid outward movement	Rapid inward movement
1 peak per heart beat	2 peaks per heart beat

Jugular Venous Pressure

- ***Examination of venous pressure***: The venous pressure can usually be estimated by watching the degree of distension of peripheral veins, especially the neck veins. For example, **in normal, resting, sitting individuals, the neck veins are not distended**. However, when the right atrial pressure rises, as in congestive heart failure, the veins become distended.
- The pressure in the right internal jugular vein is studied to assess the jugular venous pressure.
- The **external jugular vein,** a superficial vein, begins in the parotid gland near the angle of the jaw, descends through the neck across the sternomastoid muscle to empty into the subclavian vein.
- The **internal jugular vein** (the larger of the two veins) passes down the neck, from near the ear lobe and behind the angle of the jaw, lateral to internal and common carotid arteries and medial to clavicular head of sternomastoid muscle to empty into the subclavian vein.
- Though both veins act as a manometer for the right atrium, the internal jugular vein is almost in line with the right atrium and acts as a better manometer. It reflects all atrial pressure changes, thus providing important information about this pressure, which represents the "central venous pressure". Therefore, for JVP, one should not rely on external jugular vein.
- Since the venous pulse is not usually visible or palpable, it is obliterated by finger pressure just above the clavicle. The venous pressure also rises temporarily after manual pressure on the right upper abdomen (hepatojugular reflux).

Procedure for Examination of JVP

- The subject is made to lie on his back, with the upper part of the body supported at an angle of 45° to the horizontal **(Fig. 10)**, with the chin pointing slightly to the left.
- The neck veins are then inspected carefully. Normally, slight pulsations in the neck veins are seen just above the clavicle. This level is the same as the sternal angle (angle of Lewis) whatever the position of the thorax.

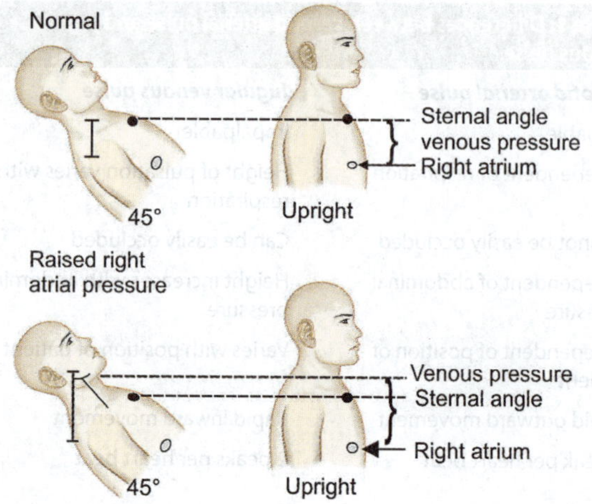

FIG. 10: Jugular venous pressure (see text for details).

- The vertical distance between the right atrium and the sternal angle indicates the mean hydrostatic pressure, which is normally 2–3 cm of water (1–2 mm Hg). The veins are then inspected in the upright position.
- Normally, no pulsations are visible. In right heart failure, however, the right atrial pressure, and thus the jugular venous pressure is raised, the veins are full and show pulsations even in the upright position.
- Identify the highest point of venous pulsation. Extend a long rectangular card/ruler horizontally from this point and a centimeter ruler vertically from the sternal angle (make an exact right angle)
- Measure the vertical height (in centimeters) above the sternal angle where the horizontal card meets the ruler.
- Add to this distance 4 cm (the distance from the sternal angle to the center of the right atrium).
- If the pulsations are not seen normally manual pressure can be applied over the right upper abdomen for 5–10 seconds **(hepatojugular reflux)**. This increases the venous return and thereby increases the right atrial pressure.
- **Normal JVP:** 6 to 8 cm above the right atrium.
- **Abnormal/elevated JVP** is >9 cm above the right atrium (>4 cm above the sternal angle).

Jugular Venous Waveform (Fig. 11)

The normal waveform consists of:

1. **Three positive waves—**
   - *"a" wave*: It is due to atrial systole. It occurs just before the first heart sound. Prominent "a" wave is seen in conditions when there is restriction of blood flow from the right atrium to the right ventricle. Cannon waves or giant "a" waves are produced when the right atrium contracts against a closed tricuspid valve, e.g. in complete heart block. The "a" wave disappears in atrial fibrillation.
   - *"c" wave*: It is due to the bulging of the tricuspid valve (atrioventricular or AV valve) toward the atrium at the beginning of isovolumetric (isometric) phase of ventricular systole.
   - *"v" wave:* The "v" wave is caused by atrial filling during ventricular systole when the tricuspid valve is closed.

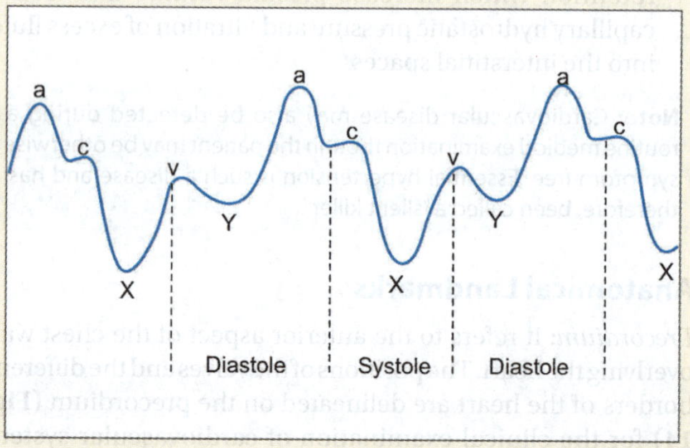

FIG. 11: The normal jugular venous pulse tracing showing three positive waves—(1) a, (2) c and (3) v and two negative waves or descents—(1) X and (2) Y.

A prominent "v" wave is characteristic of tricuspid regurgitation.

2. **Two negative waves or descents—**
   - "X" descent: The "a" wave is followed by the "X" descent which is interrupted by the "c" wave.
   - "Y" descent: The decline in atrial pressure as the tricuspid valve opens to allow ventricular filling produces the "Y" descent.

EXAMINATION OF THE PRECORDIUM

Inspection

Precordium is the area of the chest wall lying in front of the heart. The subject should be examined in the recumbent and sitting position, and in good light. The following observations are made:

A. **Shape of chest:** It is noted if there is any **deformity,** such as kyphosis (forward bending of spine), scoliosis (sideward bending of spine), or **bulging** of the precordium (enlargement of heart).

B. **Apex beat:** It is the **lowest and the outermost point of definite cardiac pulsation.** It is usually visible and palpable, and is located 8–10 cm (about 3.5–4 inches; according to body build) from the midsternal line, in the left 5th intercostal space. Normally, it is almost always within the midclavicular line (or nipple line in the male). The apex beat may not be visible in some normal persons because:
   - It may be located behind a rib.
   - The chest wall may be thick due to fat or muscle.
   - The emphysematous lung may cover part of the heart.
   - It may be hidden behind the breast.

C. **Inspection for other pulsations:** It is done in the precordium and nearby regions.
   - Arterial pulsations in the neck may be visible in hyperdynamic circulation, as in—anxiety, hyperthyroidism, aortic regurgitation, and hypertension.
   - Pulsations to the right or left of the upper sternum may be due to aortic aneurysm.
   - Enlargement of the right ventricle, or enlarged left atrium due to severe mitral regurgitation may cause pulsations in the left upper parasternal region.
   - Pulsations in the epigastrium are most commonly due to pulsations of abdominal aorta increased by emotional excitement in thin individuals, or enlargement of the right ventricle, or due to hepatic pulsations from tricuspid regurgitation.
   - Pulsations in the superficial arteries of thorax may be visible in coarctation of aorta.

Palpation

Position of the Trachea

Refer chapter—Examination of Respiratory System

Apex Beat

- For locating the position of the apex beat by palpation, the flat of the hand is placed over the heart to feel for the apical impulse.

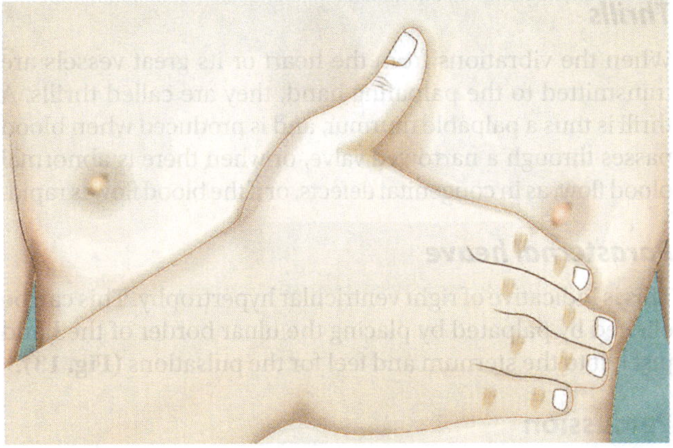

FIG. 12: Apex beat.

- Once the cardiac pulsation is felt, the ulnar border of the hand and then the tip of the index finger is used to locate and confirm the point of apex beat already defined by inspection **(Fig. 12)**. The apex beat should then be marked by a marker pen.
- **Position of apex beat:**
  - The apex beat is located 8–10 cm from the midsternal line, in the left 5th intercostal space. To locate the 5th space, the sternal angle (angle of Lewis)—the junction between manubrium sterni and body of sternum— is first located.
  - The second costal cartilage articulates with sternum at this level; the 2nd intercostal space is below the 2nd rib. The 5th space can now easily be counted downward and located.
  - If the apex beat is not palpable, the patient is then turned over to the left side, or sits up and bends forward. However, despite all efforts the apex beat may still not be palpable for the reasons already mentioned.

Note: One should always make it a habit, especially if the apex beat is not palpable in its usual place, to palpate the chest on both sides, with hands placed on either side, so as not to miss **dextrocardia**.

- **Character:** In normal persons, the apex beat gently raises the palpating finger. The strength of this thrust increases after exercise, in nervousness, in hyperthyroidism, or in left ventricular hypertrophy.

Significance of Palpating the Apex Beat

- Enlargement of the heart due to hypertrophy or dilatation may shift the apex beat.
- Pulling or pushing of the mediastinum due to lung disease may shift the position of the apex beat.
- Diffuse, sustained and more forceful thrust indicates left ventricular hypertrophy or hyperkinetic circulation.
- A "tapping" or "slapping" apex beat may be seen in mitral stenosis.
- If the apex beat is not palpable the causes may be: obesity, apex lying under a rib, dextrocardia, shift of the mediastinum to the right, pneumothorax, pericardial effusion, left sided pleural effusion.

Thrills

When the vibrations from the heart or its great vessels are transmitted to the palpating hand, they are called thrills. A thrill is thus a palpable murmur, and is produced when blood passes through a narrowed valve, or when there is abnormal blood flow, as in congenital defects, or if the blood flow is rapid.

Parasternal heave

This is indicative of right ventricular hypertrophy. This can be elicited by palpated by placing the ulnar border of the hand just left to the sternum and feel for the pulsations **(Fig. 13)**.

Percussion

- The ***upper border of the liver*** is first demarcated by starting the percussion downward along the midclavicular line till the resonance changes to dullness. Then, starting in the midaxillary line, two or three spaces above the liver dullness, percussion is carried out toward the right sternal margin.
- Normally, the **right border of the heart,** which is formed by the **right atrium,** lies behind the sternum **(Fig. 14)**.
- **Left border of the heart:** The position of the apex beat is first located. Percussion is done in the 5th, 4th, and 3rd intercostal spaces, starting in the left midaxillary line and going toward the heart till the notes change from resonance to dullness. Each point where dullness appears is marked with ink, and when these points are joined, the left border is marked.
- The area of cardiac dullness increases in pleural effusion, while it may be decreased in emphysema.
- It is of little significance and carried out sometimes to demarcate the extent of cardiac dullness in conditions like pericardial effusion. Nowadays, it has been replaced by the chest X-ray and echocardiography.

Auscultation

- It is good practice to palpate the carotid artery while listening to the heart sounds because the carotid pulse coincides with the first sound.

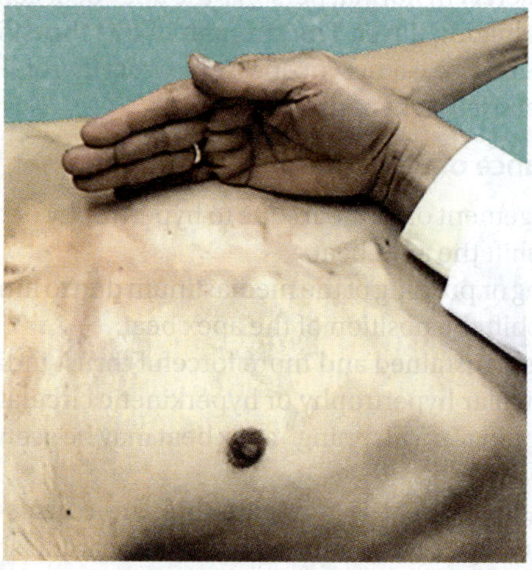

FIG. 13: Parasternal heave.

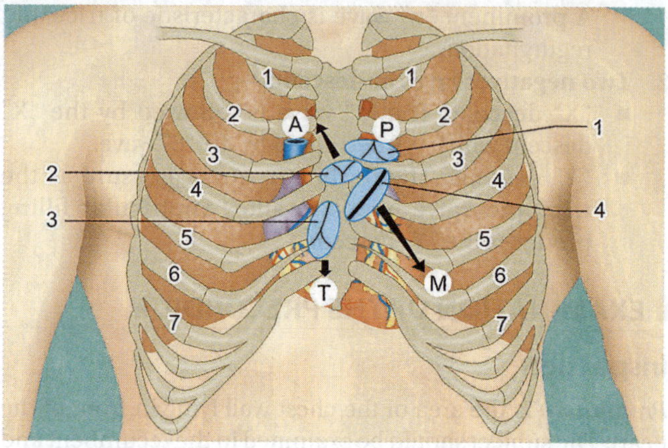

FIG. 14: Diagram showing the location of heart valves and the auscultatory areas. (1) Pulmonary artery valve, P—pulmonary area, (2) aortic valve, A—aortic area, (3) Tricuspid valve, T—tricuspid area, (4) Mitral valve, M—mitral area. The ribs are numbered from 1 to 7 on each side.

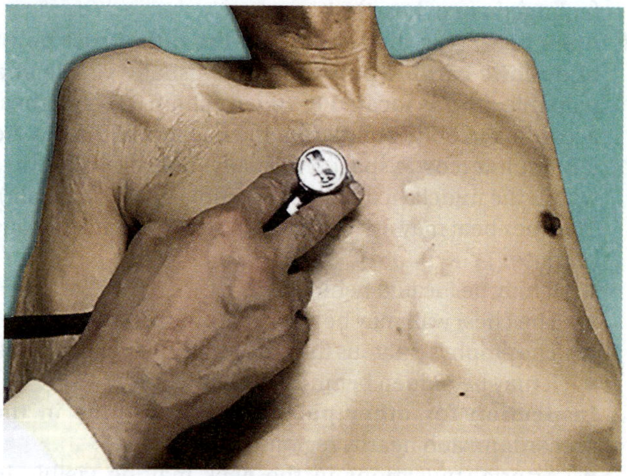

FIG. 15: Auscultation.

- As a routine, the four cardiac areas, **named according to the valves from which sounds arise (Fig. 15)**, are auscultated first. This is followed by auscultation in between these areas. The different areas are:
  i. **Mitral area:** The mitral area corresponds to the apex beat, i.e. 5th intercostal space about 8–10 cm from the midsternal line.
  ii. **Tricuspid area:** This area lies just to the left of the lower end of the sternum.
  iii. **Aortic area:** It lies to the right of the sternum in the 2nd intercostal space.
  iv. **Pulmonary area:** It lies to the left of the sternum in the 2nd intercostal space.

> **Note:** The corresponding valves of the heart do not lie under these areas; only the sounds produced by these valves are heard best over these areas.

- Over all these areas of auscultation, both the first and the second heart sounds are heard clearly, though the first sound is heard better in mitral and tricuspid areas while the second sound is heard better in aortic and pulmonary areas.

Differentiation between Heart Sounds

1. The heart sounds are **always** timed with the simultaneous palpation of carotid artery pulsation. The **1st sound coincides with the carotid pulse.** The 2nd sound follows a little later.
2. The **1st heart sound,** which is due to the simultaneous closure of the atrioventricular valves, is prolonged (0.1–0.17 sec), of low pitch (20–40 Hz) and booming in character. Phonetically, it is likened to the syllable *"LUB".* It coincides with the R-wave of the ECG and is best heard over the mitral area.
3. The **2nd heart sound,** which is due to the closure of aortic and pulmonary valves, is shorter, abrupt and clear, and of high pitch. Phonetically, it resembles the spoken sound *"DUP".* It may precede, coincide, or follow the T-wave of the ECG, and is best heard over aortic and pulmonary areas.
4. The time interval between the 1st and the 2nd heart sounds is shorter than the time interval between the 2nd sound and the next 1st sound. The sequence is thus: LUB DUB pause, LUB DUB pause, and so on as shown in **Figure 16.**
5. **3rd and 4th sounds:** These sounds occur during early and late diastole. They can best be heard with the bell of the stethoscope, with the patient leaning slightly forward. The 3rd sound is normally heard in children and in adults with hyperdynamic circulation. It is associated with rapid distension of the ventricles in early diastole. The 4th sound; whenever present is pathological. It is usually heard if the atrial systole is particularly forceful.

Note: The opening of the heart valves does not produce any sounds; only their closure produces sounds; e.g. clapping of the hands produces a sound, opening the palms does not.

Deviations of Heart Sounds from the Normal

a. **The intensity of the sounds** may be different. 1st heart sound may be accentuated in exercise, hypertension, anemia and beriberi (hyperkinetic). It may be diminished in shock, myocardial infarction and pericardial effusion. 2nd heart sound may be increased in systemic and pulmonary hypertension and diminished in aortic and pulmonary stenosis.

b. **The sounds may be split,** the two elements being very close together, which is a very important feature of split sounds. Splitting may be imitated by the syllables—*"LUB"* and *"DUP".* Split sounds may be audible in some normal young persons, though in the elderly, they may be pathologic as in bundle branch block.

c. **A triple rhythm** (gallop rhythm when the heart rate is above 100 beats/min) may be present. Splitting of heart sounds must be differentiated from triple rhythm which is produced by the addition of 3rd or 4th heart sounds to the normal 1st and 2nd sounds, and which may be imitated by *"LUB-DUP-DUP".* (Though phonocardiography shows that a 3rd and a 4th (atrial) sounds are generally present, they are difficult to hear with a stethoscope. When either of these are prominent and audible, they produce a triple rhythm, as in left ventricular failure).

d. **Adventitious or extra sounds:** These sounds may occur along with or replace the heart sounds.
- **Murmurs,** which are longer than heart sounds and may be systolic or diastolic, have a "blowing" or "swishing" quality. Their time of occurrence, region of maximum intensity, direction of propagation, and their character should be noted. They are caused by turbulent flow and eddie currents within the heart or great vessels. Valvular defects (change in size, deformities) are the usual causes of murmurs.
- **Thrill** is a palpable murmur.
- **Pericardial friction** or rub gives an impression of two pieces of dry leather being rubbed together. It occurs in pericarditis.
- **Opening snap** is commonly heard in mitral stenosis.
- **Ejection clicks** are produced due to stenosis of the aortic or pulmonary valve.
- **Mid-systolic clicks** are heard in mitral valve prolapse.

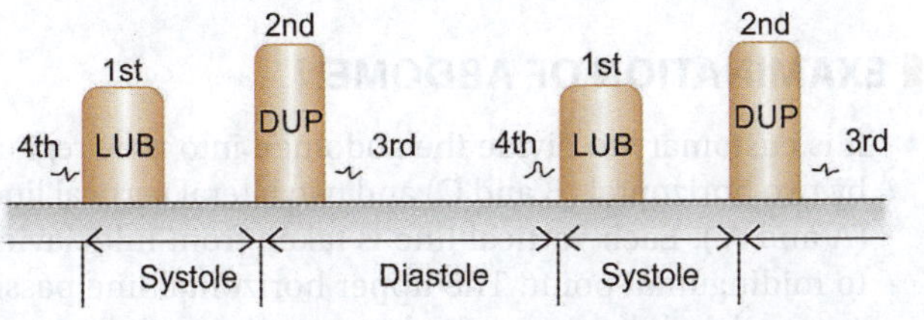

FIG. 16: Diagrammatic representation of heart sounds. LUB and DUP—phonetic representation of 1st and 2nd heart sounds respectively. The diagrammatic representation of 3rd and 4th heart sounds is to indicate that they have a lower frequency than the 1st and 2nd sounds.

QUESTIONS

Q.1. How would you proceed to examine the cardiovascular system?

Q.2. What is jugular venous pressure? How is it measured?

Q.3. Define the apex beat. What is its significance?

Q.4. What are the different heart sounds? Differentiate between first and second heart sound.

Refer text for answers to Q.1 to Q.4.

OBJECTIVE STRUCTURED PRACTICAL EXAMINATION-I

Aim: To locate the apex beat of the subject provided.

Procedural steps: See text above

Checklist:
1. Stands on the right side of the subject and exposes the chest completely and inspects the precordium to see if there is any cardiac pulsation. (Y/N)
2. Places the flat of the hand over the precordium, its base on the base of the heart and fingers toward the apex. (Y/N)
3. Uses the ulnar border of her hand to locate the apex beat. (Y/N)

4. Uses the tip of her forefinger to confirm the apex beat and marks it. (Y/N)
5. Counts the intercostals spaces and reports the exact position of apex beat. (Y/N)

OBJECTIVE STRUCTURED PRACTICAL EXAMINATION-II

Aim: To auscultate the mitral area for the heart sounds.

Procedural steps: See text above

Checklist:

1. Stands on the subject's right side and completely exposes the chest. (Y/N)
2. Checks for the correct functioning of the stethoscope. (Y/N)
3. Locates the apex beat and marks its position. (Y/N)
4. Applies the stethoscope to her ears and places its diaphragm on the mitral area. (Y/N)
5. Listens to the heart sounds and checks these with carotid artery pulse. (Y/N)

3.4: CLINICAL EXAMINATION OF THE GASTROINTESTINAL TRACT AND ABDOMEN

STUDENT OBJECTIVES

After completing this practical, the student should be able to:

- Indicate the different abdominal regions for clinical purposes.
- Name the important signs and symptoms of GIT disease.
- Palpate the abdomen for spleen, liver, and kidneys.
- Percuss the abdominal regions and demonstrate the presence of free fluid in the abdominal cavity.
- Auscultate the abdomen for bowel sounds and correlate these with intestinal dysfunction.

PY4.10: Demonstrate the correct clinical examination of the abdomen in a normal volunteer or simulated environment.

- The gastrointestinal tract (GIT) (about 7–8 m in length), along with its associated secretory glands, controls the processing of ingested material—its digestion, absorption and elimination.
- It should be noted that the signs and symptoms of GIT disease are commonly few and vague until the disease is advanced.
- The liver and pancreas are embryologically part of GIT, and for the sake of systematic examination, kidneys are considered as part of GIT.

IMPORTANT SIGNS AND SYMPTOMS OF GASTROINTESTINAL TRACT DISEASE

- Dysphagia—difficulty in swallowing
- Hematemesis—vomiting of blood
- Dyspepsia—indigestion
- Loss of appetite
- Burning sensation behind sternum or in epigastrium
- Flatulence
- Distension and tenderness of abdomen
- Nausea and Vomiting
- Diarrhea, constipation, rectal bleeding, melena ("black" stools)
- Jaundice, loss of weight and fever. Disorders of GIT are quite common in our country. Loss of appetite, indigestion, diarrhea, abdominal pain, etc. are the common complaints.
- The underlying causes of these complaints are easy to identify if proper history has been taken and physical examination carried out. The examination of the abdomen constitutes a major part of the clinical examination of GIT (alimentary system).
- Since the location of abdominal viscera is more or less anatomically exact, it is easy to identify the viscera involved in a particular patient.

Note: Oral cavity should always be checked for the health of the teeth and gums, tongue, tonsils and oropharynx.

Examination of the Gastrointestinal Tract

This is to be done as under the following headings:

1. **General physical examination:** Any systemic examination is preceded by general physical examination. Already discussed in the previous chapter.
2. **Systemic examination:** This is to be done under the following headings:
   - **Inspection**
   - **Palpation**
   - **Percussion**
   - **Auscultation**

Prerequisite for GIT Examination

- The subject should be lying flat on his back, arms by the sides, on a firm bed.
- The subject should be relaxed, with hips and knees flexed and head turned to one side.
- The subject is asked to take deep breaths through the mouth.
- The subject is examined from the right side.
- Before palpating the abdomen, the patient is asked about any pain or tenderness (pain on pressure) and such areas are the last to be palpated.
- Palpation is generally started in the left iliac fossa and worked anticlockwise to end in the suprapubic region.

EXAMINATION OF ABDOMEN

- It is customary to divide the abdomen into nine regions by two horizontal (B and C) and two lateral vertical lines (A and A'). Each vertical line is taken from midclavicle to midinguinal point. The upper horizontal line passes across the abdomen at the lowest points on the costal margin (10th costal arch). The lower horizontal line joins the tubercles of iliac crests.
- **Abdominal regions:** The regions marked by these lines are shown in **Figure 17**.

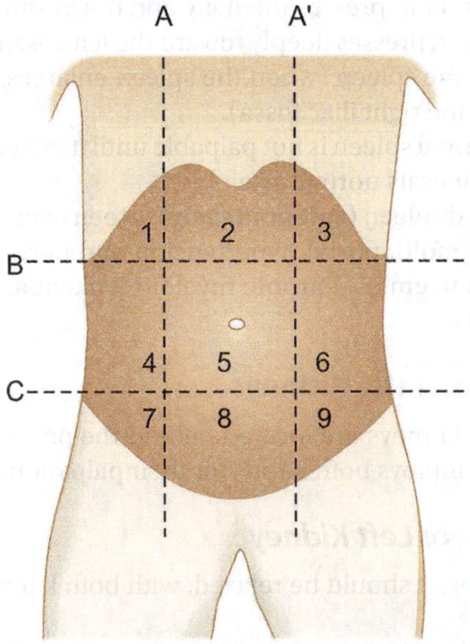

FIG. 17: Abdominal regions (see text for details).

- In the upper abdomen: (1) right hypochondrium; (2) epigastrium; (3) left hypochondrium.
- In the middle abdomen: (4) right lumbar; (5) umbilical; (6) left lumbar.
- In the lower abdomen: (7) right iliac fossa; (8) hypogastrium; (9) left iliac fossa.

- The value of these regions in clinical practice is to describe the position of pain, tenderness, rigidity, tumors, and so on. Since some of the viscera are mobile and constantly change position, these zones are not used as anatomical landmarks for them.

INSPECTION

On inspection of the abdomen the following are observed:

1. **State of the skin:** Whether stretched; presence of scars (previous operations) and striae (due to gross stretching); and pigmentation. Presence of prominent veins on the abdomen which is abnormal and is seen in obstruction of vena cava.
2. **Contour or shape:** There are three main types of abdominal contours:
   i. **Flat abdomen:** The rib margins and the abdominal wall are at about the same level.
   ii. **Globular or round abdomen:** A generalized and symmetrical fullness (i.e. a forward convexity) may be due to fat (obesity), fluid (ascites), flatus (gas), fetus (pregnancy), or feces (chronic constipation)—the five classical features. There may be sagging of the abdominal wall due to loss of muscle tone.
   iii. **Scaphoid abdomen:** The scaphoid, boat-shaped, or sunken abdomen shows a forward concavity. It is seen in extreme starvation, wasting diseases, carcinoma, especially of esophagus and stomach, and sometimes in very thin individuals.
3. **Abdominal asymmetry:** The normal abdomen is symmetrical. Asymmetric localized distention or bulging may be due to gross enlargement of liver, spleen, or ovary or due to tumors.
4. **State of umbilicus:** Normally, the umbilicus is slightly retracted and inverted or level with the skin surface. It may be everted or ballooned out in umbilical hernia, raised intra-abdominal pressure, or it may be transversely stretched in ascites (fluid in the peritoneal cavity).
5. **Movements of the abdominal walls with respiration:** The abdomen moves freely with respiration, rising gently during inspiration, and falling during expiration. (In females, the respiratory movements are mainly thoracic). The abdominal movements may be restricted in generalized peritonitis, inflammation of diaphragm, or injury to the abdominal muscles, and intense ascites.
6. **Visible pulsations:** Epigastric pulsations of abdominal aorta are frequently visible in nervous, thin individuals. Pulsations from a pulsating liver or from the right ventricle may also be seen in the epigastrium.
7. **Visible peristalsis:** Peristalsis may be visible as movement of a shadow on the abdomen in persons with thin abdominal wall, in malnourished children, and cachexia. Except for these examples, visible peristalsis may be an indication of pyloric, and small and large intestinal obstruction. One has to observe the abdomen from several angles to detect peristalsis. It may be induced by gentle kneading of the abdomen, or by applying a cold stimulus to the skin.
8. **Hernial sites:** The hernial sites in the groin should be checked for any swelling with straining or coughing.
9. **Presence of prominent veins:** Presence of prominent veins on the abdomen and chest wall is seen in obstruction of vena cava. Presence of prominent veins around the umbilicus (caput medusa) is seen in portal hypertension.

PALPATION

Palpation of the Abdomen for Liver (Fig. 18)

Note: Before palpating the abdomen, the patient is asked about any pain or tenderness (pain on pressure), and such areas are the last to be palpated.

The subject should be relaxed, with hips and knees flexed, and head turned to one side. The subject is asked to take deep breaths through the mouth. Palpation is generally started in the left iliac fossa, and worked anticlockwise to end in the suprapubic region.

Protocol

- The right hand is placed flat on the abdomen, with the wrist and the forearm in the same horizontal plane (one may have to bend down or kneel).
- The relaxed hand is "molded" to the abdomen, not held rigidly, with the fingers almost straight with slight flexion at the metacarpophalangeal joints (Fingers are never "poked" in the abdomen).
- On palpation the normal abdomen is soft and there is no tenderness.

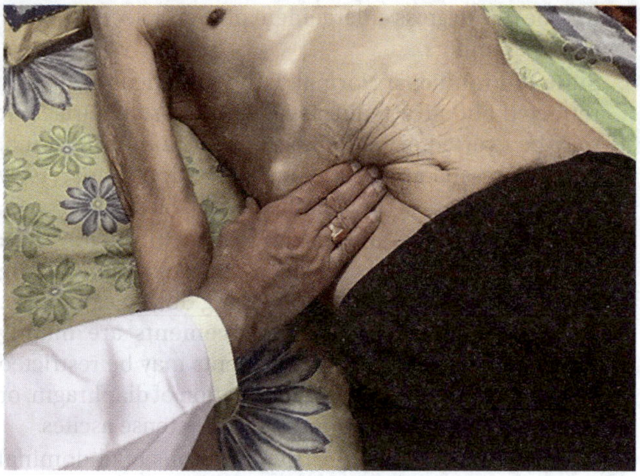

FIG. 18: Palpation for liver.

Palpation for Liver

- The palpation for the liver starts in the right iliac fossa and then gradually worked up to the right costal margin **(Fig. 18)**.
- As the patient inspires deeply, the fingers are pressed firmly inwards and upwards.
- If the liver is palpable, it meets the radial aspect of the index finger as a sharp regular border. It is sometimes palpable in children and adults, but generally it is palpable only when it is enlarged.
- If palpable, the character of its surface is noted—whether soft and smooth, very firm, or hard and irregular.
- The liver is enlarged **(hepatomegaly)** in congestive heart failure, amebic hepatitis, liver abscess, viral hepatitis, malignancy, leukemias, and so on.

Palpation of Spleen (Fig. 19)

1. The subject is relaxed, with the arms by the side, and hips and knees flexed to relax the abdominal wall.
2. The flat of the right hand is placed on the right iliac fossa and the left hand is placed over the left lowermost rib cage posterolaterally.

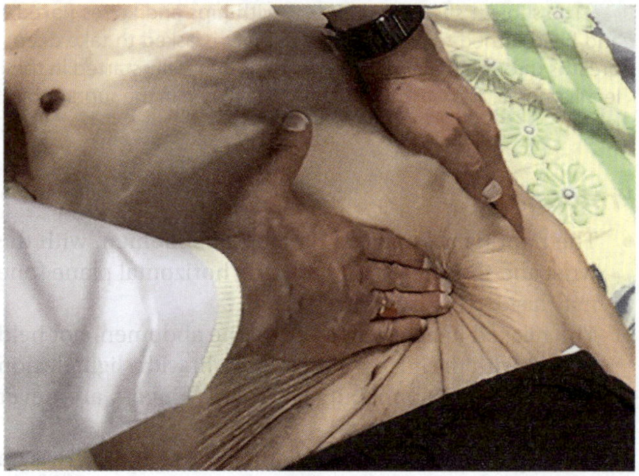

FIG. 19: Palpation for spleen.

3. The left hand presses medially and downward while the right hand presses deeply toward the left costal margin to feel for the spleen (when the spleen enlarges, it does so toward the right iliac fossa).
4. The normal spleen is not palpable until it increases two or three times its normal size.
5. Enlarged spleen **(splenomegaly)** is seen in malaria, kala-azar, typhoid, portal hypertension and portal cirrhosis, acute leukemias, chronic myeloid leukemia, and some anemias.

Palpation of the Kidneys

Since both kidneys are located behind the peritoneum, the examiner employs both hands for their palpation.

Palpation of Left Kidney

1. The subject should be relaxed, with both knees and hips flexed.
2. The right hand is placed anteriorly in the left lumbar region while the left hand is placed posteriorly under the costal margin.
3. As the subject takes a deep breath, the left hand presses forward, and the right hand presses backward, upward, and inward; and an attempt is made to feel for the kidney between the pulps of the fingers of the two hands.
4. The left kidney is not usually palpable unless enlarged or low in position.

Palpation of Right Kidney

1. The right hand is placed anteriorly in the right lumbar region with the left hand placed posteriorly in the right loin.
2. As the subject takes a deep breath, the left hand presses forward and the right hand pushes inward and upward; and an attempt is made to feel for the kidney between the fingers of the two hands.
3. The lower pole of the right kidney is commonly palpable in thin subjects as a smooth, rounded swelling which descends on inspiration.

PERCUSSION

- Using light percussion, all the nine regions of the abdomen are percussed systematically.
- A resonant (tympanitic) note is heard all over the abdomen except over the liver where the note is dull.
- The percussion note varies depending on the amount of gas in the intestines.
- Ascites, tumors, enlarged liver or spleen, enlarged glands, etc. give a dull note.
- **Clinical Significance of Percussion**
  - The principal value of abdominal percussion is to distinguish between distension due to gas, ascites, cystic or solid tumors.
  - The collection of free fluid in the peritoneal cavity is called **ascites**.
  - Approximately 500 mL of fluid must accumulate before it can be detected by physical examination.

- Ascites has to be differentiated from two other common causes of diffuse enlargement of the abdomen, namely, a massive ovarian cyst and obstruction of distal small bowel, large bowel or both.
- In the case of intestinal obstruction, the percussion note is tympanitic all over.
- In the case of a large ovarian cyst, the percussion note is resonant in the flanks and dullness with convexity upward, over the pelvis.

Test for the Presence of Free Fluid in the Peritoneum (Ascites)

Ascites has to be differentiated from two other common causes of diffuse enlargement of the abdomen, namely, a massive ovarian cyst, and obstruction of distal small bowel, large bowel or both.

Tests for Detection of Fluid (Fig. 20)

1. **Shifting dullness:**
   - Since fluid gravitates to the dependent parts, it flows into the flanks and the intestines float in the umbilical region when the patient lies on his back.
   - The abdomen is percussed first with the patient lying on his back, when both flanks show dullness, while the umbilical region shows a tympanitic note.
   - The subject is then rolled on to his left side; a resonant note is now obtained from the right flank while the left flank sounds a dull note due to shifting of fluid to the left flank and the intestines floating up to the right flank.
   - A similar procedure is repeated with the patient rolled on to his right side, when the left flank will now give a resonant note.
   - The shift of the fluid and the accompanying dullness is called "shifting dullness", i.e. dullness due to shifting of fluid with a change in the position of the subject.
2. **Fluid thrill:**
   - The patient lies supine.

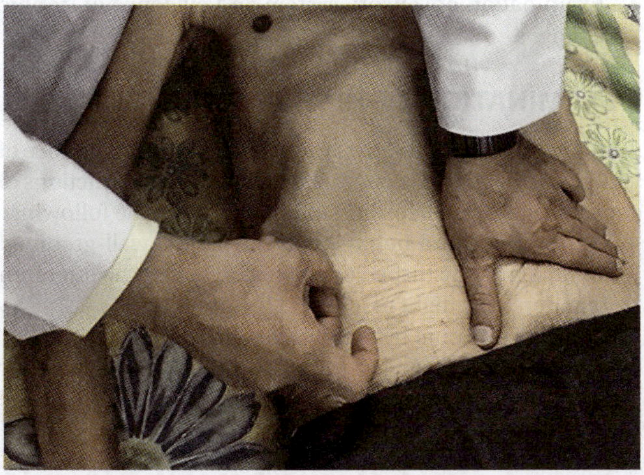

FIG. 20: Test for detection of fluid.

   - One hand is placed over the lumbar region of one side and a sharp tap or flick is given over the opposite lumbar region.
   - A *wave* or *fluid thrill* is felt by the detecting hand.
   - A similar sensation may be felt if the abdominal wall is very fat. To avoid this, the subject is asked to place the edge of his hand firmly along the midline; this damps any vibrations in the abdominal wall.
3. **Horseshoe-shaped dullness:**
   - When the amount of ascitic fluid is moderate, the fluid collects in the flanks and the hypogastric region, while the intestines float up in the upper umbilical and epigastric regions.
   - On percussion, the flanks and hypogastric regions produce dullness, whereas the epigastric and upper umbilical regions remain tympanitic.

Note: In the case of *intestinal obstruction*, the percussion note is tympanitic all over. In the case of a large ovarian cyst, the percussion note is resonant in the flanks, and dullness with convexity upward, over the pelvis.

AUSCULTATION

- ***Auscultation*** of the abdomen is done to listen for *bowel sounds* and whether they are *normal, increased or absent*, and for *detecting bruits* in the aorta and other abdominal vessels.
- The stethoscope (diaphragm) is to be placed on one site—usually just to the right of the umbilicus—and kept there until bowel sounds are heard. *It should not be moved from site to site*, and of course, there is no question of comparing the sounds on the two sides.
- *Normal bowel sounds* are heard as intermittent gurgles, low- or medium pitched, with an occasional high pitched noise or tinkle. Normal peristaltic activity of the gut create characteristic gurgling sound which may be heard from time to time by the unaided ear **(borborygmi)**.
- In *gastrointestinal obstruction*, these sounds may be greatly exaggerated, increasing in intensity with waves of pain. On the other hand, in *paralytic ileus* (intestinal paralysis) due to peritonitis or other causes, the sounds are absent—a condition called *"silent abdomen".*
- *Auscultate for peristalsis bowel sounds for at least 3 minutes before deciding that they are absent.*

QUESTIONS

Q.1. What are the important signs and symptoms of gastrointestinal tract disease?

Q.2. What is ascites? How do you test for the presence of free fluid in the peritoneum?

Q.3. How do you palpate the spleen in the subject provided?

Q.4. How do you palpate the kidneys in the subject provided?

Q.5. How do you percuss the abdomen?

Q.6. How do you auscultate the abdomen of the subject provided?

Refer text for answers to Q.1 to Q.6

OBJECTIVE STRUCTURED PRACTICAL EXAMINATION

Aim: To palpate the liver of the subject provided.

Procedural steps: See text above

Checklist:

1. Asks the subject to lie flat on the bed, relax with knees and hips flexed, and to breathe through the mouth. Asks if there is any tenderness or pain. (Y/N)
2. Bends down or kneels beside the subject's right side. Ensures that her hands are warm. (Y/N)
3. Places her right hand flat on the abdomen (with wrist and forearm in the same horizontal plane) and molds it to the abdomen. (Y/N)
4. Starting in the right iliac fossa, with fingers almost straight and slightly flexed at metacarpopharyngeal joints, presses inward and upward, works up toward costal margin. (Y/N)
5. Asks the subject to take a deep breath and at the height of inspiration, tries to feel the liver (does not poke fingers into the subject's abdomen). (Y/N)

3.5: CLINICAL EXAMINATION OF THE NERVOUS SYSTEM

STUDENT OBJECTIVES

After completing this practical, the student should be able to:

- Realize the importance of knowing the anatomy and physiology of the nervous system.
- Name the various cranial nerves, their functions, and the subjective and objective features of their lesions.
- Classify sensory receptors and sensations.
- Trace the sensory pathways.
- Name the motor pathways, their origin, course, termination, and functions.
- Elicit various superficial and deep reflexes and indicate their clinical significance.
- Test the motor and sensory functions.
- Enumerate the differences between upper and lower motor neuron (LMN) lesions.

PY10.11: Demonstrate the correct clinical examination of the nervous system: Higher functions, sensory system, motor system, reflexes, cranial nerves in a normal volunteer or simulated environment.

HISTORY TAKING

- In neurological examination, taking a careful history of illness is of great importance as the **history of progress of disease** will provide valuable leads to the specific part of the nervous system involved and the nature of underlying pathology.
- The diagnosis of a neurology patient depends primarily on correlating the signs and symptoms to the underlying disease process. The anatomical diagnosis depends on the assessment of changes in motor and sensory functions, alteration in reflexes, and subjective and objective features of lesions of cranial nerves.
- A more focused history may help in formulating a diagnosis and suggest the nature of pathology. In recent years, magnetic resonance imaging (MRI) and computed tomography (CT) scanning have transformed neurological diagnosis and refined clinical approach.

COMMON SIGNS AND SYMPTOMS OF NEUROLOGICAL DISEASE

Some of the common signs and symptoms are:

- Speech and language defects: dysarthria and dysphasia (cognitive disturbance) difficulty in communication.
- Partial unconsciousness with restlessness, or coma.
- Altered behavior and emotional state, such as confusion and disorientation.
- Motor defects such as weakness, paralysis, fits (convulsions), rigidity, tremors, involuntary movements, and alterations of gait.
- Sensory disturbances.
- Effects of involvement of cranial nerves, e.g. unilateral visual loss.

The major causes of these signs and symptoms include—vascular insults (hemorrhage and ischemic strokes), head and spinal injuries, degenerative diseases, infections (bacterial and viral), and so on.

EXAMINATION OF NERVOUS SYSTEM

This should proceed along the following lines:

- Examination of higher functions and speech
- Examination of cranial nerves
- Examination of motor system and reflexes
- Examination of sensory system and evidence of trophic changes.

EXAMINATION OF HIGHER FUNCTIONS

Apart from motor and sensory functions and maintenance of vital signs, the brain is concerned with the higher functions of consciousness, intellect, and mentation. Note the following:

- **Appearance and behavior:** Is the patient well-groomed or unkempt; disturbed or agitated; whether the attention wanders; any flight of ideas?
  - Note personal hygiene—nails, hands, and hair.
- **Emotional state:** Note, if the mood is elevated or depressed, or if there is flattening of emotions. Does he

appear confused, or does he live in a world of his own? Enquire about sleep and dreams.

- **Delusions and hallucinations:** Delusions are false beliefs, which continue to be held despite evidence to the contrary (e.g. believing that "someone is out to kill me"). Hallucinations are false impressions (visual or auditory; e.g. taking a rope to be a snake).
- **Level of consciousness:** Is there any clouding of consciousness? Ask him about events around him. Is there dementia (loss of memory), or coma (a deep state of unconsciousness from which the patient cannot be roused)?
- **Orientation in place and time:** Ask the patient about the date, month, and year; and whether he is in a hospital or at his home. Disorientation is an important sign of organic diseases of the brain and in psychiatric disorders.
- **Memory:** Test for recent and past memory by asking pointed questions. In brain injuries, for example, recent memory is affected much more than past memory.
- **General intelligence:** This will be evident during history taking. Ask for educational history and work record. One simple test is to ask her/him to continue deducting 7 from 100. Tests for reasoning and "absurdities" test can give a fair idea of the intelligence.

SPEECH (LANGUAGE) FUNCTIONS

- True speech, i.e. the **ability to understand and express in symbols,** is one of the highest functions of the human brain. For normal speech, not only the cerebral cortex must be intact but the motor mechanisms that control articulation (uttering of words) must also be perfect.
- Speech has two components—(1) a ***receiving*** or ***sensory part*** *(vision and hearing)* and (2) ***expressing or motor part*** *(spoken* and *written* speech). Thus, the disorders of speech may be **aphasias** or **dysarthria**.
- **Aphasias,** i.e. loss of the ability to understand and use symbols, may be ***sensory (or fluent)*** that are due to lesions in the Wernicke's area (area for understanding), or ***motor (or nonfluent)*** that are due to lesions in the Broca's area (area 44). The third type of aphasia is called ***global aphasia*** that is due to lesions involving both Wernicke's and Broca's areas.
- **Dysarthria** is simply the inability to utter words though the patient knows what to say.

Tests

Look for defects of articulation. Test the patient for various types of aphasias. Give him various common objects and ask him to name them, and the purpose for which they are used.

EXAMINATION OF CRANIAL NERVES

- There are 12 pairs of cranial nerves. Some of them are purely sensory (afferent), others are motor (efferent), while still others are mixed, i.e. they contain both sensory and motor fibers.
- A sound knowledge of the anatomy and physiology of cranial nerves is essential in order to understand the logic of methods employed in testing them, and the clinical significance of any abnormalities that may be detected.

1st or Olfactory Nerve (Sensory)

Origin: Olfactory epithelium

Type: Sensory

Function: Sensation of smell (olfaction)

Test the sense of smell in the subject: Consult Experiment 2.25.

2nd or Optic Nerve (Sensory)

Origin: Retina

Type: Sensory

Function: Transmission of visual sensations to the brain.

Examination of the optic nerve is done under the following headings for each eye:

1. Visual acuity (distant and near vision)
2. Field of vision
3. Color vision
4. Pupillary light reflex
5. Accommodations and near response
6. Examination of fundus.

Visual Acuity

Aim: Test the visual acuity of the subject:
Visual acuity, i.e. the ability to see objects clearly, is tested for distant as well as for near vision.

Testing for distant vision:
See Experiment 2.19.

Testing for near vision:
See Experiment 2.19.

Field of Vision

- **Confrontation test**
- **Perimetry**—(See Experiment 2.11).

CONFRONTATION TEST: Test the peripheral field of vision of the subject provided, using the confrontation test:

- It is a rough test to compare a person's visual fields with the examiner's own (presuming his own to be normal).
- The subject and the examiner sit facing each other about 3 feet apart **(Fig. 21)**.
- When testing the subject's left eye, he places his cupped right hand over his right eye, and with the left eye he fixes his gaze on the examiner's right eye, while the examiner closes his left eye.
- The subject is instructed not to move his left eye in any direction.
- The examiner then holds out his right arm to its full extent, midway between himself and the subject, and asks the subject to say "yes" when he sees any movement of the

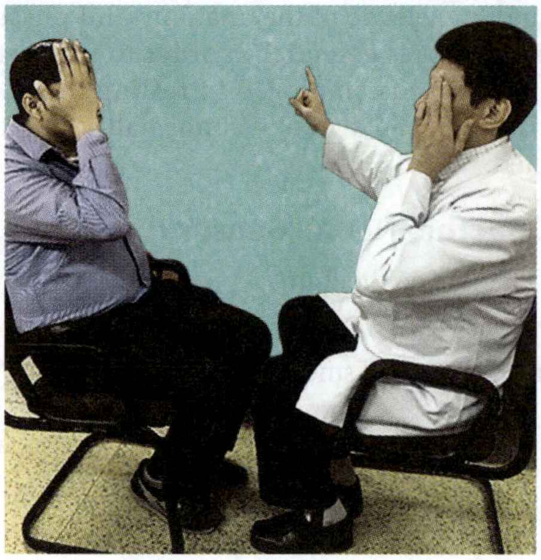

FIG. 21: Confrontation test.

examiner's finger. If no movement is perceived, the hand is moved in, kept still and the finger moved once again. In this way, the examiner compares his own *first sighting* of the movement with that of the subject.

- Using this procedure, the peripheral field is tested in all the four quadrants—(1) temporal, (2) upper, (3) lower, and (4) nasal.
- The subject's right eye is tested in a similar manner.
- The normal peripheral field of vision extends beyond 90° on the temporal side, about 50° in the vertical direction, about 55° on the nasal side, and about 65° downwards.
- Only gross changes in the field of vision can be detected with this method.
- Scotomas (blind areas within the field of vision) are impossible to locate, for which a perimeter is employed.
- When testing vision for color and visual fields, it is essential to ensure that any refractive error is corrected and that no other disease affecting acuity of vision or visual fields is present.

Color Vision

Aim: Test the color vision of the subject:
See Experiment 2.20.

Pupillary Light Reflex

Aim: Test the light reflex in the subject provided (Fig. 22).

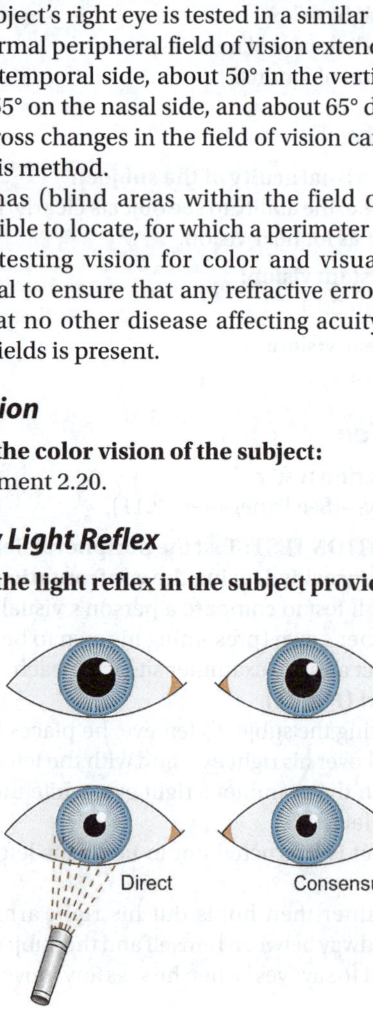

FIG. 22: Light reflex.

Direct Light Reflex

- Each eye is tested separately in a shady place. The subject is asked to look at a distance.
- A bright light from a torch, brought from the side of the eye, is shined into the eye— the result is a prompt constriction of the pupil **(Fig. 23)**.
- When the light is switched off, the pupil quickly dilates to its previous size.

Indirect or Consensual Light Reflex

- A hand is placed between the two eyes, and light is shined into one eye, observing the effect on the pupil of the unstimulated side **(Fig. 24)**.
- There is a constriction of the pupil in the other eye—a response called the *indirect or consensual light* reflex. Thus, the pupils of both eyes constrict when light is thrown into any eye.

Pathway of Direct Light Reflex

Retinal receptors—optic nerve—optic chiasma—optic tract—pretectum of midbrain—Edinger-Westphal nuclei of both sides—oculomotor nerve—ciliary ganglion—ciliary nerves—sphincter muscle of iris—constriction of pupil **(Flowchart 1)**.

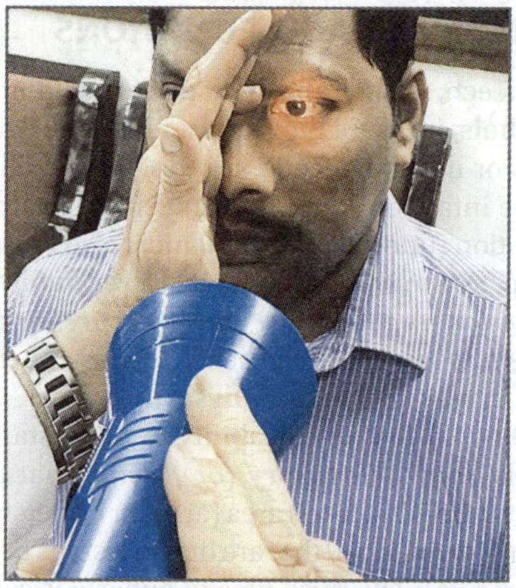

FIG. 23: Direct light reflex.

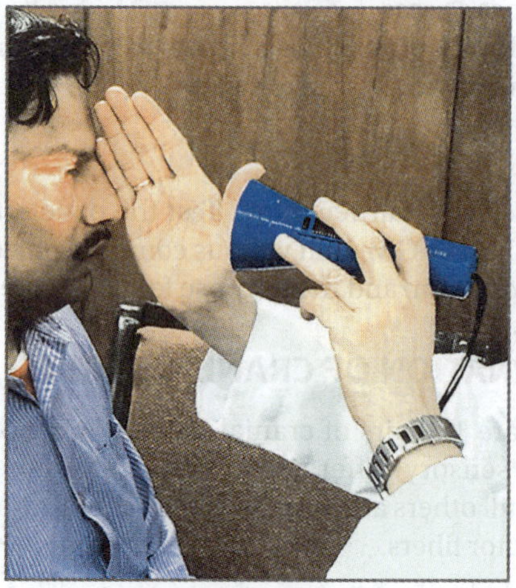

FIG. 24: Indirect light reflex.

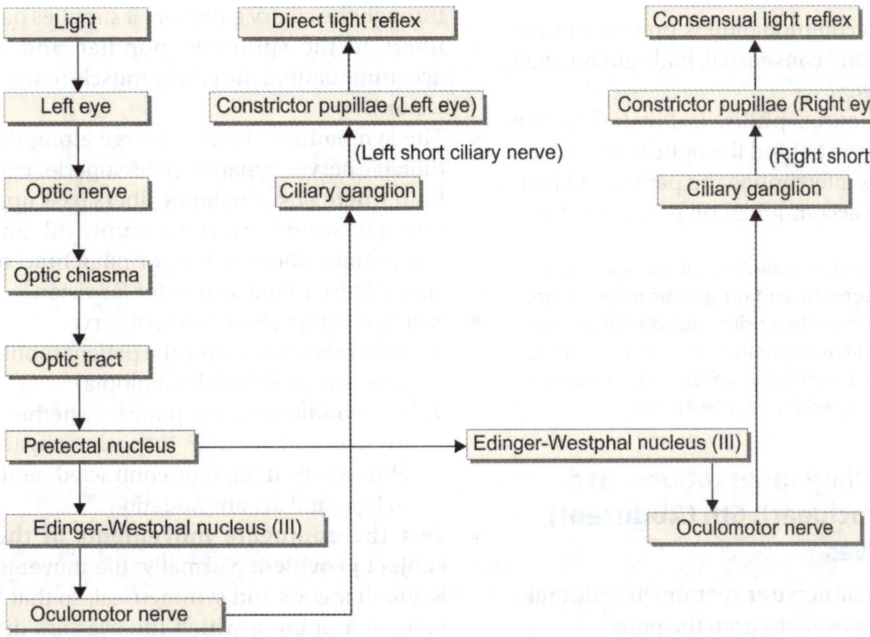

FLOWCHART 1: Pathway of light reflex.

Cause of Consensual Light Reflex

- When the retinal receptors of one eye are stimulated by light, nerve impulses pass along optic nerve, optic chiasma, optic tract, and reach the pretectal region of midbrain.
- Here, some of the fibers from each side terminate on the Edinger-Westphal nuclei of both sides. As a result, when light falls on the retina—the pupils on both sides constrict **(Flowchart 1)**.

Near Response Phenomenon

- The subject is asked to look at the far wall of the room.
- The observer then suddenly brings his finger, holding it vertically, about 15 cm in front of the subject's nose, and the subject is asked to look at it.
- When the gaze is directed at a near object—the ciliary muscle contracts. This relaxes the lens ligaments, so that the curvature of the lens increases making it more convex. The change is greatest at the anterior surface of the lens. This is called accommodation.
- In addition to accommodation, there is convergence of two visual axes and also there is constriction of pupil when an individual looks at a near object.
- This three part response—(1) accommodation, (2) convergence of visual axes, and (3) pupillary constriction is called the near response **(Fig. 25)**.

Pathway for Accommodation

The pathway for the accommodation reflex is as follows: retina—optic nerve—optic tract—lateral geniculate body—geniculocalcarine tract (optic radiation)—visual cortex (area 17)—frontal eye-field area (area 8 ap8)—Edinger–Westphal nucleus of opposite side—oculomotor nerve—ciliary ganglion—ciliary nerves—constrictor pupillae muscle. (Sympathetic system plays almost no role in accommodation) **(Fig. 26)**.

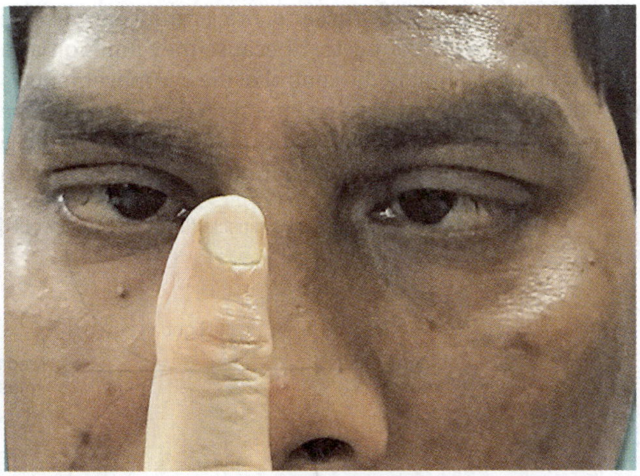

FIG. 25: Accommodation reflex.

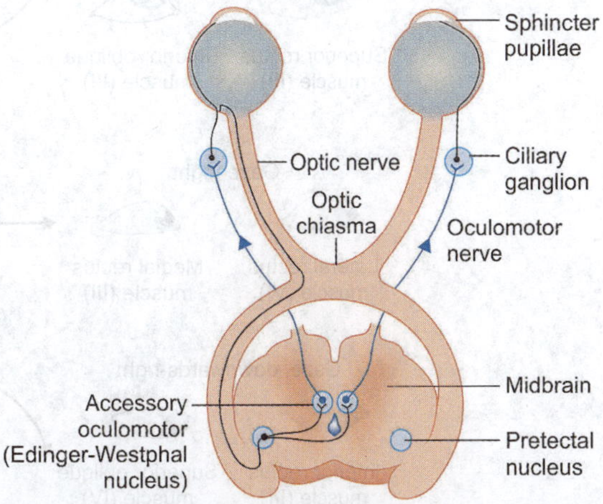

FIG. 26: Accommodation reflex pathway.

Argyll–Robertson Pupil

- A pupil in which the accommodation is present but the light reflex, both direct and consensual, is absent is called the *Argyll-Robertson pupil.*
- The lesion, usually neurosyphilis, is located in the pretectum of the midbrain behind the optic tract and the 3rd nerve nucleus, thus interrupting the pathway of light reflex while leaving the accommodation pathway intact.

Comments: Changes in the pupil in cases of head injury and cardiac arrest provide important diagnostic and prognostic information. Inequality of the pupils may indicate a rising intracranial tension due to hematoma. Dilated and fixed pupils, non reacting to light, may suggest serious and irreversible brain damage. Pupillary responses to light are also watched during anesthesia.

Oculomotor and Pupillary Innervation—3rd (Oculomotor), 4th (Trochlear), 6th (Abducent), and Sympathetic Nerves

- **Origin:** 3rd and 4th cranial nerve arises from the midbrain while the 6th cranial nerve arises from the pons.
- **Type:** Motor
- **Function:** The 3rd, 4th, and 6th cranial nerves are usually considered together because they function as a physiological unit in the control of the eye movements.
- The 6th nerve supplies the lateral rectus, the 4th nerve innervates the superior oblique, and the 3rd nerve supplies all the other external ocular muscles. It also sends fibers to the levator palpebrae superioris and through the ciliary ganglion, it supplies parasympathetic fibers to the sphincter pupillae and the muscle of accommodation, the ciliary muscle (contraction for near vision).
- The sympathetic fibers emerge along the 1st and 2nd thoracic nerves, synapse in the superior cervical ganglion, from where postganglionic fibers pass upward along the internal carotid artery to supply dilator pupillae, the involuntary fibers in levator palpebrae superioris, and ciliary muscle contraction for far vision.
- Before testing these nerves, observe:
  - If there is any squint—the patient should also be asked if he/she sees double (diplopia).
  - The condition of the pupils—whether they are equal in size and regular in outline, whether they are abnormally dilated or contracted, and their reaction to light and accommodation.
- **Test the conjugate movements of the eyes in the subject provided:** Normally, the movement of the eyes is simultaneous and symmetrical, so that the visual axes meet at a point at which the eyes are directed. This is called **conjugate movements** of the eyes **(Fig. 27)**.
- To test the eye movements, the head of the patient must be fixed with the left hand and he/she must be asked to follow the examiner's index finger to the right, to the left, upwards, and downwards as far as possible in each direction. Normally, the eyes move 50° outwards, 50° downwards, 50° inwards, and 33° upwards. The rotatory

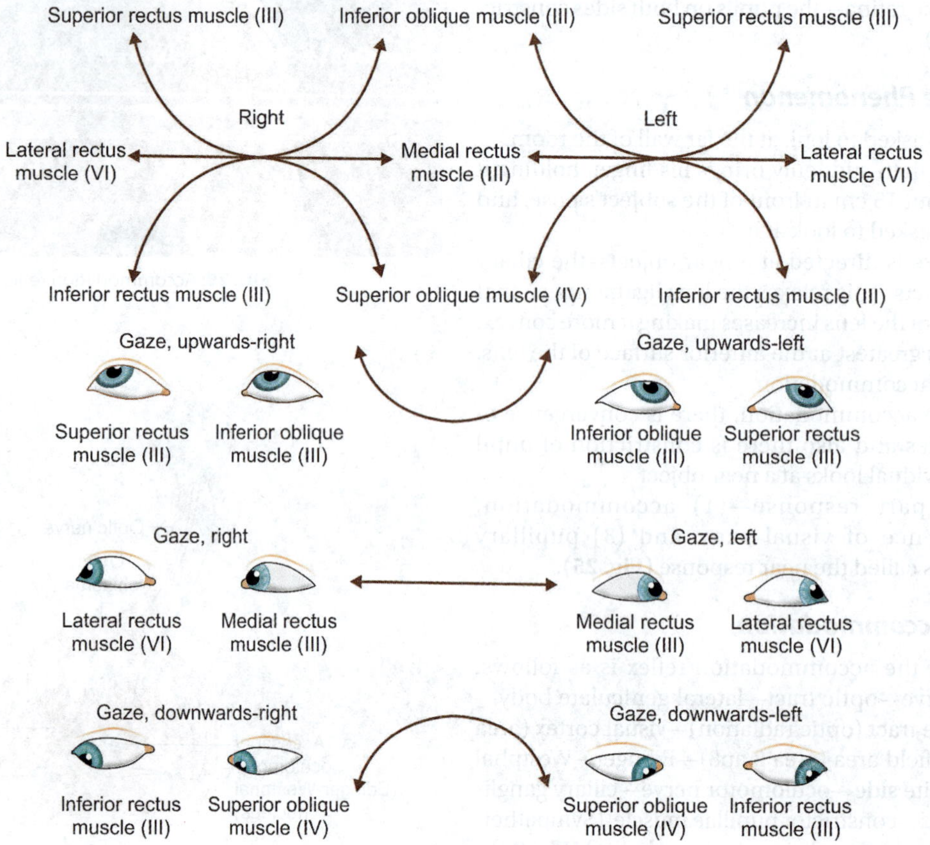

FIG. 27: Conjugate movement of eyes.

movements should also be tested. It is observed, if there is any limitation of movement in any direction.

- The brainstem centers of 3rd, 4th, and 6th cranial nerves probably control reflex movements of the eyes, while conjugate movements of voluntary origin are under the control of higher cortical centers via the corticonuclear tracts.
- **Physioclinical significance:** Changes in the pupil in cases of head injury and cardiac arrest provide important diagnostic and prognostic information.
  - Inequality of the pupils may indicate a rising intracranial tension due to hematoma.
  - Dilated and fixed pupils, non reacting to light, may suggest serious and irreversible brain damage.
  - Pupillary responses to light are also watched during anesthesia.

5th or Trigeminal Nerve (Sensory and Motor)

- **Origin:** Pons
- **Type:** Mixed (Sensory and Motor).
- **Functions:**
  - ***Sensory functions:***
    - **Demonstrate the corneal reflex:** Light wisp of absorbent cotton is twisted to a fine hair. The subject is asked to look at the far wall and, approaching from the side, the **lateral edge of the cornea** is lightly touched with the cotton. (The cornea should never be wiped with the cotton and the central cornea should never be touched, because ulceration may occur if there is corneal anesthesia).
    - The response is bilateral blinking; and the two sides should be compared. The afferent path of this reflex is ophthalmic division of the 5th nerve, the efferent path is 7th nerve, while the center is in the nuclei of these nerves in the pons.
    - The **conjunctival reflex,** also a superficial reflex, is elicited in the same manner as corneal reflex. Touching the conjunctiva with a wisp of cotton causes bilateral blinking **(Fig. 28)**. (The conjunctiva of the lower lid is supplied by maxillary division of the 5th nerve).
    - The **nasal or sneeze reflex,** i.e. sneezing when the nasal mucosa is irritated, also employs 5th nerve as its afferent path, while the motor path employs motor components of 5th to 10th cranial and upper cervical nerves.
    - *Test the general sensory functions of the trigeminal nerve*: In addition to the corneal and palpebral conjunctiva, the 5th nerve supplies a greater part of the face, forehead, temporal and parietal regions, and nasal and buccal mucosa.
    - The sensory fibers arise from unipolar cells in the semilunar or Gasserian ganglion and supply the skin and mucosa described above.
    - The nerve also contains **sensory proprioceptive fibers,** which innervate muscle spindles in the muscles of mastication, and possibly also in the external ocular muscles. The motor components supply the muscles of mastication.

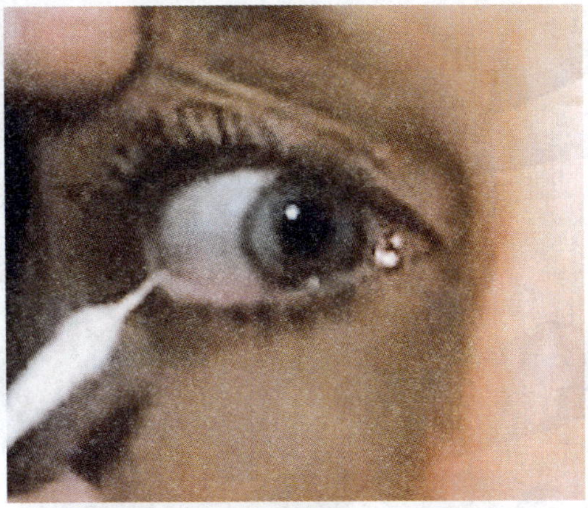

FIG. 28: Conjunctival reflex.

    - The sensations of touch, pain, and temperature over the face are tested, as elsewhere on the body as described later, with a wisp of cotton, pin pricks, and warm and cold objects.
  - ***Motor functions:***
    Aim: Test the motor functions of the trigeminal nerve in the subject provided:
    - The motor fibers of the 5th nerve, (its nucleus lies at the mid pontine level) innervate the muscles of mastication—**masseter, temporalis,** and **medial and lateral pterygoids**—and the **tensor tympani** of middle ear.
    - The subject is asked to open his mouth and show the teeth. Normally, the jaw is symmetrical. If there is paralysis on one side, the jaw deviates to the side of paralysis, the healthy pterygoids pushing it to that side.
    - The subject is asked to clench his teeth—the temporalis and masseter muscles contract and become equally prominent on the two sides. The muscles can be palpated to note, if there is any difference in the strength of contraction.
    - The subject is asked to open his mouth and move the mandible from side to side.
    - The jaw jerk (maxillary reflex) is tested by placing a finger on the chin below the lower lip, with the mouth open, and striking it with a percussion hammer **(Fig. 29)**. The response is closure of the mouth. Normally, this jerk is hardly detectable, but it is exaggerated in upper motor neuron (UMN) lesions (as are other deep reflexes). Both the afferent and efferent paths are along 5th nerve and the center is in the pons.
    - The mandibular division of the 5th nerve also supplies parasympathetic fibers to the salivary glands.

7th or Facial Nerve (Almost Purely Motor)

- **Origin**: Pons
- **Type**: Mixed
- The facial nerve supplies all the superficial muscles of the face and scalp (except levator palpebrae superioris, which

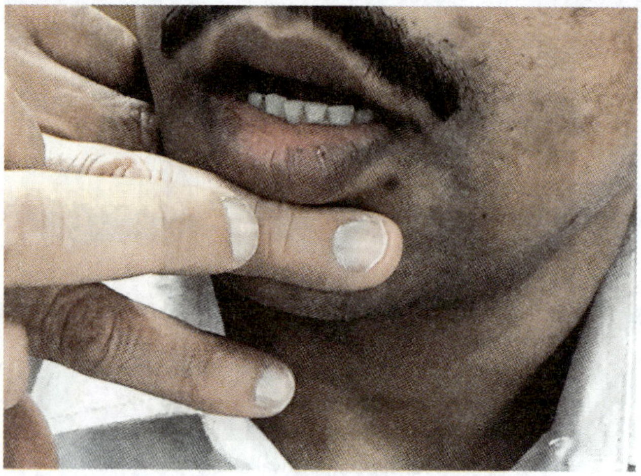

FIG. 29: Jaw jerk.

is supplied by 3rd nerve), external ear, and the stapedius in the middle ear.

- The chorda tympani runs with this nerve for part of its course. The parasympathetic fibers from the superior salivatory nucleus innervate the blood vessels and glandular cells of sublingual and submaxillary glands, and glands in the mucosa of pharynx, palate, nasal cavity, and paranasal sinuses.
- Sensation from a small medial part of the tragus of the pinna, the external auditory meatus, and tympanic membrane is relayed in the tympanic branch of the facial nerve to the geniculate ganglion.

Aim: *Test the motor functions of the facial nerve in the subject provided:*

Testing the upper face:

- The subject is asked to look up and wrinkle the skin on his forehead (occipitofrontalis muscle tested). Normally, the wrinkling of the skin is symmetrical on the two sides. By asking the subject to frown, the corrugator supercilii can be tested.
- He is asked to shut his eyes as tightly as possible. (The corners of the mouth also get drawn up). The examiner then tries to open one and then the other eye **(Fig. 30)**.

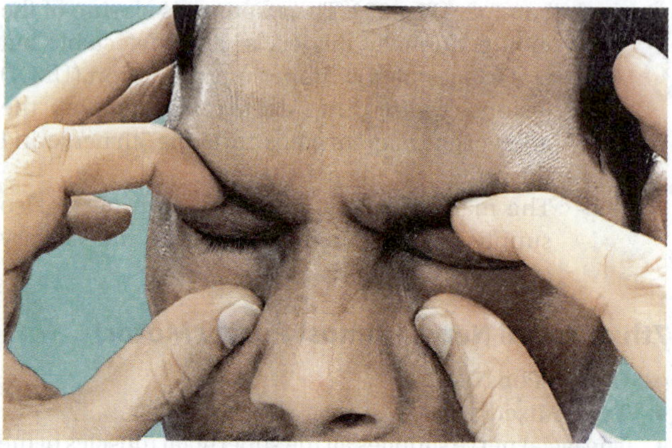

FIG. 30: Facial nerve: orbicularis oculi muscle testing.

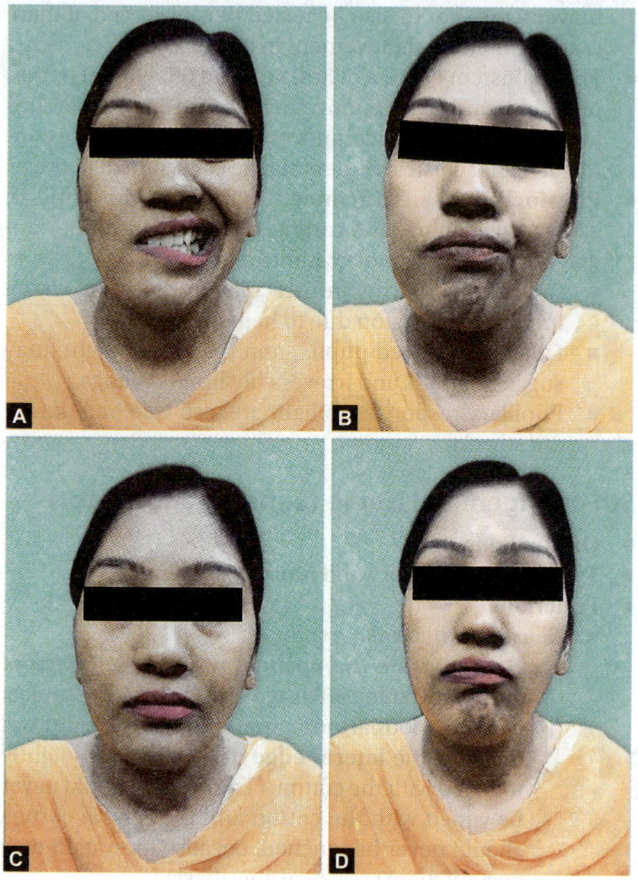

FIGS. 31A TO D: Facial nerve palsy.

Normally, it is impossible to do so against the subject's wishes. (Orbicularis oculi muscles tested).

When one tries to shut the eyes tightly, the eyeballs roll upwards, a normal response called *Bell's* ***phenomenon.*** In Bell's palsy (see below), when the patient closes his eyes, the upward movement of the eyeball becomes obvious because closure of the affected eye is not possible **(Figs. 31A to D)**.

Testing the lower face:

- The nasolabial folds on both sides are observed, which are normally symmetrical. Paralysis on one side causes flattening of the folds on that side; it also affects facial symmetry at rest or during voluntary facial movements.
- The subject is asked to smile or show his upper teeth, or to whistle. Normally, the face remains symmetrical (levator angularis muscle tested). Paralysis of one side causes the angle of the mouth to be drawn toward the healthy side, while that on the paralyzed side remains stationary. The buccinator is also involved in whistling.
- The subject is asked to inflate his mouth with air and blow out his cheeks (buccinator tested) **(Fig. 32)**. Each inflated cheek is then tapped with a finger. If there is paralysis, the air escapes easily through the angle of the mouth on the paralyzed side.
- The subject is asked to depress the lower lip (depressor labii inferioris and quadratus labii inferioris tested). In case of paralysis, the asymmetry is obvious.

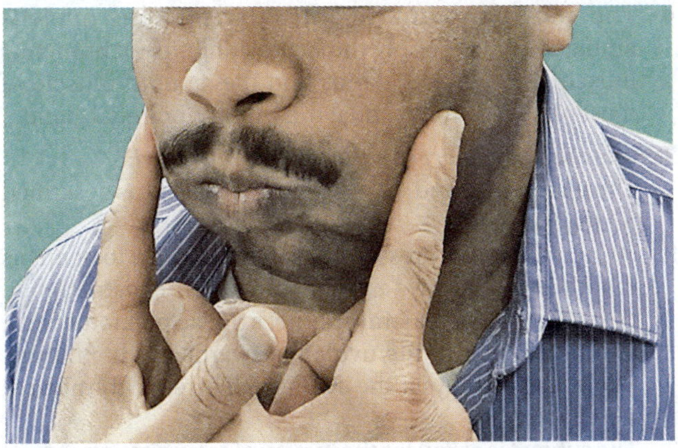

FIG. 32: Facial nerve: buccinator muscle testing.

Physioclinical Significance

- Facial paralysis results quite commonly from lesions of upper motor neurons (UMNs) or lower motor neurons (LMNs).
- To differentiate between these two, it is important to remember that 7th nerve nuclei innervating muscles of the upper face are under bilateral cortical motor control, while the facial nuclei supplying the lower face are controlled from the opposite motor cortex only.
- Therefore, in **supranuclear lesion** (upper neuron paralysis; e.g. capsular hemiplegia), only the muscles of the lower part of face are paralyzed, i.e. the forehead can be wrinkled and the eyes closed.
- In **infranuclear lesion** (LMN paralysis, i.e. lesion of facial nucleus or facial nerve—as in Bell's palsy), both the upper as well as the lower parts of the face are equally affected (paralyzed). If paralysis is complete, the whole side of the face is smooth and free from wrinkles. The lower eyelid droops, the angle of the mouth sags, and saliva may dribble. Bell's phenomenon is present.
- The taste sensation from the anterior two thirds is lost (**taste is not affected in supranuclear lesions**), and sounds seem unusually loud (hyperacusis) due to paralysis of stapedius, which normally attenuates loud sounds. Listening to a shrill whistle will test the stapedius.
- Since the 7th nerve is related to many cranial nerves and other structures during its course, involvement of some of these helps in localizing the site of lesion.

Test the taste function of the facial nerve: Consult Experiment 2.24.

The patient should always be asked about any abnormal taste sensations or hallucinations of taste, which may form the aura of an epileptic fit, particularly in temporal lobe epilepsy.

8th or Vestibulocochlear Nerve (Composite Sensory Nerve)

- **Origin**: Pons (Cerebellopontine angle)
- **Type**: Sensory
- The 8th cranial nerve has two components—
  1. **The cochlear nerve**
     - The cochlear nerve supplies the cochlea and subserves hearing, while the vestibular nerve supplies the semicircular canals (SCC; for dynamic equilibrium) and the labyrinth (otolith organ, utricle, and saccule; for static equilibrium) and subserves equilibrium, balance, and sensation of bodily displacement.
     - The symptoms of cochlear nerve involvement include tinnitus (ringing, buzzing, hissing, singing, or roaring noises in the ear); deafness; hearing scotomas (selective deafness to certain pitches and noises); and sensory aphasia in supranuclear lesions.
  2. **The vestibular nerve**
     - The vestibular nerve supplies the semicircular canals and the labyrinth and subserves equilibrium, balance and sensation of bodily displacement.
     - The symptoms of vestibular nerve damage include vertigo (a feeling of giddiness); nystagmus (a rhythmic to and fro movement of the eyes); and some general symptoms like nausea, vomiting, tachycardia and low blood pressure.

Tests for Hearing

- **Watch test**
- **Whisper test**
- **Tuning fork tests**
  - **Perform the Rinne test on the subject provided.** Consult Experiment 2.21.
  - **Perform the Weber test on the subject provided.** Consult Experiment 2.21.
  - **Demonstrate the Schwabach test of hearing.** Consult Experiment 2.21.
- **Watch test:** A watch, which the examiner can hear at a specific distance from his ear, is placed next to the patient's ear. Ask him to note when the watch sound disappears. Note that the examiner has to have normal hearing to do this exam (in at least one ear).
- **Perform the whisper test in the subject provided:** The simplest way of testing for hearing loss is the use of human voice. A conversational voice is generally heard at a distance of 10–12 feet in each ear, separately. The whisper test is the simplest test for assessing gross defects in hearing.
- The examiner stands on one side of the subject and closes the subject's opposite ear with his own finger. He then asks the subject's name, nature of his work, etc. by gently whispering into his ear from a distance of 12–14 inches. The procedure is repeated on the other side.

Tests for Vestibular Function

- In the **Barany caloric test,** the subject's head is tilted back 60°, and his external auditory meatus is irrigated with 250 mL of water at 30°C (7° below body temperature) for 40 seconds. The test is repeated with water at 44°C (7° above normal). The endolymph in the horizontal canal (which becomes vertical with head tilt) moves due to convection currents, thus stimulating the receptors in the crista ampullaris.

- The normal response to caloric stimulation is nausea, horizontal nystagmus, past pointing, and falling to the stimulated side. In vestibular dysfunction, these reactions to stimulation are diminished.
- In the **Barany chair test,** the subject is seated in a special chair, which can be rotated at a definite speed, with the subject's head tilted to specified positions to stimulate a particular pair of SCC. The effects of acceleration and deceleration, i.e. nystagmus, vomiting, past pointing, and tendency to fall, can then be observed.

9th or Glossopharyngeal Nerve (Mixed Nerve)

- **Origin:** Medulla
- **Type:** Mixed
- The 9th nerve is motor to the middle constrictor of pharynx and stylopharyngeus, and sensory for the posterior third of the tongue (both general and taste sensations), and mucous membrane of the pharynx.
- Parasympathetic fibers from inferior salivatory nucleus, after relaying in the otic ganglion, innervate the parotid gland. This nerve is rarely involved alone, but generally with the 10th and 11th nerves.

Test the 9th Cranial Nerve

- **Testing the motor function of 9th cranial nerve:**
  1. **Gag reflex (Pharyngeal reflex):**
     - Touch each side of the pharynx lightly with a wooden spatula.
     - Response is constriction and elevation of the pharynx.
     - The afferent path is 9th nerve; the center is in medulla; and the efferent path is 10th nerve. The reflex is absent when there is damage to its afferent arc.
  2. **Palatal reflex:**
     - A soft touch is applied on the soft palate.
     - The response is elevation of the soft palate.
     - The reflex arc is the same as in the gag reflex described above.
- **Testing the sensory function of 9th cranial nerve:** The sensation of taste over the posterior one-third of the tongue is tested as discussed above for the 7th cranial nerve.

10th or Vagus Nerve (Mixed Nerve)

- **Origin:** Medulla
- **Type:** Mixed Nerve
- The vagus nerve is the motor for the soft palate, pharynx, and intrinsic muscles of the larynx. **Somatic sensory fibers** from unipolar cells in the jugular ganglion supply external auditory meatus and part of the ear.
- The **visceral sensory fibers** of unipolar cells in ganglion nodosum innervate pharynx, larynx, trachea, and thoracic and abdominal viscera.
- The **parasympathetic fibers** arise from nucleus ambiguous and supply the heart (inhibitory), bronchial muscle and glands, glands and the smooth muscle of most of the gastrointestinal tract, and suprarenal gland.

Testing the vagus nerve in the subject provided:

1. The *pharyngeal* and *palate reflexes* are tested as described for the 9th nerve.
2. Using a tongue depressor, the subject is asked to open his mouth wide and say "ah". The response is constriction of posterior pharyngeal wall (Vernet's rideau phenomenon), and movement of the uvula backwards in the midline. But in vagal paralysis, the uvula is deflected to the normal side.
3. The subject is asked for the history of regurgitation of food through the nose, which is due to total paralysis of the vagus; a nasal voice may also be noted.
4. Laryngoscopy is done to note the position and movement of the true vocal cords.

11th or Accessory Nerve (Motor Nerve)

- **Origin:**
  - **Cranial part:** Arises from the medulla
  - **Spinal part:** Arises from spinal cord
- **Type:** Motor nerve.
- This purely motor nerve innervates some muscles in the pharynx and larynx (internal or medullary branch, arising from nucleus ambiguus), as well as sternomastoid and the trapezius (external or spinal branch arising from the anterior horn cells of upper 5 or 6 spinal cord segments).

Test the spinal part of the accessory nerve in the subject provided:

- The examiner presses on the shoulders from behind and asks the subject to shrug his shoulders (this tests the upper part of trapezius) **(Fig. 33)**. If the 11th nerve is damaged, shrugging is weaker on that side; the shoulder also droops. The subject is asked to approximate his shoulder blades against the examiner's resistance (this tests the lower part of the muscle).
- A hand is placed against the right side of the subject's face and he is asked to rotate the head to the right. The left

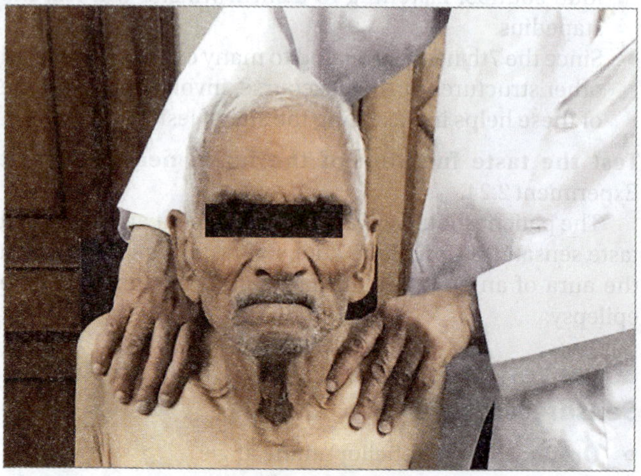

FIG. 33: Spinal accessory nerve testing.

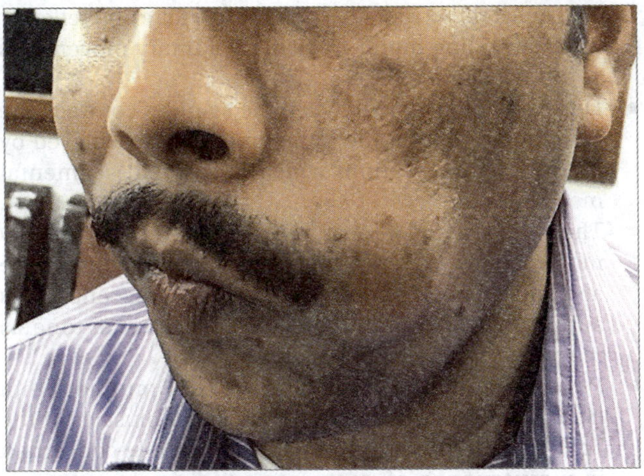

FIG. 34: Hypoglossal nerve testing.

sternomastoid is seen to become prominent. The procedure is repeated on the left side also. In case of a unilateral lesion, the head cannot be rotated to the healthy side.

- The examiner places a hand on the subject's forehead and asks him to bend his head forwards against resistance. Normally, both sternomastoids become prominent.

12th or Hypoglossal Nerve (Motor Nerve)

- **Origin:** Medulla
- **Type:** Motor
- The motor fibers arise from the hypoglossal nucleus in the lower part of the floor of the 4th ventricle. The fibers innervate the muscles of the tongue and depressors of the hyoid bone. A few proprioceptive fibers from the tongue probably run in this nerve.

Test the hypoglossal nerve in the subject provided (Fig. 34):

- The subject is asked to push out his tongue as far as possible. Normally, it remains in the midline (genioglossus tested). If the 12th nerve is paralyzed, the tongue is pushed over to the side of the lesion by the healthy muscles on the opposite side. The affected side is also wasted, wrinkled, and may show fasciculation, which indicates LMN lesion.
- The subject is asked to move the tongue from side to side over the lips and against the walls of the cheeks (extrinsic and intrinsic muscles of the tongue tested). A finger is placed against the cheek while the subject is asked to press against it with his tongue through the wall of the cheek. The strength of contraction is compared on the two sides.
- The subject is asked to touch the tongue to the palate (palatoglossus tested), and to depress the tongue in the floor of the mouth (hypoglossus tested).

OBJECTIVE STRUCTURED PRACTICAL EXAMINATION-I

Aim: To test the 5th cranial nerve in the subject provided.
Procedural steps: See text above
Checklist:

1. Makes the subject sit on a stool and explains the procedure. (Y/N)
2. Asks the subject to look at a distance, and touches his/her conjunctiva with a wisp of cotton, and notes the response. (Y/N)
3. Tests the sensations of touch and pain with a wisp of cotton and a pin on identical points on the two sides of the face. (Y/N)
4. Asks the subject to show his/her teeth and then to clench his/her teeth. Watches and feels the masseter and temporalis muscles contracting. (Y/N)
5. Asks the subject to open his/her mouth and move the mandible from side to side then tests the mandibular reflex. (Y/N)

OBJECTIVE STRUCTURED PRACTICAL EXAMINATION-II

Aim: To test the 7th cranial nerve in the subject provided.
Procedural steps: See text above.
Checklist:

1. Explains the procedure to the subject. Looks for facial symmetry, furrows on the forehead, and the width of the palpebral fissure. (Y/N)
2. Asks the subject to look up and wrinkle his/her forehead, and then to shut his/her eyes as tightly as possible against the examiner's resistance. (Y/N)
3. Asks the subject to show his/her upper teeth and to smile. (Y/N)
4. Asks the subject to inflate his/her mouth with air and to blow out his/her cheeks. Then taps his/her cheeks, on either side with his/her finger, to see if air escapes from the angle of the mouth. (Y/N)
5. Asks the subject to depress his/her lower lip. (Y/N)

OBJECTIVE STRUCTURED PRACTICAL EXAMINATION-III

Aim: To test the 11th cranial nerve of the subject provided.
Procedural steps: See text above.
Checklist:

1. Asks the subject to sit comfortably and explains the procedure. (Y/N)
2. Stands behind the subject and places his/her hands on his/her shoulders. Then asks him/her to shrug his/her shoulders against his/her resistance. (Y/N)
3. Places his/her hand on the right side of the subjects face and asks him/her to rotate his/her head to the opposite side. Watches the left sternomastoid. (Y/N)
4. Repeats the procedure on the left side and asks him/her to rotate his/her head to the left, and watches the right sternomastoid muscle. (Y/N)
5. Places his/her hand on the subject's forehead and asks him/her to bend his/her head forwards against resistance. (Y/N)

OBJECTIVE STRUCTURED PRACTICAL EXAMINATION-IV

Aim: To test the 12th cranial nerve in the subject.
Procedural steps: See text above.

Checklist:

1. Explains the procedure to the subject. (Y/N)
2. Asks the subject to push out his/her tongue as far as possible, then inspects its position, evidence of wasting and fasciculation. (Y/N)
3. Asks the subject to move his/her tongue from side to side over the lips and against the walls of the cheeks. (Y/N)
4. Places his/her finger over the subject's cheek and asks him/her to push against it. Repeats on the opposite side. (Y/N)
5. Asks the subject to touch the tongue to the palate, and then to depress it into the floor of the mouth. (Y/N)

MOTOR SYSTEM

The motor system is concerned in the execution of the following motor activities:

- Muscle tone and reflexes; mostly spinal mechanisms (involuntary)
- Gross and fine, skilled movement (voluntary)
- Semiautomatic movements (e.g. chewing, swallowing, swinging of arms while walking). There is, however, no clear cut demarcation between voluntary and involuntary movements, one activity often merging into another.

Components of the Motor System

- The motor system consists of—motor areas of cerebral cortex, subcortical structures (basal ganglia, cerebellum, reticular formation, vestibular nuclei, etc.), descending motor tracts (the so-called UMN, LMN, and the skeletal muscles.
- **Figure 35** shows the components of the motor system.

Muscles

- The skeletal muscles can contract only in response to signals received from their motor nerves. The input to the motor neurons is through two sources:

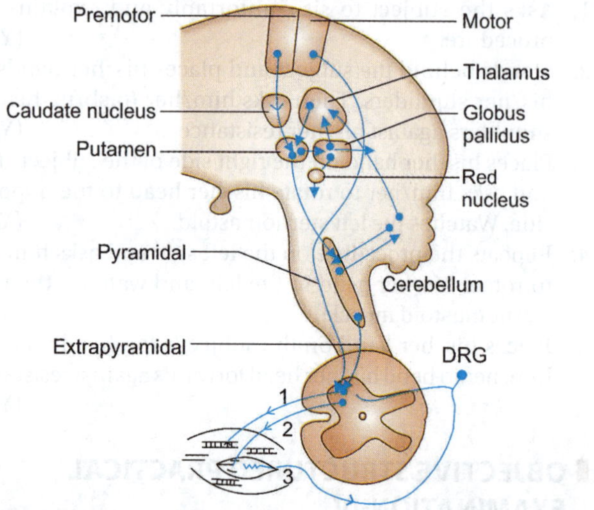

FIG. 35: Components of the motor system: 1: alpha motor neuron supplying extrafusal muscle fibers; 2: gamma motor neuron supplying intrafusal muscle fibers; 3: afferent fiber from muscle spindle).

1. Dorsal nerve root fibers for muscle tone and reflexes.
2. Descending motor tracts for voluntary movements and postural reflexes.

- During any movement, when the agonists contract, the antagonists relax at the same time. This is achieved by reciprocal innervation, which is a spinal segmental mechanism.
- The role of a stable posture is very essential in every movement. Every movement begins in a certain posture and ends in another posture. There is thus a continuous adjustment of posture by changes in muscle tone as movements progress.
- *Proximal group of muscles*: The axial muscles (hip, trunk, and shoulders) and the proximal muscles of the limbs make up this group. They are mainly concerned in **maintenance of posture, equilibrium, and gross movements.**
- *Distal group of muscles*: This group includes the muscles of the distal parts of the limbs (fingers, hands, and wrists). They are involved in **voluntary, fine, and skilled movements** such as those during writing, typing, playing on a musical instrument, etc. (i.e. manipulative behavior).

Lower Motor Neurons

- The anterior horn cells of the spinal cord and the motor cranial nuclei in the brainstem that directly innervate the skeletal muscle fibers are called LMN. Their axons leave the CNS via ventral roots (or motor cranial nerves) and eventually become the motor supply to the muscles.
- In the spinal cord, the most medially located motor neurons ***(the medial motor system)*** innervate the proximal group of muscles (for posture), while the laterally located neurons ***(the lateral motor system)*** innervate the distal group of muscles (for fine skilled movements).
- The LMNs constitute the "final common pathway" for all motor signals that leave the CNS on their way to skeletal muscles.
- The lesions of LMN cause flaccid paralysis, muscle atrophy, and absence of deep (stretch) reflexes.

Upper Motor Neurons

- These fibers arise in the cortex and brainstem and that activate the LMNs. Traditionally, the descending motor fibers are classified into **pyramidal** and **extrapyramidal**.
- The **pyramidal tract** includes all fibers (irrespective of their site of origin) descending in the pyramids of the medulla. In lower medulla, the majority of the fibers cross over to the other side to descend as the **lateral (crossed) corticospinal-pyramidal system** in the lateral funiculus of the cord **(Fig. 36)** to end on the LMN.
- Only about 3% of the fibers remain on the same side and descend as **the anterior (uncrossed) pyramidal system** to finally end on the LMN.
- The **extrapyramidal system** is a widely used term for those tracts (from basal ganglia, etc.) that indirectly control LMN but are not part of the direct corticospinal-

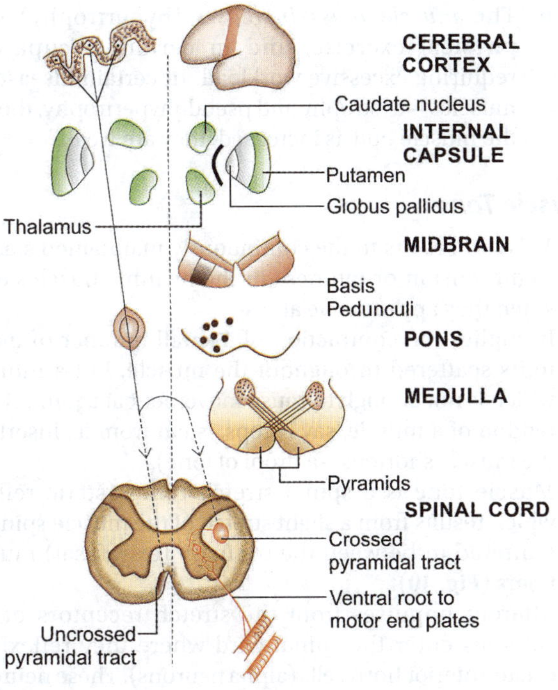

FIG. 36: Diagram showing the origin, course, and termination of corticospinal–pyramidal system. The location of the tract at each level is shown on the right. The majority of fibers cross to opposite side in lower medulla to descend as lateral corticospinal tract. Along with rubrospinal tract that lies in front of it, it forms the lateral motor control system that controls distal group of muscles.

pyramidal system. This term is now being less frequently used clinically and physiologically.

- The *lesions of UMN* cause spastic paralysis and exaggerated deep reflexes without muscle atrophy. However, three types of UMN need to be considered because:
  - Lesions in posture regulating pathways produce spastic paralysis.
  - Lesions in corticospinal and corticobulbar fibers cause weakness rather than paralysis.
  - Cerebellar lesions cause incoordination.

Present Concept

The two motor control systems are:

1. ***The lateral motor system:*** The lateral corticospinal (crossed pyramidal) tract plus rubrospinal tract that lies anterior to it, make up the lateral motor system that controls the distal groups of muscles concerned with fine, skilled movement. The red nucleus thus functions in close association with the lateral corticospinal tract.
2. ***The medial motor system:*** It includes ventral (anterior) corticospinal (uncrossed pyramidal) tract plus the medially located descending tracts from the brainstem (vestibulo-, reticulo-, olivo-, tectospinal tracts) **(Fig. 37).** This system controls the proximal group of muscles (described above) for posture and gross movements.

Note: Phylogenetically, the medial motor pathways are old, while the lateral motor pathways are new.

Planning and Execution of Movements

The motor command, planning, and execution of movements **(Fig. 38)** are now believed to occur in the following manner:

- **Planning:** The "desire" to make a movement is processed in the cortical association areas. The process of parallel processing of the sequence of movements occurs in the cerebral cortex, neocerebellum, and basal ganglia.

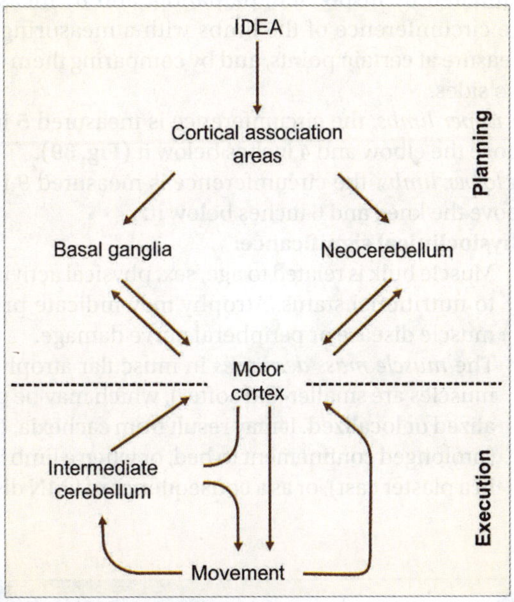

FIG. 38: The planning and execution of voluntary movements.

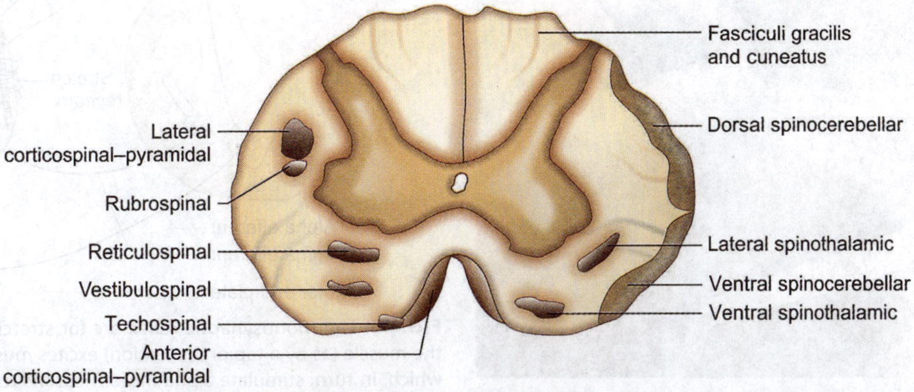

FIG. 37: Transverse section of spinal cord showing the ascending tracts (right side) and descending pathways (left side).

- **Commands:** The motor commands originate in the premotor and motor cortical areas, and pass down in the UMNs or the LMNs that make up the "final common pathway".
- **Execution:** Motor commands go from cortical and premotor areas to the LMN for execution.
- **Feedback information**—about the status of a movement is sent back from proprioceptors to cerebellum, which compares actual performance with intended movement and adjusts signals from cortical areas to smoothen out errors, if any.

Testing the Motor Functions

- Bulk of muscle
- Muscle tone
- Power or strength
- Coordination of muscular activity
- Reflexes
- Presence of abnormal movements
- Gait.

Bulk of Muscles

- **Testing the bulk of muscles:** This can be easily estimated by inspection, palpation, and by measuring the circumference of the limbs with a measuring tape; measure at certain points, and by comparing them on the two sides.
- In *upper limbs,* the circumference is measured 5 inches above the elbow and 4 inches below it **(Fig. 39)**.
- In *lower limbs,* the circumference is measured 9 inches above the knee and 6 inches below it.
- **Physioclinical significance:**
  - Muscle bulk is related to age, sex, physical activity and to nutritional status. Atrophy may indicate primary muscle disease or peripheral nerve damage.
  - The *muscle mass decreases* in muscular atrophy (the muscles are smaller and softer), which may be generalized or localized. It may result from cachexia, disuse (prolonged confinement to bed, or when a limb is kept in a plaster cast), or as a consequence of LMN disease.
  - The *muscle mass increases* (hypertrophy) with physical exercise, and in certain occupations requiring excessive workload. In certain diseases of muscles—dystrophy and pseudohypertrophy, though the muscle bulk is increased, they are weak.

Muscle Tone

- This term refers to the continuously maintained state of slight tension or tautness in the healthy muscles even when they appear to be at rest.
- It implies the contraction of a small number of motor units scattered throughout the muscle, but a number which is not enough to cause movement at a joint. (If the tendon of a muscle, say biceps, is cut from its insertion, the muscle shortens—a proof of tone).
- Muscle tone is a spinal stretch reflex (static reflex), which results from a slight stretch of the muscle spindles scattered in between the ordinary (extrafusal) muscle fibers **(Fig. 40)**.
- Afferent impulses from the stretch receptors of the spindles enter the spinal cord where they reflexively excite anterior horn cells (alpha neurons). These neurons, in turn, discharge *out of step and at a low rate,* which leads to contraction of a certain number of muscle fibers; and this is manifested as muscle tone. Damage to any part of the reflex arc abolishes muscle tone.
- Though muscle tone is a spinal reflex mechanism, it is mainly regulated by supraspinal pathways—the pyramidal (corticospinal) and extrapyramidal tracts. The anterior cerebellum, via the subcortical structures, has a facilitatory effect on muscle tone.
- This continuously maintained state of slight tension (muscle tone) does not produce fatigue because only a small number of muscle fibers contract at a time; these fibers relax and another group takes up activity.
- **The cause of stretching of the muscle spindles to start with:** From the time of early growth, the bones grow longer at a rate faster than that of muscles. This maintains a slight stretch on the muscles, and therefore, on the

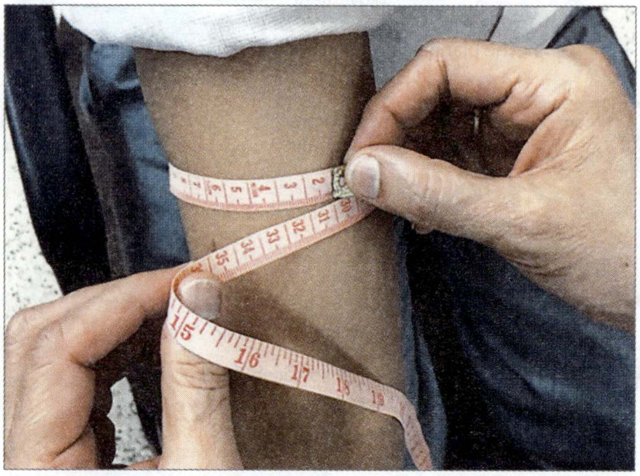

FIG. 39: Testing bulk of muscle.

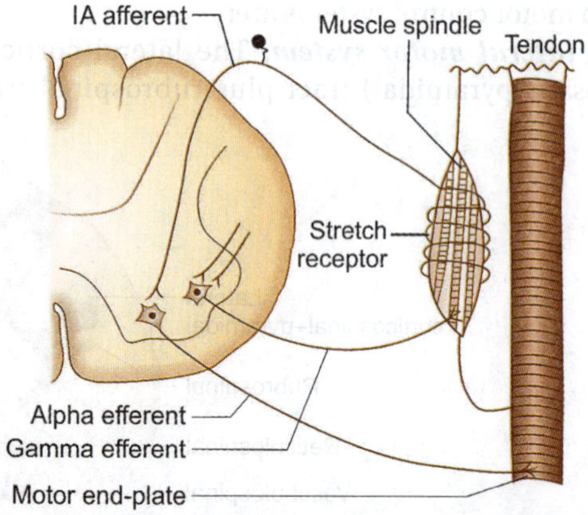

FIG. 40: The monosynaptic reflex arc for stretch reflexes. Stretching the muscle (as by a tap on its tendon) excites muscle spindle receptors, which, in turn, stimulate alpha motor neurons to cause a brief muscle contraction.

spindles, throughout the lifetime of an individual, so that the muscles remain in a state of tone.

- An increase in tone is called **hypertonia**, while a decrease in tone is called **hypotonia**. Complete loss of muscle tone is known as **atonia**.
- **Testing muscle tone:** This is tested by noting the resistance offered to passive movements done by the examiner on various joints of the subject/patient.
  - **Principle:** The examiner holds the limb on either side of a joint to be tested, and passively moves the limb through the full range of its movements. The ease or difficulty with which a limb can thus be moved is noted and compared with the similar joint on the opposite side.
  - **In the upper limbs at elbow joint:** The examiner holds the arm of the subject with one hand, and alternately flexes and extends the forearm at the elbow joint with the other hand.
  - Tone at the **fingers, wrist, and shoulder** is tested in a similar manner **(Fig. 41)**.
  - **In the lower limbs**, passive movements are done at the ankle, knee, and hip comparing these on the two sides.
  - In **hypertonia**, the patient's muscles resist the passive movements, while in **hypotonia** the movements become free and the joints can be hyperextended.
- **Physioclinical significance:**
  - ***Hypertonia:*** This occurs in lesions of UMN.
    - ***Spasticity:*** The term refers to hypertonia resulting from *lesions in many of the posture regulating pathways*. The increased tone is of *clasp-knife type*, i.e. when the limb is moved, maximum resistance is offered at once, but it suddenly gives way after some effort on the part of the examiner. It is sensitive to stretch, i.e. *"stretch-sensitive"*. It is usually maximum in flexors of the arms and extensors of the legs.
    - ***Rigidity:*** The hypertonia of rigidity results from *diseases of the basal ganglia* (e.g. Parkinsonism). It may be of *"cog-wheel"* type in which the resistance to passive movement decreases in jerky steps (probably a combination of tremor and rigidity), or of **"lead-pipe"** type in which resistance is felt throughout the passive movement. The rigidity of Parkinsonism is commonly accompanied by akinesia, i.e. poverty of movement.
  - ***Hypotonia*** is seen in LMN disease and cerebellar lesions (in humans). Passive movement is unusually free and frequently through a greater range than normal.
  - Atonia is a complete loss of muscle tone.

Strength/Power of Muscles

- ***Test the muscle strength in the upper limbs of the subject provided***: A preliminary observation of how a subject, (but especially a patient), walks, or stands up from the sitting or supine position, shakes hands, or performs other everyday movements such as buttoning a shirt or combing the hair, can provide a quick and reliable means for assessing muscle weakness, or paralysis, if any.
- The muscle power at big and small joints is then tested by asking the subject first to move parts of the body, and then against resistance of the examiner's hand, and compared with similar muscles on the opposite limb **(Fig. 42)**.
  - **Abductor pollicis brevis:** The subject is asked to abduct his thumb in a plane at right angles to the palmar aspect of the index finger, against the resistance of the examiner's own thumb. The muscle can be seen and felt to contract. This muscle is supplied by the median nerve, which is sometimes damaged by compression in the carpal tunnel at the wrist (carpal tunnel syndrome).
  - **Opponens pollicis:** The subject is asked to touch the tips of all his fingers with the tip of his thumb. The examiner opposes each movement with his index finger or thumb.
  - **First dorsal interosseous:** The subject is asked to abduct his index finger against resistance.
  - **Other interossei and lumbricals:** The subject's ability to flex his metacarpophalangeal joints and to extend the distal interphalangeal joints is tested. The interossei also adduct and abduct the fingers.

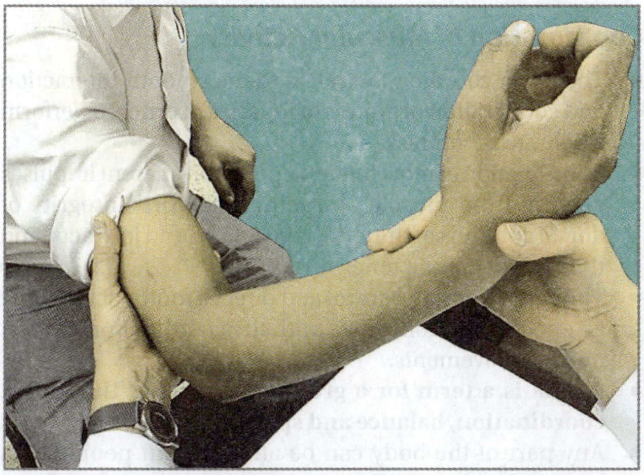

FIG. 41: Testing for muscle tone in upper limb.

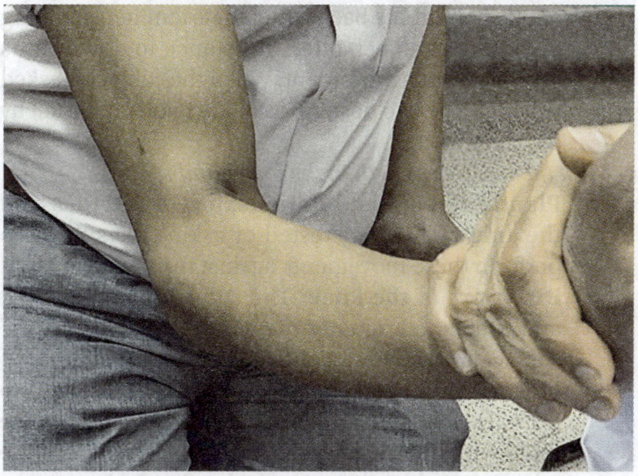

FIG. 42: Testing of muscle power in upper limb.

- **Flexors of fingers:** The subject is asked to squeeze the examiner's index and middle fingers to assess the force of grip.
- **Flexors of the wrist:** The subject is asked to bring his fingers toward the front of the forearm, while the examiner opposes this movement with his fingers.
- **Extensors of the wrist:** The subject is asked to make a fist (both flexors and extensors contract), while the examiner tries to flex the wrist against the subject's effort to maintain that position.
- **Brachioradialis:** The subject's arm is placed midway between pronation and supination, and then asked to bend the forearm up, while the examiner opposes this movement by grasping the subject's hand. The muscle can be seen and felt to stand out in its upper part.
- **Biceps:** The subject is asked to bend up the forearm against resistance in full supination. The muscle stands out clearly.
- **Triceps:** The subject is asked to straighten out his forearm against resistance.
- **Supraspinatus:** The subject is asked to lift his arm straight out at right angles to his side. The first 30° of this movement is brought about by supraspinatus and the rest 60° is carried out by the deltoid.
- **Deltoid:** The arm is held out, in abduction, straight out. The subject offers resistance, while the examiner tries to depress the elbow. The anterior and posterior fibers help to draw the abducted arm forwards and backwards, which can also be tested against resistance.
- **Infraspinatus:** With the forearm flexed to a right angle, the subject is asked to tuck his elbow into his side. Then he is asked to rotate the limb outward against resistance.
- **Pectorals:** The subject is asked to stretch the arms out in front of him and then to clasp his hands while the examiner tries to hold them apart.
- **Serratus anterior:** The subject is asked to push forward with his hands against resistance, such as a wall. When this muscle is paralyzed, the scapula is "winged".
- **Latissimus dorsi:** The subject is asked to clasp his hands behind his back while the examiner, standing behind the subject, offers resistance to downwards and backwards movement. When the subject is asked to cough, the two posterior axillary folds can be felt by the examiner.

- *Test the muscle strength in the lower limbs*:
  - **Plantar flexion and dorsiflexion of the toes and the ankle:** These are tested by asking the subject to perform these movements against resistance.
  - **Extensors of the knee:** The subject's knee is bent and while the examiner presses against his shin, the subject is asked to straighten out the leg again.
  - **Flexors of the knee:** The subject's leg is raised up from the bed, and while the examiner supports the thigh with one hand and holding the ankle with the other hand, the subject is asked to flex the knee joint.

Table 2: Grading of muscle power.

Grade 0	Complete paralysis
Grade 1	A flicker of contraction only
Grade 2	Muscle power is detected only when gravity is excluded by suitable postural adjustment
Grade 3	The limb can be held against the force of gravity, but not against resistance
Grade 4	Some degree of weakness is there, which is commonly described as poor, moderate, or fair strength, i.e. movements are possible against the examiner's resistance but are weak
Grade 5	The muscle power is normal both without load and with the examiner's resistance

  - **Extensors of the hip:** With his knee extended, the subject lifts the foot from the bed, and is asked to push it down against resistance.
  - **Flexors of the thigh:** With his leg extended, the subject is asked to raise the leg off the bed against resistance.
  - **Abductors of the thigh:** The subject's legs are placed together and he is asked to separate them against resistance.
  - **Adductors of the thigh:** The limb is abducted and then the subject is asked to bring it back toward the midline against resistance.
  - **Rotators of the thigh:** With the limb extended and resting on the bed, the subject is asked to roll it outward or inward against resistance.
- ***Testing the muscles of the trunk:***
  The subject is asked to sit up in bed from the supine position without the help of his arms (abdominal muscles tested).
  The subject lies on his face and tries to raise his head by extending the neck and back. The muscles can be seen to become prominent (extensors of the back tested).

Grading of muscle power: See **Table 2**.

- **Physioclinical significance:** Overall muscle power is a good indication of motor nerve function. The pattern of weakness varies according to the location of the lesion. It is impractical to assess every muscle group in the body.

Coordination of Muscular Activity

- This term coordination refers to the smooth interaction and cooperation of groups of muscles in order to perform a definite motor task.
- Coordination of movements depends on afferent impulses coming from muscle and joint receptors, integrity of dorsal columns of the cord, cerebellum and its tracts, and the state of muscle tone.
- Though vision can control and direct a motor act to some extent, it is not concerned with the coordination of most normal movements.
- **Ataxia is a term for a group of disorders that affect coordination, balance and speech.**
- Any part of the body can be affected, but people with ataxia often have difficulties with balance and walking,

speaking, swallowing, tasks that require a high degree of control, such as writing and eating, vision.
- If coordination of movements becomes impaired ***(ataxia),*** the carrying out of motor activities becomes difficult and sometimes even impossible.

Tests for Coordination

In the upper limbs:
- ***"Finger-nose" test*:** The subject is asked to extend his arm to the side and then touch the tip of his nose with the tip of his index finger, first with the eyes open and then with the eyes closed. The other limb is tested similarly. A normal subject is able to perform these acts accurately, both slowly and rapidly.
- The subject is asked to touch each finger in turn with the tip of the thumb.
- The subject is asked to draw a large circle in the air with his forefinger.
- The subject is asked to make fists, flex the forearm to right angles, tuck the elbows into his sides, and then to alternately pronate and supinate his forearms as rapidly as possible. An inability to perform such rapid movements is called **dysdiadochokinesia**. It is an important sign of cerebellar disease where the movements on the affected side become very clumsy or even impossible to carry out.
- Watching a patient dressing or undressing, picking up pins from a table, handling a book, etc. can provide useful information about muscle coordination.

In the lower limbs:
- The subject is asked to walk along a straight line. The examiner watches carefully as the subject turns to walk back. The subject may also be asked to walk along a line, placing the heel of one foot immediately adjacent to the toes of the foot behind (tandem walking). If incoordination is present, the subject soon deviates to one or the other side and takes a zigzag course like that of a drunk.
- ***"Heel-knee" test*:** The subject lies on his back, and is asked to lift one foot high in the air, to place its heel on the opposite knee, and then to slide the heel down the leg toward the ankle. The test is done first with the eyes open and then with eyes closed, and it is repeated on the other side.
- The subject is asked to draw a large circle in the air with his toe.

Romberg's sign: This sign is a test for the **loss of position sense** (sensory ataxia) in the legs. It is not a test for cerebellar function.
- The subject is asked to stand with the feet as close together as possible. He is then asked to close his eyes. A normal person remains steady with eyes closed.
- However, if the Romberg's sign is present, the patient starts to sway from side to side as soon as he closes his eyes. Thus, the patient becomes unsteady when his eyes are closed.
- In **sensory ataxia** (lesion of dorsal columns of cord or dorsal roots, as in tabes dorsalis) the sensory information from the legs is lacking; therefore, the patient becomes unsteady without the help of vision.
- In **cerebellar ataxia**, the patient is unsteady on his feet whether the eyes are open or closed.

***Perform any three cerebellar function tests in the subject provided*:**
1. Test the "finger-nose test" in the upper limbs. In cerebellar disease, as the finger approaches the nose, it shows tremor (called "intention" tremor, i.e. tremor appears when a movement is performed and is not present at rest) and may undershoot or overshoot the mark.
2. Test the coordination in the lower limbs by asking the subject to walk along a straight line.
3. Test the muscle tone in the upper and lower limbs. There is hypotonia in cerebellar disease. (Hypotonia also explains the pendular or swinging response when the knee jerk is elicited with the legs hanging freely over the edge of a chair).

- **Physioclinical significance:** Although incoordination is primarily a symptom of cerebellar disease, it can also be seen from other causes such as:
  a. *Sensory dysfunction*-loss of large myelinated sensory axons serving proprioception. This causes a **sensory ataxia**. Key distinguishing feature for this type of problem are a positive Romberg and loss of position sense on the sensory exam.
  b. *Vestibular dysfunction*. Key distinguishing feature is vertigo.
  c. *Corticospinal tract disease* can cause incoordination of the distal extremities. Key distinguishing features are the UMN signs.

Reflexes

***Definition*:** A **reflex**, or **reflex action**, is an involuntary contraction of a muscle or a group of muscles (or secretion of a gland) in response to a specific stimulus, and which involves some part of the central nervous system (CNS).

***Clinically tested reflexes*:** These include—*superficial reflexes* (from skin and mucous membranes), *deep reflexes* or *tendon reflexes* and *visceral reflexes*.

For each reflex, the student should know:
- The method of its elicitation
- The response (normal and abnormal)
- The receptors and the afferent (sensory) path
- The center (site of integration)
- The efferent (motor) path, and
- The clinical significance of the reflex or reflexes, i.e. their value in localization of the site of lesion, assessing the integrity of the sensory and motor pathways, the influence of higher centers, and in differentiating between the UMN and LMN lesions.

Table 3 shows a summary of clinically tested reflexes.

Superficial Reflexes

- These include the plantar response; the epigastric and abdominal reflexes; cremasteric, gluteal, and anal reflexes; the ciliospinal reflex; and the various mucous membrane reflexes described earlier with cranial nerves.

Table 3: Summary of reflexes tested clinically.

Reflexes (1)	How Elicited (2)	Response (3)	Afferent Path (4)	Center (5)	Efferent Path (6)
Superficial reflexes:					
(A) *Skin reflexes:*					
1. Plantar	Scratch on medial aspect of sole	Plantar flexion of toes (in Babinski, dorsiflexion of toes)	Tibial	L5,S1	Tibial
2. Abdominal	Scratch on abdominal wall	Contraction of the abdominal muscles	Th-7-12	Th 7-12	Th-7-12
3. Cremasteric	Scratch on upper medial thigh	Drawing upwards of the testicle	Femoral	L-1,2	Femoral
4. Gluteal	Scratch on buttock	Contraction of gluteus muscle	L-4,5	L-4,5	L-4,5
5. Anal	Scratch on skin near anus	Contraction of anal sphincter	Pudendal	S-4,5	Pudendal
(B) *Mucous membrane reflexes:*					
1. Corneal or conjunctival	Touch on cornea or conjunctiva with cotton	Closure of eye	Cranial V	Pons	Cranial VII
2. Pharyngeal	Touch on pharynx	Constriction of pharynx	Cranial IX	Medulla	Cranial X
3. Palate	Touch on soft palate	Elevation of palate	Cranial IX	Medulla	Cranial X
Deep reflexes:					
1. Jaw jerk	Tapping on middle of jaw	Closure of mouth	Cranial V	Pons	Cranial V
2. Biceps jerk	Tapping on biceps tendon	Flexion at elbow	Musculo-cutaneous	C-5,6	Musculo-cutaneous
3. Triceps jerk	Tapping on triceps tendon	Extension at elbow	Radial	C-6,7	Radial
4. Supinator jerk	Tapping on styloid process of radius	Flexion and supination of forearm	Radial	C-5/6	Radial
5. Knee jerk	Tapping on patellar tendon	Extension at knee	Femoral	L-2,3,4	Femoral
6. Ankle jerk	Tapping on Achilles tendon	Planter flexion of foot	Tibial	S-1,2	Tibial
Visceral reflexes:					
(A) *Pupillary reflexes:*					
1. Light (direct)	Shining of light on retina in one eye	Constriction of pupil on that side	Cranial II	Midbrain	Cranial III
2. Light (indirect or consensual)	Shining of light on retina in one eye	Constriction of pupil on other side	Cranial II	Midbrain	Cranial III
3. Accommodation	Subject looks on finger held in front of one eye	Constriction of pupil in that eye	Cranial II	Occipital cortex	Cranial III
4. Ciliospinal	Pinching of skin on back of neck	Dilatation of pupil	Sensory nerve	Th-1,2	Cervical sympathetic
(B) *Oculocardiac reflex*	Pressure over eyeball with thumb	Slowing of heart and fall in blood pressure	Cranial V	Medulla	Cranial X
(C) *Carotid sinus reflex*	Pressure over carotid sinus on one side	Slowing of heart and fall in blood pressure	Cranial IX	Medulla	Cranial X
(D) *Bulbocavernosus reflex*	Pinching dorsum of glans penis	Contraction of bulbocavernosus	Pudendal	S-3,4	Pelvic autonomic

(E) *Sphincter reflexes:* These reflexes include swallowing, micturition, and defecation. They depend upon complex muscular movement excited by increased tension in the wall of the viscera concerned.

- **Swallowing:** The subject is asked whether he has any difficulty in swallowing (dysphasia). If present, ask him whether he has difficulty in swallowing liquids or solids. As a rule patients with neurological disorders causing dysphasia complain of difficulty in swallowing liquids, whereas in mechanical esophageal obstruction they find difficulty in swallowing solids.
- **Defecation:** The patient should be asked if he has any difficulty in passing stools. He should also be asked whether he can feel rectal sensation.
- **Micturition:** The subject should be asked whether he has any difficulty in controlling or initiating micturition. He should also be questioned for retention and incontinence of urine.

- **Response:** In all the skin reflexes, there is contraction of the underlying muscles when a particular area of the skin is stimulated by scratching, stroking, or pinching.
- **Reflex arcs:**
  - The reflex arcs for the skin reflexes appear to be long and complex, and include a number of interneurons between the sensory and the motor neurons of the reflex arc. The afferent impulses appear to be carried up by dorsal columns and spinothalamic tracts and end somewhere in the midbrain, thalamus, or cerebral cortex.
  - From here, impulses are carried by corticospinal and extrapyramidal tracts to the anterior horn cells innervating the muscles involved in the reflex. *This is*

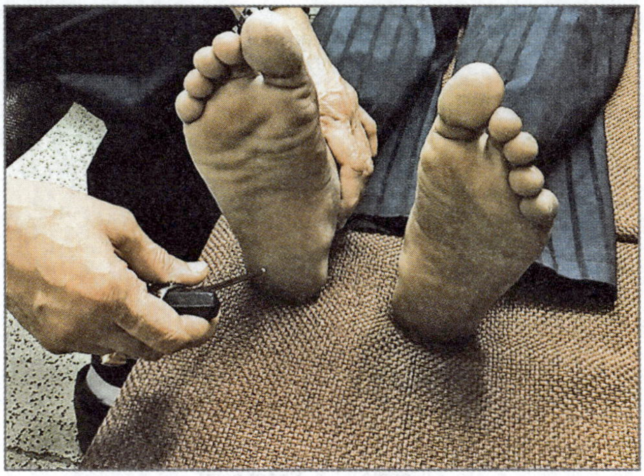

FIG. 43: Plantar reflex.

the reason why the skin reflexes are absent in the UMN lesions.

- **Flexor plantar reflex (plantar flexor reflex):**
  - The subject is asked to relax the muscles of the legs. A light scratch is given with a thumbnail (it should always be tried first), a key, or the blunt point of the patellar hammer, along the **outer edge of the sole of the foot, from the heel toward the little toe, and then medially along the base of the toes up to the 2nd toe (Fig. 43).**
  - The response to this stimulation of the skin in healthy adults is—plantar flexion and drawing together of the toes, often including the big toe, dorsiflexion, and inversion of the ankle, and sometimes, contraction of the tensor fascia lata.
  - With stronger stimuli, the limb may be withdrawn (flexed at the knee and hip) and adducted at the hip. This is the normal response in the adults, and is called the flexor plantar reflex (or the plantar flexor reflex).
  - It is never completely absent in healthy individuals. Afferent (tibial nerve): L-5, S-1,2; center: S-1,2; efferent (tibial nerve): L-4,5 segments of the spinal cord.
- **Extensor plantar reflex (plantar extensor reflex):**
  - In infants, the response is a dorsiflexion of the big toe and retraction of the foot and occasionally dorsiflexion and fan-like spreading of the other toes. In adults, such a response (first described by Babinski in 1896) is seen in lesions of the corticospinal system.
  - This abnormal response is called the **extensor plantar reflex** or the **Babinski sign.** In this response, the dorsiflexion of the toes (the big toe dorsiflexes first) is followed by dorsiflexion of the ankle and flexion of the knee and the hip. (The stimulus must be applied over the lateral region of the sole because the medial region may give a normal response).
  - In some cases with Babinski sign, the reflexogenic area (i.e. the region from which it is obtained) spreads out over a large area so that the same response is obtained by squeezing the calf muscles by a firm downward movement over anterior tibia **(Oppenheim's sign)**, by pinching the Achilles tendon **(Gordon's reflex)**, or by stroking the lateral malleolus **(Chaddok's sign)**. [The clawing movement of the fingers and the thumb upon flicking the terminal phalanx of the index finger is called the **Hoffmann's sign** (the equivalent of Babinski in the upper limb)].
- **Physioclinical significance:** The Babinski sign is perhaps the most important single physical sign in clinical neurology. It has great significance in differentiating between an organic lesion and a functional disorder (e.g. psychoneurosis) because it never occurs in the latter conditions.
- **Babinski sign is seen in the following:**
  - Infants below the age of 1 year, i.e. until the corticospinal tracts get myelinated and become functional. The plantar response becomes flexor in the next 6–8 months when the child learns to walk.
  - Upper motor neuron (corticospinal or pyramidal) lesions such as cerebral vascular disease (e.g. capsular hemiplegia), disseminated sclerosis, etc.
  - Spinal cord tumors—the pyramidal fibers are very sensitive to pressure, hence their early involvement in such cases.
  - Deep narcosis, coma due to any cause, and following an attack of grand mal epilepsy when the patient becomes unconscious. (It is temporary in some forms of coma and after epileptic fits).
  - Biochemical disturbances, such as hypoglycemia, in which convulsions may occur.
  - **Babinski sign appears in corticospinal tract lesions:** *Explanation of Babinski sign:* Any movement of a limb or part of a limb, which **increases the length of the limb is physiologically an extension movement,** and any movement, which **decreases the length of the limb is a flexion movement.**
  - The normal plantar response to stimulation is plantar flexion (downward movement) of the toes, which is **physiologically an extensor response** though brought about by muscles, which are called flexors in **anatomical** terms.
  - The Babinski response, i.e. extensor plantar reflex, was named extensor because the **upward movement of the big toe is caused by a muscle which the anatomists call extensor hallucis longus, though physiologically it is a flexor muscle.**
  - The older extrapyramidal system is concerned with controlling primitive spinal cord activities such as flexion (like an animal crawling into a hole), and the protective *nociceptive flexor withdrawal reflex* described by Sherrington in a decerebrate animal (application of a painful stimulus to a paw leads to withdrawal of that limb as a whole; this **mass flexor withdrawal reflex** can be better shown in a spinal animal or spinal man, because **"isolated" spinal cord favors flexor activity**).
  - The newer control system controls higher order of motor activity including the downward movement of the toes in response to a scratch on the sole of the

foot—a response, which helps us to walk (e.g. when an infant learns to walk, the contact with the ground acts as a stimulus and the resulting plantar flexion of the toes helps to propel the body forward).

- Therefore, as long as the corticospinal system is intact, it keeps the primitive activities under check; but when it is damaged, the older activities are released from its inhibitory effect, and this is expressed as the nociceptive flexor withdrawal reflex, a part of which is the Babinski response. Thus, the Babinski sign is a release phenomenon.

- **Abdominal reflex:** The subject should be relaxed and in supine position with the abdomen uncovered.
  - A light scratch, with a key or blunt point, is given across the abdominal skin, directed toward the umbilicus, in the upper, middle, and lower regions. The response is a brisk ripple of contraction of the underlying muscles. The centers for these reflexes are: upper abdominal—Th-8,9,10; middle—Th-9,10,11, and lower abdominal—Th-10,11,12 segments of the spinal cord.
  - These reflexes are absent in UMN lesions above their segmental level in the spinal cord. They may indicate the segmental level of thoracic spinal cord lesion by their absence.
  - The abdominal reflexes are sometimes difficult to elicit in obese or elderly, in anxious people.
- **Elicit the ciliospinal reflex:**
  - The skin of the neck of the subject is pinched; the response is dilatation of the pupil. The pathways in the spinal cord and the sympathetic trunk must be intact. Afferent path—skin of the neck region; center—Th (thoracic)-1,2; efferent—cervical sympathetic.
  - *Loss of ciliospinal reflex is used as a measure of depth of coma; it is also one of the criteria of brain death.*
- The **epigastric reflex** can be demonstrated by giving a scratch downwards from the nipple on the front of the chest; the response is a drawing of the epigastrium on that side. The center is in T -7,8 segments.

Deep Reflexes

- The deep reflexes are also called the **tendon reflexes,** or **tendon jerks** or simply **"jerks"** because when the tendon of a lightly stretched muscle is given a single, sharp blow with a rubber hammer (patellar or percussion hammer), the muscle contracts briefly and then relaxes, i.e. it gives a "jerky" response.
- **Patellar (knee) hammer (Figs. 44 and 45)** is a simple device employed for eliciting deep or tendon reflexes. It has a long metallic handle that bears a triangular rubber piece. The rubber is employed for delivering a sharp blow on the tendon of a slightly stretched muscle under study.
- The sudden stretch of the muscle causes a reflex contraction of the muscle. When using it, the hammer should be held between the thumb and fingers and the swing should be at the wrist and not at the elbow or shoulder.
- The upper part of the hammer, which can be unscrewed, has a sharp point for eliciting superficial reflexes.

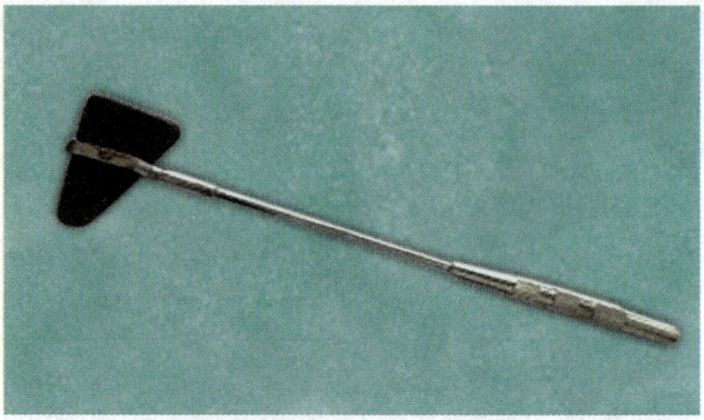

FIG. 44: Knee hammer (patellar or percussion hammer).

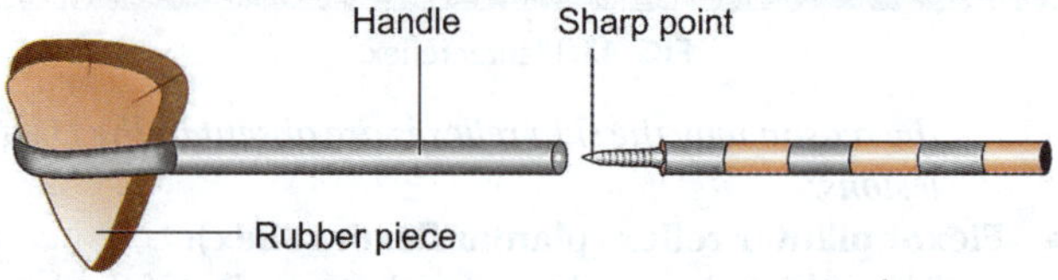

FIG. 45: Percussion (knee) hammer and its parts.

- **Stimulus:** The **stimulus** that initiates a deep reflex is the sudden **stretching of the muscle spindles,** which sends a synchronous volley of impulses from the primary sensory endings into the spinal cord. In the cord, these impulses directly (monosynaptically) stimulate the anterior horn cells, which innervate the stretched muscle **(Fig. 40)**. Thus, these reflexes are monosynaptic stretch reflexes.

Important:

- ❑ It may be noted that it is the spindle receptors and not the tendon receptors, which are stimulated though the hammer is struck on the tendon and not on the muscle belly. All muscles are somewhat excitable to direct mechanical stimulation, which is a direct response and not a stretch reflex. (The tendon receptors respond to excessive stretch—as in inverse stretch reflex, when the muscle relaxes suddenly).
- ❑ It is a simple device employed for eliciting deep or tendon reflexes. It has a long handle that bears a triangular rubber piece. The rubber is used to deliver a sharp blow on the tendon of the slightly stretched muscle under study.
- ❑ The sudden stretch of the muscle causes a reflex contraction of the muscle. The hammer should be held between the thumb and the index finger. The movement should be free and at the wrist while striking the tendon. The upper part of the handle, which can be unscrewed, has a sharp point for eliciting superficial reflexes.

Knee jerk

- **Supine position:**
  - The subject is asked to relax his legs, and is reassured that the patellar hammer will not cause injury. His legs are semiflexed and the observer supports both knees by placing a hand behind them.
  - The patellar tendon is then struck midway between the patella and the insertion of the tendon on the tibial tuberosity. (The tendon is located by palpation before striking it).

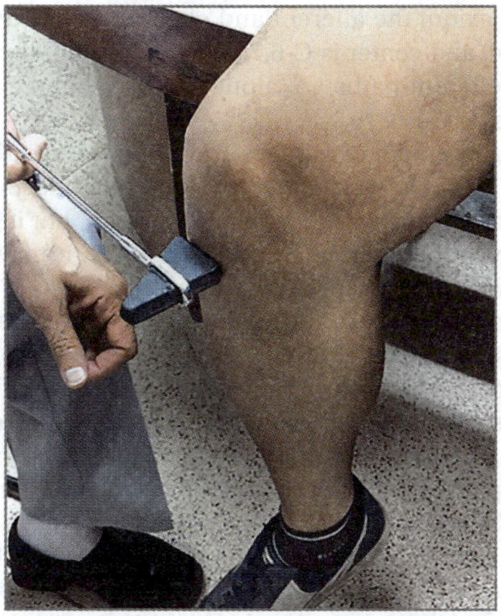

FIG. 46: Knee jerk in sitting position.

- The response is extension of the knee due to contraction of the quadriceps femoris muscle. Afferent and efferent paths—femoral nerve; center—lumbar 2,3,4 segments.

- **Sitting position:**
  - The subject is seated in a chair and is asked to cross one leg over the other, and then the reflex is elicited. The leg can be seen to kick forwards; the muscle can also be felt to contract, if the observer places his hand on the lower front of the thigh **(Fig. 46)**.
  - A better way to elicit this reflex is to ask the subject to sit with both legs dangling loosely over the edge of the chair. It permits a more rapid comparison of the two knee jerks.
    The knee jerk may be pendular in acute cerebellar disease and present on the side of the lesion. It may be sustained in chorea. In hypothyroidism, there may be delayed return of the leg to the resting position. In hyperthyroidism, the jerks are brisk.

Ankle jerk

- The subject lies supine, the knee is semiflexed, and the hip externally rotated. Then with one hand, the examiner slightly dorsiflexes the foot so as to stretch the Achilles tendon (tendo calcaneus), and with the other hand, the tendon is struck on its posterior surface.
- The response is plantar flexion of the foot due to contraction of the calf muscles **(Fig. 47)**.
- Another method is to ask the subject to kneel over a chair, so that he faces the back of the chair and his ankles lie over its edge. The ankle jerks are then tested as described above. Afferent and efferent—tibial nerve; center—sacral 1,2 segments **(Fig. 48)**.

Biceps jerk

- The subject's elbow is flexed to a right angle and the forearm semi pronated and supported on the examiner's arm. The examiner then places his thumb on the biceps tendon and strikes it with the hammer **(Fig. 49)**.

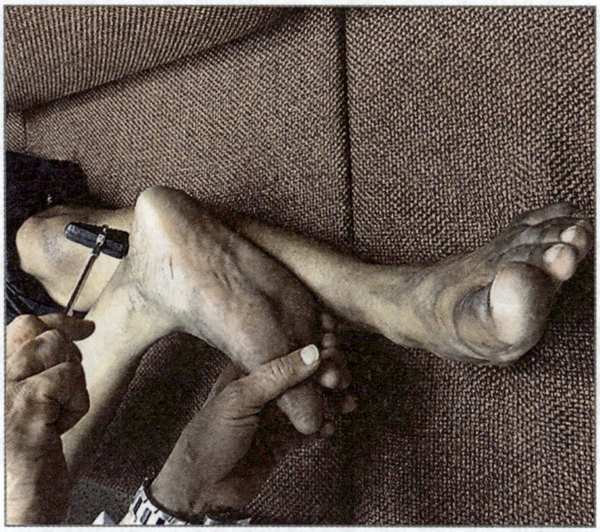

FIG. 47: Ankle jerk in supine position.

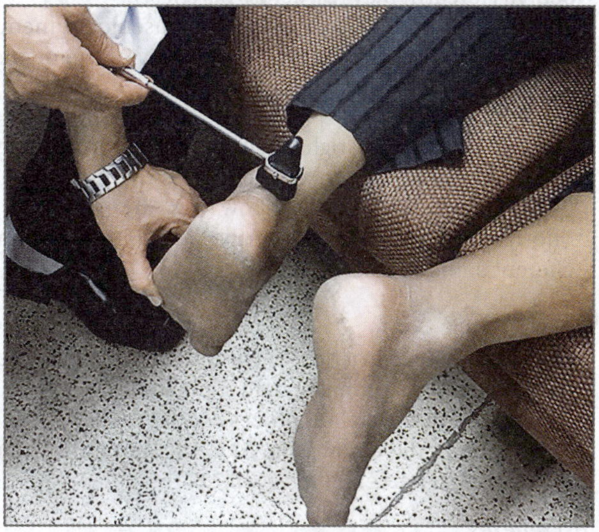

FIG. 48: Ankle jerk in kneeling down position.

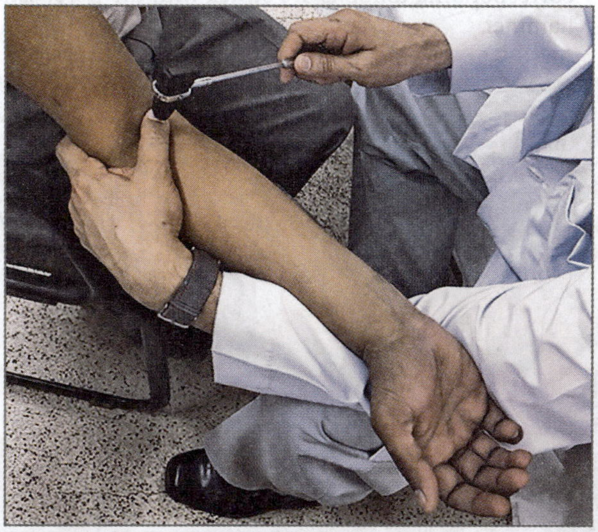

FIG. 49: Biceps jerk.

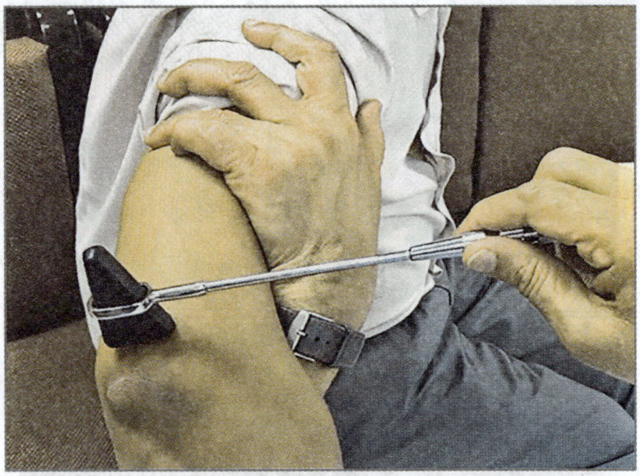

FIG. 50: Triceps jerk.

- The response is contraction of the biceps causing flexion and slight pronation of the forearm (if the patient is in bed, his forearm may rest across his chest).
- The afferent and efferent paths are musculocutaneous nerve and the center is in 5th and 6th cervical segments.

Triceps reflex

- The arm is flexed to a right angle and is supported on the examiner's arm. The triceps tendon is then struck just proximal to the point of the elbow **(Fig. 50)**.
- The response is extension at the elbow. Afferent and efferent paths—radial nerve; center—C-6,7.

Supinator reflex

- The arm is placed to a right angle and the forearm placed midway between pronation and supination.
- Upon striking the styloid process of the radius, there is supination at the elbow **(Fig. 51)**. Afferent and efferent paths—radial nerve; center—C-6,7,8.

Wrist reflexes

- There is flexion or extension at the wrist when the corresponding tendons are struck with the percussion hammer.
- For flexion, the afferent and efferent paths are median nerve, and center is C-6,7,8. For extension, the afferent and efferent paths are along the radial nerve, and the center is C-7,8.
- **Reinforcement of reflexes and when is it required:**
  - The briskness of knee jerk (and other deep reflexes) varies greatly from person to person, but it is hardly ever absent in health. Occasionally, it may be very weak or even appear to be absent.
  - In such cases, **reinforcement (Jendrassik maneuver)** is employed **(Fig. 52)**. This is done by asking the subject to perform some strong muscular effort, such as clenching the teeth, or locking the fingers of both hands as hard as possible and then trying to pull them apart while the examiner strikes the patellar tendon. The reflex generally becomes evident.
  - Reinforcement acts by increasing the excitability of the anterior horn cells due to "spilling" over of impulses from the neurons involved in reinforcement effort to the motor neurons of the reflex. In addition, gamma motor neuron activity increases the sensitivity of the spindle receptors to stretch. It also, perhaps, acts by distracting the subject's attention.
- **Physioclinical significance:**
  1. **Deep reflexes are *diminished or absent* in the following conditions:**
     - Lesions involving the afferent pathways (e.g. tabes dorsalis)
     - Lesions of the anterior horn cell (e.g. poliomyelitis), or the efferent pathways
     - In peripheral neuropathies or peripheral nerve injuries, both sensory and motor fibers are affected.
     - The tendon jerks are also abolished by spinal shock, e.g. severe injury to the cord. (In fact, all motor and sensory functions are lost below the site of lesion for the duration of the spinal shock).
     - Tendon reflexes are also lost bilaterally in coma.
     - As mentioned earlier, the deep reflexes may be sluggish or appear to be abolished in some

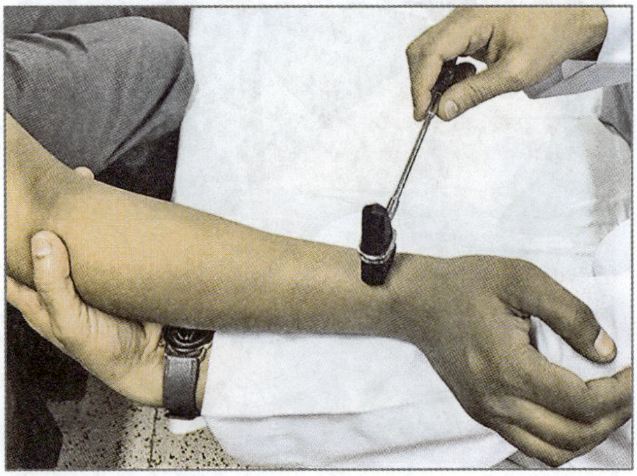

FIG. 51: Supinator reflex.

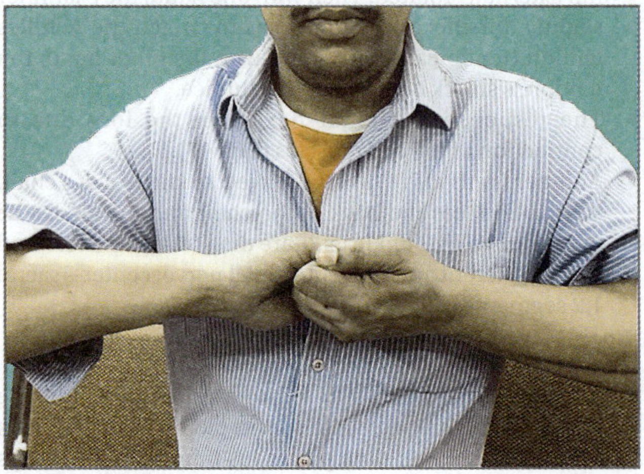

FIG. 52: Jendrassik's maneuver.

healthy individuals; reinforcement is employed in these cases.

2. **Deep reflexes are exaggerated (hyperreflexia) in the following conditions:**
   - Upper motor neuron lesions above the anterior horn cells, especially when the hyperreflexia is unilateral, or accompanied by other signs of UMN disease.
   - Anxiety or nervousness.
   - Hyperexcitability of the nervous system, as in hyperthyroidism, and tetanus.
   - The cause of exaggeration of deep reflexes in lesions of corticospinal system is the hypertonia (spasticity) resulting from overactivity of the stretch reflexes; this system keeps these reflexes under check. When this inhibition is lost, the deep reflexes are more easily elicited. Exaggeration of reflexes is thus a "release" phenomenon—as is the Babinski response.

- **Clonus:** It is a series of involuntary contractions of certain muscles in response to stretch. This phenomenon is closely allied to deep reflexes and can often be demonstrated at the ankle when these reflexes are exaggerated. It is of greater importance when it is increased by maintaining and increasing the stretch on the muscle.
  - **Eliciting ankle clonus:** The subject's knee is slightly flexed and the leg is held up by supporting it with a hand placed behind the knee. The examiner then suddenly dorsiflexes the foot after grasping its forepart. The sudden stretch of calf muscles results in their alternate contraction and relaxation. There may be two or three oscillations ("pseudo", "spurious", or "exhaustible" clonus) in normal persons who are very tense or anxious, but "true", "sustained", or "inexhaustible" clonus is present only in UMN lesions (the plantar reflexes are flexor in normal persons).
  - **Eliciting patellar clonus:** The subject's leg is placed in extension. The examiner holds the patella from its sides with his thumb and fingers and then presses it sharply and firmly downwards. If clonus is present, the patella shows a rapid up and down movement, which continues as long as the stretch is maintained.
  - **Grading of tendon reflexes:** Tendon or deep reflexes are usually graded as follows:
    - Grade 0—absent
    - Grade 1—present (as a normal ankle jerk)
    - Grade 2—brisk (as a normal knee jerk)
    - Grade 3—very brisk
    - Grade 4—clonus.

Visceral Reflexes

- The visceral reflexes include—pupillary reflexes, reflexes from the heart and lungs (sinoaortic, Hering-Breuer, etc.), deglutition, vomiting, defecation, micturition, and sexual reflexes. Those which are tested clinically are—pupillary, oculocardiac, carotid sinus reflex, bulbocavernosus, and sphincter reflexes. The tests employed for assessing autonomic function are based on some visceral reflexes.
  - **Pupillary reflexes:** The light reflex, accommodation reflex, and ciliospinal reflexes may be demonstrated.
  - **Oculocardiac reflex:** While the examiner feels the pulse of the subject with one hand, a gentle pressure is applied on the eyeball with the thumb of the other hand. The response is a slowing of the heart. Afferent—trigeminal nerve; center—medulla; efferent—vagus nerve.
  - **Carotid sinus reflex:** Pressure with the thumb on the carotid sinus in the neck (on one side only, never on both sides) causes slowing of the heart. Afferent—glossopharyngeal; center—medulla; efferent—vagus. This reflex is hyperactive in some persons with marked vasomotor instability; slight stimulation of this type may cause fainting (carotid sinus syncope).

Motor Neuron Lesions

Lesions of lower motor neurons

- The LMNs may be interrupted by lesions in the anterior horns (e.g. poliomyelitis; effects purely motor), in the anterior nerve roots (trauma; compression), in the peripheral nerves (trauma; neuropathies), or at their terminations in the muscles (motor end plates).
- The trophic changes often associated in diseases involving LMN are mainly due to associated damage to sensory nerves and autonomic systems.

Lesions of upper motor neurons

- These neurons may be damaged anywhere along their course from the cerebral motor cortex to their termination in the brainstem and spinal cord.
- Lesions restricted purely to pyramidal tracts cause muscle weakness, while lesions of extrapyramidal system alone cause spastic paralysis, tremors, and abnormal movements or posture.
- Clinically, the typically UMN lesion in the internal capsule involves both pyramidal and extrapyramidal fibers and causes hemiplegia.
- Lesions of UMN in the brainstem usually involve various cranial nerves, which help in the localization of the lesion. Thus, used unqualified, the term UMN lesion may sometimes be confusing.
- **The main features and differences between upper and lower motor neuron lesions are given in Table 4.**

Presence of Involuntary Movements

- The abnormal movements that may be seen in neurological diseases consist of various types of muscle contractions. First note whether the abnormal movements are ***localized*** or ***widespread***. Also they may be present ***at rest*** or ***during motor activity.***
- The term ***spasm*** refers to any exaggerated and involuntary muscle contraction. If the contraction is continuous, it is called ***tonic contraction.*** If there is a series of short

Table 4: Differences between upper and lower motor neuron lesions.

	Features	Upper motor neuron (pyramidal and extrapyramidal)	Lower motor (anterior horn cell type including peripheral nerve injuries)
1.	Loss of power	Incomplete	Complete
2.	Extent of paralysis	More extensive and equal involvement of muscles of a limb	Less extensive and unequal involvement
3.	Atrophy and wasting	None or slight; generalized; due to disuse	Marked, focal. May involve 70–80% of muscle mass
4.	Muscle tone	Increased (rigidity)	Decreased (flaccidity)
5.	*Reflexes:* (a) Deep (b) Superficial, abdominal	Exaggerated Absent or diminished on the side of involvement	Absent or diminished Unaffected unless thoracic anterior horn cells are affected
6.	Pathological reflexes Babinski, Gordon's, Oppenheim's, Hoffman's sign	All are present	All are absent
7.	Muscle fasciculation and fibrillation	Absent	Often present
8.	Electrical changes in muscle	Normal reactions to Galvanic and Faradic current	Partial or complete reaction of degeneration in the involved muscles
9.	Vasomotor phenomena	Mild	Marked
10.	Associated movement, e.g. Strumpell's sign	Present	Absent

contractions with partial or complete relaxations in between, it is called ***clonic contraction.***

- *Localized involuntary movements*: These include:
  - ***Fibrillation:*** They are due to contraction of a single muscle fiber. Usually, they cannot be seen though they can be recorded as electromyography (EMG).
  - ***Fasciculation:*** These are due to contraction of one or more motor units and are visible on the skin.
  - ***Myoclonus:*** It is a sudden shock like contraction of a single muscle or a group of muscles.
  - ***Tremor:*** It is an involuntary, regular, rhythmic, and purposeless movement due to alternate contraction and relaxation of agonists and antagonists. Fine tremor is seen in anxiety and hyperthyroidism. Coarse tremor is seen in Parkinson's disease, cerebellar lesions, alcoholism, barbiturate, and heavy metal poisoning.
- *Generalized involuntary movements*:
  - ***Chorea:*** These involuntary movements, seen in degeneration of caudate nucleus, are jerky, rapid, irregular, and unpredictable.
  - ***Athetosis:*** These involuntary movements are relatively slow, writhing contractions of arms. They are sometimes combined with choreiform movements.
  - ***Ballism:*** These movements are flinging, intense, and violent, usually involving peripheral parts of limbs. The lesion is in the nucleus of Luys.
  - ***Tics:*** These are sudden, rapid, repeated movements, usually in the form of blinking of eyes, or wriggling of shoulders.

Gait

- The term "stance" refers to the way of "standing on one's two feet"; while the term "gait" refers to the manner, style, or pattern of walking.
- The biped stance of man requires the integration of a large amount of sensory information, (proprioceptors from feet, legs, trunk, and neck muscles and joints), which is synthesized with visual and vestibular information. The overall picture of posture (position in space) occurs unconsciously in the middle cerebellum, basal ganglia, and cerebral cortex. If there is any tendency to sway to one or the other side, it is adjusted by muscles of the legs and trunk, and even arms.
- Gait is dependent on the same vestibular, proprioceptive, and integrative systems as stance and balance. However, it requires direction from the central gait mechanism in the frontal lobes, basal ganglia, brainstem, and descending motor systems. There is a continuous adjustment of muscle tone during walking and other movements.
- From the above, it is evident that stance and gait may be affected by a variety of neurological conditions.
- To examine the stance and gait, exclude diseases of the bones and joints, and the legs and feet should be exposed. Some forms of abnormal gait are the following:
  - ***Spastic (hemiplegic) gait:*** The patient walks on a narrow base. Since the knee cannot be flexed and the foot properly lifted off the ground, he drags his foot on the ground and tends to describe a semicircle with the affected leg, the toes scraping the ground.
  - ***Stamping gait:*** The patient raises each foot suddenly and brings it down on the ground with a thump. It is seen in sensory ataxia (e.g. tabes dorsalis). He may be quite steady as long as he can see the ground and the position of his feet.
  - ***Drunken or reeling gait:*** This ataxic gait is seen in cerebellar lesions, the patient walks on a broad base, with the feet apart. The gait is clumsy and zigzagging like the gait of a drunkard. The ataxia is equally severe whether the eyes are closed or open.
  - ***Festinant gait:*** This is seen in Parkinson's disease. Walking is usually slow and the patient takes short and shuffling steps. Sometimes, there is an uncontrolled acceleration while walking, a process called festinant gait. When gently pushed forward, the patient may be unable to stop as he chases his own center of gravity (propulsion). Similarly, when pushed back, he is unable to stop (retropulsion).

OBJECTIVE STRUCTURED PRACTICAL EXAMINATION-I

Aim: To assess the muscle tone in the upper limb of the subject provided.

Procedural steps: See text above

Checklist:

1. Explains the procedure to the subject and seats him comfortably. (Y/N)
2. Holds the forearm of the subject and alternately flexes and extends his wrist with her other hand. (Y/N)
3. Performs similar passive movements at the fingers, elbow, and shoulder. (Y/N)
4. Compares the muscle tone on the opposite side by passive movements. (Y/N)
5. Notes down the results. (Y/N)

OBJECTIVE STRUCTURED PRACTICAL EXAMINATION-II

Aim: To assess the muscle strength in the right upper limb of the subject provided.

Procedural steps: See text above

Checklist:

1. Explains the procedure to the subject. (Y/N)
2. Asks the subject to shake her hand with full force and then to cause active movements of the fingers and wrist against resistance. (Y/N)
3. Asks the subject to flex and extend the elbow against resistance and watches the prominence of biceps and triceps. (Y/N)
4. Asks the subject to move his shoulder in different directions against resistance. (Y/N)
5. Compares the strength of identical muscles on the opposite side. (Y/N)

OBJECTIVE STRUCTURED PRACTICAL EXAMINATION-III

Aim: To elicit the knee jerk in the subject provided.

Procedural steps: See text above

Checklist:

1. Seats the subject on a stool and asks him to cross one leg over the other. (Y/N)
2. Gives instructions about the procedure and assures him that the hammer will not cause any pain. (Y/N)
3. Places her hand on the subject's quadriceps muscle. (Y/N)
4. Locates the patellar tendon and then strikes it between the patella and the tibial tuberosity, holding the hammer between thumb and fingers and swinging it from the wrist. (Y/N)
5. Watches/feels the contraction of quadriceps muscle, and the kicking forward of the leg. Compares the response with the opposite side. (Y/N)

OBJECTIVE STRUCTURED PRACTICAL EXAMINATION-IV

Aim: To elicit the ankle jerk in the supine position in the subject provided.

Procedural steps: See text above

Checklist:

1. Gives instructions about the procedure and assure that the hammer will not cause pain. (Y/N)
2. Asks him to lie supine on the examination couch, and place the right knee semiflexed and externally rotated. (Y/N)
3. Sightly dorsiflexes the foot with her hand to stretch the Achilles tendon. Holding the patellar hammer between the thumb and fingers, strikes the tendon with a movement at the wrist. (Y/N)
4. Watches the plantar flexion of the foot, toes, and ankle with contraction of calf muscles. (Y/N)
5. Elicits the ankle jerk on the other side for comparison. (Y/N)

OBJECTIVE STRUCTURED PRACTICAL EXAMINATION-V

Aim: To elicit the right plantar reflex on the subject provided.

Procedural steps: See text above

Checklist:

1. Explains the procedure and asks the subject lie supine on the examination couch. (Y/N)
2. Stands on the subject's right side, asks him to relax the leg and foot, and flex the knee slightly. (Y/N)
3. Supports the foot by placing her hand on the medial malleolus. (Y/N)
4. Gives a light scratch with the blunt point of the patellar hammer along the outer edge of the sole of the foot, starting from the heel toward the little toe and then medially along the base of the toes. (Y/N)
5. Watches the response carefully. Repeats once more, if required. (Y/N)

SENSORY FUNCTIONS

Classification of Sensations

- Sensations can be divided as **superficial** (arises from the skin) and **deep** (arises from somatic structures below the skin).
- Superficial sensations are touch, pain, and temperature. Deep sensations are deep pain, pressure, and proprioception (sensation arising from in and around the joints).
- The sensations are also classified as follows:
  - **General sensations:** These are further divided into three groups:
    1. ***Cutaneous sensations:*** Touch, cold, warmth, pain, and possibly itch.
    2. ***Deep sensations:*** Proprioceptive, pressure pain from bones, joints, tendons, and muscles.

3. ***Visceral sensations:*** Sensation of distension, tightness, and pain from the viscera.

- **Special sensations:**
  - Vision, hearing, taste, smell, and equilibrium senses are traditionally grouped together as special sensations.
  - Testing of special sensations is discussed in Section 2: Unit III.

Note: Sensations can also be classified as peripheral and cortical sensations. Peripheral sensations are touch, pain, temperature, position, passive movements, and vibrations. Cortical sensations are tactile localization, two-point discrimination, stereognosis, and graphesthesia. Cortical sensations are interpretative sensory functions that require analysis of individual sensory modalities by the parietal lobes to provide discrimination. Individual sensory modalities must be intact to measure cortical sensation.

Components of Sensory System

The sensory system has the following components, as shown in **Figure 53**.

Receptors

- A sensory receptor may be formed by the naked, bare or free (non medullated) terminal part of an afferent nerve fiber, or the nerve endings may be associated with non neural cells, the two together making up organized receptors called ***sense organs.***
- The sensory receptors possess a very important property called ***functional specificity,*** i.e. each type of receptor responds best only to one particular type of stimulus (the adequate stimulus) for which it has the lowest threshold.
- Sensory receptors act as ***peripheral analyzers*** or ***biological transducers.*** They transduce (convert) a given form of energy [e.g. electromagnetic (light), mechanical, thermal, chemical, etc.] into electrical potentials (APs; signals).

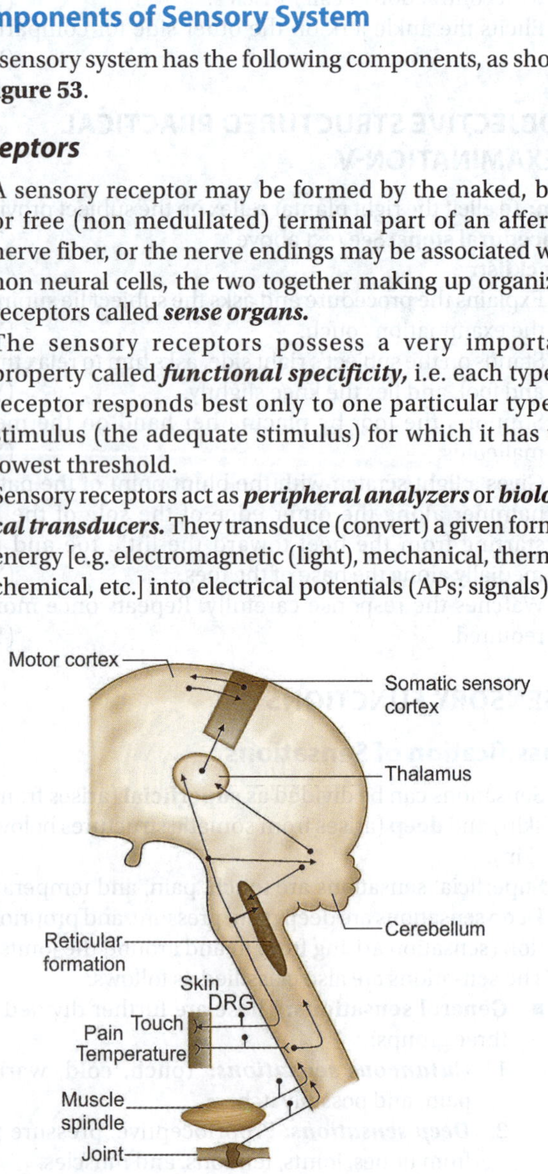

FIG. 53: The components of the sensory system. (DRG: dorsal root ganglia)

Peripheral Pathways

All afferent or sensory information (APs) concerned with sensory (and motor) functions is carried to the CNS via the unipolar primary afferent neurons (the main sensory neurons) that have their cell bodies in the dorsal root ganglia (DRG) of the spinal cord or the equivalent ganglia of sensory cranial nerves.

Central Pathways

The afferent information is then carried to the higher parts of the CNS through a chain of neurons (one synapsing on the next), which may be called *first order, second order, and third order neurons,* though one or more neurons may be interposed between them.

Thalamus

It is an important relay station for all sensations, except smell, on their way to the cerebral cortex.

Cerebellum, Reticular Formation, Etc.

These structures, though not directly concerned with our conscious perception of senses, do receive afferent information that is concerned with coordination of movements.

Sensory Areas of Cerebral Cortex

- There is a functional localization of sensations, each being represented in a specific ***primary area,*** as shown in **Figure 54**. Thus, there are areas for general somatic sensations (areas 3, 1, 2), vision (area 17), hearing (areas 41, 42), taste (lower part of 3, 1, 2), and smell (uncus).
- The cortical areas around these primary areas are called *association areas* where sensory signals are further analyzed.

"Labeled Line Principle"

- This principle, also called ***"Muller's law of specific nerve energies",*** forms the cornerstone of sensory physiology.
- It states that the pathways for each sensation, from the receptors to the cerebral cortex are clear cut and fixed. Thus, whether a touch stimulus is applied to touch receptors, or its pathway is stimulated anywhere along its course, the sensation produced is always touch.
- This principle also answers the question that if all sensory signals are carried as APs, then how we experience

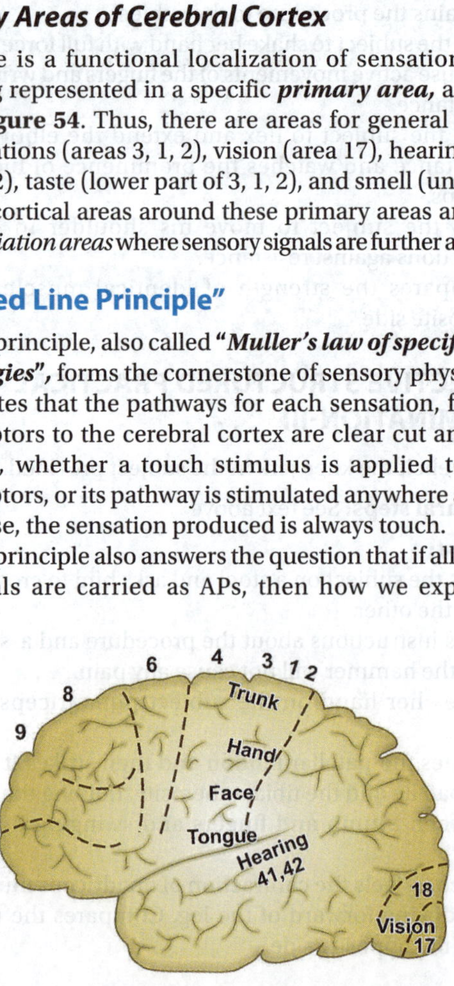

FIG. 54: Diagram showing the cortical receiving areas for sensations.

different modalities of sensations. It appears that this is still an unknown cognitive function of the cerebral cortex.

Pathways for General Sensations

- Sensory information that reaches our consciousness is carried by two main ascending tracts:
  1. ***Dorsal column-medial lemniscal system (DC-MLS)***
  2. ***Anterolateral spinothalamic system.***
- ***Nonconscious afferent information*** is carried to subcortical structures by various ascending tracts.

Dorsal Column–Medial Lemniscal System

- The two myelinated tracts—(1) the fasciculi gracilis and (2) cuneatus (tracts of Goll and Burdach) in the dorsal white columns of the spinal cord **(Fig. 55)** are formed by the central processes of first order DRG neurons.
- These tracts ascend to lower medulla where they synapse on second-order neurons in the nuclei gracilis and cuneatus.
- The axons of second order neurons cross to the opposite side in the medial lemniscus (sensory decussation), reach the thalamus, relay in the nucleus ventralis posterolateralis, from where third order neurons project to somatic sensory areas 3, 1, 2.
- *Functions*: This system carries mechanoreceptive sensations i.e. fine touch, pressure sense, proprioception and vibration sense.

Anterolateral Spinothalamic System

(The anterior and lateral spinothalamic tracts)

- The first order neurons (of DRG) synapse on the cell bodies of second order ***spinothalamic neurons*** whose cell bodies are located in substantia gelatinosa of Rolando and nearby areas of dorsal gray columns of the spinal cord.
- Most axons of these neurons cross to the opposite side at successively higher levels to form the ***anterolateral spinothalamic tract*** **(Fig. 55)**. It continues up through the brainstem as the spinal lemniscus to join the medial lemniscus in upper pons, the two lemnisci terminate in the thalamus from where third-order neurons project to the somatosensory cortex.
- *Functions:* The ***anterior spinothalamic tract*** carries crude touch (the localization of which is poor). The ***lateral spinothalamic*** tract carries: Pain and temperature sensation (warm and cold), tickle and itch, sexual sensations.

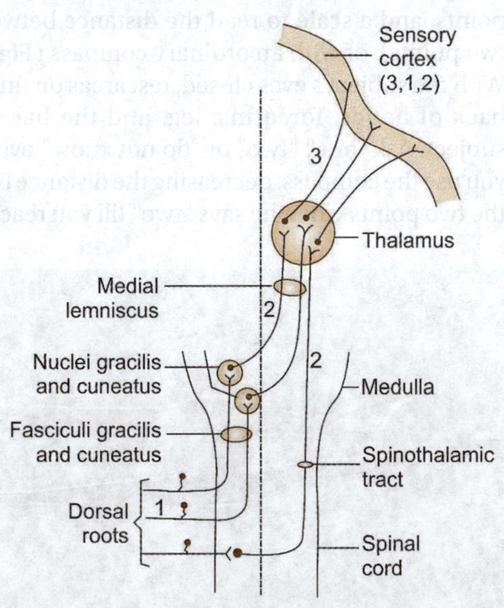

FIG. 55: The dorsal column–medial lemniscal system and the anterolateral spinothalamic system for the general sensations.

Terminology

- ***Hypoalgesia*** means decrease of cutaneous sensations, especially pain sensation. The term ***analgesia*** refers to loss of pain sensation.
- ***Hyperalgesia*** is exaggerated sensitivity to pain, so that a mild stimulus that was painless before now evokes pain.
- ***Hyperesthesia*** refers to increased sensitivity to cutaneous sensations.
- ***Paresthesia*** refers to abnormal sensations, e.g. pricking, numbness, sense of insects crawling on the skin (esthesia = perception).
- Complete loss of touch is called ***anesthesia.***

Clinical Testing of General Sensations

- Before starting the sensory examination:
  1. Ensure that the subject has been informed about the test.
  2. The subject should close his eyes or turn his face to the other side during the test.
  3. Always compare the corresponding dermatomes on both sides.
- The clinically tested general sensations include:
  - Touch*:* It includes—light touch, pressure, touch localization, and two-point discrimination
  - Proprioception
  - Vibration sense
  - Pain
  - Temperature*:* Cold and warmth
  - Stereognosis.
- **For each sensation, the student should know**—the receptors involved, and the peripheral and central pathways, i.e. the chains of neurons, which carry the sensory signals from the receptors to the thalamus, and thence to the somatosensory cortex.
- ***Equipment required:*** Pins, cotton, compass, hot and cold water in test tubes. Von Frey's hair esthesiometer **(Fig. 56)** may be used for touch perception and localization. It has a sliding graduated tube bearing a hair that fits into an outer barrel. It can record the pressure at which the hair will bend to produce a perception of touch. You can mark out touch spots with this instrument.

Touch (Tactile) Sensation

- The sensation of touch is aroused by a **mechanical deformation (indentation, stretching) of the skin.** The stimulus is not pressure but *nonuniform change in pressure with time,* which deforms the skin or deeper somatic tissues.

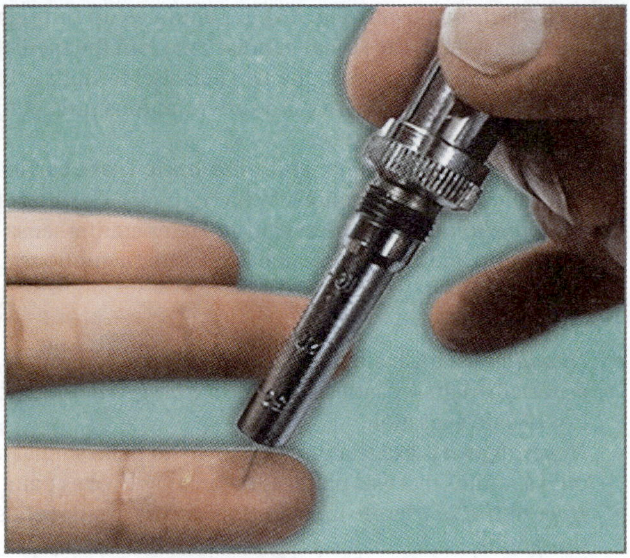

FIG. 56: Von Frey's esthesiometer.

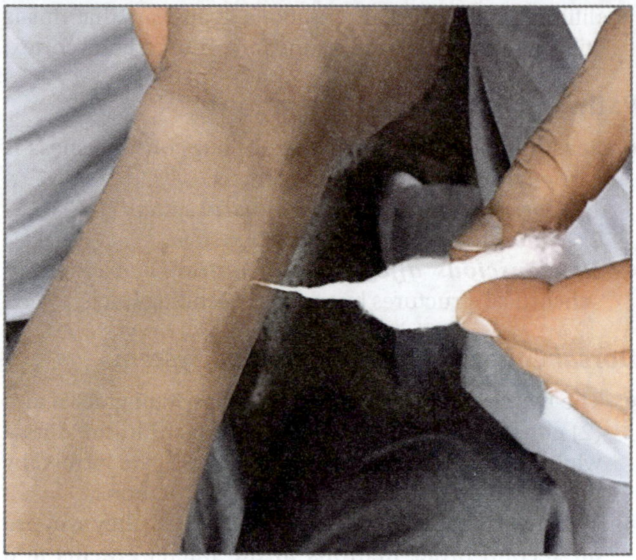

FIG. 57: Testing for fine touch.

- The receptors include—type I and type II cutaneous mechanoreceptors (Merkel disks and Ruffini corpuscles), and naked nerve endings.
- Touch is a very rapidly adapting sensation, i.e. it persists for only a very little longer than the stimulus.

Note: Because of the rapid adaptation of touch receptors the person is not aware of what he/she is wearing. In contrast, the sensation of pain does not show adaptation.

- *Fine touch and crude touch*: Fine touch (epicritic), a more critical type of sensation, of precise location, and low threshold, helps to localize the stimulus. It is also concerned with fine gradations of intensity. These aspects of touch are carried by Aβ and Aγ-fibers into the CNS and then by the DC-MLS. Crude touch (protopathic), concerned with poorly localized diffuse pressure, is carried by A8 and C fibers into the CNS and then by the anterior spinothalamic tract.
- *Test the sensation of light touch, touch localization, and two-point discrimination in the upper limbs of the subject provided*:
  - The subject should be alert and attentive, and the procedure should be explained to him. The subject is asked to close or cover his eyes.
  - A wisp of cotton wool **(Fig. 57)** is used to gently touch the skin on the fingertips, palms, back of the fingers, and hand (nonhairy areas; movement of a single hair with a pin can arouse this sensation), and arms.
  - Ask the subject to raise his finger or say "yes" when he feels the sensation of touch. The response is occasionally checked without the stimulus. If an area of anesthesia is found in the patient, it should be carefully compared with the corresponding area on the opposite side.
- **Touch localization:** Ask the subject to close his eyes. Lightly touch the skin with a colored sketch pen on different areas on fingers, arms, and back (choose areas which the subject can easily reach), one at a time, and ask him to mark the respective spots with a different colored pen.
- **Adaptation time for touch:**
  - Touch sensation is a rapidly adapting sensation. Ask the subject to close his eyes. Using the point of a pencil or a pin, very gently and carefully displace one hair on his forearm and maintain the displacement.
  - Ask the subject to report the moment he is aware of displacement (i.e. perception of touch) and the moment the touch sensation is no longer present though the hair is kept displaced. This may be tested at five different places and the results recorded in your workbook.
- **Two-point discrimination:**
  - The ability to distinguish two simultaneously applied touch stimuli as separate can be tested with a Weber's compass (it has two sharp points and two blunt points, and a scale to read the distance between the two points), or with an ordinary compass **(Fig. 58)**.
  - With the subject's eyes closed, test areas on fingertips, back of hands, forearms, leg, and the back of the subject. Ask "one", "two", or "do not know" every time you use the compass, decreasing the distance between the two points when he says "two" till you reach "one".

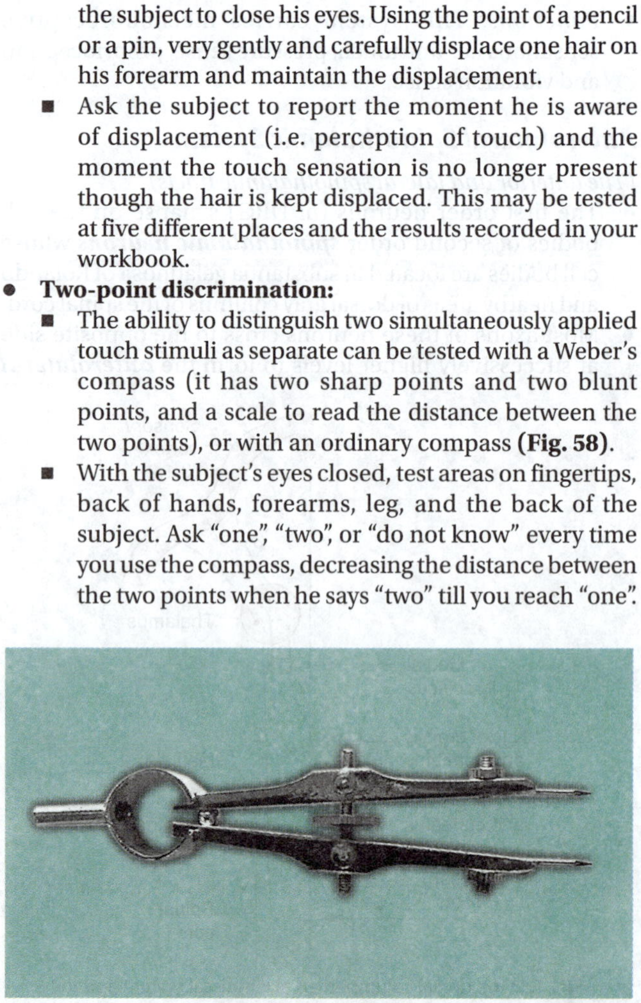

FIG. 58: Weber's compass.

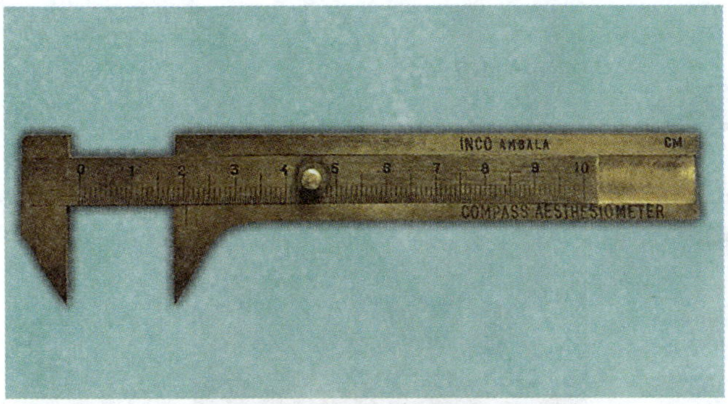

FIG. 59: Esthesiometer.

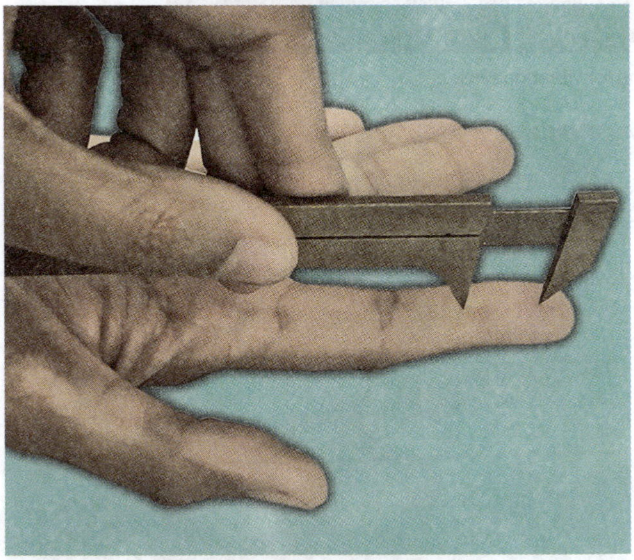

FIG. 60: Testing two-point discrimination.

- It will be seen that the distance varies at different points—2 mm at fingertips, a few mm on forearms and legs, and many cm at the back **(Figs. 59 and 60)**. It is related to the density of the touch spots.
- **Touch-pressure (pressure is sustained touch):** This is tested by applying pressure over the skin in different regions with a fingertip or the blunt end of a pencil.

Proprioception

- The proprioceptive sensations arise from the stimulation of receptors within the body tissues (proprius = self) and include sense of position and movement.
- While ***static proprioception*** is concerned with awareness of location of different parts of the body (body image), ***kinesthetic sensation*** **(kin- = motion; -esthesia = perception)** is concerned with perception of the rate of movement of different parts of the body.
- *Conscious and nonconscious proprioception*: Part of the proprioceptive information reaches consciousness at primary and association somatic sensory areas via the DC-MLS. Nonconscious proprioceptive information from muscle spindles, Golgi tendon organs, and nerve endings around joints (joint kinesthetic receptors) is carried via spinocerebellar, spinoreticular, spinal vestibular and, other similar tracts, and is meant for subcortical structures where it aids in the coordination of motor activity.
- *Test the proprioceptive sensation in the subject provided*:
  - **Position sense:**
    - The subject is told that his finger (or of an elbow, ankle, etc.) will be moved up or down and he is asked to indicate in which direction it has been moved. He is asked to close or shield his eyes.
    - Then the examiner gently moves the terminal phalanx of a finger or toe in one or the other direction. A normal person is able to appreciate displacement of only a few degrees at various joints.
    - When a limb is placed in a certain position, the subject should be able to place his opposite limb in a similar position.
  - **Sense of movement:** (Kinesthetic sense; kinema = movement):
    - A digit, finger, toe, or other joint is gradually moved to a new position, and the subject is asked to say "yes" as soon as he perceives the movement.
    - Part of proprioceptive information reaches consciousness (conscious kinesthetic) while the rest reaches the cerebellum, where it aids it in coordinating muscular activity.

Vibration Sense

- Vibration is a phasic sensation caused by repeated mechanical simulation of touch receptors and pacinian corpuscles, the frequency for the two being 6–40/second and 40–400/second, respectively.
- *Test the sense of vibration*: The foot of a low frequency tuning fork is placed over bony prominences, such as knuckles, head of radius, elbow, patella, malleoli, iliac crest, etc. **(Figs. 61A and B)**. The subject is normally conscious of a vibratory tremor, and not just the sensation of touch. The subject is asked to tell when the feeling of vibration stops; the examiner then confirms it on his own knuckles.
- Vibration sense is affected in peripheral neuropathies (diabetes mellitus), tabes dorsalis, and dorsal column disease.

Pain

- The stimulus for pain is actual or potential damage to the tissues. Though pain is an unpleasant sensation, it is said to be a "cry for help" as it is commonly the first symptom that brings a patient to the doctor.
- The receptors are naked nerve terminals of AS and C fibers, and the APs are carried up the CNS by spinothalamic tract, as described above.
- Pain has both *epicritic* and *protopathic* components, and there is no adaptation to pain sensation (otherwise it would lose its protective function).
- *Stimuli of pain*: Intense chemical, thermal, or mechanical stimuli can stimulate pain receptors. Injury to tissues releases kinins, prostaglandins, and potassium ions that stimulate pain endings.

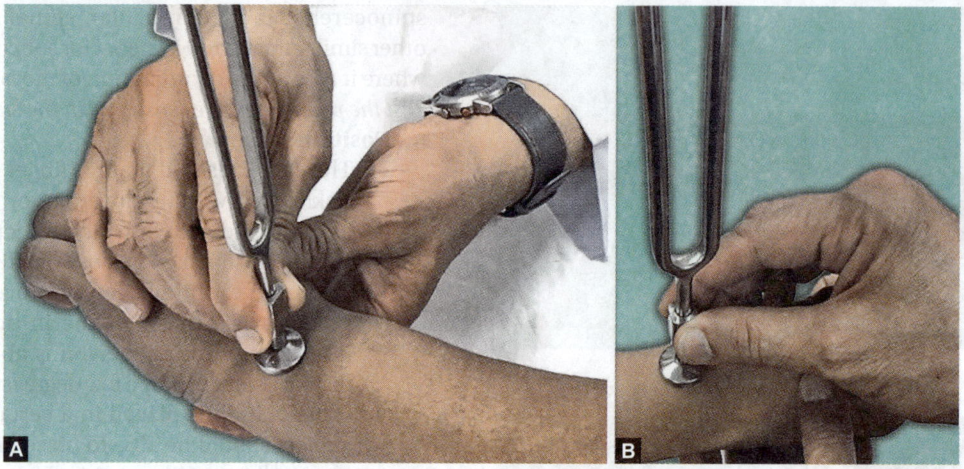

FIGS. 61A AND B: Testing for vibration sense.

- *Visual analog scale of pain*:
  - The intensity of pain is difficult to describe and assess. However, one can bypass the patient's cognitive level of pain perception by using the visual analog scale (VAS) for pain.
  - The patient is asked to point out a number on a 10-cm scale, with 0 (no pain) on its left end, and 10 (intolerable pain) at its right end, with annoying, uncomfortable, dreadful, and horrible pain in between these two ends **(Fig. 62)**.
  - *Test the sensations of pain in the upper limbs of the subject provided*: This sensibility may be tested either with a *cutaneous stimulus,* such as the prick of a pin, or by *pressure* on deeper tissues, such as muscles and bones **(Fig. 63)**.
  - The procedure is explained to the subject/patient. He is asked to close his eyes, and corresponding points on the nail bed, pulp of fingers (this is less sensitive to pain), palms and back of the hands, and arms are tested with an ordinary pin.
  - Pressure pain is tested by squeezing the arm muscles, or a pressure applied on the wrist bones (calf muscles and Achilles tendon in the lower limbs). Loss of pain sensation is called analgesia. There may be analgesia without loss of touch sensation (anesthesia) in a patient.

Temperature

- *Test the sensation of temperature in the upper limbs of the subject provided:* This sensation is tested by using two test tubes containing cold and warm (not hot) water. The tubes should be interchanged at random. The patient is asked to report "cold" or "warm" **(Fig. 64)**.

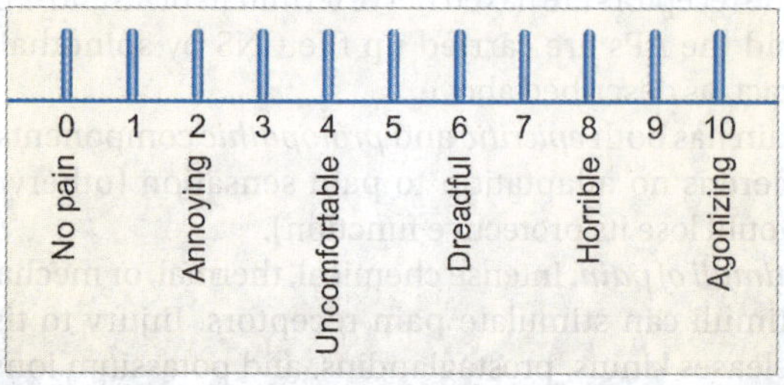

FIG. 62: The visual analog scale of pain. The patient is asked to point out a number on the scale to indicate the intensity of her pain.

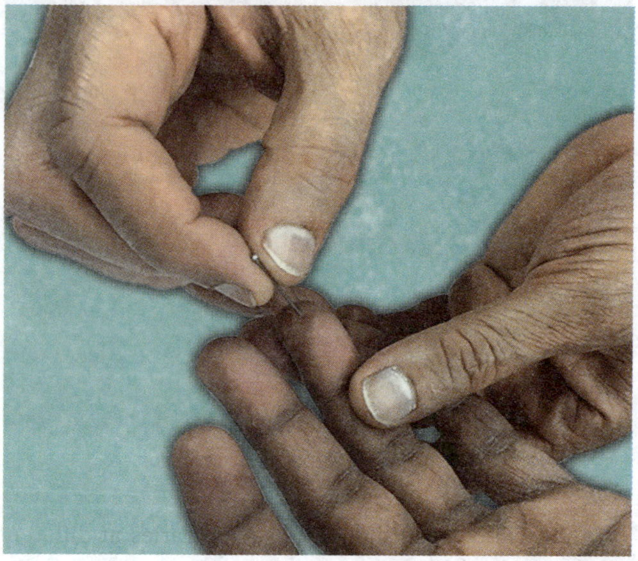

FIG. 63: Testing pain sensation.

Note: The gross features of temperature (and pain) are perceived at the level of thalamus, while their further analysis occurs at cerebral cortical level.

Stereognosis

- *Stereognosis,* i.e. the ability to identify common objects by feeling them, with eyes closed, is a complex sensation based on the synthesis of many sensations, such as touch, pressure, temperature, etc. Certain features of an object—its size, shape, form, weight softness or hardness, roughness or smoothness (e.g. the milled edge of a coin), dryness or wetness—help us to identify an object.
- The subject is asked to close his eyes, and common objects like a coin, pencil, key, matchstick, etc. are placed in his hand, one after the other. He has to name each object and the purpose for which it is used. (If a patient cannot name them, he is asked to describe these).

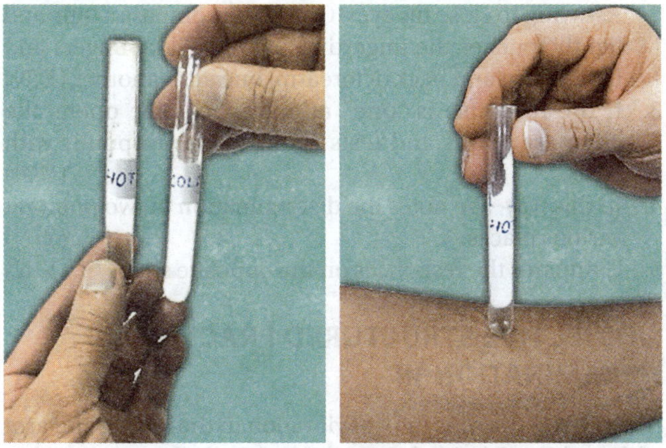

FIG. 64: Testing for temperature sense.

Note: The parietal cortex plays an important role in the process. Stereognosis is thus a "synthetic sense"—synthesized in the cerebral cortex from the information received from many sources. Loss of this faculty is called **astereognosis** that may result from lesions of the parietal lobe, or of the dorsal columns of spinal cord.

QUESTIONS

For all answers refer to the text above.

Cranial Nerves

Q.1. Test the sense of smell in the subject provided. What is the pathway for smell?

Q.2. Test the visual acuity of the subject provided.

Q.3. Test the color vision of the subject provided.

Q.4. Test the peripheral field of vision of the subject provided, using the confrontation test.

Q.5. Test the conjugate movements of the eyes in the subject provided.

Q.6. Demonstrate the light reflex in the subject provided. What is the pathway of this reflex?

Q.7. What is the cause of consensual light reflex?

Q.8. Demonstrate the reaction of the pupil to accommodation for near vision.

Q.9. What is the pathway for accommodation reflex?

Q.10. What is Argyll-Robertson pupil?

Q.11. Demonstrate the corneal reflex.

Q.12. Test the general sensory functions of the trigeminal nerve.

Q.13. Test the motor functions of the trigeminal nerve in the subject provided.

Q.14. Test the motor functions of the facial nerve in the subject provided.

Q.15. Test the taste function of the facial nerve.

Q.16. Perform the Rinne test on the subject provided.

Q.17. Perform the Weber test on the subject provided.

Q.18. Demonstrate the Schwabach test of hearing.

Q.19. Perform the whisper test in the subject provided.

Q.20. How will you test the vestibular function in the subject provided?

Q.21. How will you test the 9th cranial nerve?

Q.22. How will you test the vagus nerve in the subject provided?

Q.23. Test the spinal part of the accessory nerve in the subject provided.

Q.24. Test the hypoglossal nerve in the subject provided.

Motor System

Q.1. Test the state of nutrition in the upper and lower limbs of the subject provided.

Q.2. Test the tone of the muscles in the upper limbs.

Q.3. Test the muscle strength in the upper limbs of the subject provided.

Q.4. Test the muscle strength in the lower limbs.

Q.5. How is muscle strength graded?

Q.6. Test the muscular coordination in the upper limbs of the subject provided.

Q.7. Test the muscle coordination in the lower limbs.

Q.8. Test the subject provided for Romberg's sign.

Q.9. Perform any three cerebellar function tests in the subject provided.

Q.10. Elicit the flexor plantar reflex in the subject provided.

Q.11. Why does Babinski sign appear in corticospinal tract lesions?

Q.12. Demonstrate abdominal reflexes in the subject provided.

Q.13. Elicit the ciliospinal reflex.

Q.14. Demonstrate any three superficial reflexes.

Q.15. Demonstrate the knee jerk in the subject provided.

Q.16. Elicit the ankle jerk.

Q.17. Test the biceps jerk in the subject provided.

Q.18. Elicit the triceps reflex.

Q.19. Test the radial supinator and wrist reflexes.

Q.20. What is reinforcement of reflexes and when is it required?

Q.21. When are the deep reflexes diminished or absent?

Q.22. When are the deep reflexes exaggerated?

Q.23. What is clonus? Demonstrate this phenomenon in the subject provided.

Q.24. Demonstrate some visceral reflexes in the subject provided.

Q.25. What is meant by the terms upper motor neurons and lower motor neurons? What are the chief distinguishing features of the lesions of these neurons?

Sensory System

Q.1. Test the sensation of light touch, touch localization, and two-point discrimination in the upper limbs of the subject provided.

Q.2. Test the proprioceptive sensation in the subject provided.

Q.3. Test the sense of vibration.

Q.4. Test the sensations of pain in the upper limbs of the subject provided.

Q.5. Test the sensation of temperature in the upper limbs of the subject provided.

Q.6. Test the sensation of stereognosis in the subject provided.

OBJECTIVE STRUCTURED PRACTICAL EXAMINATION-I

Aim: To test the sensation of fine touch on the frontal aspect of the subject's left forearm.

Procedural steps: See text above

Checklist:

1. Makes the subject sit on a stool and explains the procedure. (Y/N)
2. Asks her to bare her forearms and put them on the table in front. Tells her to close his eyes. (Y/N)
3. Takes a piece of cotton and twists it into a pointed "wisp". Then lightly touches the skin on the fingertips, palms, and forearm and asks "now?" and the subject responds with a "yes", "no", or "do not know". (Y/N)
4. Checks the responses occasionally without the stimulus. (Y/N)
5. Compares the responses on the opposite forearm. (Y/N)

OBJECTIVE STRUCTURED PRACTICAL EXAMINATION-II

Aim: To test two-point discrimination on the anterior forearm of the right side.

Procedural steps: See text above

Checklist:

1. Explains the procedure to the subject and asks him to respond "one", "two", or "do not know" when she touches his skin with the compass points. (Y/N)
2. Asks him to close his eyes. Opens the compass a little and lightly touches the fingertips, palm, back of fingers and hand, front and back of forearm, one after another. (Y/N)
3. If the response is "one" at any place, she opens the compass points and tests again, till he responds with "two". (Y/N)
4. In this way, she notes the discrimination of two points at various places. (Y/N)
5. Compares the responses on the opposite side. (Y/N)

OBJECTIVE STRUCTURED PRACTICAL EXAMINATION-III

Aim: To test the sensation of vibration in the left leg and arm of the subject provided.

Procedural steps: See text above

Checklist:

1. Explains the procedure and assures him that no pain will be caused. (Y/N)
2. Selects a tuning fork of 128 Hz, strikes one prong against the edge of her hand to set it into vibration. Then places its base on his knuckle to familiarize him with the "vibrating tremor". (Y/N)
3. Tests the vibration sense on his knuckles, head of radius, elbow, patella, and medial malleolus. She occasionally tests with her finger tip or a pencil. (Y/N)
4. Notes the response in each case with a "yes", "no", or "do not know", if the response is "no" or "do not know", she tests on another bony prominence. (Y/N)
5. Compares the responses on the other side. (Y/N)

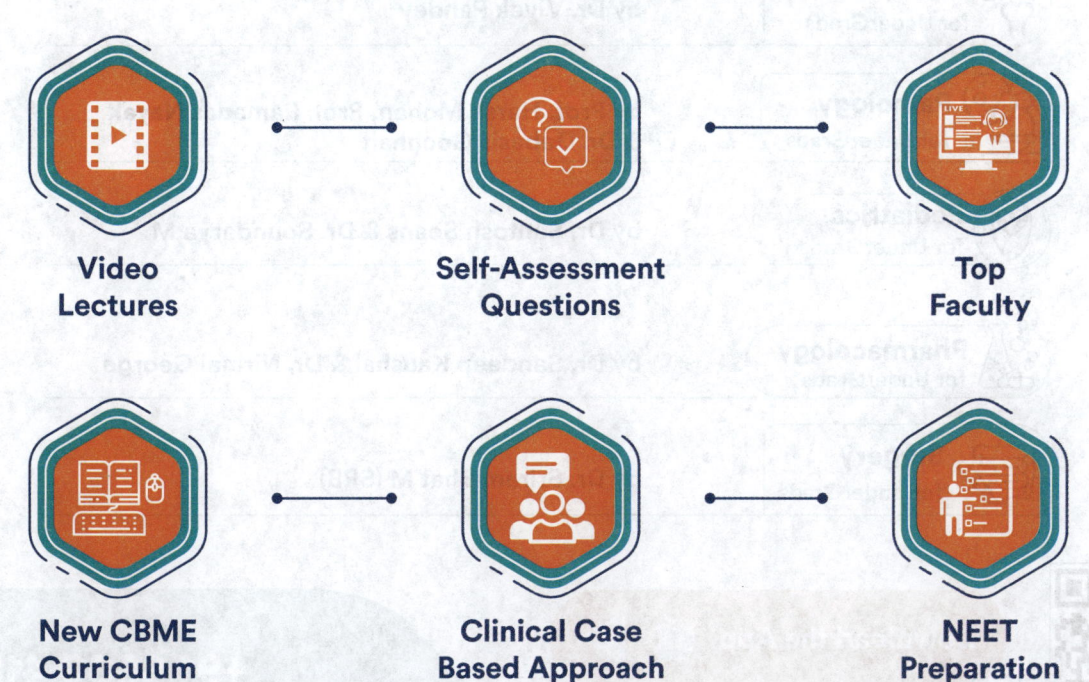

SECTION 4

Experimental Physiology

UNIT I: AMPHIBIAN EXPERIMENTS

STUDENT OBJECTIVES

After completing this experiment, the student should be able to:

- Name and describe the uses of different apparatuses used in Experimental Physiology.
- Name the various types of stimuli and the advantage of electrical stimuli in animal experiments.
- Indicate the advantages of using frog and mammalian tissues in these experiments. How would you see–oversee the care being taken of these animals?
- Name the precautions you will take while using these animals.
- Enumerate some of the properties of frog nerve and muscle tissues.
- Dissect and expose the frog's heart and show its properties, especially its refractoriness.

PY3.18: Observe with computer assisted learning (i) amphibian nerve - muscle experiments and (ii) amphibian cardiac experiments.

INTRODUCTION

- To study the response of a living tissue to a stimulus three things are required:
  1. Living tissue
  2. Stimulating device, and
  3. Recording device.
- In amphibian experiments, the living tissue, which is used, is either nerve muscle preparation or the cardiac tissue.
- The student usually begins the experimental work on the amphibian nerve and muscle tissues after removing them from the frog's body. The great advantage of the living tissues from frog is preferred because:
  - They can function as isolated preparations for many hours when handled carefully and kept moist with a suitable solution.
  - The tissues get their oxygen from the atmosphere air and therefore no oxygenation is required.
  - Frogs are cold blooded animals, so no temperature control is required.

FROG NERVE–MUSCLE PREPARATION

- The Frog's *gastrocnemius muscle-sciatic nerve preparation,* first employed by Jan Swammerdam, a Dutch physiologist, in the latter half of the 17th century, is a simple preparation for the study of many features of skeletal muscle contraction and nerve function. Frog's *sartorius* is another muscle employed for such studies.
- However, the gastrocnemius muscle has a much greater cross-sectional area than that of sartorius and hence develops much greater force required for moving the lever system during isotonic contractions.
- Within the body, the skeletal muscles are activated by trains of action potentials in their motor nerves. In the isolated preparation, the muscle can be made to contract by either stimulating its nerve, or by directly stimulating its belly.

FROG HEART

- Many properties of cardiac muscle can be demonstrated on the frog's heart either within or outside the animal's body.
- The **high-voltage mains** are supplied by high-voltage current—220 volts; AC 50 Hz—is potentially lethal. Handle the electric kymograph with utmost caution. Ensure that it is properly earthed. Uninsulated wires or improperly earthed kymographs and other apparatuses may produce a burn and/or severe shock. If in doubt, call the electrician on duty in the laboratory.
- ***Low-voltage mains*** are supplied by low-voltage current—6 volts produced by step-down transform connected to high-voltage mains.

4.1: INTRODUCTION TO AMPHIBIAN EXPERIMENTS

EXCITABILITY

- It is the property or faculty of living cells due to which they respond to stimuli. Though all cells are excitable, this property is best developed and demonstrable in nerve and muscle cells, called "excitable tissues".
- Thus, muscle cells respond by contracting, nerve cells (neurons) respond by generating and transmitting action potentials, and gland cells respond by producing a secretion.

STIMULUS

- A stimulus is defined as a change in the environment of an excitable tissue, which causes the tissue to respond in its own particular fashion.
- **Types of Stimuli:** The different types of stimuli are:
  - **Physical:** Drying, cooling, and warming.
  - **Mechanical:** Tapping, pinching, cutting, and crushing.
  - **Chemical:** Dilute acids and alkalis, and other chemicals.
  - **Osmotic:** Strong salt solutions, glycerin (it is hygroscopic).
  - **Electrical:** The different types of electrical stimuli are—Galvanic current (continuous, or direct current—DC); Faradic or induced current; rectilinear (rectangular), and sine wave (AC or alternating current).
- **Choice of Stimulus:**
  Of all the types of stimuli mentioned above, electrical stimuli are chosen for experimental work for the following reasons:
  - Their strength (in volts) and duration (in ms) can be easily controlled.
  - Since their duration is very short, they do not cause any damage to the tissues. Thus, they can be applied repeatedly, if required, without producing any harmful effects.
  - They resemble the natural mode of excitation of the tissues, i.e. the phenomena of resting potentials, and action potentials are electrical in nature.
- **Type of Electrical Stimuli Employed:**
  - Of the different types of electrical stimuli, the **induced** or **Faradic current** is generally employed for student work; it is very short-lived, does not cause damage, and can be applied repeatedly. Rectilinear (rectangular) current is obtained from an electronic stimulator.
  - The voltage rises immediately to the desired level and is maintained there for the desired duration (measured in milliseconds). Thus, the strength (volts) and the duration (ms) can be preselected.
  - The Galvanic current is the usual form of electrical stimulus, which is employed for neurophysiological studies, and in clinical situations (e.g. in testing for reaction of degeneration). The usual household

electric supply, alternating current, AC, 220 volts, 50 Hz is lethal as such, and is never employed without modifying it, such as converting it to DC-low volts.

- **Degrees of Stimuli:**
  - A **threshold** (minimal or liminal) stimulus is the minimum strength of stimulus that is just sufficient to produce a response.
  - A **subthreshold** (subminimal or subliminal) stimulus is weaker than a threshold stimulus and is unable to produce a response.
  - A **maximal** stimulus produces a maximum response and **submaximal** and **supramaximal** stimuli are weaker or stronger than a maximal stimulus, respectively.

4.2: STUDY OF APPARATUS

PY3.18: Observe with computer assisted learning (i) amphibian nerve - muscle experiments and (ii) amphibian cardiac experiments.

The different apparatus the students will be using include the following:

1. **Source of Current:**
   - ***Two-pin plug point (low voltage mains):***
     - In order to get induced current, a constant current of low voltage is fed into the primary coil of the induction coil.
     - It is supplied by 6 voltage DC from a step-down transformer having a rectifier plugged to the 220 V high voltage mains.
   - ***Three-pin plug point (high voltage mains)***
     - It is supplied with 220 V AC mains and it is used exclusively for running the kymograph.
     - The **high voltage mains** is potentially lethal. Handle the electric kymograph with utmost caution.
2. **The Keys:** A key is used as a switch to complete ("make") or interrupt ("break") an electrical circuit. The different types of keys are:
   - **Simple key/primary key (Fig. 1):**
     - It is used to open or close the primary circuit. An ordinary electrical "on-off" switch is mounted on a wooden or vulcanite base.
     - The two poles of the switch are connected to two adjustable screw terminals. Other types of simple keys include metal blocks, morse key, and unspillable mercury key.

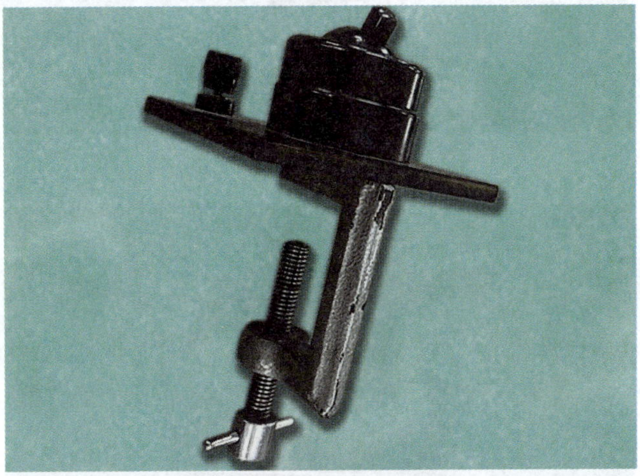

FIG. 1: Simple key.

     - The simple key is included in the primary circuit, as shown in **Figure 1**.
   - **Short-circuiting key/secondary key (Fig. 3):**
     - It is connected in parallel in the secondary circuit. It is kept closed to prevent accidental passage of current into the tissues.
     - In the open position, the current passes to stimulate the tissue. It is included in the secondary circuit **(Fig. 2)** to prevent accidental passage of current into the tissues. It also prevents unipolar induction.
   - **Reversing key (Fig. 4):** It is used where two electrodes are required. It is used to shunt the current from one electrode.

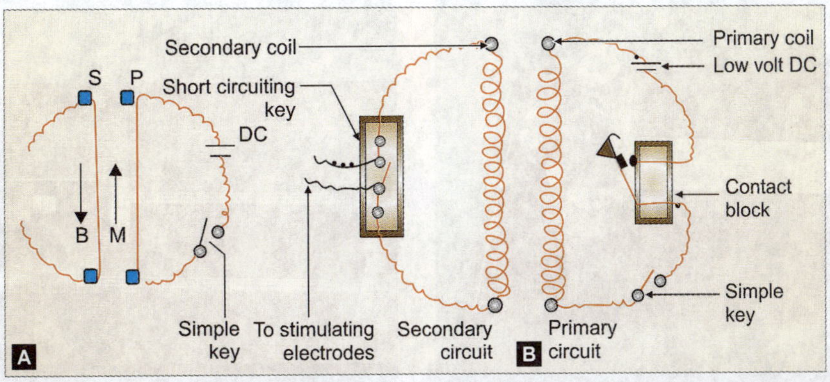

FIGS. 2A AND B: (A) Genesis of induced current. Flow of direct current (DC) in wire P causes induced (Faradic) current in a nearby wire (S—secondary) only at make or break of DC. Arrows show the direction of induced current at make (M) and break (B) of direct current; (B) Circuit for electrical stimulation of frog's nerve or muscle. The contact block makes and breaks the primary circuit by the striker of the rotating drum. The circuit can also be completed by tapping the spring with a finger.

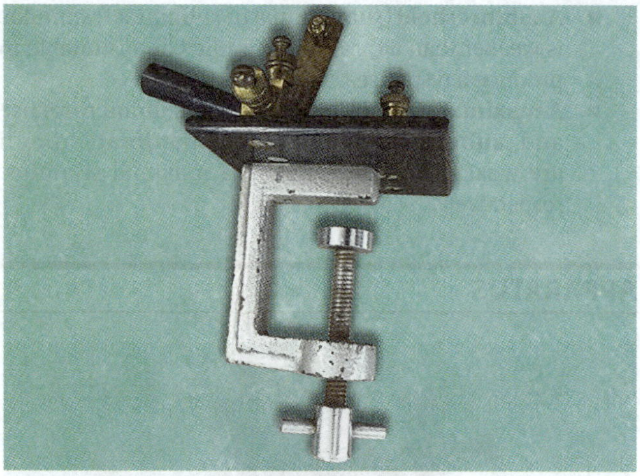

FIG. 3: Secondary key.

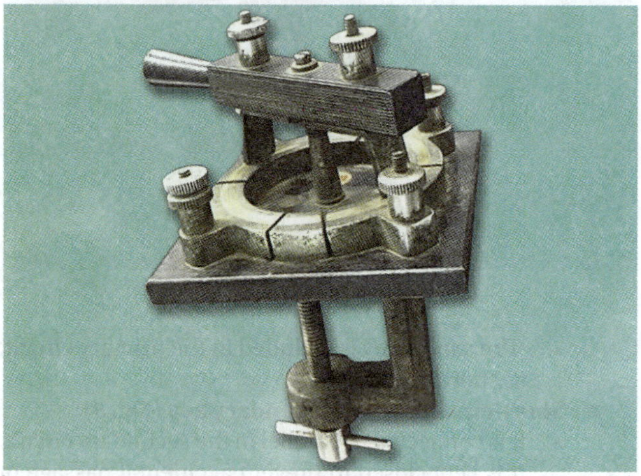

FIG. 4: Reversing key.

- **Tapping key (Fig. 5):** It is used to make or break the circuit for a limited time as and when required by gently tapping the key and releasing it suddenly. It is connected in series with the low voltage mains in the primary circuit.

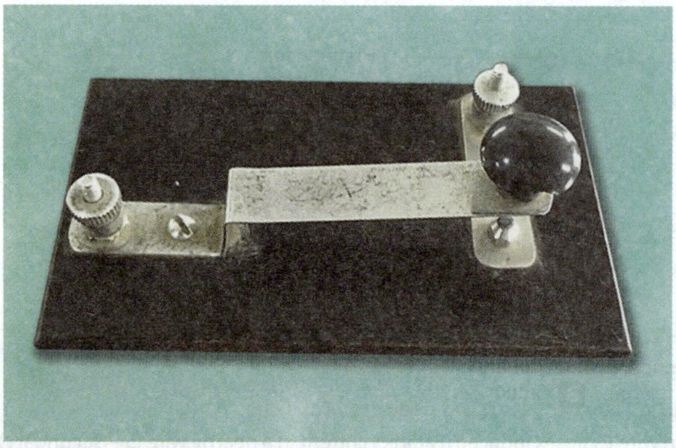

FIG. 5: Tapping key. It enables interruption of the primary circuit at a wider range of frequency which is more precisely adjustable than in the Neef's hammer.

3. **Induction Coil**
   - *Du Bois-Reymond Induction Coil, 1849* **(Figs. 6 and 7)**: It is a simple device to convert galvanic (low voltage, direct) current into the faradic (induced, high voltage phasic) current.
   - ***Principle:***
     - A flow of current in a wire (or a coil) produces a magnetic field in the space around it, which, in turn, can induce a current in another wire or coil placed nearby. In other words, a change in the magnetic field around a wire or a coil induces an electric current in it.
     - It *consists of two coils:* **Primary** and **secondary coils** which are made up of well insulated copper wire wrapped around a soft iron core. The secondary coil has a much larger number of turns than the The primary coil terminals are connected to the DC source (2-pin plug point) and the secondary coil is connected to the stimulating electrodes.
       - The **primary coil** consists of 250–300 turns of relatively thick, cotton-covered, copper wire wound round a wooden reel, which contains a bundle of soft iron wire pieces in its core (they increase the induction effects by their magnetization).
       - The **secondary coil** has 7,000–8,000 turns of thin enameled, copper wire wound round another wooden reel which is hollow. There is no connection between the two coils. However, the distance between the two coils can be increased or decreased, i.e. the secondary coil may lie over the primary, or be moved away from it.
     - *Factors affecting strength of induced current:*
       - The number of turns of wire in the two coils—this is, of course, fixed.
       - The strength of direct current fed into the primary coil—it can be increased or decreased.
       - The distance between the primary coil and the secondary coil—greater the distance and weaker the induced current.

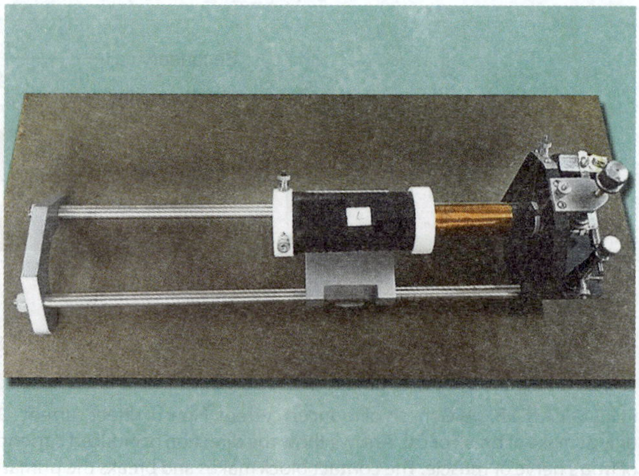

FIG. 6: Du Bois–Reymond induction coil.

- ✦ The angle between the two coils—when the secondary coil is at right angle to the primary, there is no induced current; as the angle decreases, the strength increases.

- ***"Break-induced" Current versus "Make-induced" Current:***
  - The strength of the induced current depends not only on the voltage in the primary coil, but also on the rate of change of current in this coil—whether from zero to a certain level (at "make") or from that level to zero (at "break").
  - When the Galvanic current starts to flow in the primary coil, it induces current not only in the secondary coil, it also induces current in the adjacent turns of wire in the primary coil itself, but in a direction opposite to the original current.
  - This self-induction effect impedes and slows down the rate of rise of the original Galvanic current from zero to the preselected level. However, at "break", the rate of change of Galvanic current (fall to zero) is sudden, as there is no self-induction effect.
  - As a result, the change in the magnetic field is greater at "break" than at "make". Therefore, the "break-induced" current is stronger than the "make-induced" current.
- ***Neef's Hammer:*** It is fitted on the side of the induction coil (**Fig. 7**) and is included in the primary circuit when multiple, repeated stimuli are required. It consists of an electromagnet and a horizontally mounted T-shaped iron bar with a spring. When the current is switched on, the iron bar vibrates up and down, thus repeatedly "making" and "breaking" the primary circuit at a rate of 30-40 per second.

4. **Electric Kymograph (Fig. 8):** It is a machine for recording graphically the time course of events in tissues manifesting movement (i.e. muscle contractions).
   a. ***Electric motor:*** It runs on the mains 220 volts AC current.
   b. ***Shaft:***
   - Two switches operate as ON/OFF switches—the **mains switch** labeled ON/OFF—this should always be put "ON".
   - It is connected to the motor and can be rotated at different speeds. The speed is selected by means of a calibrated **speed setting lever.** It has a groove on one side and a screw at the top.
   - A small rectangular plug mounted on the screw inside the shaft butts out through the groove. It can be raised or lowered along the groove by rotating the screw at the top.
   - It supports the weight of the drum and prevents it from sliding down. The level of the drum can therefore be adjusted by the top screw.

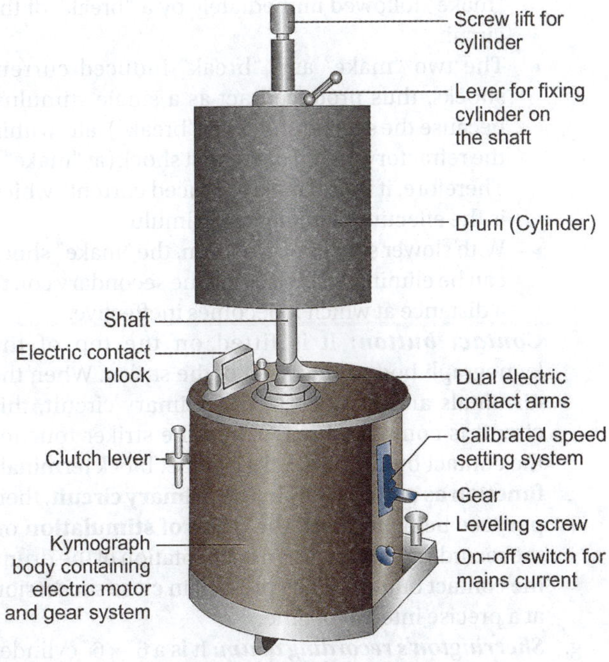

FIG. 8: Electric kymograph.

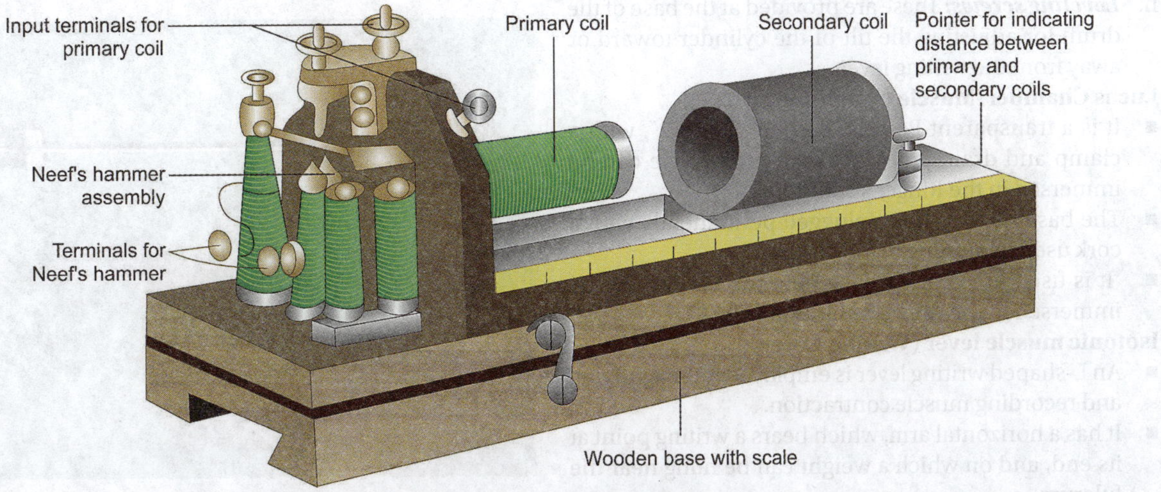

FIG. 7: The Du Bois–Reymond induction coil.

c. ***Gear:*** A **variable speed lever** permits speed between 2.5 mm/s (slowest) and 640 mm/s (fastest). It is used to change the speed of the shaft.

d. ***Clutch lever:*** Which engages or disengages the gears. This is used as an ON/OFF switch to prevent damage to the gears. The cylinder may be rotated easily by hand when the clutch lever is in the horizontal (OFF) position. There is one slot marked "N" (neutral) where the gears get disengaged from the motor.

e. ***Dual electric contact arms* (also called the "striker")**:
   - They are fitted, one over the other, at the base of the vertical shaft and rotates along with it. The two arms of the striker can be drawn apart, as and when two stimuli, one after the other is required.
   - As the shaft rotates at a fast speed, each time the striker touches the contact spring (thus completing the primary circuit), there is an instantaneous "make" followed immediately by a "break" of the circuit.
   - The two "make" and "break" induced current shocks, thus produced act as a single stimulus, because the second shock (at "break") falls within the refractory period of the first shock (at "make"). Therefore, it is the "make-induced current" which is the effective (stimulating) stimulus.
   - With slower speeds of the drum, the "make" shock can be eliminated by moving the secondary coil to a distance at which it becomes ineffective.

f. ***Contact button:*** It is fitted on the top of the kymograph body at the level of the striker. When the terminals are included in the primary circuit, this circuit is completed only when the striker touches the contact button. Thus, the contact block terminals **function as a simple key in the primary circuit**, their purpose being to **mark the point of stimulation** on the recording surface. As on each rotation of the drum, the contact button will be pressed in close succession at a precise interval of time.

g. ***Sherrington's recording drum:*** It is a 6″ × 6″ cylinder with a glazed paper wrapped around it, is firmly fixed on the shaft with the locking lever.

h. ***Leveling screws:*** These are provided at the base of the drum for adjusting the tilt of the cylinder toward or away from the writing lever.

5. **Lucas Chamber/Muscle trough:**
   - It is a transparent Perspex bath, 6″ × 4″ × 2″, with a clamp and drain pipe, in which the muscle can be immersed in the Ringer's solution.
   - The base has two holes plugged permanently with a cork used in pinning of the tissues.
   - It is used in experiments where the tissues can be immersed in the Ringer's solution **(Fig. 9)**.

6. **Isotonic muscle lever (Writing Lever):**
   - An L-shaped writing lever is employed for magnifying and recording muscle contraction.
   - It has a horizontal arm, which bears a writing point at its end, and on which a weight can be hung near the fulcrum.

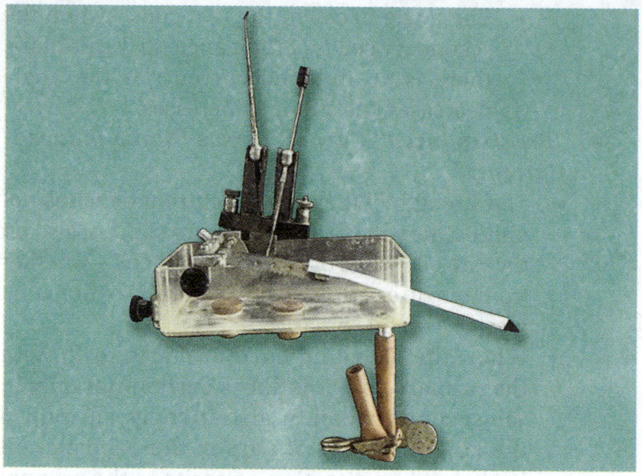

FIG. 9: Lucas moist chamber; muscle trough.

   - The vertical arm of the lever has a hook, which descends into the trough, and to which the tendon of the muscle is tied via a thread. (When properly set up, there should be no laxity in the thread).
   - The two arms of the lever must remain firmly fixed to the spindle, and at right angles to each other to get maximum leverage.
   - An **afterload screw** fitted in the frame supports the vertical arm (for afterloading), or it can be withdrawn away from it (for freeloading) **(Fig. 10)**.
   - *Ink-writing Lever:* An ink-writing stylus (filled with ink) can be fitted on the writing lever. It can then directly inscribe on the glazed paper without the need of "smoking" its surface.

7. **Starling Heart Lever:**
   - This lever is more sensitive than the writing lever and is used for recording the contractions of the frog's heart which are relatively weaker than skeletal muscle contractions.
   - It is used for recording the mechanical events of the frog's heart. The frame of the lever carries a light, flat lever arm with a finely adjustable tension spring,

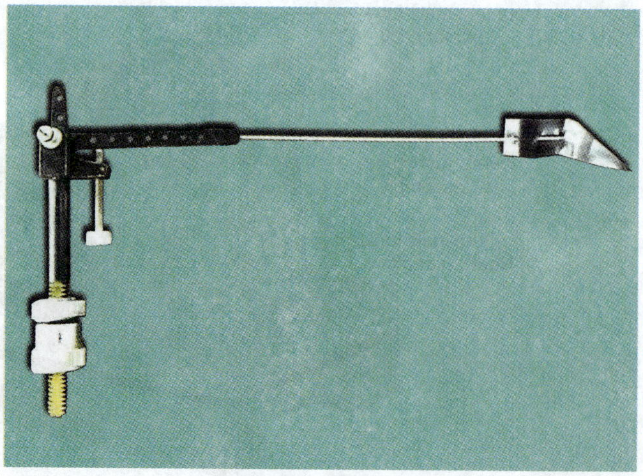

FIG. 10: Writing lever.

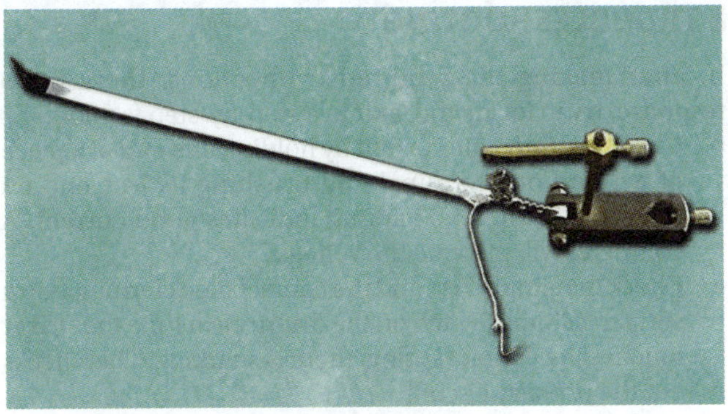

FIG. 11: Starling heart lever.

which supports the writing lever in the horizontal position.

- A piece of thread tied to the writing lever carries a bent pin, which can be hooked through the apex of the ventricle when its contractions are to be recorded.
- When the heart contracts, it pulls the lever down; when it relaxes, the spring pulls the lever back to its horizontal position **(Fig. 11)**.

8. **Isometric Lever:** It consists of a holder, which carries a steel tension spring and a flat writing lever. This lever is used for recording isometric contractions.
9. **Variable Interrupter:**
   - It enables interruption of the primary circuit at a wider range of frequency which is more precisely adjustable than in the Neef's hammer.
   - It works on the same principle as the Neef's hammer.
   - The variable frequency can be set with an adjusting screw. **(Fig. 12)**.
   - Variable interrupter when used is connected in series with the induction coil.
10. **Time Marking:** A time marking, or a time tracing, is required on the recording surface in most experiments. The following types of time markers are employed:
    - **Tuning fork:** A tuning fork of 100 is used for fast events such as muscle contraction. The tuning fork, carrying a stylus on one of its prongs, is set into vibration, and the stylus is gently touched to the smoked surface,

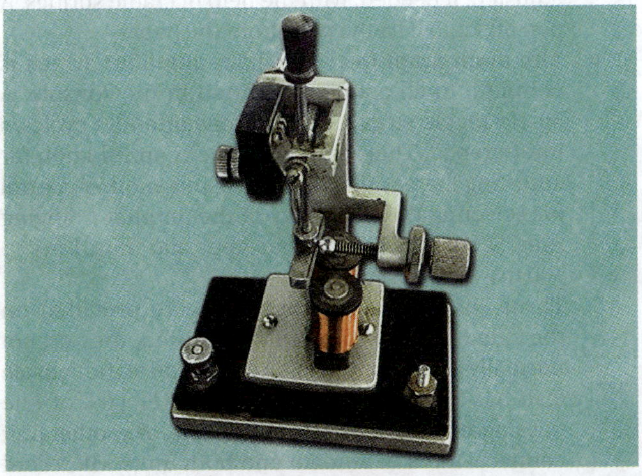

FIG. 12: Variable interrupter.

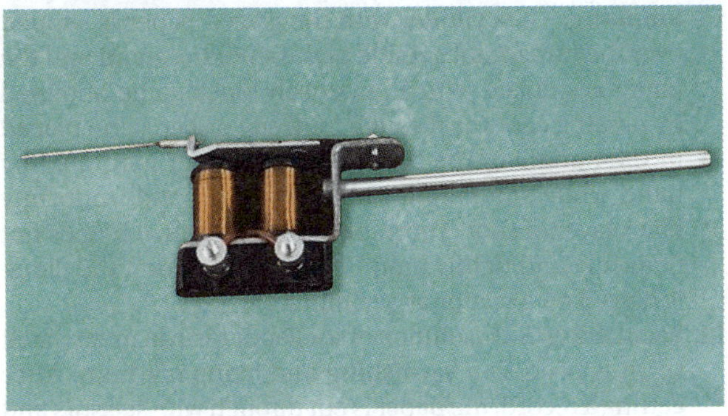

FIG. 13: Signal marker.

below the graph obtained. The time interval between two crests (or two troughs) represents 0.01 second (n = 100).

- **Spring time marker:** It is used primarily for heart experiments. It usually gives time tracing for half seconds or quarter seconds. The writer makes vertical strokes at the desired time intervals.
- **Electromagnetic time marker/signal marker: It is used in the primary circuit. The lever of the signal marker moves with every make or break of the primary circuit and a vertical line is recorded.** It can provide "make-break" contacts at intervals of 1, 2, 5, and 10 seconds **(Fig. 13)**.

11. **Stimulating Electrodes:**
    - These are employed for delivering electrical stimuli to the tissues.
    - It consists of two insulated copper wires passing through a plastic body with a central hole for fixing it to the myograph board. The ends of the wire are bared of their insulation. They are quite simple to use.
    - The usual type supplied with the muscle chamber consists of ball-and-socket-mounted silver electrodes fitted over one side of the chamber. Wooden electrodes, which consist of two copper wires fitted in a thumb-sized block of wood or vulcanite block, are quite simple to use **(Fig. 14)**.
12. **Student Stimulator:** Electronic stimulators with a DC output of 0–15 volts are now available. Each of the main stimulus parameters, i.e. volts, pulse duration, pulse frequency, mode of operation (single; repetitive, 1–100/second; or an external trigger), is controlled by knobs provided for the purpose. The "external trigger" is for use with the contact block of the kymograph.

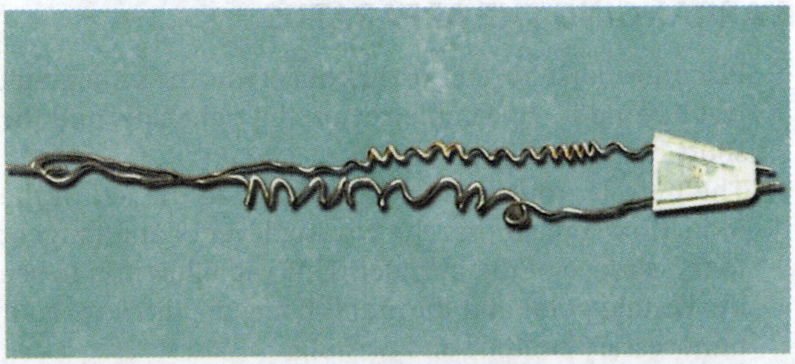

FIG. 14: Stimulating electrodes.

13. **Smoking:** The cylinder with the glazed paper is slipped over the horizontal spindle of the smoking stand and the paper is smoked with an intensely black flame obtained by passing coal gas through benzene or kerosene placed in the handle of the burner. The cylinder is rotated by hand while smoking it to obtain a thin and uniformly black layer of soot. The paper will get burnt, if it does not fit evenly and tightly around the cylinder, or if the flame is played on a stationary cylinder.
14. **Varnishing:** A 2% solution of shellac or resin in methylated spirit is used as a varnishing and fixing medium. After getting a record, the paper is cut through with scissors and the paper, with the graph side up, is passed once through the solution taken in a tray. After draining the excess solution, the paper is put on the pegs of the drying board and allowed to dry at room temperature. After it dries, a fine coat of shellac or resin remains on the paper, making it a permanent record.

ELECTRICAL CONNECTIONS

Figure 2 illustrates the connections required for obtaining induced current stimuli (induction shocks). Low-resistance cotton-covered copper wire, or ordinary flex wire, is wound round a pencil to give coiled wire pieces.

- **Circuit for single "make" and "break" stimuli:**
  - ***Primary circuit:*** Low voltage mains, simple key, and primary coil connected in series.
  - ***Secondary circuit:*** Secondary coil, short-circuiting key, and stimulating electrodes are connected as shown in **Figure 2.**
- **Taking kymograph in circuit:**
  - ***Primary circuit:*** Low-voltage mains, simple key, primary coil, and contact block of drum are connected in series.
  - ***Secondary circuit:*** The drum terminals are taken in the primary circuit when one wants to mark the point of stimulation, or when two successive stimuli are needed.
- **Taking Neef's hammer, variable interrupter, or vibrating reed in circuit:**
  - ***Primary circuit:*** Low-voltage mains, simple key, Neef's hammer of induction coil, or vibrating reed or variable interrupter, and primary coil.
  - ***Secondary circuit:*** This circuit is used for getting repeated stimuli, such as for producing tetanus, or for stimulating the vagus nerve.

ARRANGING THE APPARATUS

- Place the induction coil just in front of you, the kymograph just beyond it, the simple key on the right side, and the short-circuiting key on the left.
- The muscle trough should be placed to the left of the induction coil, so that the writing lever is at a tangent to the surface of the cylinder. This will allow you to see the writing point and the graph being obtained without unnecessary bending and twisting.

TROUBLESHOOTING

If, after making the required connections, there is no response, try to locate the fault in a step-by-step fashion.

- Check the Galvanic current by holding one end of a piece of wire on one terminal and brushing its free end on the other terminal. Sparking indicates good current. A voltmeter will indicate the voltage.
- Check the simple key, and the contact block terminals in a similar fashion. Switch on the drum; each time the striker touches the contact spring, there is sparking. This checks out the primary circuit.
- **Secondary circuit:**
  - Place the severed leg from the frog on the secondary coil terminals; if it twitches with each induction shock (as the spindle rotates), the fault lies beyond this point. "Open" (i.e. switch off) the short-circuiting key and place the "leg" on the electrodes, and switch on the drum.
  - If the leg muscles twitch with each shock, the stimuli are, evidently, reaching the electrodes. If the stimulation of the nerve does not give a response, put the electrodes directly on the muscle belly; if the muscle contracts with each shock, the nerve has been damaged. Replace the preparation with the one kept in reserve for such a contingency. If all efforts fail, seek the help of the electrician and your tutor.

STUDENT PHYSIOGRAPH

The "student physiograph" consists of the following components (Fig. 15):

1. **The main console:** The main console has the following:
   - **Chart drive:** The multi speed chart drive can provide paper speeds ranging from 0.25 mm/s to 100 mm/s through the use of a range selector knob and push buttons. The paper, 70 mm in width, is fed through a slot under the writing pens.
   - **Pen recording system:** Two recording pens are provided, the upper for the main recording channel and the lower for synchronized time/event recording. The pen is 120 mm in length to minimize arc distortion. The contact tension of the pens on the paper can be adjusted, if needed, with the help of cradle springs. A pen lift knob lefts the pens from the paper.
   - **The main amplifier:** The main amplifier, which is common to all couplers, is fitted in the console. A 50-Hz toggle switch cuts off unwanted 50 cycles/s interference. There is a "baseline" control knob for adjusting the position of the pen and another control for selecting the sensitivity of the amplifier ranging from 50 μV to 500 μV in four steps and from 1 mV to 100 mV in seven steps.

     Three screw-driver adjustments are provided on the side of the console. Once adjusted, they do not normally require adjustments. The side of the console also has IN and OUT jacks. The OUT jack of one physiograph connected to the IN jack of another unit connects them in tandem and both units will record

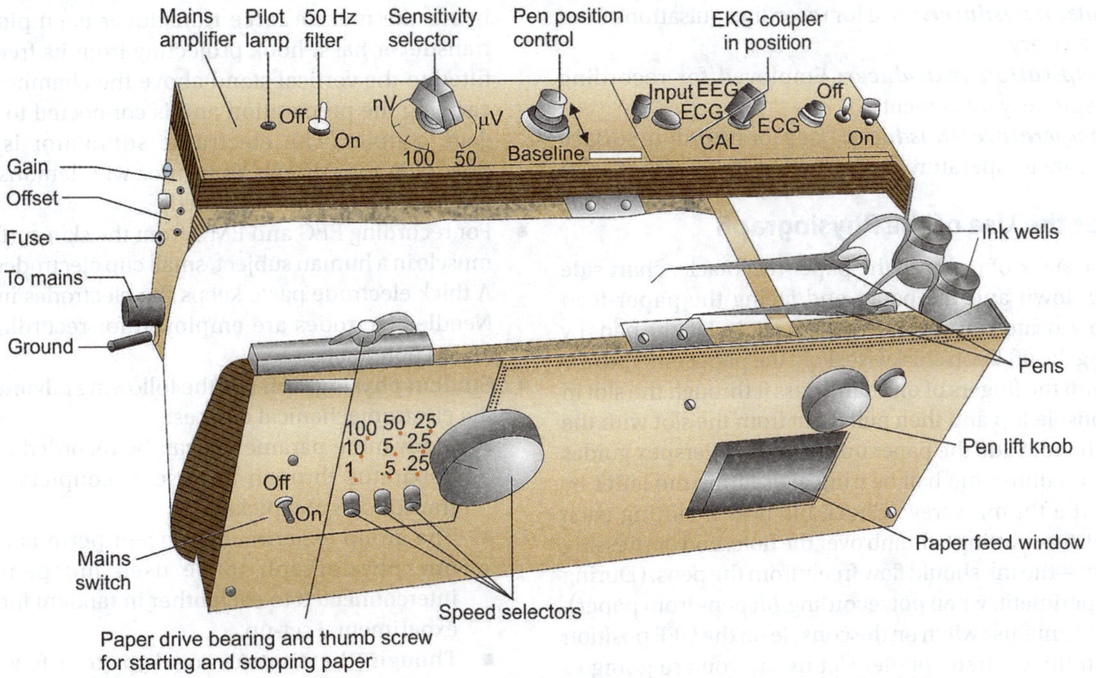

FIG. 15: Student physiograph.
(ECG/EKG: electrocardiogram; EEG: electroencephalography)

simultaneously from the same experimental set-up. Another input jack takes the synchronized event/time marker of the electronic stimulator.

- **Coupler housing:** Different interchangeable couplers can be plugged into the coupler housing. An appropriate transducer is to be connected to the coupler in use.

2. **Couplers:** The following couplers are available for use with the physiograph:
   - **Biopotential coupler:** The biopotential coupler is designed to record any AC phenomenon like **electrocardiogram (ECG),** electroencephalogram (EEG), **electromyogram (EMG), sensory and motor nerve conduction velocities in humans, movements of the eyes** (electronystagmogram), and so on. A control knob selects the phenomenon to be recorded. It has a CAL position for the checking of calibration for which a push button is provided.
   - **Electrocardiogram (EKG):** The coupler is used for recording clinical EKG (ECG). There is a knob for selecting various leads—I, II, III, aVR, aVL, aVF, V, CR, CL, and CF. There is another knob for calibration.
   - **Strain gage coupler:** This coupler records activity from various strain gage transducers (pressure-volume, volume, and muscle-force transducers). The experimental applications of this coupler include—arterial and venous pulse, blood pressure in cannulated dog or rabbit, plethysmography, experiments on frog's gastrocnemius muscle sciatic nerve preparation (simple muscle twitch, strength of stimulation, effect of two successive stimuli, effect of temperature and load, tetanus, fatigue, isometric contraction, etc.) experiments on frog's heart, experiments on isolated tissues (intestine, uterus, rat diaphragm, etc.), experiments on isolated perfused rabbit's heart, effect of load on finger movements, and so on. Springs of different tensile strength are available with the force transducer.
   - **Pulse-respiration coupler:** This coupler is employed for recording arterial pulse with a photoelectric pulse transducer and respiratory movements with a respiration belt transducer. A toggle switch selects pulse or respiration mode.
   - **Temperature coupler:** This coupler is used for recording rectal or surface temperature. For such recordings the transducer has to be calibrated within the desired temperature range using a water bath.
3. **The Stimulator:** The electronic stimulator can be used in two modes:
   i. To energize either a time base or act as an event marker.
   ii. To provide electrical stimuli of up to 30 volts as a single pulse, or as two successive stimuli with predetermined intervals ranging from 5–250 ms, or as repeated stimuli with frequencies ranging from 0.5–100/s. The electrical stimuli provided by the stimulator are rectilinear with a fixed pulse width of 0.5 ms.
4. **Transducers:** The wide range of transducers converts one form of energy into another, electrical energy, in this case:
   - ***Pressure-volume transducer*:** It is used for recording pressures from –50 mm Hg to 250 mm Hg, and small changes in volume.
   - ***Volume transducer*:** It is used for recording minute changes in volume.
   - ***Muscle-force transducer*:** Employed for recording all muscle, activity, heart activity, force, etc.

- ***Pulse transducer***: Used for recording pulsations from any artery.
- ***Respiration transducer***: Employed for recording respiratory movements.
- ***Temperature transducer***: Used for recording surface or core temperature.

Steps for the Use of the Physiograph

- Put the stack of paper in the paper receptacle, chart side facing down and the paper end facing the paper-feed window located on the front of the console. Lift the pens by turning the lift knob clockwise. Fold the paper end into a V and with the fingers of one hand pass it through the slot in the console top and then pull it out from the slot with the other hand. Slide the paper under the two Perspex guides and then under the ball bearing after lifting the latter by using the thumb screw. Check ink flow by lifting each inkwell top, putting a thumb over the hole, and depressing it down—the ink should flow freely from the pens. (During the experiment, when not recording, lift pens from paper).
- From the mains switch on the console on the OFF position plug in the desired coupler (let us say you are going to record the ECG in a subject). It is important to remember that a coupler should not be plugged in or removed while the mains switch is ON. Select the standard speed on 25 mm/s.
- Apply the electrodes on the subject's arms and legs. Connect the electrodes through lead wires to the 5-pin junction box and the latter to the EKG coupler.
- Switch ON the mains console and then the coupler. Adjust the sensitivity on the main amplifier to 1 mV. Adjust pen position to center. Put the lead selector control on the coupler to CAL position for calibration. Run the paper and press and release the CAL push button on the coupler three or four times while adjusting the CAL control so that 1 mV may produce a deflection of the pen by 1 cm. Stop paper.
- Move the lead selector control to lead I position and record 6–8 ECG complexes. Stop paper; move the control to lead II and take recording. Continue this process till all the leads have been obtained.
- For experiments on the frog's nerve-muscle preparation and for recording the mechanical activity of the frog's heart, the muscle force transducer is employed. This transducer has a hook projecting from its free end. It is fitted to the vertical stand above the chamber or board carrying the preparation and is connected to the strain gage coupler. The electronic stimulator is used for providing the stimuli. Your tutor will demonstrate how the recording is to be obtained.
- For recording EEG and EMG from the skin surface over a muscle in a human subject, small cup electrodes are used. A thick electrode paste keeps the electrodes in position. Needle electrodes are employed for recording muscle action potentials.
- **Student physiograph** has the following **advantages** over the electromechanical devices:
  - Many more parameters can be recorded on a single apparatus through the use of couplers, matching transducers and pickups.
  - The group experiment concept permits more than one physiograph to be used independently or interconnected to each other in tandem for the same experimental set-up.
  - Though, the controls are kept to a few, only the sensitivity and accuracy of these devices are high.

QUESTIONS

Q.1. Why are frogs preferred for amphibian experiments?

Q.2. What is the function of the primary and secondary key?

Q.3. What is the difference between primary and secondary coil?

Q.4. Name the various keys and their functions.

Q.5. What is the function of an induction coil?

Q.6. Name the various types of stimuli.

Q.7. What are the characteristics of an ideal stimulus?

Q.8. Why induced current is used to stimulate the living tissue?

Q.9. What is the function of Neef's hammer?

Q.10. What are the factors affecting the strength of induced current?

Q.11. How is time interval calculated from time tracing?

Q.12. What are the various functions of student physiography? Name the various couplers used.

Refer text above for all the questions.

4.3: DISSECTION OF GASTROCNEMIUS NERVE MUSCLE PREPARATION

STUDENT OBJECTIVES

After completing this experiment, the student should be able to:

- Stun the frog properly.
- Do pithing with the help of a pithing needle.
- Recognize the gastrocnemius muscle and sciatic nerve.
- Do proper mounting of the preparation correctly in the myograph board.

PY3.18: Observe with computer assisted learning (i) amphibian nerve - muscle experiments and (ii) amphibian cardiac experiments.

Initially your tutor will demonstrate the dissection steps for obtaining the nerve-muscle preparation. Keep the preparation moist with Ringer during and after dissection. Do not use a scalpel during dissection **(Fig. 16)**.

APPARATUS

1. Pithing needle, scissors, forceps, bone cutter,
2. Wooden dissection board, amphibian Ringer's solution, and cotton wool.

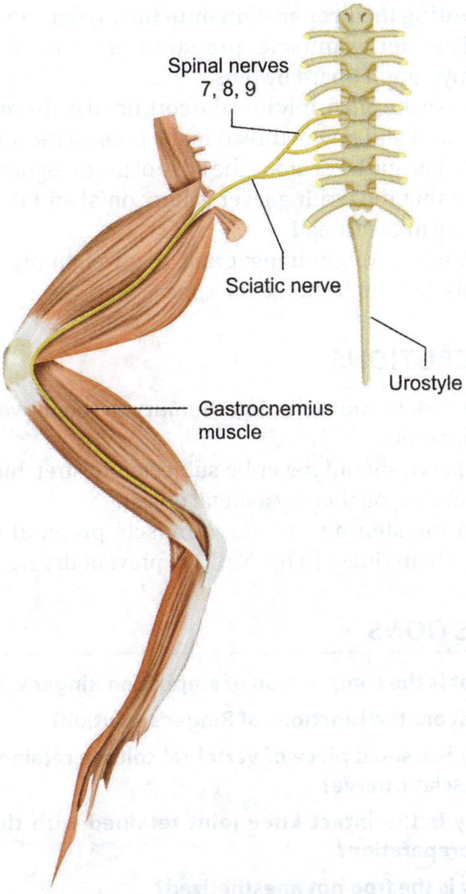

FIG. 16: Nerve–muscle preparation.

Amphibian Ringer's Solution

- This solution is isotonic with the frog's tissues and has optimal ionic constituents.
- **Sodium chloride (0.6%):** The isotonic saline for frogs is 0.6% NaCl, while for mammals—it is 0.9% NaCl solution. The composition of Ringer is given in **Table 1**.
- **Calcium chloride (0.012%):** Maintains the excitability of the living tissue.
- **Potassium chloride (0.014%):** Maintains the resting membrane potential.
- **Sodium bicarbonate (0.02%):** Maintains optimal pH

Caution: The frog must be properly "stunned" and "pithed" for smooth dissection.

PROCEDURE

1. **Stunning:** The animal is stunned to render it unconscious (anesthesia is not suitable). Hold the frog, gently but firmly, by its waist, in a duster cloth. Give a good blow on its head with a wooden mallet; one or two blows should suffice.

Table 1: The composition of Ringer's solution.

Sodium chloride	0.6 g
Calcium chloride	0.01 g
Potassium chloride	0.0075 g
Sodium bicarbonate	0.01 g
Distilled water	To 100 mL

Note: No anesthesia is used as it may suppress the excitability of the nerve, neuromuscular junction or muscle.

2. **Pithing:** The purpose of pithing is to destroy the brain and the spinal cord, so that the animal feels neither pain nor there are any reflex or voluntary movements during the dissection.
   - Hold the animal in your left hand and flex its head with your index finger. With the other hand, push a long and sharp-pointed ***pithing needle*** firmly through the skin and bone into the spinal canal, at a point where a line joining the posterior borders of tympanic membranes cuts the middle line.
   - Push the needle anteriorly into the skull and rotate it to destroy the brain. Withdraw the needle and direct it backwards into the spinal canal to destroy the spinal cord. As the cord is being destroyed, the muscles of the limbs are thrown into convulsions due to irritation of the spinal motor neurons.
   - Once the cord has been properly destroyed, the limbs will hang down loosely and limply, and pinching a toe with a forceps will not cause reflex withdrawal of that limb.
   - The animal is now "dead" in the sense that it is no longer conscious, does not "feel" any pain, and there are no voluntary or reflex movements. But the various organs, such as heart, muscles, etc. are still "alive" and can be used for experimental work.
3. **Dissection:**
   - Cut through the skin with scissors completely all around the trunk just below the forelimbs. Seize the skin in a duster and strip this "trouser" of skin right down to the toes. Place the skin and other waste tissue in the tray.
   - Place the frog on its abdomen, pick up the urostyle with a forceps, and give a cut under it with scissors. Cut through the muscles on its either side, taking care not to injure the underlying nerves. Extend these lateral cuts forwards, and using bone forceps, cut through the hip girdle on either side.
   - Lift up the urostyle and see the sciatic and other nerves emerging from the vertebral column and running parallel to the urostyle. Cut the vertebrae above and below the exit of sciatic nerves. Do not attempt to separate these nerves at this time.
   - Now there is a piece of vertebral column, and the three trunks of sciatic nerves are still attached to it on either side. Using bone forceps, make a slightly oblique cut, divide this piece into two pieces. Lift each piece with forceps and snip away the nerves going to nearby tissues, taking care not to injure the sciatic nerves, which can be seen disappearing into the thigh muscles.
   - Cut through the fascia covering the thigh muscles, and gently separate them with a blunt glass probe. The

sciatic nerves will now become visible on both sides. Holding the vertebral piece with a forceps, and free the nerves to about 2 cm above the knee joints. As you snip their branches, the thigh muscles show twitch-like contractions due to mechanical stimulation of the motor fibers.

Note: Do not directly pick up a nerve with forceps but lift it up by the vertebral piece. Once the nerve is damaged by mishandling, the muscle may continue to twitch occasionally, thus making it difficult to carry out any experiment.

- Separate the tendon of the gastrocnemius from its insertion with scissors and strip the muscle from the bones right up to the knee joint.
- Tie a stout thread around the tendon just above the sesamoid bone (which is buried in the tendon). Repeat on the other side.
- With a bone forceps, cut off the tibia-fibula below the knee joint and the thigh bone just above the point to which the sciatic nerve has been freed. Trim away any excess muscle tissue from around the knee joint.
- The dissection is now complete and there are two nerve–muscle preparations ready.
- Pass a stout all-pin through each knee joint (in-between the bones and not through the muscle tissue). The pin will be required to fix one end of the muscle firmly while the other end pulls on the hook of the writing lever.
- Keep the nerve muscle preparation immersed in Ringer's solution till the commencement of the experiment.
- Carefully lift up the preparations and transfer them to a myograph board.

4. **Mounting the preparation onto the myograph board:**
   - The nerve-muscle preparation is fixed on the myograph board by pins.
   - Push the pin firmly into the cork fitted in the myograph board and tie the thread to the hook of the lever.
   - Adjust the lever along the edge of the myograph board, so that the writing lever is horizontal and there is no slag in the thread.
   - Apply a weight hanger and 10 g weight on the lever about 3 cm from the fulcrum.

PRECAUTIONS

1. Take care to cause minimum injury to the nerve muscle preparation.
2. The nerve should never be subjected to stretching or be repeatedly touched by a metal object.
3. Keep moistening the nerve muscle preparation with amphibian ringer (0.6% NaCl) to prevent drying.

QUESTIONS

Q.1. What is the composition of amphibian Ringer's solution?

Q.2. What are the functions of Ringer's solution?

Q.3. Why is a small piece of vertebral column retained at the end of a sciatic nerve?

Q.4. Why is the intact knee joint retained with the nerve muscle preparation?

Q.5. Why is the frog not anesthetized?

Q.6. What is the purpose behind stunning and pithing frogs?

Refer text above for all the questions.

4.4: SIMPLE MUSCLE TWITCH (EFFECT OF A SINGLE STIMULUS)

STUDENT OBJECTIVES

After completing this experiment, the student should be able to:

- Dissect a frog's nerve–muscle preparation and demonstrate its excitability.
- Record the muscle response to a single stimulus applied to its nerve.
- Explain, which is the effective stimulus in this experiment, make-induced or break-induced current.
- Record the time tracing below the graph and indicate various phases and periods.
- Explain the cause of latent period, and true latent period.
- Differentiate between tension and load.
- Define isotonic and isometric contractions.
- Describe the process of excitation–contraction coupling.

PY3.18: Observe with computer assisted learning (i) amphibian nerve - muscle experiments and (ii) amphibian cardiac experiments.

INTRODUCTION

- A single adequate stimulus applied to the sciatic nerve results in a sharp, momentary contraction of the muscle, followed immediately by its relaxation. This response is called a ***simple muscle twitch (SMT)***.
- The contraction does not begin immediately upon application of the stimulus. A period between the point of stimulus and the onset of contraction is called the **latent period (LP)**.
- The **contraction period (CP)** is the period between the onset of contraction to the point that corresponds to the peak of contraction.
- The **relaxation period (RP)** is the period from the peak of contraction to the end of relaxation.
- The wave obtained at the end of the response is called the **physiological curve**. It is due to the inertia of the lever.
- **Causes of latent period:** The latent period is due to the time taken by:
  1. Action potential to travel along the nerve to the neuromuscular junction.
  2. Release of neurotransmitter (acetylcholine) and its binding to the receptors.
  3. Excitation contraction coupling.
  4. Viscosity of the muscle.

5. Inertia of the lever system, which has to be overcome before contractions can be recorded.

APPARATUS

1. Dubois-Reymond induction coil, simple key and short circuiting key.
2. Kymograph (drum); cylinder with smoked paper or glazed paper with ink-writing stylus.
3. Myograph board, stimulating electrodes, hooks and weights.
4. Tuning fork (100 Hz), dividers, pins, thread, amphibian
5. Ringer's solution and nerve-muscle preparation.

Speed of the drum: 640 mm/sec (fastest)
Strength of the stimulus: Minimal (threshold).

PROCEDURE

1. Set up the primary and secondary circuits. **Include the drum in the primary circuit** to obtain single induction shocks with every revolution of the cylinder.
2. Mount the preparation in the muscle chamber and tie its thread to the hook. Adjust the lever so that it is horizontal, and has a weight hung on it about 3 cm from the fulcrum. Support the vertical arm of the lever with the afterload screw. (This screw will support the load until the activated muscle exerts a force sufficient to lift the load).
3. Reposition the cylinder, so that the record will be obtained about 4 cm above its lower edge, and just ahead of the overlapping part of the paper. Keep the writing point 2–3 cm away from the cylinder.
4. Set the clutch on the OFF (horizontal) position, engage the gear lever at the fastest speed (640 mm/s), and place the nerve on the electrodes. Switch on the mains current. Switch OFF the simple key, and switch ON the short-circuiting key.
5. Put the clutch ON, close the simple key and open the short-circuiting key. Every time the striker touches the spring contact, thus completing the circuit, the muscle contracts. Watch 2–3 contractions to verify the suitability of the height of lever movement. Adjust, if necessary. Stop the drum with the clutch, close the short-circuiting key, and open the simple key.
6. When ready to record, bring the writing point (or the ink-writing stylus) in contact with the paper, at a tangent; and rotate the cylinder *by hand* to draw a baseline all around the paper.
7. **Marking the point of stimulus:** Bring the striker in contact with the contact spring (the induction shock will pass at this point) and steadying its position with the left hand, raise the writing point with a finger 5-6 cm above the baseline, as shown in **Figure 17**.
8. Release the clutch and let the drum speed become uniform. Switch on the simple key. The moment the striker passes the contact block, "open" the short-circuiting key but close it as soon as the muscle has contracted. Stop the drum, put the gear lever at "N" (neutral), switch off the simple key, and move the lever away from the cylinder.

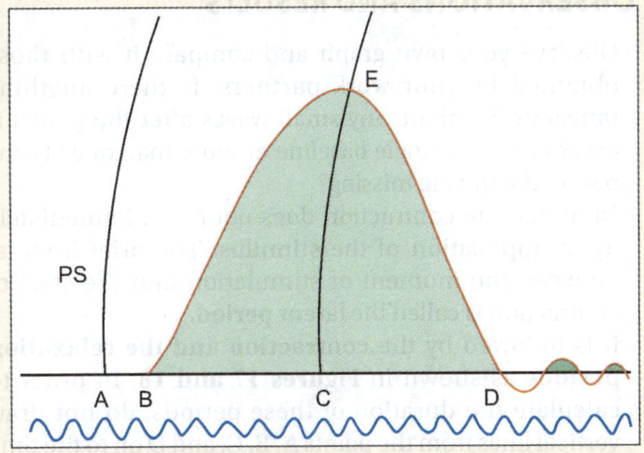

FIG. 17: Simple muscle twitch. PS: point of stimulation; AB: latent period; BC: contraction period; CD: relaxation period; BE: contraction phase; ED: relaxation phase. Tuning fork = 100 Hz. The waves at the end of the response (physiological curve) are due to bouncing of the lever on the afterload screw and have no significance.

Note: The points to be marked manually are: Point of stimulus, point of onset of contraction, point of beginning of relaxation, point of completion of relaxation before removing the drum from the circuit. In order to divide the baseline into contraction and relaxation periods, take the writing point to the summit of the curve with your hand and draw a line from this point to the baseline in one continuous smooth motion. Do not attempt to draw a vertical line from the summit to the baseline, because the writing point does not move vertically up and down but in an arc-like fashion.

9. **Recording the time trace:** Set a tuning fork into vibration by striking one of its prongs on the heel of your hand (both prongs will vibrate). Holding the fork from its base, and keeping it horizontal (so that the stylus vibrates up and down), bring the stylus in gentle contact with the revolving cylinder, below the baseline, moving the stylus slightly downwards to avoid overlapping of the waves being recorded. (The time tracing must be recorded at the same speed at which the muscle contraction was recorded).
10. Remove the cylinder from the spindle, discuss your graph with your tutor, and if it is okay, get it signed. Cut along the overlapping part of the paper with scissors (always avoid recording your graph on this part of the paper), and remove it carefully without smudging the smoked surface. Lay the paper flat, face up, on a table, and enter the following data:
    - The title of the experiment (e.g. simple muscle twitch).
    - Preparation used (frog's gastrocnemius muscle–sciatic nerve preparation).
    - Frequency of the tuning fork (n = 100).
    - Your name and the date on which the experiment was done.
    - Label the various parts of the graph.
11. Fix your graph and allow it to dry at room temperature. Cut out and trim your graph neatly; then paste it in your workbook.

OBSERVATIONS AND RESULTS

- Observe your own graph and compare it with those obtained by your work partners. Is there anything unusual? Are there any small waves after the twitch is over? Is there a single baseline or more than one? Is any part of the tracing missing?
- Note that the contraction does not begin immediately upon application of the stimulus. The brief interval between the moment of stimulation and the start of contraction is called the **latent period.**
- It is followed by the **contraction and the relaxation periods** as shown in **Figures 17 and 18**. In order to calculate the duration of these periods, do not draw vertical lines from the points A, B, C, and D on to the time tracing. Instead, use a pair of dividers; open up its points as required, place these on the time trace, and count the number of waves for each period. For example, if there is one wave for latent period, its duration will be 0.01 second (with n = 100).
- The two phases of the muscle curve are called **contraction phase** (BE) and **relaxation phase** (ED).
- The calculated durations of various periods in this experiment are given in **Table 2.**
- Compare your results with the expected durations of the twitch, and its various periods, and if these vary greatly, try to find out the reason.

Correlation of Simple Muscle Twitch and Action Potential on the Same Time Scale

When the muscle action potential and the simple muscle twitch are plotted on the same time scale the twitch starts

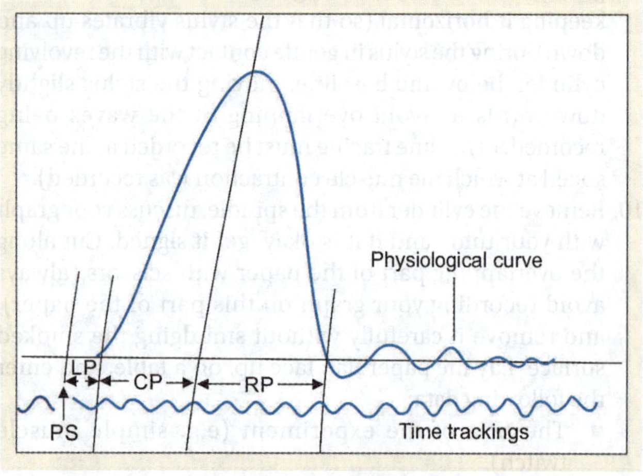

FIG. 18: Simple muscle twitch.
(PS: point of stimulation; LP: latent period; CP: contraction period; RP: relaxation period)

Table 2: The calculated durations of various periods in simple muscle twitch.	
Latent period	0.01 second
Contraction period	0.04 second
Relaxation period	0.05 second
Total twitch duration in the frog's gastrocnemius muscle	0.1 second

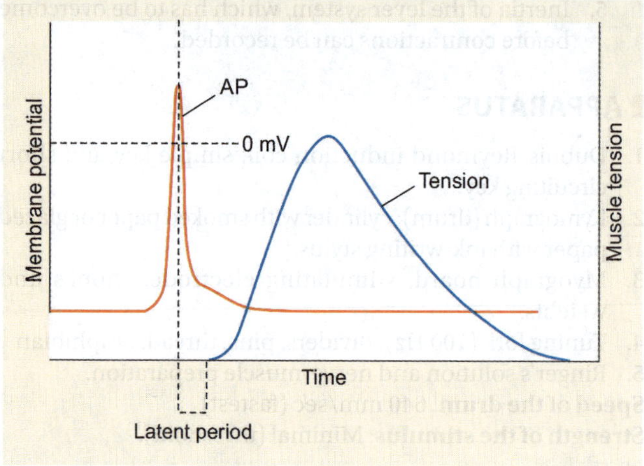

FIG. 19: Correlation of simple muscle twitch and action potential on the same time scale.
(AP: Action potential)

2 msec after the start of depolarization of the membrane before repolarization is complete **(Fig. 19).**

PRECAUTIONS

1. The nerve muscle preparation should be stimulated briefly a single induction shock.
2. Care should be taken to mark the point of stimulus.
3. Time tracing should be taken just below the graph.

QUESTIONS

Q.1. What type of nerve is the sciatic nerve? Why does its stimulation cause muscle contraction? Is the muscle twitch recorded by you a normal physiological event?

- The sciatic nerve is a mixed nerve carrying motor or efferent fibers (axons of anterior horn cells; lower motor neurons) to the muscle fibers, and sensory or afferent fibers from the sensory receptors, such as muscle spindles, joint, and tendon receptors, etc. to the spinal cord.
- Experimentally, a single supramaximal stimulus applied to the nerve simultaneously activates all the motor fibers, and action potentials (APs; nerve impulses), so generated travel to the neuromuscular junctions of all the muscle fibers where they release acetylcholine.
- This transmitter generates muscle action potentials in almost all the muscle fibers, which is followed by near-simultaneous, short-lived contraction of the muscle fibers called a muscle twitch.
- A twitch of all the muscle fibers can also be produced by direct stimulation, provided the muscle is reasonably small, because in large muscles, it is rather difficult to apply sufficient current. The sensory fibers of the sciatic nerve are also stimulated, but they have no effect on the twitch.
- ***The twitch recorded in this experiment is almost certainly not a physiological event,*** because the nervous system never stimulates all the motor neurons supplying

a muscle simultaneously, except perhaps in the case of a tic.

- The usual repetitive stimuli come sufficiently close together, so that the muscle does not relax between APs, and each fiber produces a sustained contraction called **tetanus**. The twitch, however, is much simpler to study especially in an isolated preparation since it is less likely to undergo fatigue.

Q.2. Why is the kymograph included in the primary circuit?

The drum is taken in the primary circuit for two reasons—

1. Firstly, to obtain a single induction shock (the "make"-induced current is the effective stimulus)
2. Secondly, to mark the point of stimulation.

Q.3. What is the cause of the latent period? How can this period be increased or decreased? What is "true" latent period?

A. **Cause of latent period:**

The latent period is due to a chain of events, including:

1. The time taken by the APs to travel from the point of stimulation to the motor endplates.
2. Release of acetylcholine.
3. Binding of acetylcholine to the receptors, sodium influx, and generation of muscle action potential, which lead to contraction (excitation-contraction coupling).
4. Viscosity of the muscle.
5. Inertia of the lever system, which has to be overcome before contraction can be recorded.

The latent period can be **increased** by:

1. Stimulating the nerve near its vertebral end.
2. Immersing the muscle in cold Ringer at about 5°C, which slows down various electrochemical events; it also increases the viscosity of the muscle.
3. Applying more load on the lever, which makes the lever "heavier", thus increasing its inertia.

The latent period can be **decreased** by:

1. Stimulating the nerve as close to the muscle as possible.
2. Immersing the muscle in warm Ringer at about 45°C, which speeds up various chemical processes; it also decreases the viscosity of the muscle.
3. Decreasing the load on the muscle, which decreases its inertia.

B. **True latent period:** If the muscle is directly stimulated (to exclude the time spent in conduction of APs in the motor fibers), and if an optical recording system is employed (to exclude the inertia of the mechanical lever), the latent period is much reduced, which is called the true latent period.

Q.4. What is meant by the terms "tension" and "load"?

- Contraction is the active process of shortening of a muscle during which force is generated. **Tension** is the force exerted by a contracting muscle on an object.
- **Load** is the force exerted by the weight of an object on a contracting muscle, i.e. it is the resistance offered to muscle shortening.
- Thus, muscle tension and load are opposing forces. To lift a load, the muscle tension must exceed the load. If the load is greater than the muscle tension, the load will not be lifted and no external work will be done.

Note: It is important to note that the muscles show only two types of mechanical responses—shortening and development of force or tension, and both usually occur together.

Q.5. What type of muscle contraction is recorded in this experiment?

- The muscle contraction recorded in this experiment is the *isotonic* (same tension) type.
- The distance the lever moves indicates the degree of shortening, i.e. the strength of contraction. The muscle does external work since it moves the load to a certain distance, the tension remaining the same.

Comments

Since a load is moved, it involves the phenomenon of inertia and momentum. In the beginning, the inertia of the lever slightly delays its upward movement (though the tension is rising), but then the muscle contracts and the lever starts to move up and continues to move (or jerk up) due to momentum, even after the contraction has ended. Therefore, an isotonic contraction tends to last longer. Furthermore, the height of the recorded tracing is not a true indicator of the strength of contraction because of the "jerking up" of the lever. For these reasons, isometric recordings are preferred for studying various features of muscle contraction, such as length–tension relation and force–velocity and work–velocity relations.

Q.6. What is isometric contraction? Do such contractions occur in the body?

- Muscles consist not only of *contractile components* (contractile proteins) but also *elastic* and *viscous elements* (elastic fibers, tendons, connective tissue sheaths, blood vessels, etc.), which are arranged *in series* with the contractile components.
- Therefore, if both the ends of a muscle are rigidly fixed, it is possible for the muscle fibers to contract without an appreciable shortening of the *muscle as a whole,* though there is development of tension.
- Such a contraction is called *isometric* ("same measure" or length). (The myofibrils contract and shorten, and in doing so, they stretch the in-series elastic elements. There are "parallel" elastic elements also in the muscle).
- A recording system in which one end of the muscle is attached to a force transducer, and the other to an isotonic lever, will record both tension and shortening.

Note: Even during isotonic recording of an afterloaded muscle, there is an initial period of isometric contraction during which the tension is rising, until it exceeds the load and shortening of the muscle occurs and the load is lifted.

- Both isotonic and isometric contractions occur in the body, and even in the same muscles. For example, in attempting to lift a car, muscles generate great tension or force but they cannot shorten. However, the same muscles can lift a lighter load.
- Similarly, antigravity muscles (i.e. muscles, which maintain our posture against gravity), such as extensors

of the back, hips, and knees contract isometrically to maintain the erect posture, but they can shorten to cause movements at these joints.

Q.7. What is meant by "afterloaded" and "freeloaded" contractions?

See Experiment 4.11.

Q.8. How would you ascertain whether a twitch has been recorded in the "afterloaded" or "freeloaded" condition?

- After the muscle twitch is over, a few waves or oscillations are recorded. These are not a part of muscle contraction, but a result of muscle elasticity and jerking of the lever on the "stop screw" due to its momentum.
- These waves are called *physiological* or *shatter waves.* If the muscle is in the afterloaded state, the shatter waves appear mainly above the baseline, but if it is freeloaded (or preloaded), the waves are recorded mainly below the baseline.

Q.9. What are the factors, which determine the height of the simple muscle curve?

1. **Strength of stimulus**
2. **Initial length of muscle fibers (preload)**
3. **Type of loading**
4. **Temperature**
5. **Type of muscle fibers in the muscle**
6. **Inertia of the lever system:** Greater is the instrumental inertia, and lower is the height of the twitch curve.
7. **Magnification of the lever:** The magnification by the lever depends on the ratio of the lengths of the vertical and horizontal arms. This is, of course, fixed in a given lever. A longer horizontal arm will cause greater magnification.

Note: The frequency of stimulation, whether two or more successive stimuli, determines the force of contraction. In the present context, however, we have employed a single stimulus.

Q.10. Which properties of muscle are demonstrated in this experiment?

The important properties demonstrated in this experiment include excitability, contractility, relaxation, and conductivity (the sarcolemma conducts action potential in both directions from the motor endplate, which is usually located about the middle of the fiber).

Q.11. What is excitation–contraction coupling? What is the sliding filament theory of muscle contraction?

- **Excitation–contraction coupling:** It is the process by which excitation, which is an electrical event, leads to contraction of the muscle, which is a mechanical phenomenon. Usually, one does not occur without the other. What is the link between excitation and contraction? The linking or the coupling agent is calcium, which, as a result of depolarization, is released from a highly specialized system of internal membranes, as described below.
- The arrival of action potential at the motor endplate leads to depolarization of the sarcolemma, which is transmitted, via the T-tubules, into the very interior of the muscle fiber to all the myofibrils.
- This releases large amounts of calcium from the terminal cisterns (lateral sacs) of the triads into the sarcoplasm.
- The calcium ions bind to troponin C (TnC), cause a change in its shape which, in turn, physically pushes the tropomyosin strands laterally, thereby exposing the "active" sites ("binding" sites for myosin heads) on the actin filaments. The adenosine triphosphate (ATP) is then split.
- The knob-like heads (cross-bridges) of myosin filaments now immediately bind to the active sites, and tilt back (i.e. they straighten out; this is called the *"power stroke"*), thus resulting in sliding of thin (actin) filaments over the thick (myosin) filaments. (Seven myosin binding sites are uncovered for each molecule of TnC that binds a calcium ion). Since the myosin heads attach to, tilt, and detach from successive binding sites on the thin filaments, this process has been called the *"walk along" mechanism of muscle contraction.*

Q.12. Which factors are responsible for muscle relaxation?

The following factors are involved in relaxation:

- After the contraction is over, the calcium is actively pumped back into the sarcoplasmic reticulum by a pump called the Ca^{2+}–Mg^{2+} ATPase. Once the concentration of Ca^{2+} in the sarcoplasm has fallen sufficiently low and Ca^{2+} is removed from troponin, the chemical interaction between actin and myosin ends, and the muscle relaxes.
- In resting muscle, the troponin–tropomyosin complex functions as a relaxing protein that prevents interaction between myosin and actin filaments.
- Finally, it may be pointed out that ATP provides the energy both for contraction as well as relaxation.

Q.13. Can you get an idea about the speed of muscle contraction from your graph?

Since the muscle curve shows displacement of the writing point (or pen) against time, a tangent drawn to the curve at the point of maximum slope can give an idea about the velocity of muscle shortening, i.e. steeper the slope, faster the speed of shortening.

Q.14. Can the duration of different phases of simple muscle twitch (SMT) be determined if no time trackings are taken?

Yes, this can be determined, if we know the speed of the drum accurately.

Q.16. Which properties of muscle are demonstrated in this experiment?

The important properties demonstrated in this experiment include excitability, contractility, relaxation and conductivity.

Q.17. What is a physiological curve?

See text above

Q.18. Can the duration of different phases of simple muscle twitch be determined, if no time trackings are taken?

Yes, this can be determined, if we know the speed of the drum accurately.

Q.19. What is the function of the load suspended from the lever?

- It prevents the overshooting of the lever from the drum so that the complete graph is recorded on the drum.
- It also overcomes the inertia of the lever.
- It keeps the lever horizontal.

Q.20. What are the criteria of an ideal lever?

An ideal lever should not have any momentum. It should be weightless so that there is no resistance.

4.5: EFFECT OF TEMPERATURE ON MUSCLE CONTRACTION

STUDENT OBJECTIVES

After completing this experiment, the student should be able to:

- Demonstrate the effect of change of temperature on the amplitude and different phases on simple muscle twitch.
- Explain the changes in amplitude and different phases of simple muscle twitch seen with change in temperature.

PY3.18: Observe with computer assisted learning (i) amphibian nerve - muscle experiments and (ii) amphibian cardiac experiments.

INTRODUCTION

- When there is change in the surrounding medium (Ringer's solution), there is change in amplitude and duration of different phases of simple muscle twitch (SMT).
- These changes are seen because of the changes in the viscosity and the metabolism of the muscle.
- There is also a change in the conduction velocity of the sciatic nerve.
- Keeping the point of stimulation unchanged, single contractions are recorded, first at room temperature, then at about 38°C, and finally at about 16°C. The effect of temperature on the amplitude of contraction, and on various periods is noted.

APPARATUS

- Same as in SMT except Lucas chamber is used instead of myograph board (*Refer* Experiment 4.4).
- Cold (10–15°C) and warm (38–40°C) Ringer's solution
- Thermometer.

Speed of the drum: 640 mm/sec (fastest)
Stimulus: Maximal

PROCEDURE

1. Arrange the same apparatus as used for recording SMT, except that Lucas chamber is used in place of myograph board. With the muscle immersed in Ringer at room temperature (note the temperature with a thermometer), record a SMT.
2. Replace the solution with Ringer at 38–40°C, wait for about 5 minutes, and record another contraction, taking care that the point of stimulus, strength of the stimulus and the baseline remains the same.
3. Replace the hot Ringer with cold Ringer at 10–15°C, and record another twitch after waiting for about 5 minutes.
4. Using the writing point of the lever, draw lines from the summit of each curve to the baseline.
5. Record a time tracking with a tuning fork below the graph.
6. Remove the paper and label your graph appropriately indicating the temperature for each twitch.
7. Tabulate your results, indicating the height of each curve in cm, and the durations of various periods.
8. Enter these data in your workbook.

PRECAUTIONS

1. The muscle must be immersed in the Ringer solution at various temperatures for at least 5 minutes before taking the recording.
2. Temperature of warm Ringer should not exceed 42°C as the proteins get denatured beyond this temperature.
3. Effect of warm Ringer solution should be recorded before that of cold Ringer solution. Cold Ringer slows down the metabolic activity of the muscle thereby delaying the recovery process.
4. Baseline, the point of stimulus and strength of stimulus should be the same in all the three tracings to facilitate comparison.

OBSERVATION (FIG. 20 AND TABLE 3)

Compare the three muscle curves recorded at three different temperatures with respect to durations of latent period, contraction phase, relaxation phase and height of contraction.

PHYSIOLOGICAL SIGNIFICANCE OF THIS PRACTICAL

- The warm up exercises performed before any athletic activity enhances the performance.

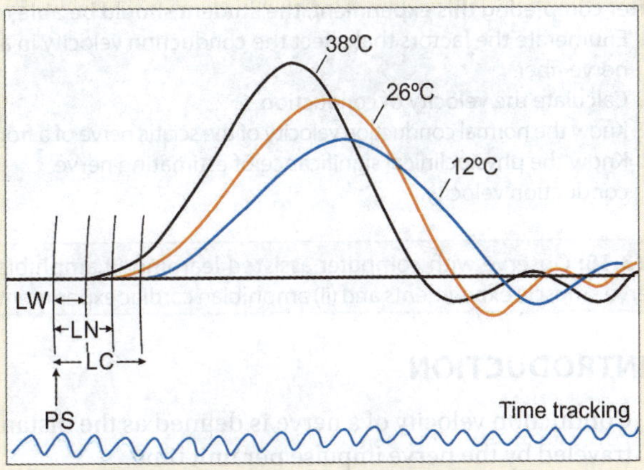

FIG. 20: Effect of temperature on simple muscle twitch (SMT).

Table 3: Recording of effect of temperature on simple muscle twitch.

Temperature	*Amplitude*	*Latent period*	*Contraction period*	*Relaxation period*
Normal				
Warm (38°)				
Cold (16°)				

- Also if the environmental temperature is increased within the physiological limits, the efficiency of skeletal muscle contraction increases (especially during exercise).

QUESTIONS

Q.1. What is the effect of moderately high temperature on the muscle twitch?

- Warm Ringer (40°C) increases the excitability and hastens various metabolic processes in the muscle; it also decreases the viscosity. The total twitch duration decreases with decrease in latent period (LP), contraction period (CP), and relaxation period (RP). The *speed of contraction* increases, as is evident from the steep slope of the contraction phase; relaxation is also faster. Also due to the increase in enzymatic and chemical activities inside the muscle the height of contraction increases. (Isometric recording would give a true indication of the force of contraction).
- High temperature, (say, 45–50°C and above) causes coagulation of muscle proteins, the muscle shortens, and goes into an irreversible state called **"heat rigor"**. Heat rigor does not occur in the body as such a high temperature is incompatible with life, though another type of rigor, called rigor mortis, is seen after death.

Q.2. What is the effect of low temperature on muscle contraction?

- Cold has opposite effects due to slowing down of chemical processes and increase in viscosity. If the temperature is reduced to 0°C or below, the excitability is lost.
- However, if the muscle is gradually rewarmed, excitability is regained. In hibernating mammals, the body temperature falls *naturally* to around 15°C without any ill effects on arousal.
- *Induced hypothermia* produced by cooling the skin or blood, where the core temperature can be reduced to about 25°C, is frequently employed in patients during operations on the brain or heart. Rats can be cooled to 0–1°C for short periods and then revived. But formation of ice crystals damages the tissues by dehydration, if such hypothermia is prolonged.

Q.3. What is rigor mortis and what is its importance?

- ***Rigor mortis,*** in which there is shortening and rigidity of muscles, occurs some hours after death. The rigidity is due to loss of all the ATP, which is required for detachment of cross-bridges, which are fixed to actin filaments in an abnormal and resistant manner.
- Depending on the environmental temperature and other factors, the rigidity disappears after some hours due to destruction of muscle proteins by enzymes released from cellular lysosomes. The appearance and disappearance of rigidity and other factors help a forensic expert in fixing the time of death.

Q.4. Is "all-or-none law" being violated in this experiment?

- No, in this experiment, the temperature is changing hence the law is not valid.
- It is valid only when environmental temperature is kept constant.

4.6: VELOCITY OF NERVE IMPULSE

STUDENT OBJECTIVES

After completing this experiment, the student should be able to:

- Enumerate the factors that affect the conduction velocity in a nerve fiber.
- Calculate the velocity of conduction.
- Know the normal conduction velocity of the sciatic nerve of a frog.
- Know the physioclinical significance of estimating nerve conduction velocity.

PY3.18: Observe with computer assisted learning (i) amphibian nerve - muscle experiments and (ii) amphibian cardiac experiments.

INTRODUCTION

- Conduction velocity of a nerve is defined as the distance traveled by the nerve impulse per unit time.
- The conduction velocity varies from nerve to nerve, but as a general rule, the myelinated nerves conduct faster than the unmyelinated nerves.
- Estimating nerve conduction velocity in humans has many physioclinical significance.
- Two most important determinants of nerve conduction velocity are:
  - Diameter of nerve fiber
  - Myelination of nerves.
- In frogs, the nerve conduction velocity is recorded by a simple experiment. By keeping the point of stimulation unchanged, the sciatic nerve is stimulated first near the knee joint, and then at its vertebral end. The difference in the two latent periods and the length of the nerve allow calculation of the velocity of nerve impulses.

PRINCIPLE

- The conduction velocity is calculated by dividing the distance between the two points of stimulation with the difference in the latent period of the two simple muscle twitches (SMTs).
- **Conduction velocity of a nerve** = Distance traveled/ Time taken by nerve impulse to travel from one point to another.

APPARATUS

1. Same as in SMT
2. Reversing key (instead of short-circuiting key).
3. Two pairs of electrodes

Speed of the drum: 640 mm/s (fastest)
Strength of stimulus: Minimal

PROCEDURE

1. Set up the nerve–muscle preparation as used to record a SMT.
2. The sciatic nerve is first stimulated at the muscle end (labeled as A curve) and the SMT is recorded.
3. Record the point of stimulus and the point of onset of contraction is recorded.
4. Shift the electrodes to the vertebral end of the nerve and, keeping the point of stimulation unchanged, record another contraction (labeled as B curve). Run a time trace, preferably with a tuning-fork of frequency 100 Hz. The distance is measured between the midpoints of the two pairs of electrodes (d in cm).
5. The muscle responds with a shorter latency when the nerve between the vertebral and muscle end is measured.
6. The difference in the two latent periods determines the time taken for the impulse to be conducted from the vertebral end of the nerve to the muscle end (**Fig. 21**).

Calculation of Velocity

Conduction velocity of a nerve

$$= \frac{\textbf{Distance ("d") travelled in cm}}{\textbf{Time ("t") taken by nerve impulse to travel from one point to another in seconds}}$$

Express the nerve conduction velocity as m/s.

Note: The normal conduction velocity of frog's sciatic nerve = 38–40 m/s.

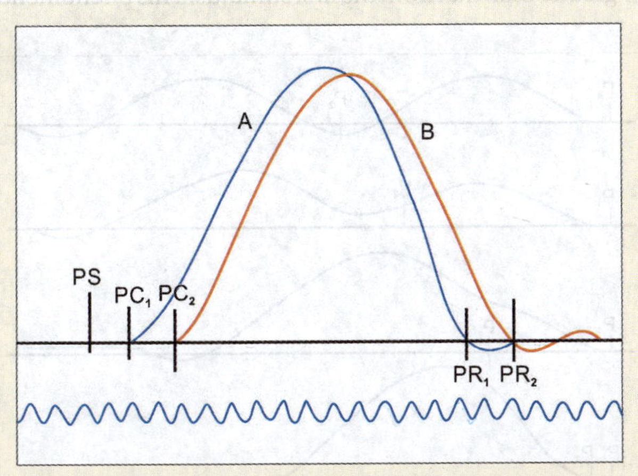

FIG. 21: Determination of nerve conduction velocity in frog (A-curve: simple muscle twitch following stimulation of the nerve near the muscle end; B-curve: simple muscle twitch following stimulation of nerve near vertebral end). PS-point of stimulus, PC_1-point of contraction for A curve, PR_1-point of complete relaxation for A curve, PC_2-point of contraction for B curve, PR_2-point of complete relaxation for B curve.

PHYSIOCLINICAL SIGNIFICANCE

Determination of conduction velocity helps in assessing:
1. Extent of damage to the nerve fiber.
2. Recovery of the nerve fiber after damage.

PRECAUTIONS

1. Same as for SMT.
2. The baseline, point of stimulation, and strength should be the same for all the recordings.
3. The distance between the points of stimulation of the vertebral end and the muscular end should be measured carefully.
4. The difference in the latent period should be measured accurately.

QUESTIONS

Q.1. What is the normal conduction velocity of Frog's sciatic nerve?
Normally, it is around 38 to 40 metres/sec.

Q.2. What conclusions would you draw from this experiment?
One can conclude that the conduction of nerve impulses is not an instantaneous phenomenon (unlike conduction of electricity, which is almost instantaneous, about 300,000 km/s). Considering that the electrical and chemical changes in the muscle are identical in the two contractions, the difference in the latent periods must be due to transmission of the impulses from the vertebral end of the nerve to the other.

Q.3. What are the factors which affect the velocity of conduction of nerve impulses?
1. **Diameter of nerve fiber:** In general, the greater the diameter of the nerve fiber, the greater is its conduction velocity.
2. **Presence of myelin sheath:** In myelinated fibers, the nerve impulse jumps from one node of Ranvier to the next, a process called salutatory (jumping) conduction. (Ionic fluxes occur only at the nodes).
3. **Temperature:** It also affects the conduction velocity, warming increases it and cooling decreases the velocity.
4. **Species differences:** Compared to mammals, the velocity is lower in amphibians.

Q.4. Why is the distance traveled by nerve impulse measured from the midpoints of the two electrodes?
As the electrode has two limbs and it is not known which limb is anode or cathode. Thus, the distance is measured from the midpoints of two limbs of the electrodes.

Q.5. What is a nerve impulse (action potential)? How is it transmitted?
See Experiment 5.5.

Q.6. How are nerve fibers classified?
See Experiment 2.27 Table 15.

Q.7. What is the physioclinical significance of this practical?
See text above.

4.7: EFFECT OF TWO SUCCESSIVE STIMULI (OF SAME STRENGTH)

STUDENT OBJECTIVES

After completing this experiment, the student should be able to:

- Define absolute and relative refractory period (RRP).
- Show the effect of two successive stimuli on muscle contraction.
- Explain the mechanism of beneficial effect.

PY3.18: Observe with computer assisted learning (i) amphibian nerve - muscle experiments and (ii) amphibian cardiac experiments.

INTRODUCTION

- When two successive stimuli (maximal/supramaximal stimuli) are applied to the skeletal muscle, the response to the second stimulus depends upon how soon it has been given after the first stimulus.
- Since the contractile machinery does not have a refractory period, the effects in response to two successive stimuli can be added up.
- The magnitude of the contraction in response to the second stimulus is greater than the first. This phenomenon is called the **"Beneficial Effect"** as the first stimulus becomes beneficial for the second one.
- The interval between the two stimuli can be varied by appropriately separating the two prongs of the "striker".
- **Dual electric contact arm ("striker"):** The dual electric contact arm, or the striker, fitted at the bottom of the spindle, has two prongs; the lower prong is firmly screwed to the spindle (shaft), while the upper prong can be moved back as much as desired.
- Thus, two successive stimuli can be applied *during one complete revolution of the cylinder;* the first stimulus (with the lower prong) arriving at the same point of stimulation, while the second stimulus (with the upper prong) can be made to fall during the latent, contraction, or the relaxation periods of the twitch resulting from the first stimulus, or after the first twitch is over.

Note: It is important to note that the muscles show only two types of mechanical responses—shortening and development of force or tension, and both usually occur together.

APPARATUS

- Same as in simple muscle twitch (SMT)
- **Speed of the drum: 640 mm/s (fastest)**
- **Strength of stimulus: Maximal/supramaximal.**

PROCEDURE

1. Set up a nerve-muscle preparation, and a stimulation unit to supply maximal/supramaximal stimuli (to avoid quantal summation); include the drum in the primary circuit.
2. Draw a baseline, mark the point of stimulation (PS), and record a single twitch, and label it SMT.
3. Separate the projecting strikers, so that they strike the contact button in close succession. Adjust the distance between the strikers, so that the 2nd stimuli would fall during:
   - First second half of the latent period of the first twitch
   - Second half of latent period
   - In the contraction period
   - In the relaxation period
   - Immediately after the RP of the first SMT.
4. Record the all above muscle contractions using the same stimulus strength.
5. Write your observation in terms of whether the response of the two stimuli is fused or discrete and what is the change in the height of contraction.

OBSERVATION (FIGS. 22 AND 23)

- The interval between the two stimuli can be varied by appropriately separating the two prongs of the "striker".
- Record your observations as separate curves.
- Describe the observations in terms of the fact whether the responses of the two stimuli are fused or discrete. Also Note the heights of contraction.

PHYSIOCLINICAL SIGNIFICANCE

Beneficial Effect

- When the response obtained from a successive stimulus is greater than that from the first stimulus. This phenomenon

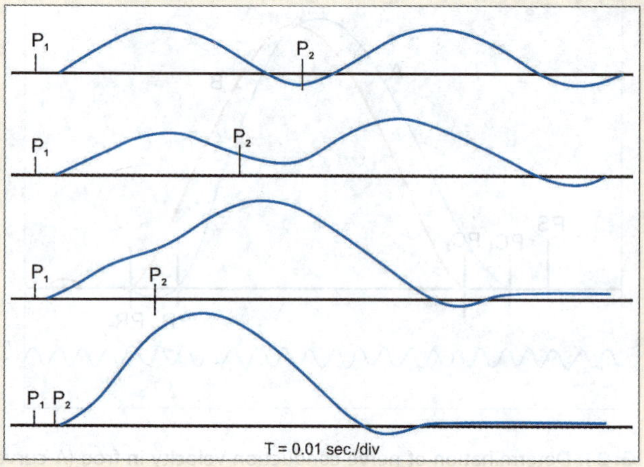

FIG. 22: The effect of two successive stimuli on muscle contraction. Four responses are shown. The first stimulus (P_1) in each case falls at the point of stimulation, the second stimulus (P_2) arriving:
A. After the first simple muscle twitch (SMT) is over
B. In the relaxation period of the first SMT
C. During the contraction phase of the first SMT
D. Within the latent period of the first SMT.

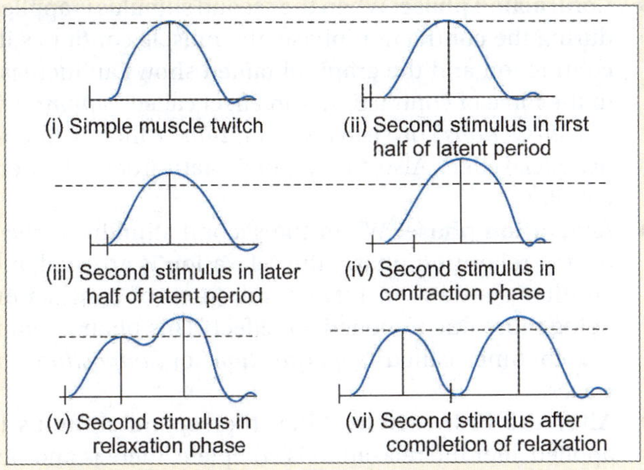

FIG. 23: Effect of two successive stimuli on muscle contraction given during different phases of muscle contraction (i to vi).

is called a beneficial effect. The second contraction gets benefited from the changes produced in the muscle due to the first stimulus.

The causes of this effect are:

1. In a single twitch, the Ca^{2+} released from the terminal cisterns into the sarcoplasm is rapidly mopped up during relaxation. When there is no relaxation, or incomplete relaxation, some Ca^{2+} remains in the sarcoplasm for a longer time, and this, together with additional Ca^{2+} released by the second stimulus, increases the *duration of the active state.* The prolonged active state increases the amount of stretch on the series elastic elements of the muscle, so that more force is transmitted to the recording system (or to the bones in the intact animal), thus increasing the height of the curve.
2. Decrease in the viscosity of the muscle resulting from the first contraction decreases the elastic inertia of the muscle, which may contribute to beneficial effect.
3. Some increase in H^+ ion concentration may be contributing to the beneficial effect.
4. A slight increase in temperature also contributes to the beneficial effect.

PRECAUTIONS

1. Care should be taken to gradually increase the distance between the contact arms (strikers).
2. The point of stimulus should be marked for both the SMT.
3. The applied stimuli should be of maximal/supramaximal strength.

QUESTIONS

Q.1. What is the refractory period? Is it the same in all the excitable tissues?

- After a tissue has responded to an effective stimulus, there is a very brief interval of time, called the *refractory period,* during which the tissue loses its excitability, i.e. it does not respond to a second stimulus.
- It is divided into **Absolute refractory period (ARP)** and **Relative refractory period (RRP)**. During ARP, the tissue does not respond to another stimulus however strong it may be; while during RRP, the tissue responds to a stronger than usual stimulus.
- The muscle and nerve tissues are refractory during their action potentials (APs).
- The ARP corresponds to most of the spike potential, while the RRP coincides with its later part (activation and inactivation of sodium channels. The AP in skeletal muscle **(Figs. 24A to C)** lasts only for 3–5 ms (i.e. early half of latent period of a twitch), but the mechanical response, which starts just before the end of AP, lasts much longer (300–400 ms). Since the contractile machinery has no refractoriness, the effect of two or more stimuli can be added up.
- In contrast, the cardiac muscle is refractory throughout its contraction phase, which lasts almost as long as its action potential (i.e. 200–300 ms). A second stimulus applied during the contraction phase, is, therefore, ineffective. The muscle must start relaxing before it can respond to another stimulus **(Fig. 25)**.
- In nerve fibers, the refractory period, which corresponds to the spike potential, lasts for 0.3–0.4 ms.

NOTE: Absolute refractory period (ARP): *When two successive stimuli are given in such a way that the second stimulus falls during the latent period of the muscle, there is no additional response seen. The muscle is said to be in ARP.*

Relative refractory period: *When the second stimulus falls a little later (either in the contraction/relaxation period) leading to a response. The muscle is said to be in the RRP.*

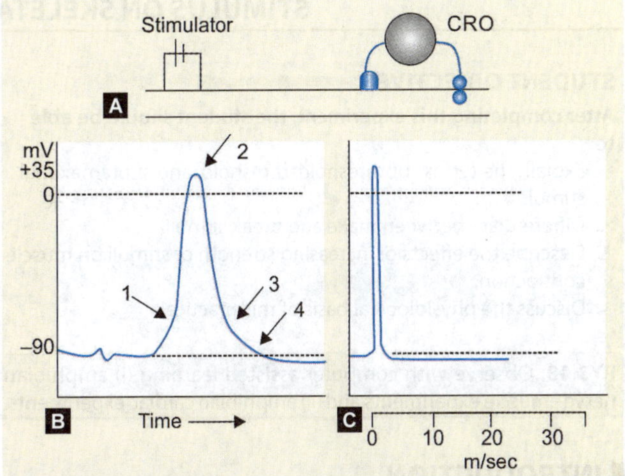

FIGS. 24A TO C: Diagram of action potential in a thick mammalian myelinated nerve fiber. (A) Method or recording monophasic action potential; (B) Action potential drawn with time distortion to show its various components. Arrows 1—firing level, 2—overshoot and start of repolarization (positive part of action potential), 3—repolarization slows down, 4—beginning of after-depolarization; (C) Action potential drawn without time distortion, showing the typical spike.

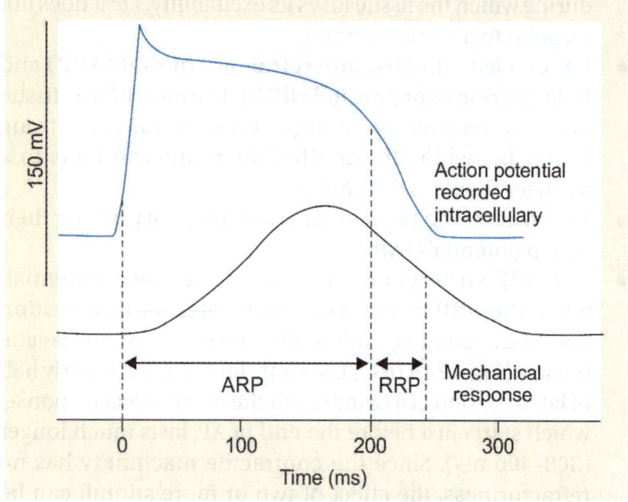

FIG. 25: Relationship between mechanical response and action potential in cardiac (ventricular) muscle.

Q.2. Describe the graphs obtained when the second stimulus is applied during different phases of the simple muscle twitch resulting from the first stimulus.

- **Latent period:** As the early half of this corresponds to ARP, a second stimulus applied during this period has no effect. The muscle responds only to the first stimulus and the graph obtained is similar to that obtained with a single stimulus. If the second stimulus falls during the latter half of the latent period, the effects of the two are added up and the graph obtained is of higher amplitude.
- **Contraction phase:** When the second stimulus is applied during the contraction phase, the muscle continues its contraction and the graph obtained shows an increase in the force of contraction—an effect called *"summation of contractions"* or *"wave summation",* which is due to beneficial effect. Also, the response starts from a "higher" baseline.
- **Relaxation phase:** When the second stimulus arrives during relaxation phase, the relaxation is arrested and another contraction results, the force of contraction being more due to beneficial effect. This phenomenon is sometimes called *"superposition"* or *"imposition"* of waves.
- **After the first twitch:** When the second stimulus is applied after the relaxation is complete, there is another response and two twitches are obtained, the second being more forceful. The increase in the height of the second curve is due to beneficial effect.

Q.3. What is beneficial effect and what is its mechanism?

- **Beneficial effect:** See text above.
- **Mechanism of beneficial effect:** See text above.

Q.4. Why are maximal/supramaximal stimuli employed for this experiment?

Supramaximal stimuli are employed to avoid quantal summation, because with such a stimulus, all the motor fibers in the sciatic nerve are stimulated. Thus, the second stimulus cannot bring more motor fibers into action and thereby increase the force of contraction.

Q.5. In this experiment, do we see summation of stimuli or summation of effects?

It is the summation of effects that we see here.

4.8: RECORDING THE EFFECT OF INCREASING STRENGTH OF STIMULUS ON SKELETAL MUSCLE CONTRACTION

STUDENT OBJECTIVES

After completing this experiment, the student should be able to:

- Explain the terms subthreshold, threshold, and supramaximal stimuli.
- Differentiate between make and break stimuli.
- Describe the effects of increasing strength of stimuli on muscle contraction.
- Discuss the physiological basis of this practical.

PY3.18: Observe with computer assisted learning (i) amphibian nerve - muscle experiments and (ii) amphibian cardiac experiments.

INTRODUCTION

- Single "make" and "break" stimuli of successively increasing strength, from subthreshold to supramaximal, are applied to the sciatic nerve and their effect on force of muscle contraction is recorded separately on a stationary drum.
- The different types of stimuli that can be applied to an excitable tissue are:
  - **Subthreshold stimulus:** This stimulus does not produce a response.
  - **Threshold stimulus:** It is defined as the minimum strength of stimulus that is required to produce a response (also called the **minimal stimulus**).
  - **Maximal stimulus:** The stimulus that produces maximum response.
  - **Supramaximal stimulus:** The stimulus that is stronger than the maximal stimulus, which when applied causes no further increase in the magnitude of contraction.
- By stimulating a muscle with increasing strength of stimulus, more and more motor units are recruited leading to increase in amplitude of contraction.
- Supramaximal stimuli are generally avoided in physiological studies because they are susceptible to cause disturbances in the state of living tissues.

APPARATUS

Same as for simple muscle twitch (SMT)

Speed of the drum (exclude it from the primary circuit): stationary

Strength of the stimuli: variable

PROCEDURE

1. Set up a nerve-muscle preparation and a stimulation unit for obtaining single "make" and "break" stimuli. **Exclude the drum from the primary circuit,** and do not connect it to the mains AC supply.
2. Engage the gear at the "N" position, and, with the writing point clear of the cylinder, move the secondary coil away from the primary to a point just beyond the threshold level, by testing with "make" and "break" stimuli.
3. Draw a baseline and start with subthreshold stimuli **(Fig. 26)**. Shift the secondary coil toward the primary, in steps of 3 cm, and pass "make" and "break" stimuli at each position of the coil. Record the responses, in pairs, at each position, after rotating the cylinder by hand, and noting the distance of the secondary coil until it slips over the primary coil.
4. With subthreshold stimuli, mark the point of stimulation *below* the baseline, otherwise it will be mistaken for a weak contraction, as shown in **Figure 26**.
5. Label the response "M" (for "make" stimulus) and "B" (for "break" stimulus), and the position of the secondary coil, in cm, under each pair of responses.

Note:

- One should wait for at least 15 seconds between make and break shocks. This is to avoid the beneficial effect.
- **Summation of effect in response to subminimal stimuli:** Move the secondary coil to just beyond the threshold position then rapidly switch the simple key ON and OFF a few times until the effects of these stimuli are summated and a contraction results. (This is not shown in **Figure 26**).

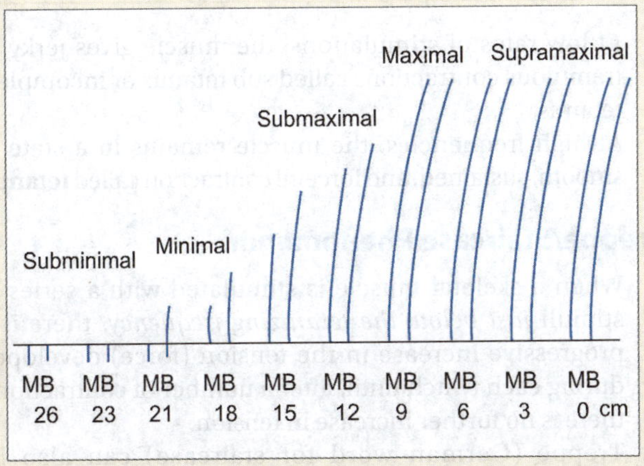

FIG. 26: Effect of increasing the strength of stimulus on the force of contraction of skeletal muscle. The points of stimulation of subthreshold stimuli are marked below the baseline. The first response appeared with a **break stimulus,** with the secondary coil 21 cm away from the primary coil.

Table 4: Measurement of amplitude of contractions and distance between primary and secondary coil in centimeter.

Sl. No.	*Distance between primary and secondary coil (in cm)*	*Amplitude of contraction (in cm)*
1.		
2.		
3.		
4.		
5.		
6.		

OBSERVATION AND RESULTS

Measure the amplitude of contractions in cm and note down the findings in **Table 4**.

PRECAUTIONS

1. The writing point should not be removed from the cylinder during the experiment, so that it presses on the paper with the same force each time a stimulus is applied.
2. The tilt of the cylinder should be so adjusted that the writing point remains in contact with the paper throughout its upward movement.

PHYSIOCLINICAL SIGNIFICANCE

The results of this experiment helps in understanding the gradation of muscle activity. Voluntary movements, which depend on the activity of many different efferent pathways (pyramidal and extrapyramidal) converging on the anterior horn cells, are very weak at times and very powerful at other times. This *gradation of muscular activity* is brought about in the following ways:

1. **Number of motor units in operation:** With minimum activity, only a few motor units are in action. With increasing effort, more and more motor units from the "motor neuron pool" of a muscle are recruited into activity, a phenomenon called *"multiple motor unit summation".*
2. **Frequency of nerve impulses:** Varying the frequency of muscle stimulation is the other major method used by the motor control system to vary the force of muscle contraction. As the impulse frequency increases, its effects are summated (wave summation), and the muscle tension increases. Though the sarcoplasmic Ca^{2+} concentration does not increase beyond a certain limit, the *duration of the active state* is increased due to the repetitive release of Ca^{2+} from the terminal cisterns.
3. **Synchronization of impulses:** Different motor units are, at any one time, in different phases of activity— some contracting and others relaxing; algebraic summation occurs and the muscle gives a steady but weak pull. With increasing synchronization, the force increases.
4. **Initial length of muscle fibers:** Up to an optimal limit, greater the initial length of muscle fibers (i.e. before they contract), greater is the force of contraction. This, however, is not the usual method of varying the force of contraction in the body.

5. **Warming up:** It is a complex mechanism, which increases muscle performance.

QUESTIONS

Q.1. What is a motor unit?

A single anterior horn cell, its axon and all its branches, and all the muscle fibers innervated by this neuron (alpha motor neuron) are called a *motor unit.*

Q.2. What are the different grades or degrees (in terms of strength) of stimuli?

Refer to chapter 4.2.

Q.3. Which stimulus is the threshold stimulus in your experiment?

- The "break"-induced shock with the secondary coil at 21 cm is the threshold stimulus, i.e. the minimum intensity of stimulation that would activate enough motor units to cause contraction of the muscle.
- It is also obvious that this stimulus is stronger than the "make"-induced shock for the reasons already discussed in chapter 4.2.

Q.4. Why does the force of contraction increase when the strength of stimuli, in the submaximal range, is gradually increased?

- The sciatic nerve contains motor fibers of varying excitability. Subthreshold stimuli fail to excite any, while a threshold stimulus excites a few motor units and the muscle gives a weak contraction.
- As the strength of the stimuli is increased, more and more fibers are recruited into activity and the force of contraction goes on increasing. This phenomenon is called *quantal* or *multifiber summation.*

Q.5. Why does the force of contraction not increase after the strength of stimulus is increased beyond the maximal level?

- A maximal stimulus is that which excites all the motor fibers, and therefore, all the motor units are already contracting to their maximum extent (all-or-none law; see below).
- As a result, any further increase in the strength of the stimuli (supramaximal stimuli) has no effect in increasing the force of contraction.

Q.6. What is "all-or-none" law? How is it applicable to excitable tissues?

- The *"all-or-none" law* (or "all-or-nothing") refers to the relationship between the *strength of a stimulus* and the *extent of response of a single unit* of excitable tissue *(unit tissue),* be it a *nerve fiber, a motor unit, a single skeletal muscle fiber,* or *the heart as a whole.*
- The law states that under the same experimental conditions, a "unit tissue" responds to its maximum possible extent (or does not respond at all, if the stimulus is subthreshold), whatever the strength of stimulus as long as it is at or above the threshold level. In the case of a nerve fiber, the height of action potential and its other features remain unchanged even when the strength of stimulus is increased.
- Similarly, a motor unit, a single skeletal muscle fiber, or the heart as a whole (because it is a functional syncytium) contracts maximally, if they respond at all; an increase in the strength of stimulus does not increase the force of contraction. However, the skeletal muscle as a whole does not obey the "all-or-none" law.
- The "all-or-none" law does not mean that the force of contraction of a unit muscle tissue cannot be increased in any way; the law only means that *this cannot be achieved by increasing the strength of stimulus.* For example, increase in the initial length of muscle fibers (called the "preload"), or increase in the frequency of stimulation increases their force of contraction (this does not go against the "all-or-none" law). Thus, the law applies to the strength of stimulus only.

Q.7. How is the force of muscle contraction graded (varied) in the intact body? How are skeletal muscles inhibited?

See text above (physioclinical significance)

4.9: GENESIS OF TETANUS

STUDENT OBJECTIVES

After completing this experiment, the student should be able to:

- Define treppe, clonus, incomplete, and complete tetanus.
- Calculate the tetanizing frequency.
- Differentiate between clinical and experimental tetanus.
- Enumerate the factors influencing the tetanizing frequency.

PY3.18: Observe with computer assisted learning (i) amphibian nerve - muscle experiments and (ii) amphibian cardiac experiments.

INTRODUCTION

- If instead of applying two successive stimuli (as was done in the last experiment), many successive stimuli are applied, the response of the muscle depends on the frequency of stimulation.
- At low rates of stimulations, the muscle gives jerky or tremulous contractions called sub tetanus or incomplete tetanus.
- At high frequencies, the muscle remains in a state of smooth, sustained, and forceful contraction called **tetanus.**

Treppe/Staircase Phenomenon

- When a skeletal muscle is stimulated with a series of stimuli *just below the tetanizing frequency,* there is a progressive increase in the tension (force) developed during each twitch until, after a number of contractions, there is no further increase in tension.
- Treppe (German word for staircase) can also be demonstrated in ***cardiac muscle,*** which, however, ***cannot be tetanized due to its refractoriness during the contraction phase.*** Treppe should not be confused with summation of contractions and tetanus.

Clonus

When repeated maximal stimulations are given and frequency is such that successive stimuli **fall in the mid relaxation phase** of the previous stimulus, the muscle relaxes but not completely. This response is called as clonus.

Tetanus

- It is defined as the continuous state of sustained contraction resulting from multiple successive stimuli.
- It results when multiple successive maximal stimuli are falling **during the contraction phase** due to the previous stimulus so that the activation of contractile mechanism occurs repeatedly before the muscle gets time to relax.
- It is a complete tetanus when there is a complete fusion of contractions without any relaxation in between. Here all the fibers contract maximally and the tension developed is approximately four times greater than that developed during individual twitch contraction.
- The tetanic contraction is said to be **incomplete** when the muscle fibers do not completely fuse but a partial relaxation is there in-between successive stimuli.

APPARATUS

1. Same as for simple muscle twitch (SMT)
2. Electromagnetic signal marker
3. Variable interrupter/Neef's hammer.

Speed of the drum: 12.5 mm/sec
Strength of stimuli: maximal

PROCEDURE

1. Exclude the drum from the primary circuit.
2. Include, in its place, either a vibrating reed or a variable interrupter to provide 5–25 stimuli/s, or the Neef's hammer to provide 40 or more stimuli/s, as required.
3. Engage the gear lever at 12.5 mm/s speed (medium speed).
4. Set up a nerve-muscle preparation and stimulate it with gradually increasing frequencies, *for a few seconds each time.*
5. Note the effects by gradually increasing the frequency of stimuli as 5, 10, 25 and 40 stimuli per second **(Figs. 27 to 29)**.
6. If a state of complete tetanus is not obtained by a variable interrupter, the Neef's hammer is used instead.
   - With such high rates (obtained with Neef's hammer), successive stimuli arrive before the muscle begins to relax, so that it remains in a state of sustained, smooth, and forceful contraction called tetanus.
   - The graph shows an increasing slope of the uninterrupted tracing, which exceeds the peaks of single twitches.
   - When the stimulation is stopped, the muscle relaxes immediately; but if it is continued, the plateau is

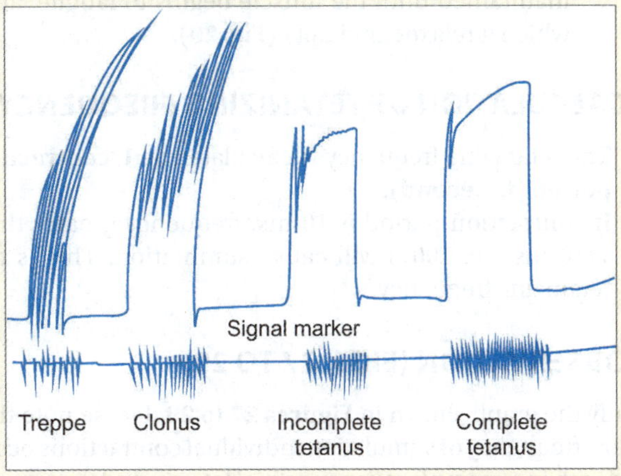

FIG. 27: Genesis of tetanus. The approximate rate of stimulation is indicated above each set of recordings. At lower rates, single contractions occur, while with increasing rates, incomplete tetanus and then tetanus (sustained contraction of the muscle) occur. Fatigue sets in, if tetanic stimulation is continued.

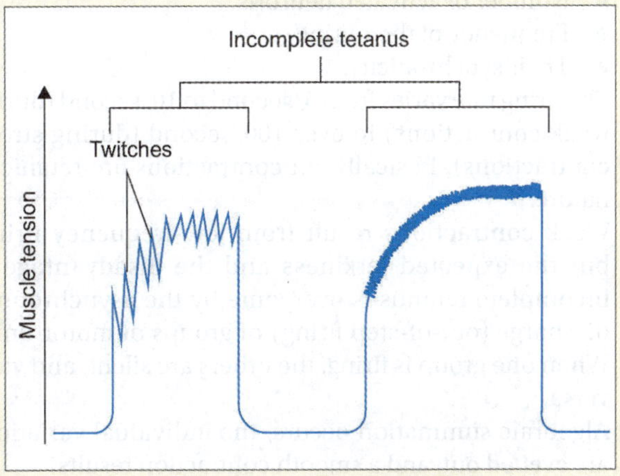

FIG. 28: Incomplete tetanus.

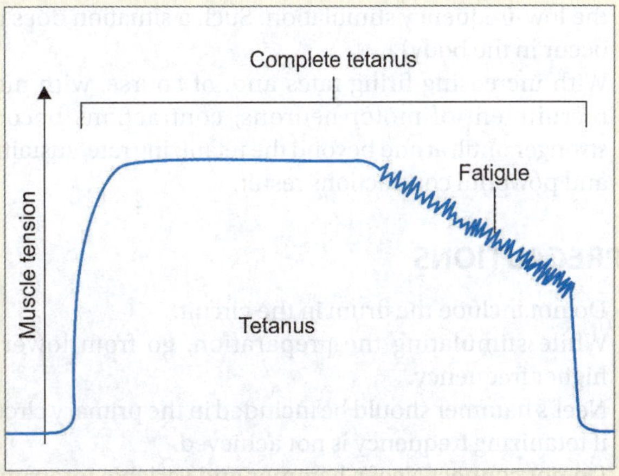

FIG. 29: Complete tetanus.

maintained until the muscle begins to fatigue, after which it relaxes gradually **(Fig. 29)**.

CALCULATION OF TETANIZING FREQUENCY

- The tetanizing frequency is calculated as **1/contraction period (in second)**.
- If contraction period is 10 ms, frequency greater than 1/10 ms, i.e. 100/s will cause summation. This is the tetanizing frequency.

OBSERVATION (FIGS. 27 TO 29)

Study the graph shown in **Figures 27 to 29**. Please note that at low frequency of stimulation individual contractions occur and with increasing frequency partial tetanus and the tetanus occur.

PHYSIOCLINICAL SIGNIFICANCE

- Voluntary and reflex movements depend on the *nature of discharge from the motor neurons* i.e.
  - Number of activated neurons
  - Frequency of their firing
  - Their synchronicity.
- The firing rate varies from 5/second to 10/second (during weak contractions) to over 100/second (during strong contractions). Basically, all contractions are tetanic in nature.
- Weak contractions result from low-frequency firing, but the expected jerkiness and the disadvantage of incomplete tetanus is overcome by the asynchronous discharge (out-of-step firing) of groups of motor units. When one group is firing, the others are silent, and vice-versa.
- Algebraic summation occurs, the individual variations are evened out, and a smooth contraction results.
- The degree, to which the motor neuron discharge is asynchronous, is related both to the force and duration of contraction. (In the sub-tetanus experiment, the muscle fibers contract and relax at the same time in response to the low-frequency stimulation. Such a situation does not occur in the body).
- With increasing firing rates and, of course, with more recruitment of motor neurons, contractions become stronger until, at and beyond the tetanizing rate, sustained and powerful contractions result.

PRECAUTIONS

1. Do not include the drum in the circuit.
2. While stimulating the preparation, go from lower to higher frequency.
3. Neef's hammer should be included in the primary circuit, if tetanizing frequency is not achieved.
4. Do not connect Neef's hammer and variable interrupter simultaneously into the primary circuit.

QUESTIONS

Q.1. What is "tetanizing" or "fusion" frequency?

- The *"tetanizing"* or *"fusion"* frequency is that rate of stimulation at which there is complete fusion of individual contractions to produce tetanus.
- In amphibian muscle and in "slow" muscle fibers, the tetanizing frequency is about 30/second, while in mammalian muscle and in "fast" fibers, it is 60 or more stimuli per second.

Q.2. What is "treppe" or "staircase effect"?

See text above.

Q.3. Why does a tetanically contracting muscle develop more tension than that developed during a single twitch?

- How much tension is *developed* by a muscle depends on the active state of the contractile components; and how much tension is *transmitted* to the recording system (or to the bone) depends on the amount of stretch (laxity or tautness) exerted on the series elastic components (SEC) of the muscle.
- During one twitch contraction, enough Ca^{2+} is released to engage all the myosin heads to the actin sites, but it is removed quickly from the cytoplasm and relaxation occurs. With repeated stimuli, Ca^{2+} remains longer in the cytoplasm, increasing the *duration of the active state* (due to continuous recycling of myosin heads).
- This increases the amount of stretch on the SEC and the tension developed rises. Up to a certain point, greater the frequency of stimulation, greater is the tension developed, the maximum being 3–4 times that of a twitch.

Q.4. What is meant by the term "genesis of tetanus"? Can you demonstrate tetanus in your body?

- The term refers to the "generation", or production, of tetanus by gradually increasing the frequency of stimulation of the nerve–muscle preparation until tetanus results.
- By definition, tetanus is a smooth and sustained contraction of a muscle, without reference to the frequency of stimulation. If you make a strong fist, your forearm muscles will contract tetanically.
- The term tetanus should not be confused with a disease called tetanus. In this condition, there are widespread convulsions in the body due to tetanus toxin released by the infecting bacteria. Vaccination is a common practice to provide immunity against this disease.

Q.5. What is the nature of muscle contractions in the body? Are they simple twitches, subtetanic, or tetanic contractions?

See Physioclinical Significance.

Q.6. How is tetanus different from tetany?

- Tetany is the condition of neuromuscular excitability, which occurs due to decrease in ionized Ca^{2+}, which in turn causes increased membrane permeability to Na.
- Skeletal muscle spasms and cramps are seen in the extremities.
- Tetanus is described above.

4.10: GENESIS OF FATIGUE

STUDENT OBJECTIVES

After completing this experiment, the student should be able to:

- Define fatigue, contracture, and contraction remainder.
- List the factors causing fatigue.
- Explain the mechanism of recovery from fatigue.
- Locate the site of fatigue in vitro.

PY3.18: Observe with computer assisted learning (i) amphibian nerve - muscle experiments and (ii) amphibian cardiac experiments.

INTRODUCTION

- Fatigue is defined as a physiological state of reduced mental or physical capability,
- ***Muscle fatigue*** is defined as a temporary decrease in maximal force or power production in response to contractile activity.
- When the muscle is stimulated repeatedly for a prolonged period of time, it loses its physiological property of contraction and there occurs a decrease in the working capacity.
- However, it regains its property of contraction after some time. It is a reversible phenomenon.
- Muscle fatigue can originate at different levels of the motor pathway and is usually divided into central and peripheral components.
  - Peripheral fatigue is produced by changes at or distal to the neuromuscular junction.
  - Central nervous system (CNS), which decreases the neural drive to the muscle.

Cause of fatigue:

1. Lack of nutrition
2. Accumulation of waste metabolites and interference with neuromuscular transmission by substances like pyruvic and lactic acids, and breakdown products of ATP.
3. Depletion of acetylcholine from the motor nerve endings.

APPARATUS

Same as in simple muscle twitch (SMT)
Speed of the drum: 640 mm/sec (fastest)
Strength of stimuli: maximal

PROCEDURE

1. Set up the apparatus and circuit as for the SMT. Draw a baseline and mark the point of stimulation. Record a single contraction and label it as "1".
2. Switch on the drum and at a speed of 640 mm/s and record the second and third contractions. Keep the point of stimulation the same.
3. Stop the drum and move the writing lever away from the drum taking care that the point of stimulation does not change.
4. Now record every 10th contraction by applying the writing lever to the drum. This should be done till the muscle contractions are too weak to be recorded **(Figs. 30A and B)**.

Note: This is done to prevent the overlap of responses.

5. Place the stimulating electrodes directly on the muscle and record the response keeping the baseline same on the clean portion of the paper. Label this contraction DS (direct stimulation) as shown in **Figure 30B**.
6. Rest the nerve muscle preparation for 5 minutes. During this time, keep pouring fresh Ringer's solution.
7. After changing the point of stimulus on the same baseline, stimulate the nerve and record the recovery of the muscle.

OBSERVATIONS

- Observe the change in amplitude and duration of the various phases of the first three contractions and the

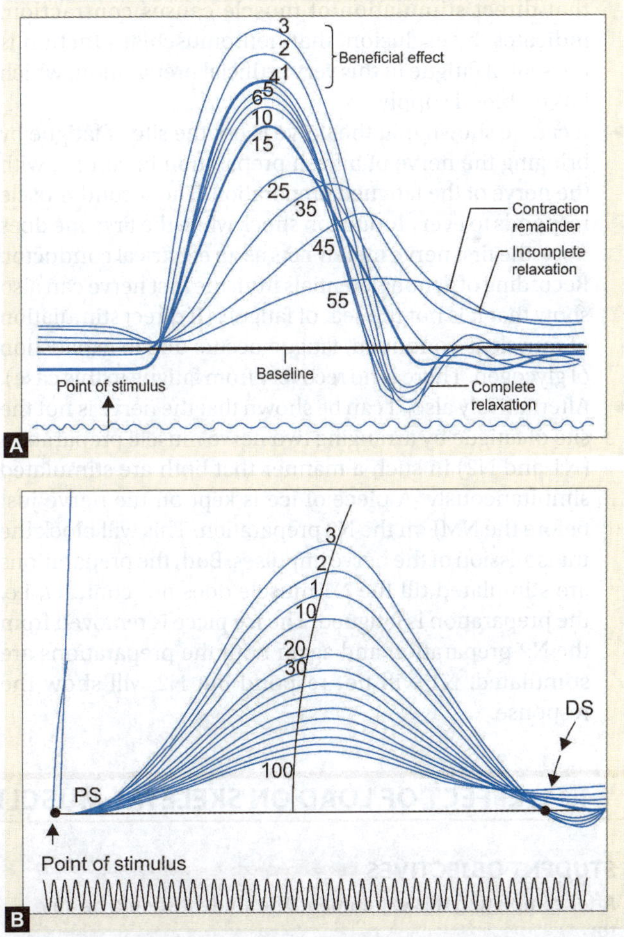

FIGS. 30A AND B: The phenomenon of fatigue. PS: point of stimulation. The record shows repeated contractions of the muscle through stimulation of its nerve. 1: First contraction, the following few contractions show beneficial effects. DS: direct stimulation of the muscle with electrodes placed on it.

following contractions. The first few contractions increase in amplitude due to ***beneficial effect***.

- As stimulation is continued, there is a progressive increase in latent period, and a decrease in amplitude. The rise of tension is slower, and relaxation is more gradual and incomplete.
- Finally, the muscle fails to contract altogether, and the lever does not return to the baseline, i.e. the muscle remains in a state of partial contraction called ***contraction remainder.***
- After the muscle undergoes fatigue through stimulation of its nerve, it responds briskly to direct stimulation. After a variable period, the muscle responds once again to stimulation of its nerve.

PHYSIOCLINICAL SIGNIFICANCE

- ***Site of fatigue:*** The only three possible sites are—
  - The nerve fibers,
  - The neuromuscular junctions
  - The muscle fibers.
- The fact that the nerve is practically unfatiguable, and that direct stimulation of muscle causes contraction, indicates, by exclusion, that neuromuscular junction is the seat of fatigue in this very artificial preparation, which has no blood supply.
- It can be shown that the nerve is not the site of fatigue by bringing the nerve of a fresh preparation in contact with the nerve of the fatigued preparation. The second muscle responds to every induction shock while the first one does not—the first nerve merely acts as an electrical conductor. Recording of action potentials from the first nerve can also show that it is not the seat of fatigue. (If direct stimulation of muscle is continued, fatigue occurs due to exhaustion of glycogen. There is no recovery from fatigue in this case).
- Alternatively also, it can be shown that the nerve is not the site of fatigue by arranging two nerve muscle preparation (N1 and N2) in such a manner that both are stimulated simultaneously. A piece of ice is kept on the nerve just before the NMJ on the N2 preparation. This will block the transmission of the nerve impulses. Both the preparations are stimulated till the N1 muscle does not contract, i.e. the preparation is fatigued. The ice piece is removed from the N2 preparation and again both the preparations are stimulated. N1 will not respond but N2 will show the response.
- ***Cause of fatigue*** is depletion of acetylcholine from the motor nerve endings and interference with neuromuscular transmission by substances like pyruvic and lactic acids, and breakdown products of ATP.

PRECAUTIONS

1. The point of stimulus and the baseline should remain unchanged for recording the fatigue curve.
2. For recording the effect of direct stimulation on the muscle, the baseline should remain the same but the point of stimulus should be changed.
3. Rest the preparation for 5 minutes and keep pouring fresh Ringer solution in order to record the response of the muscle after recovery.

QUESTIONS

Q.1. What is the site and cause of fatigue in the nerve–muscle preparation?

See Physioclinical Significance above.

Q.2. How is fatigue studied in man and what is its cause?

Fatigue in man is studied by using a *Mosso's ergograph* in which work is performed by a finger or thumb in lifting a weight.

Q.3. What is the contraction remainder and what is its cause?

- A delay in the relaxation period is an early sign of fatigue.
- When fatigue sets in, the muscle is unable to relax fully and remains in a state of partial contraction called *contraction remainder.*
- Since ATP, by removing Ca^{2+} ions from the cytoplasm, is responsible for relaxation, a decrease of ATP, and accumulation of metabolites appear to be responsible for the inability of all the myosin heads to disengage from the active sites on actin filaments (compare with Rigor mortis).

Q.4. What are the causes of recovery from fatigue?

1. Removal of waste metabolites
2. Supply of nutrition (fresh Ringer solution)
3. Resynthesis of acetylcholine helps in recovery from fatigue.

Q.5. What is the medical relevance of fatigue?

An athlete runs the initial part of the race slowly because speeding up in the initial part will lead to early setting of fatigue as anaerobic metabolism will lead to accumulation of lactic acid and waste metabolites.

4.11: EFFECT OF LOAD ON SKELETAL MUSCLE CONTRACTION (FREELOAD AND AFTERLOAD)

STUDENT OBJECTIVES

After completing this experiment, the student should be able to:

- Define preload and afterload.
- Calculate the work done in freeloading and afterloading conditions.
- Explain the physiological basis of change in force of contraction in freeloaded and afterloaded conditions.
- Physioclinical significance of this practical.
- Define Franks–Starling law and explain its physiological basis.

PY3.18: Observe with computer assisted learning (i) amphibian nerve - muscle experiments and (ii) amphibian cardiac experiments.

INTRODUCTION

- A load can act on a muscle either before it starts to contract **(freeloading/preload)** or after the contraction has started **(afterloading)**.
- Using successively increasing loads (weights), muscle contractions are recorded in these two conditions. The

work done by the muscle for each weight can then be calculated.

- Load at which maximum work is done is called **optimal load.**
- The performance of the muscle is measured in terms of work done during isotonic muscle contraction.

APPARATUS

Same as in SMT, and weights (10, 20, 30, 40, and 50 g).
Speed of the drum: Fastest/stationary
Strength of the stimulus: Minimal

PROCEDURE

Recording on a Moving Drum (Speed 640 mm/s)

1. Set up the experiment as for SMT. Draw a baseline and mark the point of stimulation. Put a weight hanger on the lever about an inch from the fulcrum.
2. **Afterloaded condition:**
   - Ensure that the afterload screw is in firm contact with, and supports, the vertical arm of the lever, so that the weight does not stretch the muscle. The weight here does not act on the muscle at rest but acts on it after the onset of muscle contraction. This is called the afterloaded condition.
   - Record a single contraction (with only the weight hanger) and label it 0 (no load).
   - Record the subsequent contractions with different weights (10, 20, 30...g); and label the curves, accordingly.
   - Repeat the procedure till the muscle is unable to lift the weight any more.
3. **Freeloaded condition (preload):**
   - Remove all the weights from the hanger, and withdraw the afterload screw right up to the frame of the lever, so that it will no longer support the vertical arm of the lever. The weight will now act freely on the muscle. This is a freeloaded condition.

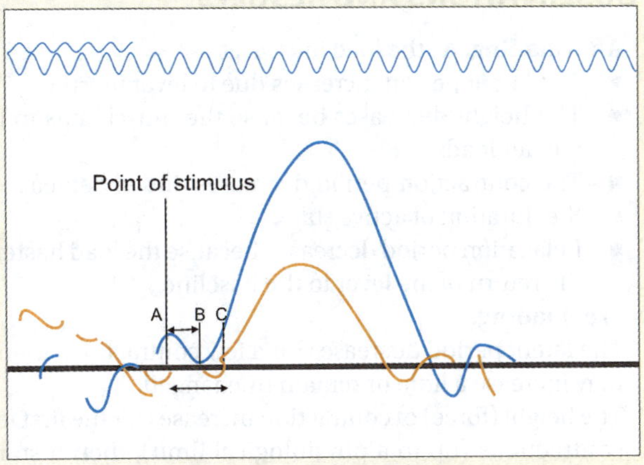

FIG. 31: Effect of load on muscle contraction on a moving drum.

- Record the first and subsequent contractions as explained above using different weights. Each time when more weight is added on the hanger, the lever sags down more and more, thus stretching the muscle more. The drum has to be lowered to bring the writing point to the same baseline.
- Repeat the procedure till the muscle is unable to lift the weight any more.

Note: On a moving drum, the free-and afterloaded contractions may be recorded separately on two locations on the paper, but on the same baseline, keeping the point of stimulus and strength of stimulus the same **(Fig. 31)**. One can record the height, the speed of shortening, and various periods of each contraction curve.

Recording on a Stationary Drum

- The freeloaded and afterloaded contractions can also be recorded on a stationary drum by rotating the cylinder forwards by hand through 2 cm after each increase of load, as shown in **Figures 32A and B**. In this case, only the height of contraction can be noted.
- Here also, the baseline shifts down more and more on adding subsequent weights in freeloaded condition.

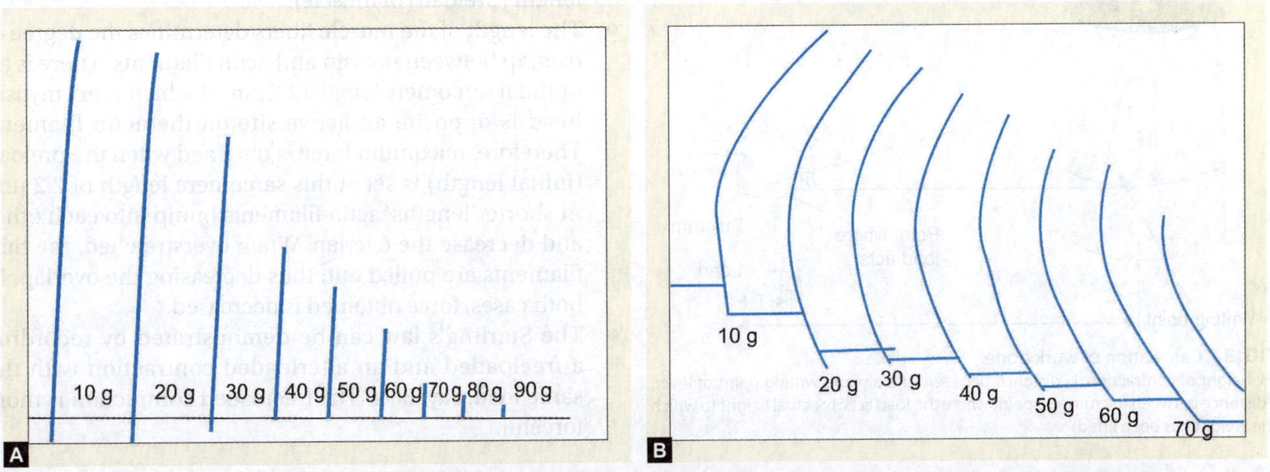

FIGS. 32A AND B: Effect of load and length on muscle contraction on a stationary drum. (A) Afterloading; (B) Freeloading.

OBSERVATIONS AND RESULTS

- **Afterloading:** As the load increases—
  - The latent period increases due to lever inertia.
  - The height decreases because the muscle has to lift greater loads.
  - The contraction period decreases due to decrease in the duration of active state.
  - Relaxation period decreases because the load hastens the return of the lever to the baseline.
- **Freeloading:**
- The latent period decreases for a few contractions then it may increase a little or remain unchanged.
- The height (force) of contraction increases for the first few contractions (up to a physiological limit), then it starts decreasing.
- The speed of contraction also increases as can be seen from the slope of the curve.
- Since the duration of the active state does not change, the contraction time does not change.
- The relaxation period decreases because the load hastens the return of the lever.

CALCULATION OF WORK DONE (FIG. 33)

- The following data are needed for calculation of the work done for each weight (load) in both freeloaded and afterloaded contractions.
- Work done = Force (W) × Displacement (h)
  W = Load lifted in g
  h = Actual height to which the weight has been lifted in cm.
  $$h = l/L \times H$$
  Where;
  l = Distance between the fulcrum and the point where the load acts
  L = Distance between the fulcrum and the writing point of lever
  H = Height of contraction curve for each load work done
- Therefore, (W) = Force (load) × l/L × H in gm cm
- Multiply with 981 to express the result in ergs.

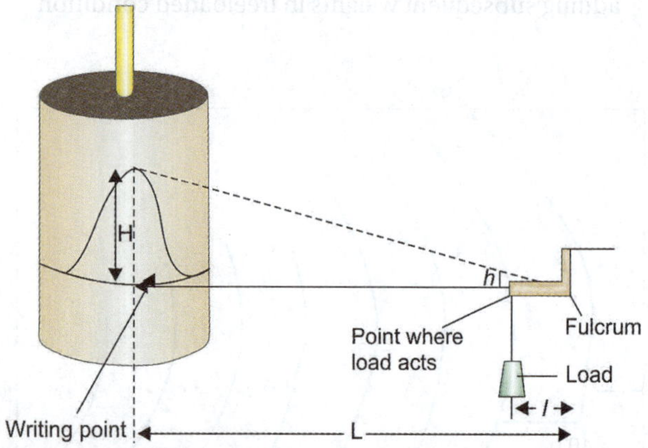

FIG. 33: Calculation of work done.
(H: height of contraction; L: distance between fulcrum and writing point of lever; l: distance between fulcrum and point where the load acts; h: actual height to which the weight has been lifted)

PHYSIOCLINICAL SIGNIFICANCE

- When some muscular work is done the muscles are slightly stretched in order to obtain maximum effect.
- Stretching and warm-up by athletes probably serve the same purpose.

See Q.2 and Q.4.

PRECAUTIONS

1. Same as for SMT.
2. Do not change the point of stimulus (for recording on a moving drum) and strength of stimulating current.

QUESTIONS

Q.1. What is meant by the terms "tension" and "load"?

See Q/A 4 and Experiment 4.4.

Q.2. Define resting length, initial length, equilibrium length and optimal length of a muscle.

- **Resting length:** The length of the muscle in the body at rest at which the active tension is maximum.
- **Initial length:** The length of the muscle just before the onset of contraction.
- **Equilibrium length:** Length of the relaxed muscle cut from its bony attachment.
- **Optimal length:** The length of a muscle at which the active tension is maximum.

Q.3. Why is the work done more in freeloaded condition than in an afterloaded condition?

The gradual stretching of the muscle during freeloading increases the initial length of the muscle fibers which increases its force of contraction and work efficiency.

Q.4. What is Starling's law and what is its basis? Can it be demonstrated in your experiment?

- Starling's **law** (or Frank-Starling law) states that "the force (or energy) of contraction, however measured, is a function of the initial length of the muscle fibers". Up to a physiological limit, *greater the initial length, greater is the force of contraction.* Though originally described for the heart, it is also applicable to the skeletal muscle. [In the case of the heart, the diastolic filling determines the initial length (preload) of muscle].
- The length of the muscle fibers determines the degree of overlap between myosin and actin filaments. There is an optimal sarcomere length (2.2 μm) at which every myosin head is opposite an active site on the actin filament. Therefore, maximum force is obtained when the preload (initial length) is set at this sarcomere length of 2.2 μm. At shorter lengths, actin filaments bump into each other and decrease the overlap. When overstretched, the thin filaments are pulled out, thus decreasing the overlap. In both cases, force obtained is decreased.
- The Starling's law can be demonstrated by recording a freeloaded and an afterloaded contraction with the same load, say, 30 g. The freeloaded contraction is more forceful.

Q.5 Do freeloaded and afterloaded contraction occur in the body?

Varying the preload (i.e. the initial length) is not an important method of varying the force of contraction of muscles because the muscle lengths generally depend on the type of motor activity being performed. But, if it is possible to stretch the muscles, more force can be obtained, as is done by weight lifters who allow the weight to stretch their muscles before they lift the weight with a sudden effort. Stretching and warm-ups by athletes probably serve the same purpose. Throwing a stone may be considered as associated with freeloading. Lifting an object from the ground involves afterloaded contractions.

Q.6. What is the physioclinical significance of this practical?

See Q.2 and Q.4.

Q.7. How would you ascertain whether a twitch has been recorded in the "afterloaded" or "freeloaded" condition?

- After the muscle twitch is over, a few waves or oscillations are recorded. These are not a part of muscle contraction, but a result of muscle elasticity and jerking of the lever due to its momentum. These waves are called physiological or shatter waves.
- If the muscle is in the afterloaded state, the shatter waves appear mainly above the baseline, but if it is freeloaded (or preloaded), the waves are recorded mainly below the baseline.

Q.8. Write the freeloaded and afterloaded conditions of cardiac muscle in vivo.

In vivo the end-diastolic volume represents the preload of the cardiac muscle and peripheral resistance constitutes the afterload.

4.12: RECORDING OF A NORMAL CARDIOGRAM OF FROG'S HEART AND EFFECT OF TEMPERATURE ON IT

STUDENT OBJECTIVES

After completing this experiment, the student should be able to:

- Record a normal cardiogram.
- Identify the different waves in a cardiogram.
- Describe the differences between amphibian and mammalian heart.
- Study the effect of cold and warm Ringer's solution on frog's heart.
- Discuss the physiological basis of the effect of cold and warm Ringer's solution on frog's heart.
- Describe the physioclinical importance of the experiment.

PY3.18: Observe with computer assisted learning (i) amphibian nerve - muscle experiments and (ii) amphibian cardiac experiments.

INTRODUCTION

- The frog's heart consists of two atria and one ventricle. **Sinus venosus** is the pacemaker of frog's heart and the impulse travels from sinus venosus to the atria and then to the ventricles.
- Electrical events in the heart precede the mechanical contractions.
- The different **mechanical events** recorded are atrial systole, atrial diastole, ventricular systole followed by ventricular diastole.
- The recording obtained of the various mechanical events of the frog's heart is known as the **Cardiogram.**

EXPOSURE OF THE FROG'S HEART

1. Stun and pith a frog and lay it on its back in a dissection tray. Using a scissors, incise the skin in the midline from xiphisternum to the jaw. Extend the lower end of this cut laterally and remove both pieces of skin. The anterior chest wall is now exposed.
2. Give a horizontal cut in the muscles at the level of xiphisternum (do not cut through the abdominal wall, otherwise the viscera will spill out). Using bone forceps and scissors, cut through the pectoral girdles and remove the chest wall in one piece. The heart will now be revealed beating in its pericardial sac. Note its size. Slit through the pericardium and remove it right up to the base of the heart. The size of the heart will be seen to increase.
3. Examine the heart carefully and note that it differs structurally from the mammalian heart **(Fig. 34)**.
   - There is **one ventricle,** separated from the **two atria** by the atrioventricular groove, and the **bulbus arteriosus,** which arises from the ventricle and divides into two aortae. Lift the ventricle up and find behind it the **sinus venosus** with the two venae cavae emptying into it.
   - A careful observation will reveal the **white crescentic line** between the sinus and the right atrium. This is the site of the Remak's and Bidder's ganglia of the vagus nerves.

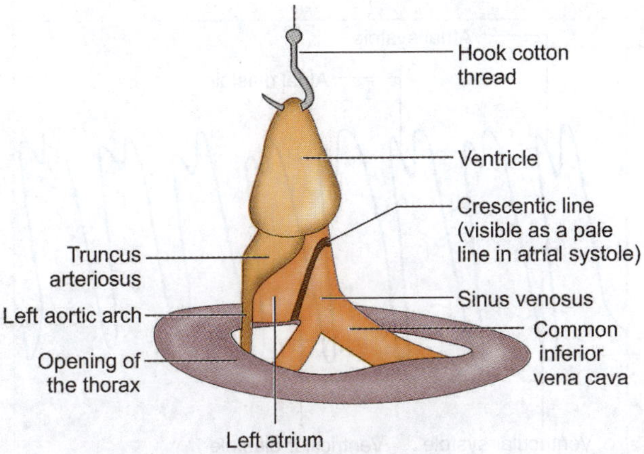

FIG. 34: Frog's heart.

- The color of the ventricle becomes pale during systole as blood is forced out of it. Feel the hardening of the ventricle when it contracts. There are no valves in the frog's heart.
- **Sequence of heartbeats:** The contractions of the **four units** of the heart are progressive. The sinus leads off, followed by the atria, ventricle, and the bulbus, in that order. The rate of the heart depends on the frequency of the sinus, as it is the pacemaker. Pour cold Ringer on the heart to slow it down in order to appreciate the pauses between the contractions of the cardiac chambers.

NORMAL CARDIOGRAM

The cardiogram is a record of the mechanical activity of the heart, while electrocardiogram is a record of the electrical activity of the heart. In this and the following experiments, the mechanical events of the heart will be recorded with a Starling's heart lever **(Fig. 35)**.

APPARATUS

1. Myograph board
2. Lucas chamber
3. Dissection apparatus
4. Amphibian Ringer's solution (cold and warm)
5. Kymograph with drum
6. Starling's heart lever
7. Time/signal marker
8. Dropper, thread, cotton wool and pins.

Speed of the drum: 2.5 mm/sec

PROCEDURE

1. Transfer the frog to the frog board or trough. Fit the Starling heart lever on the vertical rod of the stand directly above the heart, and pass the sharp hook of the bent pin through the apex of the ventricle, taking care not to puncture its cavity.
2. Lift the heart gently by raising the lever, and adjust its position, so that its movements are satisfactory, and its mean position is horizontal. Note that during systole, the lever is pulled down, while during diastole the spring of the lever pulls it back to its former position.
3. Move the stand carrying the preparation and the lever, so that the lever is at a tangent to the cylinder, and the writing point is lightly touching the cylinder surface. Record the cardiac activity for about 15 cm on the paper, with the drum moving at a speed of 2.5 mm/s.
4. Record a time tracking of 5 seconds with the time signal marker below the graph obtained. Compare your graph with that shown in **Figure 36**, and note how many peaks have been recorded. Note the rhythm of the heart, and calculate the rate of the heart (the frog's heart rate varies from 30 per minute to 50 per minute, depending on the atmospheric temperature).
5. Pour Ringer at room temperature on the heart to keep it moist; note the temperature of the Ringer. With the drum running at slow speed, pour Ringer solution warmed to about 40°C on the heart, drop-by-drop, until there is an obvious increase in its rate and force.
6. Stop the kymograph, and pour Ringer at room temperature on the heart till it resumes the previous rate and force. Then record the effect of cold Ringer at about 10°C in the same manner.
7. Record a 5-second time tracking below the graph obtained. Label your tracking, indicating with arrows, the points where hot and cold Ringer was applied. Calculate the heart rate at these temperatures and enter the data in your workbook.

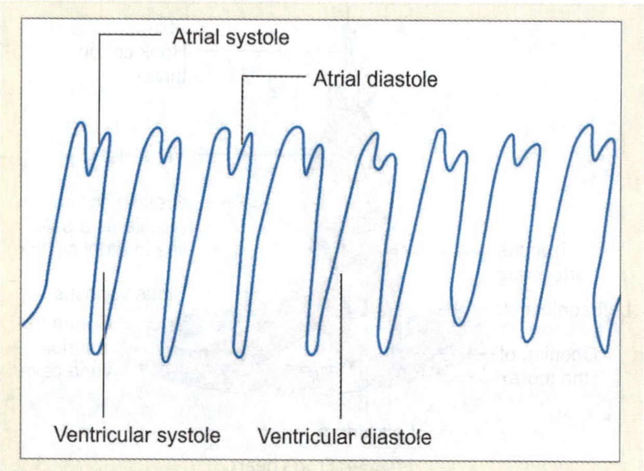

FIG. 35: Normal cardiogram.

Note:
- During systole, the lever is pulled down, while during diastole the spring of the lever pulled up to its former position.
- Normal heart rate of frog varies from 30/minute to 50/minute

OBSERVATIONS

Effect of Temperature on Frog's Cardiogram

- **At high temperature:**
  - There is an increase in the metabolic activity of the pacemaker cells, which generates more cardiac impulses per unit time (due to increase in the slope of phase 4 of the AP), thus increasing the **heart rate and height of contraction.**

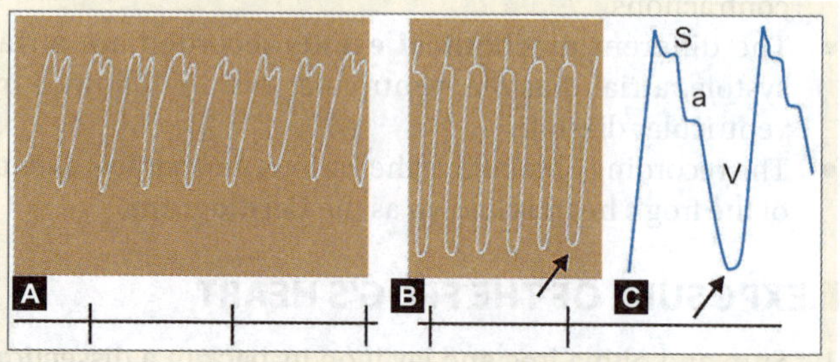

FIGS. 36A TO C: Record of spontaneously beating heart of frog. (A) In this only the atrial and ventricular events are seen; (B) In this trace, recorded from another frog, contractions of sinus (S), atria (a) and ventricle (v), followed by relaxations, can be seen as shown in the diagram; (C) Contraction of truncus arteriosus occurs just before the beginning of ventricular diastole (arrow).

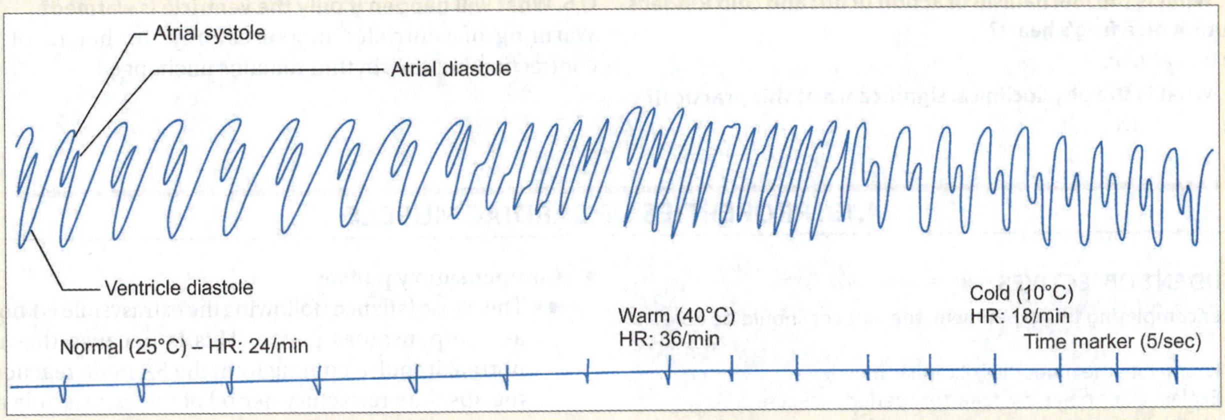

FIG. 37: Effect of temperature on cardiogram.

- Increased metabolic activity of the working cells of the atria and ventricle and decrease in the viscosity increases the **force of contraction**.
- Tachycardia due to fever is due to the effect of high temperature on the sinoatrial (SA) node, which is the pacemaker **(Fig. 37)**.
- **Cold** has the opposite effects due to decrease in metabolic activity.

Recording of effect of temperature on frog's cardiogram

	Heart rate (beats/min)	*Height of contraction (cm)*
Normal (°C)		
Warm Ringer's solution (...°C)		
Cold Ringer's solution (...°C)		

PHYSIOCLINICAL SIGNIFICANCE

- This practical shows that heart rate changes in the human body with change in internal body temperature, e.g. exercise, fever, and hypothermia.

PRECAUTIONS

1. Care should be taken not to damage the heart during dissection.
2. Pericardium should be removed before fixing the heart on the myograph board.
3. Record the normal cardiogram before recording the effect of warm and cold Ringer's solution.
4. The temperature of warm Ringer's should not be more than 42°C.
5. Effect of warm Ringer's should be recorded before the effect of cold Ringer's solution.
6. Do not puncture the ventricle while passing the pin through its apex.

QUESTIONS

Q.1. Why is frog's heart used for the study of properties of the heart?

- The frog heart is a convenient preparation because it will continue to beat after the chest is opened. It obtains an adequate supply of oxygen directly from the blood in its chambers and from the atmosphere (it has no coronary circulation). Its rate is sufficiently slow to allow observation of its sequence.
- Also, it continues to function over a wide range of temperatures. The properties, which can be studied, include excitability, automaticity, rhythmicity, contractility, conductivity, refractoriness, and all-or-none law.

Q.2. Describe the graph obtained by you.

- The downstroke of the tracing represents systole, and the upstroke diastole.
- There is atrial systole followed by atrial diastole, then ventricular systole (this is the strongest of the four contracting units) is followed by diastole (contraction of sinus may also be recorded).
- The heart rate is beats/min and the rhythm is regular.

Q.3. What is the cause of the heartbeat in the frog's heart? Can it continue to beat outside the body?

- The cause of the heartbeat lies within the heart itself, i.e. in the pacemaker, which lies within the wall of the sinus venosus.
- The pacemaker spontaneously and rhythmically generates action potentials (cardiac impulses), which pass quickly to atria, ventricle, and bulbus from muscle cell to muscle cell. There is no definite fibrous ring between the atria and the ventricle. The muscle fibers in this region run circularly around the heart and not directly from atria to ventricle. This may account for the normal delay between the atria and the ventricle.
- There is no impulse generating and conducting system such as that found in the mammalian heart.
- When removed from the frog's body and kept in Ringer placed in a petri dish, the heart will continue to beat. If the sinus, atria, and the ventricle are cut and separated from each other, each unit, in due course, will be seen to beat at its own inherent rate, the sinus rate being the fastest, and ventricle slowest (idioventricular rhythm) (heart transplantation is a life-saving procedure as the heart continues to beat in the recipient's body. But since there is no nerve supply, the heart rate cannot increase much during exercise).

Q.4. What is the mechanism of action of hot and cold Ringer's solution on a frog's heart?
See text above.

Q.5. What is the physioclinical significance of this practical?
See text above

Q.6. What will happen if only the ventricle is warmed?
Warming of ventricles increases only the height of the contraction but the rhythm remains unchanged.

4.13: PROPERTIES OF CARDIAC MUSCLE

STUDENT OBJECTIVES

After completing this experiment, the student should be able to:
- Enumerate the properties of cardiac muscle.
- Explain all-or-none law, refractory period, staircase phenomenon, extrasystole and compensatory pause.
- Explain the physiological basis of the various properties of cardiac muscle.
- Discuss why the cardiac muscle cannot be tetanized.

PY3.18: Observe with computer assisted learning (i) amphibian nerve - muscle experiments and (ii) amphibian cardiac experiments.

INTRODUCTION

The properties of cardiac muscle are:
a. Autorhythmicity
b. Extrasystole and compensatory pause
c. Refractory period
d. Summation of subminimal stimuli
e. All-or-none law
f. Staircase phenomenon.

The following properties can be studied in a **beating heart.**
a. Autorhythmicity
b. Extrasystole and compensatory pause
c. Refractory period.

The following properties can be studied in a **quiescent heart.**
a. All-or-none law
b. Staircase phenomenon
c. Summation of subminimal stimuli.

APPARATUS

1. Same as in recording of normal cardiogram
2. Induction coil
3. Wire electrodes and signal marker.

Speed of the drum: 2.5 mm/sec (Slow)

PROPERTIES IN A BEATING HEART (FIG. 38A)

- **Extrasystole:**
  - When the heart is stimulated [by an impulse other than that originates from the sinoatrial (SA) node] during late diastole (relative refractory period), the heart muscle may contract.
  - This contraction comes earlier than the normally expected contraction. This is called extrasystole.
- **Compensatory pause:**
  - The pause (silence) following the extrasystole is known as compensatory pause. This is because the next normal impulse coming from the SA node reaches in the absolute refractory period of the extrasystole and hence fails to evoke a response.
  - The response which follows the compensatory pause is of greater magnitude than the previous one because of the accumulation of calcium ions during the pause.
- **Refractory period:**
  - The cardiac muscle has a long refractory period. This is because the action potential of cardiac muscle has a long duration of about 300 ms.
  - During much of the action potential (about 250 ms), the cell is completely refractory to further stimulation, i.e. it is unable to fire no matter how strongly it is stimulated. This unresponsive state is called an absolute ***refractory period.***
  - During the latter part of action potential (about 50 ms), the cell is able to fire a second action potential provided a stronger than normal stimulus is given. This period is called the relative ***refractory period.***
  - The cardiac muscle action potential duration is almost equal to the duration of mechanical activity. Therefore, the mechanical responses of cardiac muscle cannot be **summated or tetanized.**

PROCEDURE

1. Set up the experiment as for recording a normal cardiogram.
2. Apply electrodes on the ventricle of the heart.
3. The distance between primary and secondary coil is so adjusted that a minimal stimulus is obtained.
4. Use the electromagnetic signal marker to indicate the application of stimulus.
5. A few normal beats are recorded.
6. A "break" shock is applied by opening the short circuiting key and thereafter the primary key.
7. Stimulate the ventricle during the different phases of the cardiac cycle, i.e. systole, early and late diastole and record the effects **(Fig. 39).**
8. The graph is labeled properly to show the systole and diastole in the cardiogram, point of application of extra stimulus, extrasystole and compensatory pause. A time tracking is also taken.

This experiment also shows the properties of **excitability, contractility, autorhythmicity and conductivity**

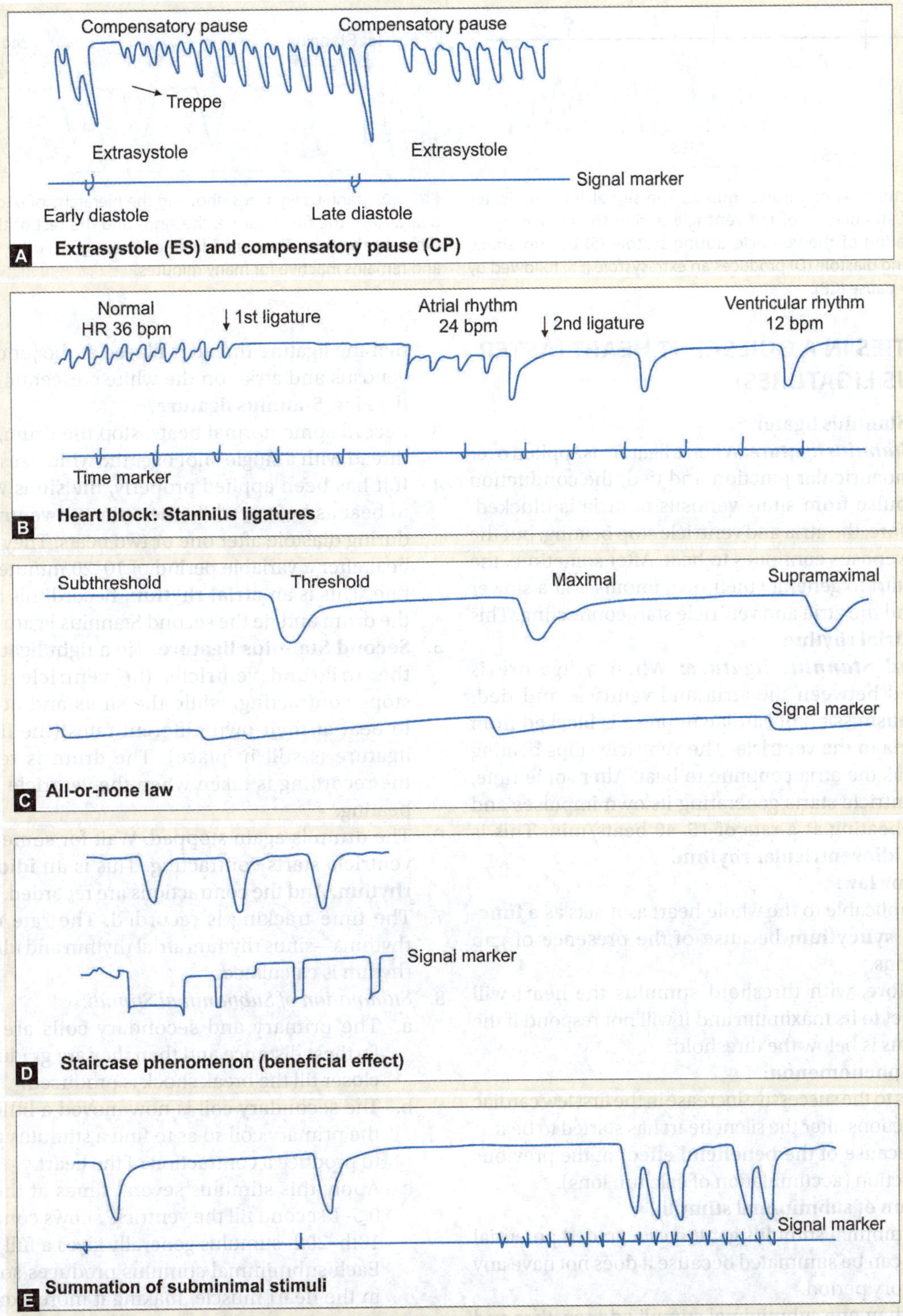

FIGS. 38A TO E: (A) Extrasystole and compensatory pause; (B) Effect of Stannius ligatures; (C) All-or-none law; (D) Staircase phenomenon (beneficial effect); (E) Summation of subminimal stimuli.
(HR: heart rate; bpm: beats per minute).

(stimulation of any part causes contraction of the rest of the heart).

Note: When the stimulus falls during any part of systole, it has no effect the heart continues to beat as before. But when the stimulus falls during diastole, the heart contracts immediately. This extra contraction is called **extrasystole or premature beat,** followed by a pause called a **"compensatory pause"**. Duration of normal contraction, the extrasystole and compensatory pause is equal to two normal cardiac cycles.

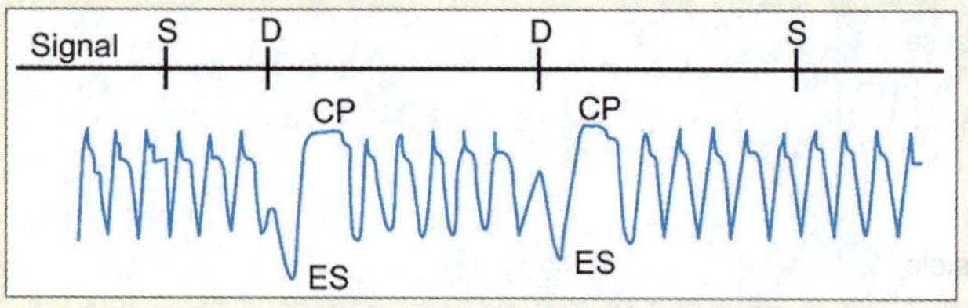

FIG. 39: Refractoriness of cardiac muscle. The signal trace indicates the moment of stimulation of the ventricle during the cardiac cycle. Outside stimulation of the ventricle during systole (S) has no effect; stimulation during diastole (D) produces an extrasystole (ES) followed by a compensatory pause (CP).

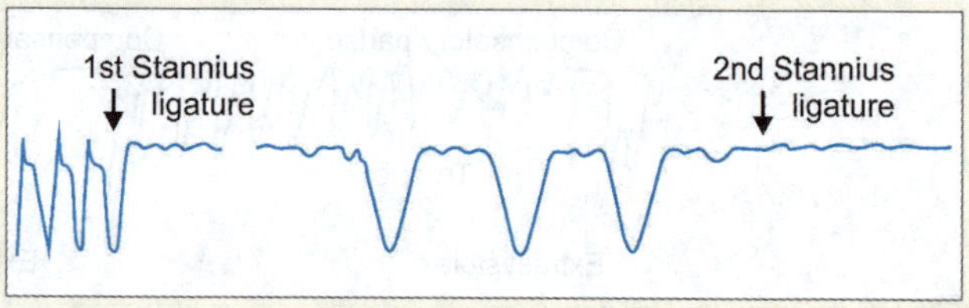

FIG. 40: Stannius ligatures, showing the hierarchy of pacemaking in the heart. After the first ligature, the sinus and the rest of the heartbeat at different rhythms. The ventricle stops beating after the second ligature and remains inactive for many minutes.

PROPERTIES IN A QUIESCENT HEART (AFTER STANNIUS LIGATURES)

- **Effect of Stannius ligature:**
  - ***First Stannius ligature:*** When a ligature is applied over the sinoauricular junction and tied, the conduction of impulse from sinus venosus to atria is blocked. Therefore, the atria and ventricle stop beating, but the sinus venosus continues to beat. After sometime, the atria start to generate their own impulses at a slower rate and the atria and ventricle start contracting. This is an **atrial rhythm**.
  - ***Second Stannius ligature:*** When a ligature is applied between the atria and ventricle and tied, the transmission of cardiac impulse is blocked from the atria to the ventricle. The ventricle stops beating whereas the atria continue to beat. After some time, the ventricle starts generating its own impulses and starts beating at a rate of 15–40 beats/min. This is called **idioventricular rhythm.**
- **All-or-none law:**
  - It is applicable to the whole heart as it acts as a **functional syncytium** because of the presence of gap junctions.
  - Therefore, with threshold stimulus the heart will contract to its maximum and it will not respond if the stimulus is below the threshold.
- **Staircase phenomenon:**
  - It refers to the successive increase in the first few cardiac contractions after the silent heart has started to beat.
  - It is because of the **beneficial effect** of the previous contraction (accumulation of calcium ions).
- **Summation of subminimal stimuli:**
  - A subminimal stimulus generates a graded potential which can be summated because it does not have any refractory period.
  - More than one subminimal stimuli add together and may take the membrane potential to the firing level so as to generate an action potential.

PROCEDURE

Effect of Stannius Ligature (Figs. 38B to E and 40)

1. Set up the experiment as for recording a normal cardiogram.
2. Pass a ligature thread under the truncus arteriosus and the atria, bring its ends to the dorsum of the heart. Ensure that the ligature thread is placed at the junction of sinus venosus and atria (on the white crescentic line). This is the **First Stannius ligature**.
3. Record some normal beats, stop the drum, then tie the thread with a single knot over the white crescentic line.
4. If it has been applied properly, the sinus will continue to beat as before, while the atria and ventricle will stop during diastole after one or two beats. They will begin to beat after a variable period of 10–20 minutes at a slower rate. This is an **atrial rhythm.** Record this activity. Stop the drum and tie the second Stannius ligature.
5. **Second Stannius ligature:** Tie a tight ligature between the atria and ventricle, the ventricle immediately stops contracting, while the sinus and atria continue to beat at their own different rates (the first Stannius ligature is still in place). The drum is restarted and the recording is taken when the ventricle has stopped beating.
6. The drum is again stopped. Wait for some time till the ventricle starts contracting. This is an **idioventricular rhythm.** And the contractions are recorded.
7. The time tracking is recorded. The rate of the three rhythms—sinus rhythm, atrial rhythm and idioventricular rhythm is calculated.
8. *Summation of Subminimal Stimuli:*
   a. The primary and secondary coils are kept at the farthest distance and then they are gradually brought closer till the break shock is produced.
   b. The secondary coil is now moved a little away from the primary coil so as to find a stimulus that just fails to produce a contraction of the heart.
   c. Apply this stimulus several times at the interval of 0.5–1 second till the ventricle shows contraction. The 10th–20th stimulus generally gives a full contraction. Each subminimal stimulus produces some changes in the heart muscle, making it more excitable to the successive stimulus. Once the summation of potential changes induced by subminimal stimuli reaches to threshold, the ventricle contracts.
9. *All-or-none Law*:
   a. Starting with subthreshold stimuli, gradually increase the strength of stimuli until there is a contraction (threshold response).
   b. Continue to apply a single stimulus of increasing strength, allowing at least 30 second intervals between each response.

c. Note that though the strength of each stimulus is successively increased but the force of contraction remains the same.

10. *Staircase Effect:*
   a. Three to four **threshold** stimuli are given one after the other at an interval of 2–3 seconds, so that a new contraction occurs immediately after the previous relaxation is over.
   b. Note the successive increase in the force of contraction of the ventricle due to **beneficial effect.**

PRECAUTIONS

1. To study the phenomena of extrasystole and compensatory pause, the stimulus has to be applied during late diastole.
2. To study the staircase phenomenon, the ventricle should be stimulated repeatedly after every 2 seconds.
3. For studying the summation of effects due to repeated subminimal stimuli, the stimuli (subthreshold) should be applied repeatedly after 0.5–1 seconds.

PHYSIOCLINICAL SIGNIFICANCE

A. **Extrasystole:** Extrasystoles are commonly seen in medical practice. The common causes are:
   1. **Physiological causes**
      a. Smoking
      b. Excessive intake of tea or coffee
      c. Anxiety
      d. Lack of sleep.
   2. **Pathological causes**
      a. Hyperthyroidism
      b. Hypoxia
      c. Electrolytes imbalance
      d. Myocardial damage
      e. Digitalis overdose, etc.
   - Some ectopic foci (from other than the normal site) in the atria or the ventricles generate an impulse, which causes an extrasystole (premature beat). About **2–4 extrasystole/minute** are considered normal in humans. If the frequency of extrasystoles is >6/min, that may indicate some **pathological condition.**

B. **Heart block:** Whenever there is a stoppage of impulse transmission from atria to ventricle, it is called heart block. Three degrees of heart block can occur in humans (I, II and III degree).

QUESTIONS

Q.1. What is the cause of compensatory pause after an extrasystole?
During the extrasystole, when the usual cardiac impulse from the pacemaker reaches the ventricle, it finds that it is already contracting (due to extrasystole) and in the absolute refractory period (ARP), so it has no effect. The ventricle has, therefore, to wait for the next impulse from the sinus to arrive before it can contract—hence the brief pause.

Q.2. What is "postextrasystolic potentiation"?
The first contraction after the compensatory pause is often more forceful than the usual heartbeat. This is due to increased availability of intracellular calcium.

Q.3. Do extrasystoles occur in humans? What is the normal frequency of extrasystole?
See text above.

Q.4. How will you differentiate between atrial and ventricular extrasystole?
Atrial and ventricular extrasystole can be distinguished with the help of an electrocardiogram (ECG).

Q.5. What is the cause of the long refractory period of the cardiac muscle? What is its advantage?
See text above.

Q.6. What is all-or-none law? Which tissues obey this law? Are all-or-none law and the Starling's law of the heart incompatible?
For the all-or-none law to be applicable, all the experimental conditions are to be kept constant. This doesn't happen in Starling's law of the heart where the initial length of cardiac muscle changes resulting in increased force of contraction.

Q.7. What is the staircase phenomenon and what is its physiological basis?
See text above.

Q.8. To demonstrate the all-or-none law phenomenon, why should the interval between the stimuli be 30 seconds?
This will prevent summation of stimuli or beneficial effect.

Q.9. With the help of a diagram describe the properties of the cardiac muscle of a frog.
See text above.

Q.10. Why cannot Stannius ligatures be employed in mammalian heart?
The Stannius ligatures cannot be employed in mammalian hearts because they would cut off the blood flow through the coronary arteries, thus depriving the musculature of oxygen and other nutrients. When the blood supply is shut off, the muscle soon undergoes necrosis (death).

4.14: EFFECT OF STIMULATION OF VAGOSYMPATHETIC TRUNK AND WHITE CRESCENTIC LINE; VAGAL ESCAPE; EFFECT OF NICOTINE AND ATROPINE ON FROG'S HEART

STUDENT OBJECTIVES

After completing this experiment, the student should be able to:

- Identify the vagosympathetic trunk.
- Explain the physiological basis of the effect of vagal stimulation on the heart.
- Demonstrate and explain the phenomenon of vagal inhibition and vagal escape.
- Identify the white crescentic line (WCL) in a frog's heart.
- Demonstrate and explain the effect of stimulation of WCL.
- Demonstrate the effect of nicotine and atropine.
- Explain the physiological basis of action of atropine and nicotine.

PY3.18: Observe with computer assisted learning (i) amphibian nerve - muscle experiments and (ii) amphibian cardiac experiments.

INTRODUCTION

- The vagosympathetic trunk contains preganglionic parasympathetic nerve fibers, and postganglionic sympathetic fibers (in mammals the two systems run separately), but there are many more vagal fibers than sympathetic. Therefore, *vagal effects usually predominate.*
- As in other locations, parasympathetic ganglia (where preganglionic fibers end and synapse on the postganglionic neurons) are situated in or near the organs supplied by this system. The ganglia, called Bidder's and Remak's, are situated in the crescentic area.
- The inhibitory effects of vagal and crescent stimulation are due to release of acetylcholine, which increases cardiac cell permeability to K^+ ions, as described in the last experiment.
- The stimulation of vagal fibers decreases heart rate and conduction, but it has no effect on ventricular contraction.
- The **white crescentic line** is formed by the postganglionic parasympathetic neurons located at the junction between sinus venosus and atria. Stimulation of WCL will have the same effect as the stimulation of vagal fibers.
- **Atropine:**
  a. It is a parasympatholytic agent.
  b. It blocks the action of ACh on the muscarinic receptors.
  c. When applied on the heart after ACh, it has no effect, but when applied before ACh, atropine blocks the inhibitory action of ACh.
- **Nicotine:**
  a. It acts through the nicotinic cholinergic receptors which are present in the neuromuscular end plates and in the peripheral autonomic ganglia.
  b. When applied to the frog's heart it acts on the parasympathetic ganglia located on the white crescentic line.
  c. ***In low concentrations***, nicotine stimulates the postganglionic parasympathetic fibers causing bradycardia.
  d. ***In high concentrations*** nicotine blocks the ganglia **by causing persistent depolarization**

APPARATUS

1. Same as in properties of cardiac muscle
2. Atropine 0.5%, Nicotine 0.5%
3. Stimulating electrodes
4. Signal marker.

PROCEDURE

1. **Exposure of vagosympathetic trunk:**
   - Expose the heart as before. Identify the narrow strip of petrohyoid muscle, which runs from the base of the skull to the hyoid bone, as it crosses a very shiny tendon.
   - Lift up the lower border of the muscle and you will find the vagosympathetic trunk and carotid vessels crossing the shiny tendon.
   - Expose the other trunk also. Put loose ligatures around them, so that they can be lifted up for stimulation.
   - Include the Neef's hammer (for repeated stimuli) and an event marker in the primary circuit.
2. **Stimulation of vagosympathetic trunk:** Record a few normal beats then stimulate the vagosympathetic trunk for 4–5 seconds with the help of Neef's Hammer. Note the stoppage of the heart during diastole **(Figs. 41A to C).** This is **vagal inhibition.**
3. **Stimulation of white crescentic line (WCL):** After normal beats are restored, stimulate the WCL for a few seconds and note cardiac inhibition as above. Repeat steps 2 and 3 on the other side.
4. **Vagal escape:** Stimulate the vagus once again, but continue the stimulation until the heart starts to beat again, i.e. it escapes the vagal effect. Test the other side as well.
5. **Nicotine:** After normal beats are restored, pour a few drops of nicotine solution on the heart. Note that there is no effect. Now perform the following experiments:
   - Stimulate the vagosympathetic trunk—there is no inhibition of the heart.
   - Stimulate the crescentic line—the heart is inhibited, as shown in **Figure 41C.**
6. **Atropine:** Wash the heart with Ringer. When normal beats are restored, pour atropine on the heart. Note that there is no effect on the heart. Now perform the following experiments:
   - Stimulate the vagosympathetic trunk—the heart is not inhibited **(Fig. 41C).**
   - Stimulate the WCL—the heart is not inhibited.

PHYSIOCLINICAL SIGNIFICANCE

- Unlike the amphibian heart, the vagal and sympathetic fibers are separate in human beings, therefore, only parasympathetic effects are seen on stimulating the vagus. On continuous stimulation of the vagus, there results vagal escape (mainly due to **idioventricular rhythm**) **(Figs. 42 and 43).**
- **Vagal tone** is the tonic inhibitory influence of the vagus on the human heart. When the heart is denervated (sympathetic and parasympathetic supply are cut) the intrinsic heart rate is 100–120/min, whereas the normal heart rate in humans is 60–100/min. This reduction in the heart rate is due to vagal tone.
- **Vagal escape:** When the vagus (it supplies the ventricle in amphibia) is stimulated, the heart at first stops, but as the stimulation is continued, the heart escapes from this inhibitory effect and starts to beat once again—a phenomenon called vagal escape. The following factors are involved:
  - ***Idioventricular rhythm:*** Due to prolonged inhibition, a new rhythm center in the ventricle causes it to start beating, though at a slower rate of about 15/min **(Fig. 41B).**

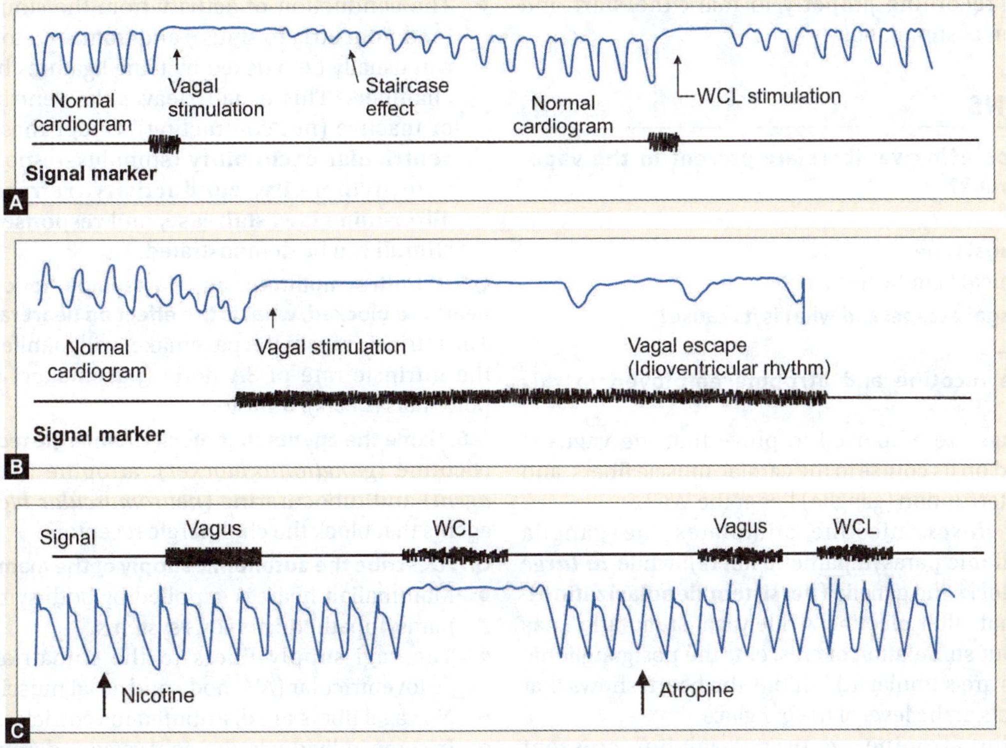

FIGS. 41A TO C: (A) Effect of stimulation of vagosympathetic trunk and white crescentic line (WCL); (B) Phenomenon of vagal escape. (C) Frog's heart treated with nicotine and atropine followed by stimulation of vagus and white crescentic line (WCL) after each drug [Using these procedures, an unknown drug (e.g. nicotine, atropine, adrenalin, and acetylcholine can be identified by the student)].

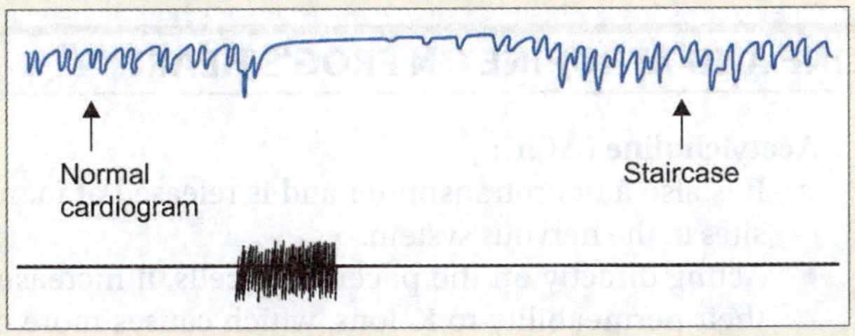

FIG. 42: Effect of white crescentic line (WCL) stimulation.

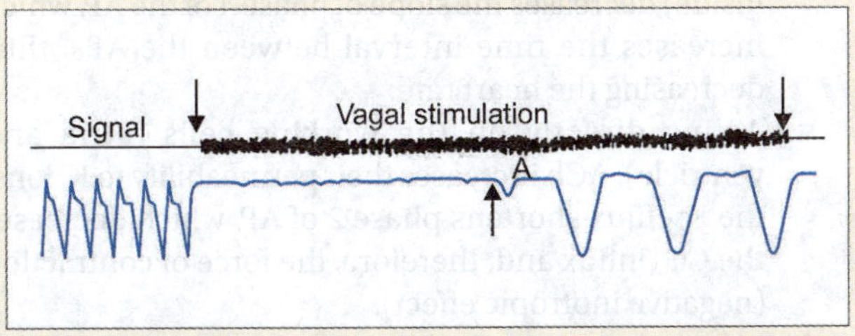

FIG. 43: Idioventricular rhythm after prolonged vagal stimulation.

- There may be exhaustion of acetylcholine from the vagal endings, or the ventricular muscle may remain depolarized (normally acetylcholine is inactivated immediately after exerting its action).
- The sympathetic effect may overpower the vagal effect, thus releasing the ventricle from inhibition.
- Strong emotions in humans may lead to vagal syncope, but the immediate vagal escape restores the heart beat (the Bainbridge effect may also be involved here).
- **Vasovagal syncope:** If there is sudden stimulation of the vagus nerve, there occurs transient and sudden loss of consciousness.

Note:

A. Nicotinic receptors:
1. They are located on all autonomic (sympathetic and parasympathetic) postganglionic neurons and also on neuromuscular end plates. These respond to low doses of nicotine.
2. Hexamethonium at autonomic ganglion and tubocurarine at neuromuscular junction block these receptors.

B. Muscarinic receptors
1. These are located on the smooth muscle cells, cardiac muscle, and glands are stimulated by mushroom poison called muscarine.
2. These muscarinic receptors are blocked by atropine.

PRECAUTIONS

1. The student should record the normal cardiogram before recording the effect of each variable.
2. The frog's heart should be rinsed with normal saline between applications of various drugs.
3. The vagosympathetic trunk should be identified by its anatomical landmark.
4. A lower strength to a higher strength of stimuli should be used to study the effect of vagal stimulation on the heart.

5. Label the recording properly to mark the start and termination of stimulation.

QUESTIONS

Q.1. What type of nerve fibers are present in the vago-sympathetic trunk?
See text above.

Q.2. What is vagal tone?
See Physioclinical Significance.

Q.3. What is vagal escape, and what is its cause?
See text above.

Q.4. Why are nicotine and atropine employed in this experiment?

- These drugs are employed to prove that the vagus is interrupted on its course to the cardiac muscle fibers, and that the interruption (ganglia) lies at the WCL.
- ***In small doses***, nicotine stimulates the ganglia (postganglionic parasympathetic fibers); while ***in large doses,*** it blocks the ganglia **(persistent depolarization)**. The fact that, after nicotine, while vagal stimulation has no effect but stimulation of crescent (the postganglionic cell bodies are stimulated) inhibits the heart, shows that nicotine acts at the level of the ganglia.
- Since, after atropine, neither vagal nor crescent stimulation inhibits the heart, one can conclude that atropine acts at the level of acetylcholine receptors on muscle cell membranes.
- The conduction of activity from the sinus to the atria (and from atria to sinus), and from atria to the ventricle, can usually be blocked by tying ligatures between these chambers. This usually leaves the ventricle quiescent or inactive (not contracting). Under these conditions, **ventricular excitability** (stimulus–response relation), **autorhythmicity, conductivity, refractory period, all-or-none law, staircase,** and **response to repetitive stimuli** can be demonstrated.

Q.5. If both sympathetic and parasympathetic nerves to the heart are blocked, what is the effect on heart rate?
The intrinsic rate of the pacemaker will manifest. In humans the intrinsic rate of SA node (pacemaker) is 100 action potentials (beats)/minute.

Q.6. Name the agents that block cholinergic receptors?
Nicotine (*ganglionic blocker*), atropine (*antimuscarinic agent*) and tubocurarine (*neuromuscular blocker*) are the agents that block the cholinergic receptors.

Q.7. Describe the autonomic supply of the mammalian heart.

- Mammalian heart is supplied by both sympathetic and parasympathetic nervous systems.
- The vagi supply fibers to the sinoatrial (SA) node, atrioventricular (AV) node and atrial muscles.
- No vagal fibers are distributed to ventricles.
- In some individuals, the right vagus is dominant, whereas in others it is the left vagus.
- The sympathetic fibers supply SA and AV nodes and muscles of atria and ventricles.

4.15: EFFECT OF ADRENALIN, ACETYLCHOLINE AND ATROPINE ON FROG'S HEART

STUDENT OBJECTIVES

After completing this experiment, the student should be able to:

- Explain the effect of adrenalin, acetylcholine and atropine on frog's cardiogram.
- Explain the physioclinical importance of this practical.

PY3.18: Observe with computer assisted learning (i) amphibian nerve-muscle experiments and (ii) amphibian cardiac experiments.

INTRODUCTION

1. **Adrenalin:**
   - It is a neurotransmitter in the brain.
   - A sympathomimetic agent, it is also released by the adrenal medulla.
   - Acting directly on the cardiac muscle cells, it increases their permeability mainly to Ca^{2+} ions and, to some extent, to Na^{+} ions.
   - Influx of Na^{+} in the pacemaker cells increases the slope of phase 4 of the AP (they reach firing level soon) and hence the increase in heart rate.
   - The large influx of Ca^{2+} in the working cells increases their force of contraction (positive inotropic effect).
2. **Acetylcholine (ACh):**
   - It is also a neurotransmitter and is released at many sites in the nervous system.
   - Acting directly on the pacemaker cells, it increases their permeability to K^{+} ions, which causes more of these ions to move out.
   - The resulting hyperpolarization (more negativity inside) decreases the slope of phase 4 of the AP, which increases the time interval between the APs, thus decreasing the heart rate.
   - Acting directly on the working cells (atria and ventricle), ACh increases their permeability to K^{+} ions; the K^{+} efflux shortens phase 2 of AP, which decreases the Ca^{2+} influx and, therefore, the force of contraction (negative inotropic effect).
3. **Atropine:**
   - It is a parasympatholytic agent and blocks the action of ACh by attaching itself to the membrane receptors of cardiac muscle cells.
   - Therefore, when applied on the heart after ACh, it has no effect, but when applied *before* ACh, atropine blocks the inhibitory action of ACh (there are no impulses coming in the vagi or sympathetic nerves, because the frog's brain has already been destroyed.

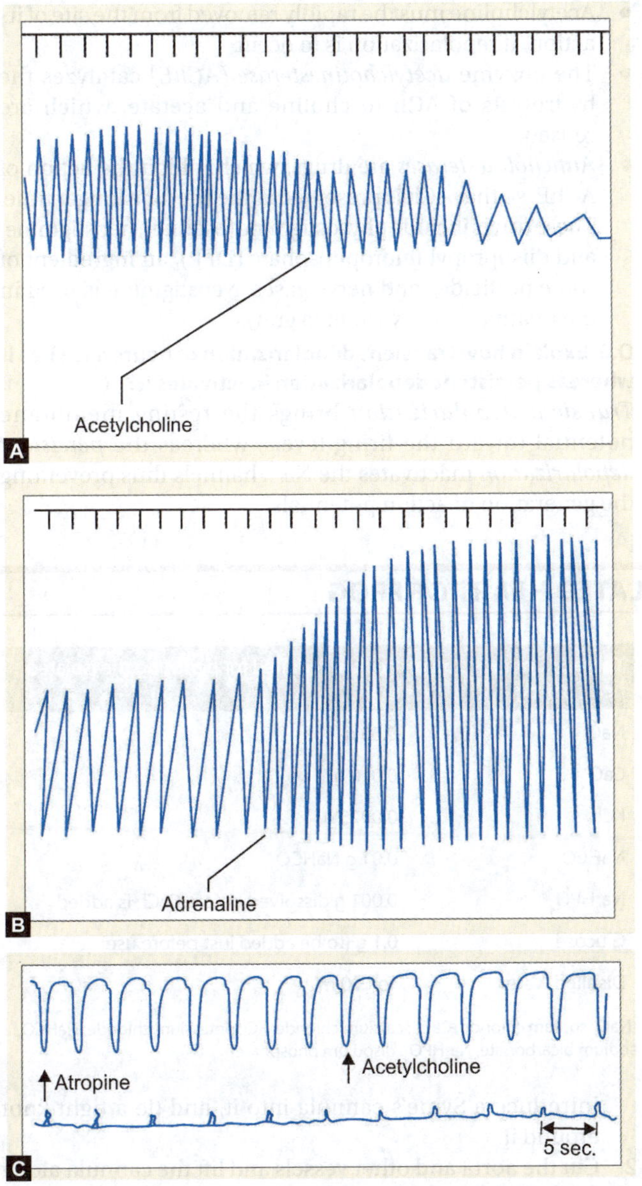

FIGS. 44A TO C: Effect of adrenalin, acetylcholine and atropine on Frog's heart.

Therefore, when applied on the heart, atropine does not increase its rate) **(Fig. 44)**.

APPARATUS

Same as the previous experiment, adrenalin (1:10,000), acetylcholine (1:100,000), and 0.5% atropine.

PROCEDURE

1. Record some normal beats. Stop the drum and pour a few drops of 1 in 10,000 solution of adrenalin on the heart. Record the increased rate and the force. Stop the drum and wash the heart with Ringer.
2. Record a few normal beats then pour a few drops of 1 in 100,000 solution of acetylcholine. Record the decrease in rate and force. As the heart is beating, apply 0.5% atropine solution. There will be no effect, i.e. the heart will remain inhibited.
3. Stop the drum, wash with Ringer, and study the effect of acetylcholine *after* applying atropine solution on the heart—the heart will not be inhibited this time. Label the graph appropriately.

PHYSIOCLINICAL SIGNIFICANCE

Refer Q.4 and Q.5 below.

PRECAUTIONS

Same as in the previous experiment.

QUESTIONS

Q.1. What is meant by the terms adrenergic, noradrenergic and cholinergic fibers?

- Adrenergic fibers (neurons) are those, which release adrenalin at their nerve terminals.
- Noradrenergic fibers release noradrenalin (all post-ganglionic sympathetic neurons, excepting a few, are noradrenergic; see below).
- Cholinergic fibers release acetylcholine at their endings.

Q.2. What are catecholamines and how are they inactivated in the body?

- Catecholamines are a group of substances, which are synthesized from tyrosine by hydroxylation and decarboxylation.
- These include adrenalin (methylnoradrenaline), nor-adrenalin, and dopamine (also a neurotransmitter).
- They are mostly taken up by the nerve endings, which secrete them, and the rest are degraded by the enzymes monoamine oxidase (MAO) and catechol-O-methyl-transferase (COMT) into vanillylmandelic acid (VMA) and others, which are excreted in the urine.

Q.3. What are the locations in the body where acetylcholine is released? How is it synthesized in the body?

Synthesis of ACh from choline and acetyl coenzyme A (CoA) is catalyzed by the enzyme ***choline acetyltransferase.***

Sites where acetylcholine is released: Acetylcholine is released at the following sites:

- Preganglionic sympathetic nerve endings (in the ganglia).
- Preganglionic and postganglionic parasympathetic nerve endings.
- Postganglionic sympathetic fibers supplying the sweat glands, pilomotor muscles, and those supplying the blood vessels of skeletal muscles are cholinergic (all others are noradrenergic).
- Neuromuscular junctions of all skeletal muscle fibers (the anterior horn cells of spinal cord and the equivalent motor neurons of cranial nerves are thus cholinergic).

- Many synapses in the CNS, and some amacrine cells in the retina.

Q.4. What are the different types of actions of acetylcholine in the body?

Acetylcholine has two main types of actions— **muscarinic** (muscarine is an alkaloid of a poisonous mushroom), and **nicotinic** (nicotine is an alkaloid of tobacco) actions.

- **Muscarinic actions:** These are the actions of ACh on cardiac muscle (inhibition), smooth muscle, and exocrine glands, including sweat glands. These actions are blocked by the drug atropine.
- **Nicotinic actions:** These are the actions of ACh on motor end-plates (blocked by curare, etc.) and on postganglionic neurons in autonomic ganglia (blocked by hexamethonium and other drugs).

Q.5. How is acetylcholine inactivated in the body? What are anticholinesterases?

- Acetylcholine must be rapidly removed from the site of its action, if repolarization is to occur.
- The enzyme *acetylcholinesterase (AChE)* catalyzes the hydrolysis of ACh to choline and acetate, which are reused.
- *Anticholinesterases* are drugs, which inhibit the action of AChE, so that ACh is preserved at the site for a longer time. These drugs include physostigmine (eserine), neostigmine, and diisopropyl fluorophosphate (DFP), an ingredient of some pesticides and nerve gases. Neostigmine is used in the treatment of myasthenia gravis.

Q.6. Explain how transient depolarization of neuron excites it whereas persistent depolarization inactivates it?

Transient depolarization brings the resting membrane potential toward the firing levels, whereas the *persistent depolarization* inactivates the Na^+ channels thus preventing the generation of action potentials.

4.16: PERFUSION OF ISOLATED HEART OF FROG

STUDENT OBJECTIVES

After completing this experiment, the student should be able to:

- Describe the effects of drugs and chemicals on normal cardiogram of frog.
- Explain the physioclinical basis of this practical.

PY3.18: Observe with computer assisted learning (i) amphibian nerve - muscle experiments and (ii) amphibian cardiac experiments.

INTRODUCTION

- The rate and force of contraction of the heart is affected by different drugs and ions.
- These agents change the ionic composition of the myocardial cells and the nodal tissue either acting directly on ion channels or on different receptors. In this practical, the effect of various drugs and chemicals are being observed in normal cardiogram of frog's heart **(Fig. 46 and Table 6)**.

APPARATUS

1. Amphibian Ringer–Locke solution
2. Mariotte (perfusion) bottle
3. Syme's cannula
4. 1% $CaCl_2$, 1% NaCl and 1% KCl
5. Adrenaline: 1:100,000
6. Acetylcholine: 1:1000,000

Composition of Ringer–Locke Solution

The fluid required for perfusing the isolated heart of frog has the composition given in **Table 5**.

Table 5: Composition of the fluid required for perfusing the isolated heart of frog.

NaCl	0.60 g
$CaCl_2$	0.010 g
KCl	0.0075 g
$NaHCO_3$	0.01 g $NaHCO_3$
Na_2HPO_4	0.001 g dissolved before $CaCl_2$ is added
Glucose	0.1 g (to be added just before use)
Distilled water	To 100 mL

(NaCl: sodium chloride; $CaCl_2$: calcium chloride; KCl: potassium chloride; $NaHCO_3$: sodium bicarbonate; Na_2HPO_4: disodium phosphate)

PROCEDURE

1. Expose the frog's heart and pass a thread around the sinus and tie a loose knot. Make a small slit in the sinus, introduce a Syme's cannula into it, and tie a tight knot around it.
2. Cut the aorta and other vessels and lift the cannula along with the heart. Fit a Starling heart lever, upside down, on a stand, and fix the cannula in a clamp directly above the heart lever. Connect the side arm of the cannula to a reservoir containing Ringer–Locke solution; and raise the reservoir about 30 cm above the heart to provide a pressure head **(Fig. 45)**.
3. Push the bent pin of the lever through the apex of the ventricle, make necessary adjustments, and record a few beats. Note that, in this case, the upstroke is systole and the downstroke diastole. After the tracing has stabilized, raise the reservoir to increase the perfusion pressure. If done properly, the force of contraction will increase, thus demonstrating the Starling's law of the heart.
4. **Add 1.0% NaCl solution** via the side tube of the cannula, and record its effects. Wash the heart with the perfusion fluid, and study the effects of **1% KCl and 1% $CaCl_2$** solutions.
5. Wash the heart well with Ringer–Locke solution and study the effects of *adrenalin* and *acetylcholine*.

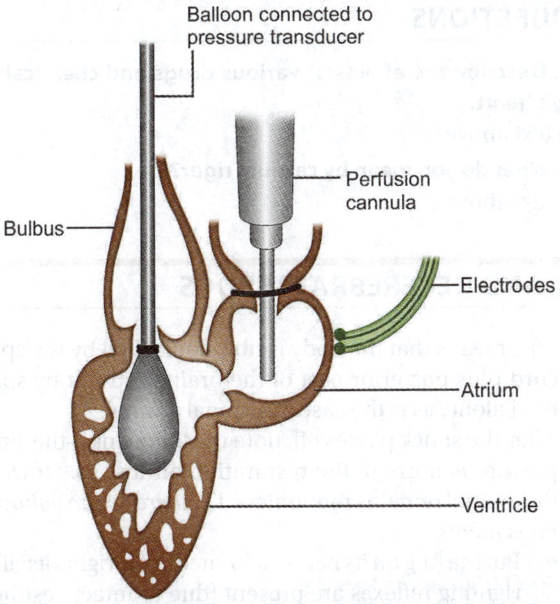

FIG. 45: Perfusion of isolated frog's heart.

OBSERVATION

- **Effect of sodium ions:**
  - Perfusion of the heart with a high concentration of Na^+ alone causes weakening and finally failure of contraction of the heart, which stops in diastole.
  - Increased extracellular fluid (ECF) sodium interferes with the action of calcium, which is the link between excitation and contraction.
- **Effect of potassium ions:**
  - Excess K^+ decreases the rate and force of contraction, the heart finally stopping in diastole.
  - A high ECF K^+ decreases the resting membrane potential of the muscle cells (because of reduction in the concentration gradient across the cell membrane), and the intensity of the action potential. As a result, the force of contraction gradually decreases and the heart stops beating.
- **Effect of calcium ions:**
  - Excess Ca^{2+} increases the force of contraction, and the heart ultimately stops in systole **(calcium rigor)**.

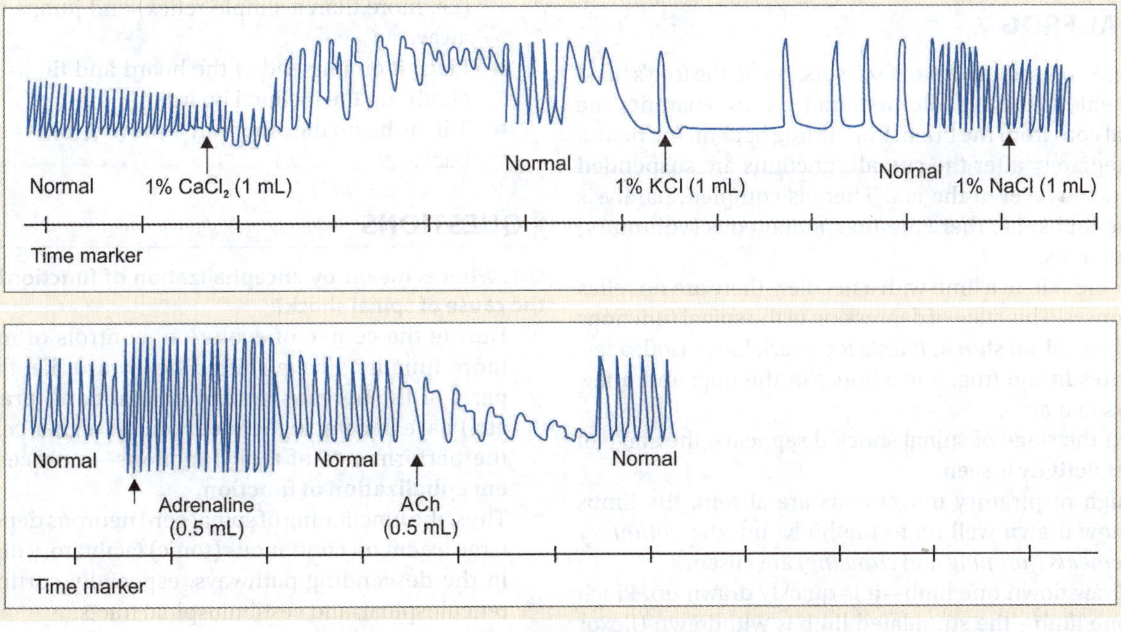

FIG. 46: Effect of variables on isolated frog's heart preparation.

Table 6: Effect and mechanism of action of variables on frogs' heart.

Agent	*Heart rate*	*Force of contraction*
1. NaCl (1%)	No effect	There may be a decrease in the contractility as Na^+ competes with Ca^{2+}
2. KCl (1%)	↓ because of decrease in RMP of nodal tissue	↓ Finally the heart stops in diastole. This is because of decrease in RMP of atrial and ventricular muscles
3. $CaCl_2$ (1%)	No effect	Increase in ECF Ca^{2+} leading to increase in intracellular Ca^{2+}. Marked increase in Ca^{2+} in ECF may cause calcium rigor
4. Adrenaline	Increases, due to increased Na^+ entry in nodal tissues	Increases due to Ca^{2+} influx in myocardial fibers
5. Acetylcholine	Decreases, HR as K^+ efflux hyperpolarizes the nodal tissues	Decreases because of decrease in Ca^{2+} influx in myocardial fibers

(ECF: extracellular fluid; RMP: resting membrane potential)

Part of the excess Ca^{2+} ions in the ECF of the T-tubules are added to the Ca^{2+} released from the terminal cisterns.

- As a result, more Ca^{2+} is made available to the contractile machinery, and the force increases. The heart stops in systole because diastole does not occur.

QUESTIONS

Q.1. Describe the effects of various drugs and chemicals on frog's heart.

See text above.

Q.2. What do you mean by calcium rigor?

See text above.

4.17: STUDY OF REFLEXES IN SPINAL AND DECEREBRATE FROGS

PY3.18: Observe with computer assisted learning (i) amphibian nerve - muscle experiments and (ii) amphibian cardiac experiments.

- Observe a frog placed on a frog board. The head is well raised on the forelimbs, the hind limbs are flexed, and respiratory movements are present.
- The frog responds to various stimuli (e.g. a prick) by jumping or crawling away.
- When put on its back, it quickly rights itself. When put in a basin of water, it swims. This indicates the presence of *righting reflexes.*

SPINAL FROG

- Using a bone cutter or stout scissors, cut off the frog's head just behind the tympanic membranes, thus separating the spinal cord from the brain. Put the frog back on the board.
- Immediately after the cut, all functions are suspended below the level of the cut. There is complete paralysis of the limbs, i.e. there are no spontaneous (voluntary) movements.
- Prick the skin of a limb with a needle—there are no reflex responses. This state of depression of the spinal functions is called **spinal shock.** It lasts for a variable period; a few minutes in the frog, a few hours in the dog; and a few weeks in man.
- When the stage of spinal shock disappears, the stage of **reflex activity** is seen.
- Though respiratory movements are absent, the limbs are now drawn well up to the body; but the *voluntary movements (jumping* and *crawling)* are absent:
  - Draw down one limb—it is quickly drawn up. Pinch one limb—the stimulated limb is withdrawn (flexor reflex).
  - Pinch with greater force; all the limbs are flexed (irradiation of impulses). Put the animal on its back—the frog cannot right itself.
  - Put it in water—it cannot swim and sinks to the bottom, i.e. the *righting reflexes are absent.*
  - Now destroy the spinal cord with a pithing needle—no reflex can be demonstrated now.

DECEREBRATE FROG

- Take another frog; cut off its head just behind the level of the eyes.
- This section separates the olfactory lobes and cerebral hemispheres from the optic lobes and the spinal cord.
- This means that the body is now controlled by the spinal cord plus posterior part of the brain, and not by spinal cord alone, as is the case in a spinal animal.
- After the shock passes off, note the following—the sitting posture is normal; the respiration almost so. However, the animal remains motionless, i.e. *there are no voluntary movements.*
  - Put the frog on its back—it immediately rights itself, i.e. righting reflexes are present (due to intact vestibular apparatus).
  - Pinch a limb—the animal makes complex movements (i.e. more than a simple reflex) and jumps or crawls away.
  - Place it on one end of the board and tilt it—the frog climbs up the inclined board.
  - Tilt the board the other way—the frog turns and crawls back.

QUESTIONS

Q.1. What is meant by encephalization of function? What is the cause of spinal shock?

- During the course of evolution, controls of more and more functions have shifted headward, i.e. the lower parts of the nervous system (spinal cord, brain stem, etc.) have become dependent on the higher centers for the performance of their functions—a process called **encephalization of function.**
- Thus, the functioning of spinal cord neurons depends to a large extent on continuous (tonic) facilitatory discharges in the descending pathways, especially corticospinal, reticulospinal, and vestibulospinal tracts.
- When the cord is suddenly deprived of these higher influences, it temporarily loses its reflex functions—a state called spinal shock. The higher the animal is on the ladder of evolution, the longer the duration of spinal shock.

Q.2. How does a decerebrate frog differ from a decerebrate higher animal?

A decerebrate frog differs from a decerebrate higher animal, say, a cat, in the following ways:

- In a *decerebrate frog,* the muscle tone and posture are almost normal, righting reflexes are present, and the animal can perform complex movements on stimulation.
- In a *decerebrate cat,* there is extensive rigidity (neck extended, back arched, and all limbs extended), the righting reflexes are absent, and the animal cannot

perform complex reflex movements. The voluntary movements are absent in both.

Q.3. What is classical decerebrate rigidity?

- When Sherrington, in 1906, transacted the brainstem in the upper pons between the superior and inferior colliculi (between red nuclei and vestibular nuclei), the cat, as soon as it came out of anesthesia, showed a marked increase in muscle tone, especially the antigravity muscles. This is called *classical decerebrate rigidity.*
- The cut blocks the normal inhibitory signals from the cortex and caudate nucleus to the descending inhibitory reticular formation of the brainstem.
- The descending facilitatory reticular formation being tonically active now, and increases the activity of the spinal stretch reflexes by stimulating the gamma efferents. As a result, the muscle tone, which is a reflex phenomenon, increases. Thus, decerebrate rigidity is a release phenomenon.

UNIT II: MAMMALIAN EXPERIMENTS

4.18: EXPERIMENTS ON ANESTHETIZED DOG

PY3.18: Observe with computer assisted learning (i) amphibian nerve - muscle experiments and (ii) amphibian cardiac experiments.

INTRODUCTION

- The rabbit and the dog are the usual mammals employed for practical class work. The dog (7–10 kg) must be quarantined for 10 days.
- Never frighten, annoy, or give pain to the animal. If scratched or bitten by the dog, thoroughly scrub the area with soap and water, then wash with alcohol and apply carbolic acid.

INSTRUMENTATION

1. **Brodie–Starling Long-paper Electric Kymograph:** It is fitted with assemblies for a manometer for recording blood pressure (BP), a Brodie, or Marey tambour for recording respiratory movements, an event marker, a time marker, a stimulating unit, and tuning knobs for speed control.
2. **Manometer:** It is a U-shaped glass tube containing mercury. One limb carries a float with a curved undersurface and a light-weight steel capillary bearing a writing point. The other limb has a side tube for connecting the manometer to an arterial cannula, and a vertical tube for connecting to a pressure bottle containing an anticoagulant. A manometric slide-adjustable scale is fitted between the two limbs for noting the BP.
3. **Pressure Bottle:** It has two tight-fitting rubber corks bearing glass tubes, one at the top for air entry, and the other near the bottom for connecting to the manometer. The bottle contains 3.8% sodium citrate solution. Pressure is created in the pressure recording system by raising the bottle. This prevents coagulation of blood and entry of blood into the manometer.
4. **Francis–Francois Arterial Cannula:** It has a nozzle, a bulb, and a side-arm bearing a short piece of rubber tube and a clamp. A clot, if any, can be removed through the side-arm.
5. **Operation Table:** The stainless steel top has two halves, with a removable drain pipe between and under them. The surface can be heated with electric lamps. Cleats are provided on the table edges for fastening the animal. A steel upright carries the instrument tray.
6. **Instrument Tray:** The instruments required include scalpels, scissors, artery forceps, bulldog clamps, retractors, tracheal cannula (Y-shaped or Z-shaped), venous cannula, arterial cannula, gauze pieces, and cotton swabs wetted with normal saline, and various drugs.

EXPERIMENTAL PROTOCOL

1. Calibrate the recording surface, in mm Hg, with the help of manometric scale and the writing point.
2. Anesthetize the animal with nembutal [pentobarbitone sodium; 35 mg/kg body weight injected in a leg vein (marginal vein of the ear in rabbit)]. Make a 7–8 cm midline cut in the neck, expose the trachea by blunt dissection, insert the tracheal cannula and tie it in position with stout thread. Connect the cannula to the tambour (the respiratory movements may also be recorded by tying a stethograph around the animal's chest).
3. Create a pressure of about 100 mm Hg in the manometer by raising the bottle.
4. Expose the femoral artery for about 4 cm in one thigh and tightly ligate it away from the heart. Place a bulldog clamp away from the ligature. Lift up the swollen segment of the artery, give a small nick in its wall, insert the arterial cannula and tie it in position.
5. Insert a venous cannula in the femoral vein in the other thigh, and connect it to a burette containing 0.9% sodium chloride solution. This route will be employed for injecting drugs.
6. Using blunt dissection on either side of the trachea, expose 3 cm of both common carotid arteries in the middle of the neck. Place loose thread ties around the arteries. Lift up the vagus. Place two loose ties around it.
7. Identify the smaller nerve, which is the cervical sympathetic trunk. Place a loose tie around it, lift it up, and place it on the electrodes of the stimulating probe. If it has been correctly identified, its stimulation will cause dilation of the pupil on that side. (In the rabbit, the nerve

fibers from the stretch receptors in the aortic arch run as a separate nerve—the aortic depressor nerve—which also runs in the carotid sheath. In other mammals, these fibers run in the vagus).

Blood Pressure Tracing

- The mercury manometer cannot record the systolic and diastolic pressures, because mercury has a high inertia and a low natural frequency. It dampens the fluctuations; the high values are less and the low values are high. As a result, the oscillations of the mercury with each beat of the heart are small.
- The recorded tracing, therefore, represents fluctuations around the *mean arterial pressure.*
- Usually, three types of fluctuations in pressure are recorded:
  1. **Cardiac waves:** These small waves are caused by successive cardiac contractions and are superimposed on the respiratory waves.
  2. **Respiratory waves (Traube–Hering waves):** These waves, which are composed of cardiac waves, represent fluctuations in BP synchronous with the movements of respiration. The waves show a rise of pressure during inspiration and a fall during expiration. The waves may be quite large, if the respiration is slow and deep. The BP rises during inspiration due to—(1) irradiation of impulses from the inspiratory center to the vasomotor center, which lies nearby, (2) the increase in intrathoracic negativity causes increased venous return and therefore cardiac output, and (3) the rise in heart rate also increases the cardiac output and hence the BP.
  3. **Meyer waves:** The Meyer waves, also called *vasomotor waves,* are small changes in BP over long periods of time, and encompassing a number of respiratory waves. These waves result primarily from baroreceptor activity, as well as of the vasomotor center. When the BP is low (50–80 mm Hg), chemoreceptors contribute mostly to generate these waves, as the influence of baroreceptors becomes very weak.

EXPERIMENT

Note the general features of the BP tracing and identify the cardiac and respiratory waves. Note the rate and rhythm of breathing. Then perform the following experiments and note the results:

1. **Carotid occlusion:**
   - Clamp both the carotid arteries, pressing on the event marker at the same time. Note the rise in BP. When the pressure has stabilized at the new level, remove the clamps from the arteries and the finger pressure from the event marker.
   - Carotid occlusion lowers the pressure in the carotid sinuses, which increases the BP due to stoppage of inhibitory discharges from them (consult Experiment 2.10 on carotid occlusion). Since the aortic baroreceptors are still functioning, the rise in pressure is not excessive.
   - Stimulation of carotid bodies by ischemia also contributes to the rise in BP.
2. **Vagal stimulation:**
   - The first example of inhibition discovered in physiology was in 1845 when Weber brothers found that weak stimulation of the vagus decreased the heart rate and force, while strong stimulation stopped the heart.
   - The cervical vagus contains afferent fibers from aortic body chemoreceptors, aortic arch mechanoreceptors, mechanoreceptors from heart, chemoreceptors from coronary and pulmonary chemoreceptors, and stretch receptors in small airways (for Hering–Breuer reflex). The efferent fibers for the heart arise form nucleus ambiguus, and terminate on clusters of neurons (nervous nuclei of Dogel, Remak, Bidder, and Ludwig) located in the sinoatrial (SA) node (mainly right vagus) and atrioventricular (AV) node (mainly left vagus). The postganglionic fibers form these ganglia innervate the atria, the nodes, and the AV bundle. There are very few fibers, if any, supplying the basal parts of the ventricles, which is the reason why the ventricles escape the inhibitory effect of continued vagal stimulation.
     - ***Stimulate one vagus and then the other,*** with weaker and stronger stimuli. In both cases, there is slowing of the heart and fall in BP, and stoppage of the heart with stronger stimuli. The respiration is usually arrested.
     - With slower beating of the ventricles, the diastolic period is prolonged, ventricular filling is more, and the stroke volume is increased. These are reflected in wide swings in the oscillations of the mercury column. If stimulation is continued after stoppage of the heart, the ventricles usually "escape" and start to beat at the slower idioventricular rhythm of 20–30 beats/min (pacemaker in the ventricles). Vagal escape perhaps also suggests that the vagus has very little direct effect on the ventricular activity.
     - ***Section of vagi:*** Cut first one vagus and then the other between the two ties. There is an increase of heart rate due to loss of vagal tone. The respiration becomes slower and deeper.

       Vagal tone: A prolonged excitation, which is not accompanied by fatigue, is called tone. There is an appreciable vagal tone and a moderate sympathetic tone in man. If vagal tone in humans is blocked with atropine, the heart rate increases from the resting value of about 70 beats/min to 150–170 beats/min. If both cholinergic and noradrenergic systems are blocked with drugs (pharmacologic denervation), the heart rate is about 100 beats/min.

- ***Stimulate the peripheral ends of the cut vagi,*** first one then the other. There is inhibition of the heart as before. There is no effect on respiration.
- ***Stimulate the central ends of the cut vagi,*** first on one side and then on the other. There is stoppage of respiration due to excitation of afferent fibers coming from the stretch receptors of the lungs (these fibers are involved in the Hering–Breuer reflex). There is no effect on the heart.

3. **Inject 5 µg of adrenalin** (1 in 10,000 solution; 1 mL = 10 µg) intravenously. There is an immediate but small and transient fall in BP (due to slight fall in total peripheral resistance), which is at once followed by a rise, due mainly to increase in cardiac output. The baroreceptor signals, which inhibit the vasomotor center, also inhibit the respiratory center located nearby. Thus, a rise in BP may depress the respiration, or even cause a temporary stoppage of respiration—a condition called ***adrenalin apnea.***
4. **Inject 5 µg of noradrenalin** into the vein. There is no initial fall in the BP, and the rise in pressure is much greater and more sustained. The mean pressure rises in spite of reduction in cardiac output by the baroreceptor mechanism. This drug causes intense vasoconstriction of almost all the systemic arterioles via alpha-1 receptors.
5. When the BP has returned to control levels, **inject 2 µg of *acetylcholine*** (1 in 100,000; 1 mL = 1 µg) intravenously. There is a marked decrease in heart rate and BP due to inhibition of the heart. When the pressure has returned to control level, repeat the dose after first injecting atropine. There will be no inhibition of the heart.
6. **Effect of asphyxia:**
   - Close the tracheal cannula to produce asphyxia, i.e. hypoxia plus hypercarbia. There is a gradual increase in the rate and depth of respiration, and a rise in BP.
   - As the asphyxia progresses, the animal makes violent respiratory efforts. Increased partial pressure of carbon dioxide (PCO_2) stimulates the vasomotor center, thus increasing the BP.
   - Acting on the respiratory center via medullary chemoreceptors, and reflexly via carotid and aortic bodies, a high PCO_2 stimulates breathing.
   - A low partial pressure of oxygen (PO_2) stimulates respiration reflexly, but its action on the medullary neurons is depressant (consult Experiment 2.1 for details).
   - The animal may be revived at this time, but if the asphyxia is continued, the toxic effects of CO_2 on the heart and the brain result in fall of BP and depression of breathing. There is generalized muscle twitching and failure of respiration. Ventricular fibrillation and cardiac arrest occur in 4–5 minutes.
7. **Effect of raised intrathoracic pressure on systemic arterial pressure:** After the BP returns to control level, simultaneously place a fingertip over the tracheal cannula and, with the other hand, squeeze the thoracic cage just below the ribs to prevent the descent of diaphragm. There is a fall in BP due to decrease in venous return resulting from raised intrathoracic pressure.
8. **Effect of hemorrhage:**
   - It depends on the *amount of blood removed* and the *rapidity of bleeding.*
   - Cannulate the other femoral artery and remove blood equivalent to 10 mL/kg body weight into a measuring cylinder (normal blood volume = 80 mL/kg body weight).
   - Note the fall in BP, which is due to decrease in venous return, and thus of cardiac output.
   - The breathing may show an increase in rate (tachypnea), which is due to poor perfusion of carotid bodies (aortic bodies are ineffective because the vagus nerves have been cut).
   - About 50% of the blood is present in the veins at any one moment. Therefore, constriction of veins is an important compensatory mechanism, which tends to restore circulating blood volume after hemorrhage; the other compensatory processes for restoring blood volume and pressure being arteriolar constriction and decreased formation and increased reabsorption of tissue fluid in the capillaries (the receptors primarily responsible for monitoring the "fullness" of the cardiovascular system and for regulating the blood volume are the low-pressure stretch receptors in the atria).

Some Important Charts and Questions

SECTION 5

This section includes idealized normal charts, figures, and graphs on which the students are quizzed/tested during their class tests and university examination. Of course, the charts on which the students are tested are not labeled. The students should, however, note that the questions/answers mentioned here are not exhaustive. It will be a good practice if they make up other related questions and try to answer them during discussions with their class fellows.

5.1: JUGULAR VENOUS PULSE TRACING

Q.1. What is meant by jugular venous pulse? How is a record of this event obtained?

- **Jugular venous pulse (JVP):** The term JVP refers to the pulsations observed in the jugular veins in the neck.
- These venous pulsations are due to the pressure changes in the right atrium that are reflected back into the large veins near the heart (**Fig. 1** and Practical 3.3).
- The JVP tracing is obtained by placing a suitable transducer over the vein and recording the pressure changes on the electronic polygraph.
- Before the days of electrocardiogram (ECG), this cardiac event is used to be recorded with the Mackenzie, ink polygraph by placing the neck receiver over the vein, and connecting it to the recording system.

Q.2. Name the various waves recorded in the jugular venous pulse (JVP) tracing.

The JVP record shows three positive waves—

1. **a**
2. **c**
3. **v**, and
4. Two negative waves or descents—(i) **X** and (ii) **Y**

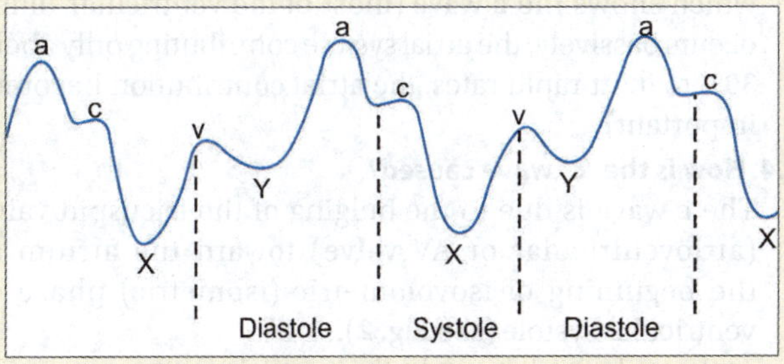

FIG. 1: The normal jugular venous pulse tracing showing three positive waves—(1) a, (2) c, and (3) v and two negative waves or descents—(1) X and (2) Y.

Note: The letters **a**, **c**, and **v** stand for: a = atrial wave, c = carotid (or ventricular wave), and v = *venous stasis* wave].

Q.3. What is the cause of "a" wave?

- The **a** wave is due to atrial systole (duration = 0.1 s).
- During atrial systole, the pressure inside, which was rising gradually, now rises suddenly and is reflected back as the

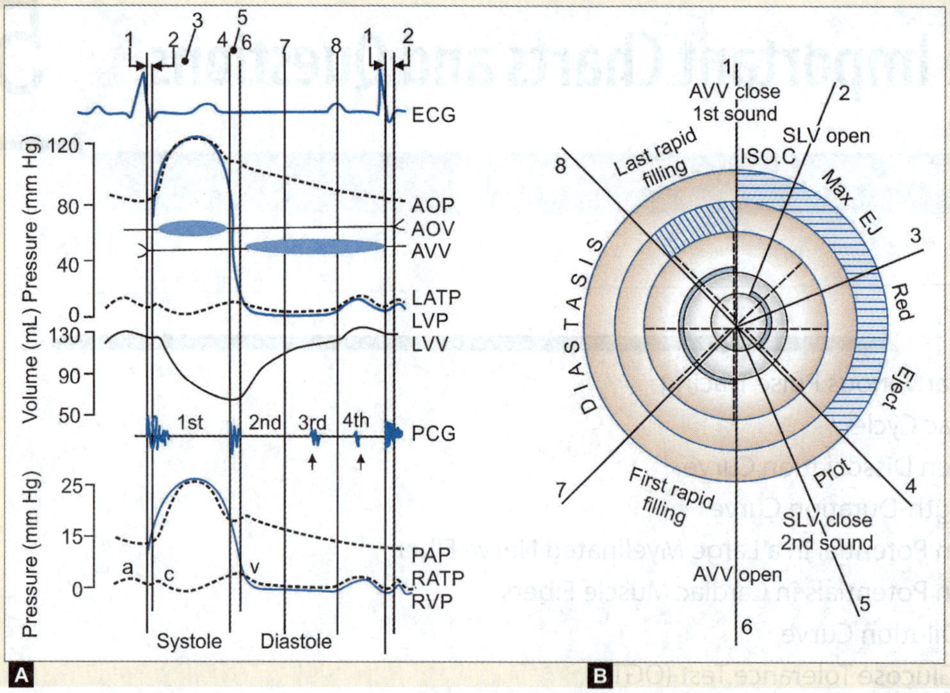

FIGS. 2A AND B: (A) Events of the cardiac cycle showing pressure changes in aorta (AOP), left ventricle (LVP), left atrium (LATP), right atrium (RATP), right ventricle (RVP), and pulmonary artery pressure (PAP). Electrical changes (ECG), sound production (PCG) are shown. The opening and closing of atrioventricular valve (AVV) and aortic valve (AOV), and changes in left ventricular volume (LVV) are also shown; (B) Cardiac cycle time = 0.8 s. Outer circle: Ventricular events, inner circle: atrial events. Dotted lines indicate the circles divided into eight equal segments, each 0.1 s. Solid lines separate various phases of the cardiac cycle. Shaded segments: Systole, unshaded segments: Diastole. Note that for half the cycle, all four chambers are in diastole (relaxing). Numbers 1–8 represent events in both diagrams: (1) start of isovolumetric systole, closure of AVV, and first heart sound, (1–2) isovolumetric systole (0.05 s), (2–3) maximum ejection (0.1 s), (3–4) reduced ejection (0.15 s), (4–5) protodiastole (0.05 s), (5–6) isovolumetric relaxation (0.1 s), (1–8) atrial diastole (0.7 s), (1–4) ventricular systole (0.3 s), and (4–1) ventricular diastole (0.5 s).

(AOP: aortic pressure; ECG: electrocardiogram; LATP: left atrial pressure; LVP: left ventricular pressure; PCG: phonocardiogram; RATP: right atrial pressure; RVP: right ventricular pressure; SLV: semilunar valve).

a wave in the JVP tracing (the contracting atrium also holds back blood in the vein).

- It corresponds with the last phase of ventricular filling (last rapid filling). The **a** wave is followed by the **X** descent which shows the **c** wave (most of the ventricular filling occurs passively, the atrial systole contributing only about 30% to it. At rapid rates, the atrial contribution becomes important).

Q.4. How is the "c" wave caused?

- The **c** wave is due to the bulging of the tricuspid valve (atrioventricular or AV valve) toward the atrium at the beginning of isovolumetric (isometric) phase of ventricular systole (see **Fig. 2**).
- At the end of atrial systole, the ventricle starts contracting isovolumetrically as a closed chamber (the pulmonary valve is still closed and will not open till the pressure in the ventricle exceeds the diastolic pressure in the pulmonary artery, and causes the valve to bulge back into the atrium which is recorded as the upstroke of the **c** wave).
- At the end of isovolumetric contraction, the pulmonary valve opens and the ventricle ejects blood into the pulmonary artery. This pulls the AV ring downward, the atrial pressure decreases, and the downstroke of the **c** wave is inscribed (the **c** wave is thus a *mechanical artifact of the valve motion*. A cardiac valve opens or closes due to a pressure gradient across it).

Q.5. What is the cause of "v" wave?

- The **v** wave represents the passive rise of atrial pressure and venous stasis in the jugular vein as venous return continues before the tricuspid valve opens at the end of isovolumetric relaxation of the right ventricle (ventricular systole continues between the **c** and the **v** waves).
- As the tricuspid valve opens, and blood rapidly enters the ventricle, the fall in atrial pressure causes the **Y** descent (once the tricuspid valve opens, the atrium and ventricle are a common chamber, and pressure in both cavities falls as ventricular relaxation continues. Thus, most of the ventricular filling occurs before atrial systole).

Q.6. What is the clinical significance of the jugular venous pulse tracing?

- The recording of the JVP tracing is not a routine clinical procedure because a simple clinical examination of the neck veins (see Experiment 3.3) can provide important information about some cardiac conditions.
- However, the procedure is noninvasive and the JVP tracing shows some characteristic changes in certain heart diseases. For example, there is a prominent **a** wave in right ventricular hypertrophy and tricuspid stenosis, while this wave is absent in atrial fibrillation. There is a sudden fall in the **Y** descent when right atrial pressure is elevated. The interval between the **a** and **c** waves is increased in heart block.

5.2: CARDIAC CYCLE (FIGS. 2A AND B)

Q.1. What is the cause of contraction of the heart?

- The cause of cardiac contraction lies within the heart itself (the autonomic nerves only modify this activity).
- The sinoatrial (SA) node spontaneously generates action potentials (cardiac impulses) which spread over the atria and then to the ventricles via the atrioventricular (AV) node and the bundle of His (the atrial muscle of the SA node is the first part of the heart to depolarize and repolarize).
- During depolarization, calcium enters the cardiomyocyte via L-type calcium channels. Calcium then activates ryanodine receptors on the SR, which triggers calcium release from the SR that further increases calcium availability in the cell (CICR).
- As the contraction ends, intracellular calcium returns to the SR via SERCA calcium channel.

Q.2. What is cardiac cycle and what are its main events? What are the durations of atrial and ventricular systole and diastole?

- The sequence of changes that occur in the heart from one beat to the next is called a cardiac cycle.
- During one cycle, there are changes in pressures, volumes, electrical potentials, opening and closure of valves, and sound production due to closure of valves. The durations of atrial and ventricular systole and diastole are:
  - Atrial systole = 0.1 s, diastole = 0.7 s
  - Ventricular systole = 0.3 s, diastole = 0.5 s.

Q.3. What is ventricular end-diastolic volume? How much is the contribution of atria to ventricular filling?

- *The ventricular end-diastolic volume* (EDV) is the amount of blood present in each ventricle at the end of diastole; it amounts to about 120–130 mL.
- The atrial contraction contributes 20–30% toward ventricular filling (atrial contribution becomes important at high cardiac rate because it is mainly the diastolic period that is cut down).

Q.4. What is ventricular end-diastolic pressure and what is its significance?

- *The ventricular end-diastolic pressure (EDP)* is the pressure in each ventricle at the end of diastole; normally it is near zero or a few (3–5) mm Hg.
- The ventricular EDV and ventricular EDP are interrelated and change together, setting the preload for the next ventricular contraction, i.e. the initial length of the muscle fibers.

Q.5. What is stroke volume?

- The **stroke volume**, or **stroke output** is the volume of blood ejected by **each ventricle separately** per beat. Normally, the stroke volume amounts to about 70–80 mL.
- Cardiac output is the amount of blood ejected per minute, i.e. stroke volume × heart rate; at rest, it amounts to about 5–6 L/min.

Q.6. What is ventricular end-systolic volume and what is ejection fraction?

- **The ventricular end-systolic volume (VESV)** is the amount of blood that remains in each ventricle at the end of systole.
- At rest, it amounts to about 50–60 mL. The ejection fraction, i.e. the percent of ventricular EDV that is expelled is about 65%.
- The ventricles do not empty out completely when they contract (when heart contracts forcefully, the ventricular ESV can fall to as low as 10–20 mL. But when there is a large venous return, the ventricular EDV can be as high as 150–180 mL in the normal heart.
- Thus, by increasing the ventricular EDV and decreasing the ventricular ESV, the stroke volume can be increased to nearly double its resting value, as happens during muscular exercise, during which the heart rate also increases).

Q.7. What are the maximum and minimum pressures in the left and right ventricles?

- The maximum pressure in the left ventricle is just above 120 mm Hg when the aortic systolic pressure is 120 mm Hg. The minimum pressure is a few mm Hg.
- The maximum pressure in the right ventricle is just above 25 mm Hg, when the pulmonary artery systolic pressure is 25 mm Hg. The minimum pressure is a few mm Hg.

Q.8. During which phase of ventricular systole is the rise in pressure maximum?

- The maximum rise in ventricular pressure occurs during *isovolumetric contraction* (the length of muscle fibers remains approximately constant) when the pressure rises from 0 to 80 mm Hg (minimum pressure in aorta).
- The ventricle contracts as a closed chamber (blood is incompressible) because blood cannot leave it until the aortic valve opens. In the right ventricle, the pressure rises from near 0 to 10 mm Hg when the pulmonary valve opens.

Q.9. During which phase of cardiac cycle does the maximum fall in ventricular pressure occur?

- The maximum fall in ventricular pressure occurs during the isovolumetric relaxation phase when the pressure falls from about 80 mm Hg to near zero. During this phase, the ventricle is a closed, isolated chamber.
- This phase lasts for 0.04 s and ends at the peak of atrial pressure **v** wave as ventricular pressure falls below atrial pressure and the bicuspid (mitral) valve opens.

Q.10. What is protodiastole? Is it part of systole or of diastole?

- During this very brief (0.02 s) phase of *protodiastole* (before diastole), the ventricular systole has ceased but relaxation has not yet started.
- When the already falling ventricular pressure (i.e. during reduced ejection) falls below that in the aorta, the transient reversal of blood flow in the root of the aorta causes the aortic valve first to float away from aortic walls and then to close abruptly.
- Thus, protodiastole ends with closure of semilunar valves and production of second heart sound.

Some workers consider protodiastole as part of diastole because muscle contraction has stopped; others consider it as part of systole because muscle relaxation has not yet started.

OTHER QUESTIONS

Q.11. What are the pressures in the aorta?

See text above.

Q.12. What are the pressures in the right ventricle and the pulmonary artery?

See text above.

Q.13. What is phonocardiography? When do the heart sounds occur during the cardiac cycle and what is their cause?

See text above.

5.3: OXYGEN DISSOCIATION CURVE (FIG. 3)

Q.1. What are the gas concentrations and pressures in the arterial and venous bloods?

- The arterial blood [hemoglobin (Hb) = 15 g%] contains about 20 mL/100 mL of oxygen (O_2) (15 × 1.34; 1 g Hb combines with 1.34 mL O_2), at a partial pressure of about 100 mm Hg [actually a little less; this partial pressure of oxygen (pO_2) is due solely to 0.3 mL O_2 dissolved in plasma]. The carbon dioxide (CO_2) content is 48%, at a partial pressure of carbon dioxide (pCO_2) of about 40 mm Hg.
- The venous blood contains about 15% O_2 at a pO_2 of 40 mm Hg (this pO_2 is due to 0.1 mL% of O_2 dissolved in plasma). The CO_2 content is 52 mL%, at partial pressure of 45 mm Hg.
- The rest of the gas pressure (760 minus O_2 and CO_2 pressures) is due to nitrogen dissolved in plasma (0.98%). Nitrogen is not present in any combined form.

Q.2. What is the difference between oxygen content and oxygen capacity?

- The term oxygen (O_2) *content* refers to the amount of O_2 actually present in a given sample of blood, while O_2 capacity refers to the total amount of O_2 that can be carried by blood when the hemoglobin (Hb) is fully saturated with O_2.

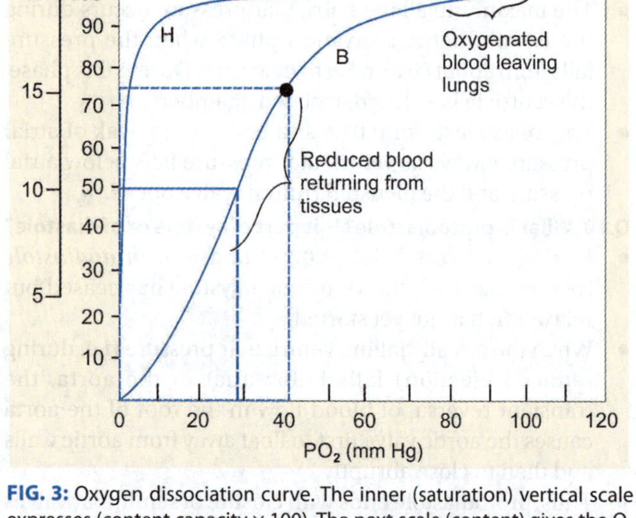

FIG. 3: Oxygen dissociation curve. The inner (saturation) vertical scale expresses (content capacity × 100). The next scale (content) gives the O_2 content (mL/dL) of blood, assuming a normal Hb concentration (15 g/dL) and combining power (1.34 mL O_2/g Hb). B: Dissociation curve of whole blood, H: Dissociation curve of simple Hb solution in water. (Hb: hemoglobin; pO_2: partial pressure of oxygen).

- The term *percentage saturation* refers to the percent of Hb that is saturated with O_2. For example, arterial blood is nearly 100% saturated, while venous blood is 75% saturated, i.e. 75% of the Hb molecules are carrying oxygen.

Q.3. What are the special features of reactions of hemoglobin and oxygen?

- The Hb molecule has 4 subunits and the heme of each subunit contains one atom of the metal iron. It is this iron (ferrous) which is the binding site for oxygen (O_2), and can combine with one molecule of O_2 (a reversible reaction).
- The oxygenation of Hb occurs in four separate steps. At first, one molecule of O_2 is taken up by Hb; this increases its affinity for the second molecule of O_2 and so on, the affinity being maximum when the third molecule of O_2 has been taken up. This *shifting affinity of Hb for O_2* is responsible for the upper part of oxyhemoglobin dissociation curve being flat.

Q.4. What does the oxyhemoglobin dissociation curve represent?

- The *oxyhemoglobin dissociation curve* or *oxygen dissociation curve*, represents the relationship between partial pressures of oxygen and the percentage saturation of hemoglobin with oxygen.
- The curve shows a sigmoidal shape because of cooperativity among the four subunits of the Hb molecule.

Q.5. How is oxyhemoglobin dissociation curve obtained?

- About 5 mL of blood is exposed to gas mixtures [oxygen (O_2), carbon dioxide (CO_2), and nitrogen (N_2)] of varying, but known composition (and thus partial pressures), in each of the 10 tonometers (these are cylindrical glass vessels, of 250 mL capacity, with nozzles and stopcocks).
- The blood samples are allowed to equilibrate with O_2 at the same tension as that present in each tonometer.
- The O_2 content, and thus the percent saturation, of each sample is then determined. The results are plotted in the form of a curve with partial pressure of oxygen (pO_2) along the abscissa (X-axis) and percentage saturation (or O_2 concentration) in the ordinate (Y-axis). The graph that is obtained is called oxyhemoglobin dissociation curve of the blood.
- Such a curve can be obtained under different conditions of temperature, partial pressure of carbon dioxide (pCO_2), and H^+ ion concentrations, not only for blood, but also for myoglobin and a simple solution of hemoglobin (Hb).

Q.6. What is P50 and what is its importance?

- The P50 is the partial pressure of oxygen (O_2) at which the blood is 50% saturated, i.e. when it has given up half of its O_2.
- The normal P50 is 25–30 mm Hg.
- It serves as an index for shifts in the curve that occur under different conditions.

Q.7. What is the significance of the sigmoid or "S" shape of the dissociation curve?

- **The "flat top" of the curve,** which is due to increased affinity of the fourth oxygenation reaction, means that the alveolar partial pressure of oxygen (pO_2) (and therefore, arterial pO_2) may fall, say, from 100 to 60 mm Hg without greatly reducing the degree of saturation of blood with O_2, the saturation decreasing from 97 to 90%. On the other hand, if pO_2 increases from 97 mm Hg to, say, 400 mm Hg, the saturation increases from 97 to 100% (though dissolved O_2 will increase). Thus, at moderately high altitudes, an individual would suffer little from impairment of O_2 uptake from the alveoli.
- **The steep part of the curve** shows that large amounts of O_2 can be given out with relatively minor falls of tissue fluid PO_2. That is, tissue fluid PO_2 does not have to fall very much for O_2 to be released from hemoglobin. In heavy exercise, extra amounts of O_2 are released with little further fall in tissue pO_2 than down to 20–25 mm Hg.
- Because of the sigmoid shape of the curve, the dissociation of oxyhemoglobin acts as a buffer for tissue pO_2. When this pO_2 falls below 40 mm Hg, extra amount of O_2 are given up; when this pO_2 tends to rise (as when one enters areas of compressed air) above 40 mm Hg, less O_2 is released from the Hb to the tissues (the curve above 60 mm Hg is flat). Thus, Hb automatically delivers O_2 to tissues at a pO_2 that is held rather tightly between 20 and 40 mm Hg (high pO_2 can be damaging to the tissues, as is low pO_2).

Q.8. What does a shift of the dissociation curve to the right signify? Name the factors that cause the "right shift".

- A shift of the curve to the right (as indicated by shift of P50) indicates a decreased affinity of hemoglobin for oxygen (O_2), i.e. the unloading of O_2 is facilitated (more O_2 is released at the same partial pressure of oxygen, though actually, the pressure gradient is increased).
- The shift of the curve to the right is caused by the following:
  - **Increase in carbon dioxide:** When tissues become active, their own carbon dioxide (CO_2) production increases, and this lowers the affinity of Hb for O_2. The resulting right shift increases the pressure gradient between capillary blood pO_2 and tissue pO_2. The CO_2 not only lowers the pH, it also causes vasodilation in active tissues.
  - **Increase in H^+ ion concentration:** This also causes a right shift. There are other sources of hydrogen ions besides CO_2. A change in pH from 7.4 to 7.2 causes a right shift by 15%.
  - **Increase in temperature:** A rise in temperature causes a right shift, i.e. more O_2 is released. The rise in temperature by itself causes vasodilation in the active tissues.
  - **Increase in concentration of 2,3-bisphosphoglycerate:** There are high concentrations of 2,3-bisphosphoglycerate (BPG), a byproduct of glycolysis in the red blood cells. It acts as a highly charged polyanion which decreases the affinity of Hb for O_2 by binding to the beta chains of reduced Hb but not to those of oxyhemoglobin. Thus, the presence of BPG favors dissociation of O_2 from the Hb. The concentration of BPG rises within 40–60 minutes of exercise, at high altitudes, in anemia, and under the influence of androgens and thyroid hormones.

Q.9. What does a shift of the dissociation curve to the left signify? Name the factors that cause a left shift.

- **Shift of the curve to the left:** It indicates increased affinity of the hemoglobin for oxygen (O_2), i.e. the O_2 remains tenaciously bound to Hb and is less readily given up.
  - The factors that cause a shift to the left and upward are: a fall in partial pressure of carbon dioxide (pCO_2)
  - Rise of pH (i.e. decreased hydrogen ion concentration)
  - Decrease in the concentration of 2,3-bisphosphoglycerate, and
  - The presence of large amounts of fetal Hb and abnormal hemoglobins.
- The fetal Hb has greater affinity for O_2 due to poor binding of BPG by the gamma chains (HbF causes increased O_2 release to fetal tissues under hypoxic conditions in which the fetus exists).

Q.10. What is Bohr effect and Haldane effect and what is it's importance?

- The **Bohr effect** describes hemoglobin's lower affinity for oxygen secondary to increases in the partial pressure of carbon dioxide and/or decreased blood pH.
- This lower affinity, in turn, enhances the unloading of oxygen into tissues to meet the oxygen demand of the tissue.
- The increased capacity of deoxygenated hemoglobin to carry CO_2 is referred to as the **Haldane effect**.
- Consequently, venous blood carries more CO_2 than arterial blood, and CO_2 uptake is facilitated in the tissues and CO_2 release is facilitated in the lungs.

Q.11. What is coefficient of utilization?

- The percent of blood that gives up its oxygen as it passes through the tissue capillaries is called the coefficient of utilization.
- At rest, it is about 25%, while during heavy exercise, the coefficient of utilization of the whole body can increase to 75–80% (in local areas of active tissues, it may be 100%, i.e. almost all of the oxygen may be extracted by the tissues).

Q.12. What are the features of oxygen dissociation curves of a simple solution of hemoglobin and solution of myoglobin in water?

- The oxygen dissociation curve of a simple solution of hemoglobin is a rectangular hyperbola (see **Fig. 3**). It means that this Hb will not give up its O_2 until the partial pressure of oxygen falls to 2–3 mm Hg, and even then little O_2 is given up.

- Also this curve does not show Bohr effect. Thus, the Hb in simple solution would not function as a suitable supplier of O_2 to the tissues.
- The dissociation curve of blood, as we have seen is S-shaped. The dissimilarity between the curves of Hb solution and blood is due to the presence of carbon dioxide (CO_2) and hydrogen ions, 2,3-bisphosphoglycerate, and electrolytes and inorganic salts in the blood, and of course the fact that Hb in the blood is confined to the red cells.
- **The dissociation curve of unimolecular myoglobin** (Mgb; it has one iron atom) is also rectangular hyperbola; it also does not show Bohr effect. Myoglobin present in the muscles takes up O_2 from blood at low pressures much more readily than blood. Even at a pO_2 of 40 mm Hg, the Mgb is still 95% saturated with O_2. It does not give up O_2 until the pO_2 falls to below 5 mm Hg. Thus, it acts as a temporary store of O_2 in the muscles, supplying O_2 during muscle contractions when their blood flow ceases (blood flow is restored when they relax).

5.4: STRENGTH-DURATION CURVE (FIG. 4)

Q.1. What does the strength-duration curve represent? How is this curve obtained?

- The strength-duration curve is a graphical representation of the relationship between the intensity of an electrical stimulus and the length of time taken to elicit a minimal contraction in that muscle or produce an action potential in a nerve fiber. Here, strength refers to the stimulus intensity on the vertical axis while duration refers to the pulse duration on the horizontal axis.
- **Strength-duration curve also called the chronaxie curve** thus represents the relationship between the *strength of a stimulating current* and the *time duration for which it must be applied* to produce an action potential in an excitable tissue.
- The strength of a stimulus must rise to its effective level within a very short time to be effective; if it rises slowly, it is ineffective; the fiber tends to accommodate to the presence of the current—due to inactivation of the sodium channels. Further, for a stimulus to be effective, it must be passed for a certain minimum time, i.e. for an adequate time).
- A stimulating and a recording unit are set up where **both strength (voltage)** of a stimulus as well as its **duration** (msec) can be preselected (in the stimulating unit) before it is applied to the tissue under study.

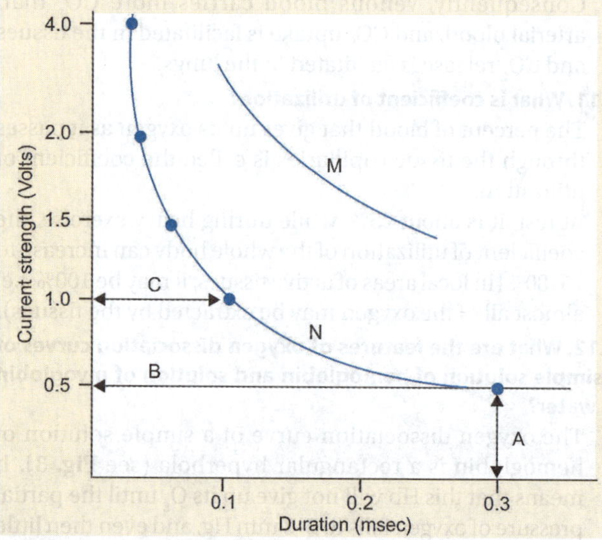

FIG. 4: Strength-duration curve. (A) Rheobase, (B) Utilization time, (C) Chronaxie, (N) Nerve, and (M) Muscle.

- Starting with a weak stimulus of a long duration, various combinations of the two are applied till a stimulus of minimum strength and of adequate duration are found that is effective. For example, in the record shown in **Figure 4**, a stimulus of 0.3 or 0.4 V was ineffective even when it was passed for more than 0.5 msec. A stimulus of 0.5 V was found to be effective when it was passed for 0.3 msec (it was ineffective when it was applied for 0.1 or 0.2 msec). Similarly, when the stimulus intensity was increased to 1 V, it had to be applied for 0.1 msec before it became effective. With further increase in strength, the duration of the stimulus decreased, but only up to a limit above which there was no further decrease in the duration of a stimulus.

Q.2. What is rheobase?

- **Rheobase:** It is the minimum strength of stimulus current (0.5 V in this case) which when passed for an adequate time (measured in msec) will produce an action potential.
- The time for which the rheobase is passed is called the utilization time (0.3 msec in this case). The utilization time decreases as strength of stimulus increases.

Q.3. What is chronaxie, and what is its significance?

- **Chronaxie:** It is the minimum duration of time for which a current twice the rheobase ($0.5 \times 2 = 1$ V in this case) must be passed to elicit a response. Thus, the chronaxie is 0.1 msec in the case cited here.
- Chronaxie is an indicator of the excitability of a tissue; shorter the chronaxie, greater is the excitability, and vice versa. Chronaxie curves are charted in lesions of nerves or muscles to assess the degree of damage and to follow the progress of recovery.

Q.4. What are the chronaxie values of different excitable tissues?

- The chronaxie values of excitable tissues are given in **Table 1**.

Table 1: Chronaxie values of different excitable tissues.

Tissues	*Chronaxie (msec)*
Large myelinated nerve fibers	0.1
Small myelinated nerve fibers	0.2
Nonmyelinated nerve fibers	0.5
Skeletal muscle fibers	0.5–1
Cardiac muscle fibers	1–3

- It is obvious that the large myelinated nerve fibers are the most excitable of the tissues, i.e. their threshold is the lowest of these tissues.

5.5: ACTION POTENTIAL IN A LARGE MYELINATED NERVE FIBER (FIGS. 5A TO C)

Q.1. What is resting membrane potential, and what is its cause? How is this potential recorded?

- **Resting membrane potential (RMP):**
  - Under resting unstimulated conditions, a potential difference exists across the cell membranes of most cells, the inside being negative relative to the outside of the cell. By convention, this RMP is indicated with a negative sign.
  - The RMP varies from tissue to tissue, ranging from –6 to –100 mV. In the excitable tissues, nerve and muscle cells, the RMP is usually between –70 and –90 mV.
  - The cell membranes are selectively permeable to various ions due to the presence of ion channels which are transmembrane proteins embedded in the bilipid cell membrane.
  - A portion of the protein molecule functions as a sort of "lid" or "gate" over the outer [extracellular fluid (ECF)] or inner [intracellular fluid (ICF)] side of the aqueous pore of the ion channel. The movements of these gates are controlled by changes in the membrane potential, i.e. these gates open or close at specific membrane potentials. Such channels are called voltage-gated channels (there are ligand-gated channels also which open when a chemical agent attaches to the ion channel).
- **Cause of resting membrane potential:**
  - The Na^+/K^+ pump (an ATPase) located in the cell membrane maintains a high concentration of K^+ ions inside the cell (ICF), and a high concentration of Na^+ ions outside the cell (ECF).
  - As a result of this concentration gradient, the K^+ ions passively diffuse out of the cell through the continuously open K^+ leak channels (they are only slightly permeable to Na^+ ions, hence they are also called K^+/Na^+ leak channels).
  - However, the K^+ ions that move out of the cell do not enter the ECF, but instead they stick to the outside of the membrane where they are balanced by the negatively charged impermeant anions (mainly proteins, also organic phosphates, and sulfates) sticking to the inside of the membrane.
  - When the amount of K^+ bound to the outside of the membrane is sufficient to cause a membrane potential (MP) that can prevent any net increase in K^+ efflux, a state of equilibrium is reached. In this state, the MP is equal to the Nernst potential for K^+ (Ek), which is -90 mV.
- **Recording of resting membrane potential:**
  - The RMP can be recorded by placing one electrode on the outside of the fiber, while a glass capillary microelectrode (tip diameter less than 0.5 urn) is inserted (pierced) into the interior of the fiber. When the electrodes are connected, through a suitable amplifier to a CRO, the RMP is recorded.
  - Another method of recording RMP is to crush a small segment of the nerve fiber so that the outside of the fiber in this region becomes equally negative as is the inside. One electrode placed on the injured part, and the other on the nearby uninjured region will record a potential difference—the so-called injury potential (a microelectrode is thus not required).

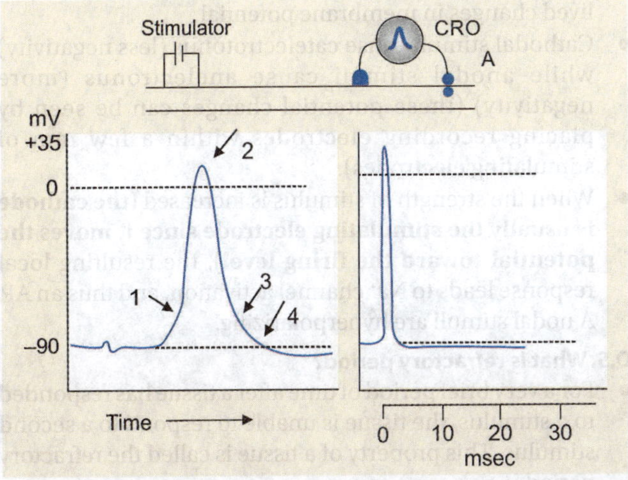

FIGS. 5A TO C: Diagram of action potential in a thick mammalian myelinated nerve fiber. (A) Method of recording monophasic action potential; (B) Action potential drawn with time distortion to show its various components. Arrows 1—firing level, 2—overshoot and start of repolarization (positive part of action potential), 3—repolarization slows down, 4—beginning of afterdepolarization; (C) Action potential drawn without time distortion, showing the typical spike.

Q.2. What is an action potential and how is it recorded? What is its practical application?

- **Action potential (AP):**
  - An AP is the rapid and sequential change in the membrane potential of a nerve (or muscle) fiber when it is conducting an impulse.
  - The AP is the "signal" that is transmitted along the cell membrane without decrement, and is the only proof of conduction of activity.
  - The AP in a nerve fiber is called a nerve impulse (nerve AP), while an AP in a muscle fiber is called the muscle AP (muscle impulse).
  - An action potential has two phases—(1) the **upstroke** or **depolarization** (excitation) which is due to sodium influx, and (2) a **downstroke or repolarization** (recovery) which is due to efflux of potassium ions.
- **Recording of action potential:**
  - The AP can be recorded by using either extracellular or intracellular electrodes.
  - The intracellular electrodes record the resting membrane potential (RMP) and AP which is monophasic, i.e. in one direction.
  - Extracellular electrodes where both the electrodes are placed on or near a nerve or muscle, record a biphasic AP, but not the resting potential.
- **Clinical application:** Extracellular recordings are useful in recording the electrical activity of the excitable tissues in clinical situations such as
  - Electrocardiogram (ECG)

- Electroencephalogram (EEG)
- Electromyogram (EMG; recordings from nerves and muscles)
- Electroretinogram (ERG), and so on.

Q.3. What are the components of an action potential and what is their ionic basis?

- The record of an action potential shown in the **Figures 5A to C** shows the following components:
  - **The stimulus artifact:** This is due to leakage of current from the stimulating to the recording electrodes, and though undesirable, it marks the point of stimulation.
  - The **latent period** (isopotential interval) extends from this point to the start of depolarization and is due to the conduction of the impulse [the slower and partial depolarization from -90 to about -75 mV produced by a marginal stimulus is called the **local response** which is a graded response (this is not shown earlier in the Figure above)].
  - The rapid depolarization from the firing level of -75 mV to the overshoot (i.e. reversal of potential to +40 mV), and the quick fall of potential to about -75 mV constitutes the **spike potential** (its shape resembles that of spike; duration = 0.4 msec) (the overshoot and reversed potential above the zero potential is called the positive part of the action potential).
  - The repolarization from -75 mV to the resting potential is termed **after depolarization (negative after potential).** After the resting membrane potential is reached, the membrane remains slightly hyperpolarized for 40–50 msec, a phase called after hyperpolarization (positive after potential).
- **Ionic basis:**
  - In addition to potassium leak channels, which are responsible for the resting potential, the cell membrane also contains voltage-gated Na^+ channels (fast channels) and voltage-gated K^+ channels.
  - The outer gate (**m gate**) of Na^+ channel is called the activation gate, while its inner gate (**h gate**) is called inactivation gate.
  - The K^+ channel has only one gate—the outer or **n gate**.
  - These gates open and/or close in response to changes in the membrane potential.
  - **Spike potential:**
    - At rest, both voltage-gated Na^+ and K^+ channels are closed (**m** and **n** gates closed, **h** gates open).
    - A slight decrease in membrane potential causes a few Na^+ channels to open, but the increased efflux of K^+ restores the RMP. However, if the depolarization causes more Na^+ channels to open, there is greater influx of Na^+ and greater depolarization (an example of positive feedback).
    - When the firing level is reached, a large number of Na^+ channels open rapidly (Na^+ channel activation, n gates open) and the membrane permeability to Na^+ ions rises by 500 to 5,000 times.
    - As a result of this, there is a massive influx of positively charged Na^+ ions, the potential rises to zero, and then overshoots to about +40 mV. The E_{Na} of +60 mV is not reached because the Na^+ channels rapidly begin to close (Na^+ channel inactivation, closure of **h** gates) during the later part of the upstroke. Increasing positivity inside also restricts Na^+ influx.
    - The rapid repolarization from + 40 mV to about -75 mV is due to K^+ efflux resulting from the opening of voltage-gated K^+ channels (**n** gates open); these channels open slowly, remain open for a longer time, and close slowly. Thus, it is the time sequence of the opening and closing of these two types of channels which is responsible for the shape of the spike (it may be pointed out that the number of ions involved in RMP and AP is very small, only a fraction of the total number of ions).
  - **After depolarization:**
    - The slowing down of repolarization from -75 mV to -90 mV is due to the slow return of K^+ channels to their closed state.
    - The net movement of positive charges (K^+ ions) restores the resting potential.
  - **After hyperpolarization:**
    - The slight increase in negativity is recorded because a few K^+ ions continue to diffuse out before all the K^+ channels close (closure of **n** gates).
    - Activation of the Na^+–K^+ pump by the Na^+ ions gained during the AP also contributes to this phase. The number of ions involved is very small relative to their total numbers. Significant gains and losses of these ions can only be shown after repeated and prolonged stimulation.

Q.4. What are electrotonic potentials?

- The electrotonic potentials are passive changes in potential as a result of subtraction or addition of charges.
- Subthreshold stimuli, though not able to produce an action potential, do cause small, localized, and short-lived changes in membrane potential.
- Cathodal stimuli cause catelectrotonus (less negativity) while anodal stimuli cause anelectronus (more negativity) (these potential changes can be seen by placing recording electrodes within a few mm of stimulating electrodes).
- When the strength of stimulus is increased (**the cathode is usually the stimulating electrode since it moves the potential toward the firing level**), the resulting local response leads to Na^+ channel activation, and thus an AP. A nodal stimuli are hyperpolarizing.

Q.5. What is refractory period?

- For a very brief period of time after a tissue has responded to a stimulus, the tissue is unable to respond to a second stimulus. This property of a tissue is called the refractory period.
- During the refractory period a cell is incapable of repeating an action potential. In terms of action potentials, it refers to the amount of time it takes for an excitable membrane to be ready to respond to a second stimulus once it returns to a resting state.

Q.6. What is absolute refractory period and what is its cause?

- **The absolute refractory period (ARP)** corresponds to the period of time from the point of firing level to about one-third of repolarization.
- During ARP, an extra stimulus, however strong it may be, will not produce a second action potential.
- The refractoriness is due to the closure of **h** gates of Na^+ channels, and these gates will not start to open until repolarization is about one-third complete.
- The ARP decides the number of impulses (APs) that can be transmitted along a nerve fiber. For example, if the ARP is 1 msec, the fiber can transmit about 1,000 impulses/sec.

Q.7. What is relative refractory period?

- **The relative refractory period** (RRP) lasts from the end of absolute refractory period (ARP) to the start of after depolarization.
- During this period, stimuli stronger than normal can cause excitation.
- The excitability of the nerve is increased during after depolarization, while it is decreased during after hyperpolarization. Thus, refractory period lasts during action potential.

Q.8. What is a compound action potential?

- In a mixed nerve containing fibers of different diameters, recordings made at some distance from the point of stimulation show a complex action potential showing many spikes. This multipeaked AP is called compound AP.
- The first spike to arrive belongs to the fastest conducting Aα fibers; this is followed by Aβ and AS spikes. If group B and C fibers are also present, their spikes will also be seen.
- To record this potential, a part of the nerve is crushed so that this region remains in a depolarized state. One electrode placed on this injured region and the other on a nearby uninjured part will record injury potential. When the nerve is stimulated at a distance, the arrival of APs will cause the injury potential to disappear, thus producing many peaks.

Q.9. How is an action potential propagated?

- The propagation of an action potential involves the generation of APs on contiguous patches of the membrane along the nerve fiber.
- The depolarized area of the membrane acts as a "current sink" which draws positive charges from the adjacent polarized regions and this result in passive current flow. Because "new" APs are being generated constantly, the magnitude of the APs does not change as it is being propagated.
- The speed of conduction of the AP is proportional to the square root of the fiber diameter.
- In a myelinated fiber, the AP propagates at a fast speed due to *saltatory conduction*, the AP jumping from one node of Ranvier to the next because the cell membrane is exposed to the extracellular fluid only at the nodes.

5.6: ACTION POTENTIALS IN CARDIAC MUSCLE FIBERS (FIG. 6)

Q.1. What type of action potentials are recorded from the cardiac muscle cells?

- There are two types of cardiac muscle fibers:
  - (1) Those present in the cardiac impulse generating and conducting system [sinoatrial (SA) and atrioventrivular (AV) nodes, bundle of His, and its branches] and
  - (2) the normal "working" or contracting cells which make up the bulk of the atria and ventricles including the subendocardial plexus of Purkinje fibers.
  - The pacemaker (P) cells of the SA and AV nodes are slow (or slow response) fibers having a slow speed of conduction,
  - The rest of the fibers are fast (or fast response) fibers. Under abnormal conditions (e.g. hypoxia due to ischemia), the fast fibers can become slow fibers and generate action potentials.
  - The pacemaker cells (p cells) of SA and AV nodes have unsteady resting potential and show pacemaker potentials, while the working cells are characterized

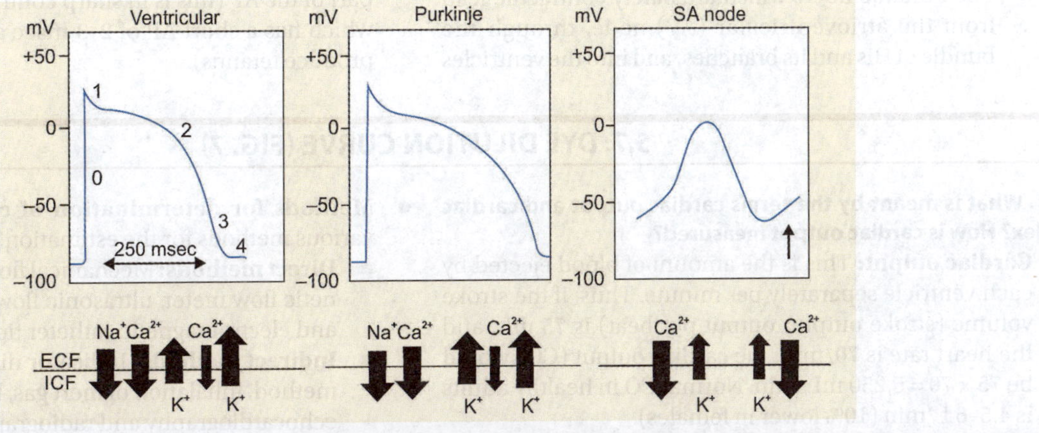

FIG. 6: Diagram showing action potentials in cardiac muscle fibers showing the duration, strength, and period of flow of ions (ionic currents) underlying the potentials. Phase 4 in SA node fiber is unsteady (arrow).
(ECF: extracellular fluid; ICF: intracellular fluid; SA: sinoatrial)

by a steady resting potential, and when excited, a 4-phase action potential that shows a plateau **(Fig. 6)**.

Q.2. Discuss briefly the course of the action potential of working myocardial cells? What is the cause and significance of the plateau?

- The sharp depolarization (upstroke—phase 0) in the action potential of the working myocardial cell is due to the activation (opening) of the fast Na^+ channels and the rapid Na^+ influx (the Na^+ current, INa^+; as in nerve, Na^+ influx is favored by the electrostatic charges across the cell membrane, i.e. positivity outside and negativity inside).
- The initial rapid repolarization (phase 1) is due to increased conductance of Cl^- and K^+ ions and inactivation of Na^+ channels. This is followed by the plateau.
  - **Cause of the plateau:** The plateau [the flat part of action potential; sustained depolarization] is due to Ca^{2+} influx through the more slowly opening voltage-gated Ca^{2+} channels (the Ca^{2+} current, ICa^{2+}; channels start to open at a potential of about –50 mV). The slow opening and the still slower closing of the Ca^{2+} channels results in a sustained depolarization—the plateau.
  - **The significance of the plateau:** Calcium enters the cell during the plateau (phase 2), and is added to the Ca^{2+} released from the terminal cisterns. The prolonged availability of the activator Ca^{2+} to the contractile machinery of the cell causes a prolonged contraction phase of the cardiac muscle. Since the AP and the period of Ca^{2+} removal from the cytoplasm are nearly equal, summation and tetanus are not possible (the force of contraction can vary with the amount of calcium entering the cell).
- The final rapid repolarization (phase 3) is due to inactivation of calcium channels, and a relatively rapid increase in K^+ permeability; the resulting K^+ efflux completes the repolarization.
- In between the APs (phase 4), the working cells show a steady resting potential of –90 mV. In the heart, these cells are excited by cardiac impulses originating in the sinoatrial (SA) node.
- **Purkinje cells:**
  - The Purkinje fibers which are barely contractile lead from the atrioventricular (AV) node, through the bundle of His and its branches, and into the ventricles where they become continuous with the ventricular muscle fibers.
  - Compared to ventricular muscle fibers which have a conduction velocity of 0.3–0.5 m/sec, the Purkinje fibers conduct APs at a speed of 2–4 m/sec.
  - The Purkinje fibers also exhibit the longest plateau phase of any cardiac fibers which also provides them with the longest refractory period (this prevents a backward conduction of depolarization).
- The various parts of the conductive system and under abnormal conditions (e.g. ischemia), parts of the myocardium are capable of spontaneous discharges.

Q.3. Describe the electrical activity of pacemaker cells.

- **Pacemaker potentials:** The rhythmically discharging cells (normally present only in sinoatrial and atrioventricular nodes) have a membrane potential of about –55 to –60 mV. After each action potential, this potential slowly declines to the firing (threshold) level. This slow diastolic depolarization (it occurs during diastole of heart), also called "pacemaker potential" or "prepotential" is the cause of automaticity.
- The APs in pacemaker cells are largely due to Ca^{2+} influx through the L (long-lasting) Ca^{2+} channels, with hardly any contribution by Na^+ influx.
- Because of this, there is no rapid depolarization, hardly any overshoot, or a sharp spike. At the peak of each AP, K^+ efflux brings about repolarization; then K^+ efflux decreases and the membrane begins to depolarize (early part of prepotential). The later part of prepotential is due to Ca^{2+} influx through the T (for transient) Ca^{2+} channels.

Q.4. How much is the absolute refractory period of cardiac muscle? What is the advantage of this period?

- The cardiac muscle fiber is absolutely refractory to a second stimulus during most of its action potential, i.e. throughout the contractile response of 0.3 seconds.
- It means that cardiac muscle fiber must begin to relax before it can respond to another stimulus, i.e. the cardiac muscle cannot be tetanized.
- Refractoriness is, therefore, a safety mechanism for the pumping action of the heart.
- This muscle fiber is relatively refractory during the last part of the AP (this is in sharp contrast to skeletal muscle which has a short AP of 2–3 msec and repetitive stimuli produce tetanus).

5.7: DYE DILUTION CURVE (FIG. 7)

Q.1. What is meant by the terms cardiac output and cardiac index? How is cardiac output measured?

- **Cardiac output:** This is the amount of blood ejected by each ventricle separately per minute. Thus, if the stroke volume (stroke output, output per beat) is 75 mL, and the heart rate is 70/min, the cardiac output (CO) would be 75 × 70 = 5,250 mL/min. Normal CO in healthy adults is 4.5–6 L/min (10% lower in females).
- **Cardiac index** is the cardiac output per m^2 body surface area. Normal: 2.4–3.5 L/min, slightly higher in males, and considerably higher in children.
- **Methods for determination of cardiac output:** The various methods for the estimation of CO are:
  - **Direct methods:** Mechanical flow meter, electromagnetic flow meter, ultrasonic flow meter, cardiometry, and electromagnetic catheter tip velocity meter.
  - **Indirect methods:** Indicator dilution methods, Fick method, inhalation of inert gas, ballistocardiography, echocardiography and radiographic methods.

Q.2. What is the basis of indicator dilution methods for determining cardiac output? Describe the dye dilution method and compare it with thermal dilution method.

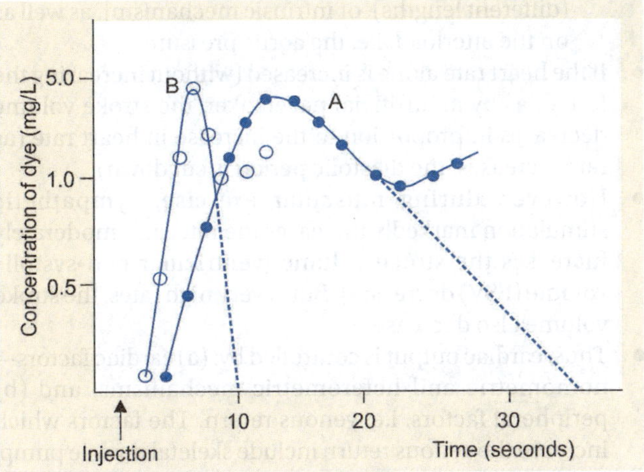

FIG. 7: Indicator dye (Evans blue) concentration curves plotted on semi-logarithmic paper. (A) Subject at rest, (B) Subject during exercise.

- **Basis of indicator dilution methods:**
  - If a suitable indicator (I = amount injected) is added to an unknown volume of fluid (V), the volume of the fluid can be estimated from the resulting concentration of the indicator (C) with the equation V = I/C (using Evans blue dye, this method is employed for estimation of the blood volume).
  - Similarly, the flow (F) of a fluid can be measured if the mean concentration of the indicator (C) is determined for the time (T) required for that indicator to pass a given site. The flow (F) is measured from the equation: F/C × T.
- **Indicators employed:** Some of the indicators are:
  - Evans blue (T-1824)
  - Cardiogreen
  - Hypotonic and hypertonic saline
  - Ascorbate
  - Cold saline, and
  - Radioactive isotopes.
- **Hamilton's dye dilution method:**
  - A known amount of the dye Evans blue is rapidly injected into the arm vein and its mean concentration in a series of samples of brachial arterial blood collected at 1–2 sec intervals, is determined photoelectrically (brachial artery puncture can be avoided by measuring the rise and fall of dye concentration in plasma by shining a light through the vasodilated ear lobe on to a photocell).
  - Usually, recirculation of the dye occurs before the passage of dye is complete, i.e. the concentration starts to rise as shown earlier in the **Figure 7**.
  - After the peak concentration is reached, the exponential decrease in dye concentration is extrapolated to zero concentration, and the mean concentration of the dye during the time period is calculated.
  - **Calculation:** Cardiac output (F) = 60 × I/C × T, where I is the amount of dye injected, C is the mean concentration of dye during first circulation in mg/L, and T is the time taken for first circulation in seconds.

In the resting state example shown in the **Figure 7:**

$$\text{Cardiac output} = \frac{60 \times 5}{35 \times 1.5} = 5.6 \text{ L/min}$$

Dye injected = 5 mg; mean concentration in 35 seconds = 1.5 mg/L

For the exercise example:

$$\text{Cardiac output} = \frac{60 \times 5}{10 \times 1.4} = 21.4 \text{ L/min}$$

Dye injected = 5 mg; mean concentration in 10 seconds = 1.4 mg/L

- **Thermodilution method:**
  - A double-lumen catheter with a thermistor at its tip is inserted into the arm vein and floated into the pulmonary artery.
  - Cold saline is injected through a proximal opening which lies within the right ventricle.
  - The temperature change of blood measured by the thermistor which lies downstream is inversely proportionate to the amount of blood flowing through the pulmonary artery.
  - It is a preferred method because the saline is harmless, there is little change in temperature of surrounding tissues, and no recirculation occurs.

Q.3. What is Fick principle and what is its application in physiology?

- **Fick principle:** The Fick principle states that the amount of substance (X) taken up (or removed) by an organ (or by whole body) is equal to the rate of blood flow (Q) multiplied by the difference between the concentration of the substance before (C_1) and after (C_2) passing through the organ, i.e. $X = Q (C_1 - C_2)$

$$Q = \frac{X}{C_1 \times C_2}$$

- The Fick principle (Adolf Fick, 1870) is an important concept which is used to measure the cardiac output as well as the blood flow through any organ (kidney, brain, liver, etc.). This is also the standard method against which all other methods of estimating cardiac output are checked.
- **Determination of cardiac output by Fick method:** By measuring the amount of oxygen (O_2) taken up per minute by the venous blood as it passes through the lungs, and the O_2 concentration difference between the arterial blood and mixed venous blood, the blood flow through the lungs can be calculated.

$$\text{Cardiac output} = \frac{\text{Oxygen consumption per minute}}{\text{Arteriovenous oxygen difference}}$$

- Since the cardiac output of the two ventricles is identical, **Figure 7** also gives the output of the left ventricle.
- **Indirect Fick method:** In this method where carbon dioxide (CO_2) excretion by the lungs is used, arterial puncture and cardiac catheterization are avoided. Arterial CO_2 is determined from alveolar air sample, while mixed venous blood CO_2 is estimated by rebreathing into a closed bag. The CO_2 in the bag comes into equilibrium with venous blood in the lungs. The rebreathing is done in an interrupted manner so that blood CO_2 is not increased.

Q.4. How is cardiac output regulated?

- **Factors affecting cardiac output:**
  - Changes in heart rate and/or stroke volume can cause changes in the cardiac output.
  - The heart rate is primarily controlled by the cardiac nerves—the sympathetic stimuli increasing it (chronotropic effect), while vagus has opposite effect.
  - The stroke volume, which depends on the strength, speed, and extent of contraction of ventricular muscle [and, of course, on ventricular end-diastolic volume (VEDV)] is determined partly by neural signals—sympathetic stimuli increasing the force of contraction (inotropic effect) at any given fiber length [homometric (same length) or extrinsic regulation].
  - The force of cardiac contraction is also dependent on its preload, i.e. the degree to which the cardiac fibers are stretched by the blood [Frank-Starling, heterometric (different lengths), or intrinsic mechanism], as well as on the afterload, i.e. the aortic pressure.
- If the heart rate alone is increased (without increasing the force), as by an artificial pacemaker, the stroke volume decreases in proportion to the increase in heart rate (as rate increases, the diastolic period is cut down).
- However, during muscular exercise, sympathetic stimulation markedly increases the rate, and moderately increases the stroke volume [ventricular end-systolic volume (ESV) decreases]. But at very high rates, the stroke volume also decreases.
- Thus, cardiac output is controlled by: (a) cardiac factors—homometric and heterometric mechanisms, and (b) peripheral factors, i.e. venous return. The factors which increase the venous return include skeletal muscle pump, respiratory pump, pressure gradient, and the volume of blood.

5.8: ORAL GLUCOSE TOLERANCE TEST (OGTT) (FIG. 8)

Q.1. How is oral glucose tolerance test curve obtained?

- **Oral glucose tolerance test (OGTT):** This test is carried out according to the following protocol:
- The patient is placed on a diet which includes 200–300 g of carbohydrates per day for 3 days prior to the test (starvation produces a diabetic type of response).
- The subject fasts for 15 h before the test which is generally done in the morning.
- Urine and fasting venous blood samples are collected for their glucose concentrations.
- The patient then drinks 75 g of glucose (50 g in children under 14 years of age) in 300 mL of water over 5 min.
- Venous blood samples are then collected after 30 min, 60 min, 90 min, 120 min, and sometimes, after 150 min and 180 min. Urine is collected after 60 min and 120 min.

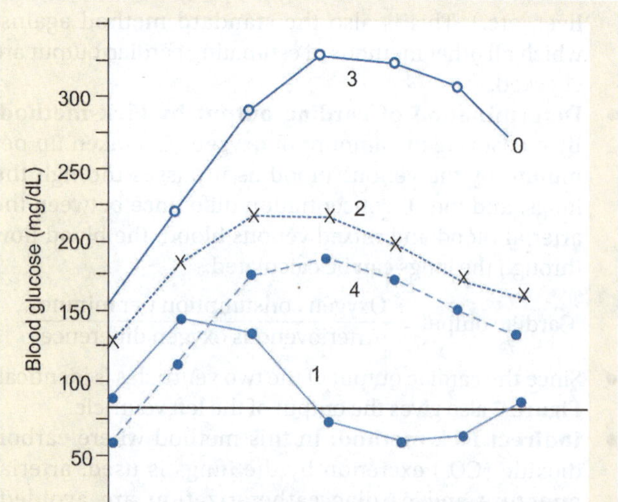

FIG. 8: Oral glucose tolerance curves. (1) Normal, (2) Mild diabetes mellitus, (3) Severe diabetes mellitus, and (4) Liver disease.

- The glucose concentrations of the blood samples are determined and plotted against time (intravenous glucose, 0.5 g/kg body weight, is sometimes used, particularly in cases of abnormalities of intestinal absorption of glucose).

Q.2. Describe the normal glucose tolerance curve.

- Normally, the fasting venous plasma glucose level varies between 80 mg% and 90 mg% (4.4–4.9 mmol/L), the upper limit of the normal being 110 mg% (6 mmol/L) [A fasting level less than 110 mg% excludes diabetes mellitus (DM)].
- After ingesting glucose, the peak level of 130–140 mg% is reached in about 30–40 min. The glucose level starts decreasing and falls back to fasting value, and then to below fasting level in about 120–150 min.
- The 120 min value is less than 140 mg% (7.8 mmol/L), and no value exceeds the renal threshold of glucose of 180 mg% (9.9 mmol/L). No sample of urine contains glucose.

Q.3. What is the renal threshold for glucose?

- **Renal threshold for glucose:** It is the *plasma level of glucose* at which glucose first appears in the urine in more than the normal minute amounts (normal urine contains a few mg of glucose which are undetectable with the usual tests).
- The renal threshold for glucose is 180 mg%. As long as blood glucose level is below this level, all the filtered glucose is reabsorbed in the proximal tubules, but when the level exceeds 180 mg%, all the excess glucose is excreted in the urine.

Q.4. Describe the glucose tolerance curve in diabetes mellitus.

- The shape of the oral glucose tolerance test curve is quite different in a patient of diabetes mellitus as compared to that of a normal person.
- The fasting blood glucose level is almost always above 110 mg%, and generally above 145 mg%; it may exceed 200 mg% (two fasting levels ≥ 145 mg% confirm the diagnosis of DM).

- The glucose levels after ingestion of glucose, and the peak value depend on whether the patient is *prediabetic* or has *mild* or *severe* diabetes. The peak value, which may cross 300 mg%, is reached only after about 90 min, and the fasting level is reached only after 4–5 h. Also, the glucose level fails to fall below the fasting level. The urine samples show the presence of glucose if the renal threshold is crossed.
- Prolonged OGTT is found in the following:
  - **Diabetes mellitus**
  - **Pituitary diabetes** (due to excess growth hormone), and adrenal diabetes (due to excess of cortisol, the chief glucocorticoid of adrenal cortex).
  - **Liver disease:** The liver is unable to handle the glucose load. The curve resembles that of prediabetes or mild DM, except that the fasting blood glucose level is *below* the normal fasting level.

Comments:

- Glucose is too large a molecule to diffuse through the cell membrane channels into the cells. However, it is transported into all cells by facilitated diffusion, which is a carrier-mediated process. In muscle, adipose, and connective tissues (they form the bulk of the body weight), the cells depend on insulin for glucose entry into them.
- Insulin facilitates this process by increasing the number of glucose transporters [glucose transporter type 4 (GLUT4); there is a family of GLUTs, numbered 1–14]. These GLUTs are different from the sodium-dependent glucose transporters [sodium glucose cotransporters 1 (SGLTs1)] responsible for the secondary active transport of glucose out of the intestinal and renal tubules (the Na^+ concentration gradient and its transport provides the energy for glucose transport). Thus, glucose entry into muscle, adipose, and connective tissue cells requires insulin, while intestine, kidneys, liver, red blood cells (RBCs), and most of the brain does not require insulin for glucose entry.
- In a normal person, the artificial hyperglycemia produced by glucose ingestion causes the release of insulin from the pancreas (glucose acts directly on the beta cells, an example of substrate control of hormone secretion). About 60% of the absorbed glucose is converted into glycogen and stored in the liver, and the rest is utilized by the peripheral tissues over the next 60–90 min. The insulin released by glucose causes a slight hypoglycemia.
- However, in DM, there is already a persistent hyperglycemia due to lack of insulin secretion from the pancreas (type I DM), or diminished responsiveness of the peripheral tissues to the actions of insulin (type II DM). A glucose load further raises the blood glucose, which also returns to the baseline much more slowly than normal. Also, there is no hypoglycemia following the return of blood glucose to the fasting level.

Q.5. What is tubular load? How much is it for glucose?

- *The tubular load* or the *filtration load*, is the amount of a substance delivered to the renal tubules per minute due to the process of filtration.
- It depends on the plasma level of that substance and the glomerular filtration rate (GFR). With a blood glucose level of 80 mg%, and a GFR of 125 mL/min, the tubular load is about 100 mg/min (80 × 125/100). When the glucose level is 180 mg% (renal threshold for glucose), the tubular load is 225 mg% (180 × 125/100).

Q.6. What is meant by transport maximum? How much is the transport maximum for glucose?

- *The transport maximum (Tm)* is the maximal rate at which substances that are actively reabsorbed (e.g. glucose, some amino acids, uric acid, phosphates, and possibly albumin) or secreted (e.g. creatinine, PAH, penicillin, etc.) can be transported across the tubular epithelial cells.
- This maximum limit is due to the saturation of the specific carrier systems—proteins or enzymes—involved in the process.
- The transport maximum for glucose (TmG) in the adult individual is about 320 mg/min (350 in males and 300 in females). This means that a maximum of 320 mg of glucose can be transported (reabsorbed), per minute, from the tubular fluid of both kidneys into the blood.
- TmG is nearly constant and depends on the number of functioning tubules. Tm is, therefore, used clinically to assess renal function.
- Substances absorbed passively do not have a transport maximum.
- Some solutes have no definite upper limit for unidirectional transport, and hence, have no Tm.
- The reabsorption of Na^+ along the nephron has no Tm, and secretion of K^+ by the distal tubules has no Tm.

Comments: As mentioned earlier, glucose and Na^+ bind to a common carrier sodium glucose cotransporter 1 (SGLT1) in the luminal membrane and as Na^+ moves down its concentration and electrical gradients, glucose is also carried into the cells. The Na^+ is then pumped out of the cell by the Na^+-K^+ pump into the lateral intercellular spaces and glucose is transported by glucose transporter type 2 (GLUT2) into the interstitial spaces via the basal cell membrane, and hence into the peritubular capillaries by simple diffusion. As in the intestine, it is the difference in the luminal and basolateral GLUTs that makes it possible for a net movement of glucose across these epithelial cells. Renal tubular transport of glucose, as also of intestinal, is not facilitated by insulin.

Q.7. If TmG is 320 mg/min, why does glucose appear in the urine when the plasma glucose level is 180 mg%, at which the tubular load is 225 mg/min?

- With a TmG of 320 mg/min, and a glomerular filtration rate (GFR) of 125 mL/min, one would predict that the renal threshold for glucose would be 256 mg% (320/125 × 100 = 256). That is, glucose would first appear in the urine at a plasma glucose level of 256 mg%.
- However, the actual renal threshold is 180 mg%, at which the tubular load is 225 mg/min.
- The reason for this discrepancy is the following:
  - The renal tubules show considerable variability in their length, filtration and reabsorption capacities.
  - Some tubules have a much lower TmG than others. In these tubules, some glucose remains unabsorbed (after saturation of the carrier system) even at a lower plasma glucose level, and is excreted in urine.
  - *This phenomenon, called splay,* refers to the curved portion observed in glucose reabsorption and excretion graphs.

- Though the affinity of the transport system is high, a finite concentration of glucose must remain in the tubular fluid to fully saturate the transport system. Some glucose may remain unabsorbed before saturation occurs.

Q.8. What are the causes of hyperglycemia and what are its effects?

- **Diabetes mellitus** is the major cause of hyperglycemia.
- Secondary forms of diabetes occur in **chronic pancreatitis, pheochromocytoma** (excess adrenalin from adrenal medulla), acromegaly (excess growth hormone), and Cushing's syndrome (excess cortisol).
- It is also present when there is excessively rapid absorption of glucose after meals, especially after gastrectomy, etc. It may also be encountered after meals in liver disease.
- **Effects of hyperglycemia:**
  - The effects are due to an increase in the osmolality (osmotic pressure) of the blood.
  - As tubular load exceeds TmG, glucose appears in the urine (glycosuria). The presence of large amounts of osmotically active glucose particles in the filtrate causes loss of large amounts of water (polyuria due to osmotic diuresis); there is also loss of large amounts of Na^+ and K^+ as well.
  - The resulting dehydration leads to excessive water drinking (polydipsia) via the thirst center of the hypothalamus.
  - The intracellular deficiency of glucose in the neurons of the feeding center of the hypothalamus causes excessive eating (polyphagia).

Comments: The long-term damaging effects of DM are primarily due not to hyperglycemia, but to abnormal lipid metabolism; the major tissues of the body switching over from the carbohydrate to fat metabolism in the absence of insulin. Excessive breakdown of fats causes hyperlipidemia, ketosis, and ketoacidosis. Atherosclerosis of retinal arteries may cause blindness, while in the coronary, cerebral, and renal arteries, it may lead to myocardial infarction, cerebral hemorrhage (stroke), or renal failure. There is loss of body weight due to the depletion of fat and protein stores. In fact, DM has been called more a disease of fat metabolism than of carbohydrate metabolism.

Q.9. What is hypoglycemia and what are its effects?

- A plasma glucose level of less than about 45 mg% is called hypoglycemia. However, the level at which symptoms appear varies markedly from person to person, especially in diabetics.
- Hypoglycemia may be fasting (no food taken), or postprandial (or reactive; after meals).
- The most common cause of fasting *hypoglycemia* is overzealous treatment (overdosage) of diabetes mellitus with insulin injection (in type I DM), or sulfonylurea (which is taken orally, in type II DM).
- It may also occur in islet cell tumors, liver failure, and pituitary insufficiency. Alcoholics on a drinking binge may forget to ingest food.
- Hypoglycemia after meals occurs after gastric surgery or vagotomy (done in cases of peptic ulcer), where rapid gastric emptying and rapid glucose absorption cause excessive release of insulin. Plasma glucose falls more rapidly than the insulin level, and hypoglycemia results.
- The symptoms of hypoglycemia include sweating, tremors, anxiety, and hunger which are due to sympathetic stimulation and release of adrenalin from adrenal medulla. The central nervous system (CNS) symptoms include dizziness, diminished mental activity, personality changes, convulsions, and coma.

Comments: The maintenance of plasma glucose within narrow limits is essential for health. Hypoglycemia is dangerous, more serious in the short run than hyperglycemia because glucose is the primary energy source of the brain. In contrast to other tissues, brain cannot utilize free fatty acids (FFAs) as energy source. Though, short-chain metabolites of FFA, such as acetoacetic acid and beta-hydroxybutyric acid, can be efficiently oxidized by the brain, ketosis requires many hours to develop. Therefore, absence of glucose, like that of oxygen (O_2), produces deranged function, tissue damage, or even death if the deficit is prolonged.

Q.10. What is renal glycosuria?

- The presence of glucose in the urine even when the renal threshold for glucose of 180 mg% is not exceeded is called *renal glycosuria*, i.e. glycosuria due to renal disease.
- It is a congenital disorder associated with a low renal threshold for glucose.

Calculations

SECTION 6

Calculations are another method of assessing the students' understanding of the subject. The calculations included in this section are based on idealized 'given' data. However, when students are tested on these, the teacher often 'manipulates' the given data. A student should be able to explain and reason out why the results are at variance with the expected normal values.

Q.1. Calculate the velocity of nerve impulse in the frog's nerve-muscle preparation from the data given below.

Data

(a) Latent period with stimulation of spinal end of the nerve = 0.01 sec

(b) Latent period with stimulation of muscle end of the nerve = 0.005 sec

(c) Length of the nerve between the two stimulated points = 7.5 cm

---

Difference in the two latent periods

= 0.01 – 0.005 sec = 0.005 sec

Distance travelled by the nerve impulses in 0.005 sec = 7.5 cm

Distance travelled by the nerve impulses in 1 sec

$$= \frac{7.5 \times 1000}{5}$$

= 1500 cm

The velocity of the nerve impulse = 15 m/sec.

Q.2. Calculate the work done by the muscle from the following data.

Data

(a) Height of recorded contraction (H) = 5 cm

(b) Long arm of the lever (L, from fulcrum to writing point) = 15 cm

(c) Short arm of the lever (l, from fulcrum to point of load) = 2.5 cm

(d) Weight (load) lifted = 15 g.

$$\text{Magnification factor} = \frac{L}{l} = \frac{15}{2.5} = 6$$

Load lifted = 15 g

Actual height through which load was lifted (h)

$$= \frac{\text{Height of contraction}}{\text{Magnification factor}} = \frac{5}{2.5} = 0.83 \text{ cm}$$

Work done = Load × Height (h) = 15 × 0.83 = 12.45 g cm

Q.3. Determine the absolute counts of neutrophils, eosinophils, and basophils from the data given below.

Data

(a) Total leukocyte count = 7800/mm³

(b) Neutrophil count = 65%

(c) Eosinophil count = 3.5%

(d) Basophil count = 0.5%

Absolute neutrophil count = 7800/100 × 65 = 4875/mm³

Absolute eosinophil count = 7800/100 × 3.5 = 273/mm³

Absolute basophil count = 7800/100 × 0.5 = 39/mm³

Q.4. Determine the mean corpuscular hemoglobin (MCH) from the data given below.

Data

(a) Hemoglobin concentration = 14.5 g/dL

(b) RBC count = 4.8 million/mm³

(c) Packed cell volume = 42%

$$\text{MCH} = \frac{\text{Hb g/dL} \times 10}{\text{RBC count in millions/mm}^3}$$

$$= \frac{14.5 \times 10}{4.8} = 30 \text{ pg } (30\ \mu\text{g})$$

Q.5. Calculate the mean corpuscular volume (MCV) from the data given below.

Data

(a) RBC count = 4.5 million/mm³

(b) Packed cell volume (PCV) = 40%

(c) Hb concentration = 14 g/dL

$$\text{MCH} = \frac{\text{PCV} \times 10}{\text{RBC count in millions/mm}^3}$$

$$= \frac{40 \times 10}{4.5} = 88\ \mu\text{m}^3 \text{ (cubic micrometers)}$$

Q.6. Calculate the mean corpuscular hemoglobin concentration from the data given below.

Data

(a) Hemoglobin concentration = 9 g/dL

(b) Packed cell volume (PCV) = 36%

(c) RBC count = 3.4 million/mm³

$$\text{MCHC} = \frac{\text{Hb g\%}}{\text{PCV}} \times 1000 = \frac{9}{36} \times 100 = 25\%$$

Q.7. Determine the color index from the data given below.

Data

(a) Hb concentration = 16 g/dL
(b) RBC count = 6 million/mm^3
(Normal 100% RBC count = 5.0 million/mm^3)
(Normal 100% Hb = 15 g/dL)

- -

1. 5.0 million/mm^3 RBC count = 100%
   6.0 million/mm^3 RBC count will be 6/5 × 100 = 120%
2. 15.0 g% hemoglobin = 100%
   16.0 g% Hb will be 16/15 × 100 = 107%

$$\text{Color index} = \frac{\text{Hb percent of normal}}{\text{RBC count percent of normal}} = \frac{120}{107} = 0.89$$

Q.8. Calculate the platelet count from the data given below.

Data

(a) Number of platelets in 80 smallest squares = 34
(b) Dilution of blood employed = 1 in 200 (1:200)

- -

Number of platelets in 80 smallest squares = 34
Volume of these 80 squares = 1/50 mm^3
(volume of 1 smallest square = 1/4000 mm^3)
Thus, 1/50 mm^3 contains = 34 platelets
∴ 1 mm^3 contains 34 × 50 = 1700 platelets
Dilution employed is 1 in 200
Number of platelets in undiluted blood = 1700 × 200 = 340,000/mm^3
The platelet count is 3.4 lacs/mm^3.

Q.9. Determine the reticulocyte count from the data given below.

Data

(a) Number of RBCs in 50 oil-immersion fields = 1500
(b) Number of reticulocytes in 100 oil-immersion fields = 45

- -

Number of RBCs in 50 oil-immersion fields = 1500
∴ Number of cells in 100 oil-immersion fields = 3000
Number of reticulocytes in 100 oil-immersion field = 45 (data)
Thus, per 3000 RBCs, there are 45 reticulocytes
∴ Per 100 RBCs, there are 45/3000 × 100 = 1.5 reticulocytes
The reticulocyte count is 1.5% of red cells.

Q.10. Find out the physiological dead space from the data provided below.

Data

(a) Tidal volume = 450 mL
(b) Alveolar air PCO_2 = 40 mm Hg
(c) Expired air PCO_2 = 26 mm Hg

- -

Physiological dead space

$$= \frac{\text{Alveolar air } PCO_2 - \text{Expired air } PCO_2}{\text{Alveolar air } PCO_2} \times \text{Tidal volume}$$

$$= \frac{40 - 26}{40} = 157 \text{ mL.}$$

Q.11. Find out the expiratory reserve volume (ERV); residual volume (RV); inspiratory reserve volume (IRV); and functional residual capacity (FRC) from the given data.

Data

(a) Total lung capacity = 5200 mL
(b) Tidal volume = 450 mL
(c) Inspiratory capacity = 3000 mL
(d) Vital capacity = 4000 mL

- -

ERV	= VC – IC	=	4000 – 3000	= 1000 mL
RV	= TLC – VC	=	5200 – 4000	= 1200 mL
IRV	= IC – TV	=	3000 – 450	= 2550 mL
FRC	= RV + ERV	=	1200 + 1000	= 2200 mL

Note: Consult **Figure 6** of Experiment 2.3 on lung volumes and capacities.

Q.12. Determine the oxygen carrying capacity and oxygen content of arterial and venous blood samples from the data provided below.

Data

(a) Percentage saturation of arterial blood with oxygen = 97%
(b) Percentage saturation of venous blood with oxygen = 75%
(c) Hemoglobin concentration = 14.5 g/dL

- -

Oxygen carrying capacity of blood (mL/100 mL)
= Hb g% × 1.34 = 14.5 × 1.34
= 19.43 mL/dL

$$\text{Formula for } O_2 \text{ content of blood} = \frac{\text{Percentage saturation} \times \text{capacity}}{100}$$

$$\text{Oxygen content of arterial blood} = \frac{97 \times 19.43}{100} = 18.84 \text{ mL/100 mL}$$

$$\text{Oxygen content of venous blood} = \frac{75 \times 19.43}{100} = 14.57 \text{ mL/100 mL}$$

Q.13. Find out the breathing reserve and the dyspnea index from the data provided below.

Data

(a) Respiratory rate = 12/min
(b) Tidal volume = 500 mL
(c) Maximal voluntary ventilation (MVV) = 130 liters
(Syn: maximal ventilatory volume)

- -

Respiratory minute volume (RMV; volume of gas expired per minute) = 500 × 12 = 6000 mL
Breathing reserve = MVV – RMV
= 130–6 = 124 liters.
(It means that the ventilation can be increased from 6 l/min to 130 l/min with maximum effort).
Dyspnea index (Breathing reserve percent)

$$= \frac{\text{MVV} \times \text{RMV}}{\text{MVV}} \times 100 = \frac{130 \times 6}{130} \times 100 = 95\%$$

(When the dyspnea index falls below 70% (dyspnea point), dyspnea is present. We are not conscious of breathing until ventilation is doubled. Breathing is not uncomfortable (i.e., dyspnea point is not reached) until ventilation increases 3 or 4 times the resting level).

Q.14. Calculate the respiratory quotient from the data given below.

Data

(a) Volume of expired air in 6 minutes = 30 liters
(b) Percentage of CO_2 in expired air = 4.2%
(c) Oxygen consumption in 6 minutes = 1470 mL

Volume of expired air in 6 minutes = 30 liters
Volume of expired air in 1 minute = 5 liters
Percentage of CO_2 in expired air = 4.2%
∴ 5000 mL of expired air in 1 minute contain = 5000 × 4.2 = 210 mL of CO_2
Oxygen consumed in 6 minutes = 1470 mL
∴ Oxygen consumed in 1 minute = 1470/6 = 245 mL

$$\text{Respiratory quotient (RQ)} = \frac{CO_2 \text{ output/min}}{O_2 \text{ consumed/min}} = \frac{210}{245} = 0.85$$

Q.15. Find out the basal metabolic rate (BMR) of the subject from the data given below.

Data

(a) Oxygen consumption in 6 minutes = 1470 mL
(b) Body surface area (BSA) of the subject = 1.6 m^2
(c) Standard BMR for the age and sex of the subject = 40 Cal/m^2 BSA/hour

---

Oxygen consumption in 6 minutes = 1470 mL
Oxygen consumption in 1 hour = 14.70 liters
When 1 liter of O_2 is consumed, 4.8 calories are released.
∴ Calories released from consumption of 14.7 liter of O_2 = 4.8 × 14.70 = 70.56

$$\text{BMR} = \frac{\text{Calories consumed/hr}}{\text{Body surface area}} = \frac{70.56}{1.6} = 70.56$$

Standard BMR for the subject = 40 cal/m^2 BSA/hour
∴ Calculated BMR is in excess by 4 calories/m^2 BSA/hour

$$\text{Percentage excess} = \frac{4}{40} = 10\%$$

Thus, the BMR of the subject is = + 10%
(Normal range = ± 15%).

Q.16. Calculate the cardiac index of the individual from his data given below.

Data

(a) Cardiac output = 5.20 liters/min
(b) Body surface area (BSA) = 1.65 m^2

(Cardiac index is the cardiac output per m^2 BSA per minute)

$$\text{Cardiac index} = \frac{\text{Cardiac output/min}}{\text{BSA}} = \frac{5.20}{1.65} = 3.15$$

Cardiac index = 3.15 liters/min.

Q.17. Calculate the heart rate from the ECG provided.

There are two methods to calculate the heart rate from an ECG.

1. Divide 1500 by the number of smallest squares between any two successive R waves:
   Assume there are 18 smallest squares between two R waves:
   Then the heart rate will be 1500/18 = 82/min.
2. Divide 60 by the time interval, in seconds, between two successive R waves:
   Assume there are 21 smallest squares between two R waves:
   21 smallest squares = 0.84 sec
   (each smallest square = 0.04 sec)
   ∴ Heart rate = 60/0.84 = 71/min.

Q.18. Calculate the stroke volume and cardiac output from the data given below.

Data

(a) Oxygen content of mixed venous blood = 14.8 mL/100 mL
(b) Oxygen content of systemic arterial blood = 19.5 mL/100 mL
(c) Heart rate = 70/min
(Mixed venous blood is collected from the right ventricle or pulmonary artery via a catheter. Systemic arterial blood can be taken from any artery)
(d) Oxygen consumption per minute = 245 mL

(The cardiac output is calculated by applying Fick principle).

$$\text{Cardiac output} = \frac{\text{Oxygen consumption}}{\text{Arteriovenous oxygen difference}} \times 100$$

$$\text{Stroke volume} = \frac{245}{19.5 - 14.8} \times 100 = \frac{245}{4.7} \times 100 = 5200 \text{ mL}$$

Comments: In the example cited above, every 100 mL blood that flow through the lungs per minute pick up 4.7 mL of oxygen. Therefore, to pick up 245 mL of oxygen, 5200 mL blood must flow through the lungs per minute. This is an example of Fick principle. Normally, the output of the two ventricles is identical, except at the start of exercise when the output of the right ventricle is higher (due to increased venous return) for a few seconds until the output becomes similar on the two sides.

Q.19. Calculate the effective filtration pressure from the data given below.

Data

(a) Glomerular capillary hydrostatic pressure = 55 mm Hg
(b) Glomerular capillary blood osmotic pressure = 30 mm Hg
(c) Bowman's capsular fluid pressure = 15 mm Hg
(d) Bowman's capsular fluid osmotic pressure = 0 mm Hg.

Effective filtration pressure

Glomer. hydro. pressure **(55 mm Hg)**	–	Glomer. osm. press. **(30 mm Hg)**	+	Bowman. caps. pressure **(15 mm Hg)** = 10 mm Hg

The glomerular hydrostatic pressure is about 55 mm Hg when the mean systemic arterial pressure is 100 mm Hg.

Thus, the effective filtration pressure = 55 – (30 + 15) = 10 mm Hg

The glomerular capillary hydrostatic pressure is about 55 mm Hg when the mean systemic arterial pressure is 100 mm Hg.

Thus, the effective filtration pressure = 55 – (30 + 15) = 10 mm Hg

Comments: The effective filtration pressure is the function of two variables: the hydrostatic pressure gradient driving fluid out of the glomerular capillaries and into Bowman's capsule, and the colloid osmotic pressure gradient bringing fluid into the glomerular capillaries. The colloid osmotic pressure of capsular fluid is near zero because it normally contains little protein—only a few milligrams of albumin which is reabsorbed in the proximal tubules.

Q.20. Calculate the glomerular filtration rate (GFR) from the data provided below.

Data

(a) Concentration of inulin in plasma (P) = 0.24 mg/mL
(b) Concentration of inulin in urine (U) = 34 mg/mL
(c) Rate of urine formation (V) = 0.9 mL/min

Plasma inulin clearance

$$= \frac{\text{Concentration of inulin in urine} \times \text{Volume of urine/min}}{\text{Concentration of inulin in plasma}}$$

$$= \frac{U_{IN} \times V}{P_{IN}} = \frac{34 \times 0.9}{0.24} = 127 \text{ mL/min}$$

Comments: The major determinant of GFR is the hydrostatic pressure within the glomerular capillaries. In addition, the renal blood flow (RBF) through the glomeruli has a great effect on GFR; when the rate of RBF increases, the GFR increases.

The term clearance refers to the volume of plasma from which a substance X is completely removed or "cleared" per unit time, i.e., the mL of plasma that "contained" the substance X that is present in one minute's urine. It is a theoretical volume rather than a volume that can be collected and directly measured. Its value can be calculated from measurable quantities. For example, inulin is only filtered and measures GFR, while p-aminohippuric acid (PAH; see below) is both filtered and secreted into the proximal tubules, and measures renal blood flow (RBF).

Q.21. Calculate the renal blood flow (RBF) from the data given below.

Data

(a) Concentration of PAH in urine (U_{PAH}) = 14 mg/mL
(b) Concentration of PAH in plasma (P_{PAH}) = 0.03 mg/mL
(c) Rate of urine flow (V) = 1.5 mL/min
(d) Hematocrit (Hct) = 43%

$$\text{Plasma clearance of PAH} = \frac{U_{PAH} \times V}{P_{PAH}} = \frac{14 \times 1.5}{0.03} = 700 \text{ mL/min}$$

This plasma clearance of PAH is the effective renal plasma flow (ERPF).

The ERPF can be converted into actual renal plasma flow (RPF):

$$\text{Actual RPF} = \frac{\text{ERPF}}{\text{Extraction ratio}} = \frac{700}{0.9} = 770 \text{ mL/min}$$

(About 90% of PAH in the arterial blood is removed during a single passage through the kidneys, i.e., its extraction ratio is 0.9)

Hematocrit = 43% (given data)

$$\therefore \text{Renal blood flow} = \frac{100}{100 - \text{Hct}} \times \text{RPF} = \frac{100}{100 - 43} \times 770$$

$$= \frac{100}{57} \times 770 = 1350$$

The renal blood flow is 1350 mL per minute.

Q.22 Calculate the urea clearance from the given data.

Data

(a) Concentration of urea in urine (U) = 20 mg/mL
(b) Concentration of urea in blood (B) = 38 mg/100 mL
(c) Rate of urine flow (V) = 1.5 mL/min

Since the urine flow is less than 2.0 mL/min, the formula of "standard" urea clearance is:

$$\frac{U \times \sqrt{V}}{B} \times 100$$

$$\text{Urea clearance} = \frac{20 \times \sqrt{1.5}}{38} \times 100 = \frac{20 \times 1.22}{38} \times 100 = 64 \text{ mL/ min}$$

Comments: It has been shown empirically that with rapid flow of urine (2 mL per minute or more), the excretion of urea is maximum—hence called "maximum" urea clearance. The formula for maximum clearance is UV/P. The value for maximum clearance is 65–100 mL per minute, while the normal value for standard clearance is 40–65 mL per minute.

Sample Problem Solving

SECTION 7

7.1: SAMPLE PROBLEM SOLVING IN HEMATOLOGY

1. Calculate mean corpuscular hemoglobin (MCH) from the following data:

- **Hb: 14 g/dL of blood**
- **RBC count: 4.2 million/cumm of blood**

Name a condition in which MCH is decreased.

Ans. MCH = 33 pg. Iron deficiency anemia (microcytic hypochromic).

2. A child aged 2 years has the following differential count:

- **Polymorphs: 25%**
- **Lymphocyte: 70%**
- **Eosinophil: 2%**
- **Basophil: 1%**
- **Monocyte: 2%**

Comment on the blood picture.

Ans. The child has relative lymphocytosis which is normal for this age.

3. The Hb count is 15 g% and RBC count is 5 million/mm^3. Calculate the MCH.

Ans. 30 pg/cell.

4. If packed cell volume (PCV) is 42% and Hb is 14 g%, find out the mean corpuscular hemoglobin concentration (MCHC).

Ans. 33 g/dL.

5. A patient comes to the OPD with presenting complaints of small bleeding points in the oral cavity and small hemorrhages. BT (bleeding time) is 8 minutes and CT (clotting time) is 4 minutes, platelet count is 270,000/mm^3, prothrombin time is 18 seconds. Give the probable diagnosis and how will you confirm your diagnosis?

Ans. Purpura (See page 83).

6. A patient's peripheral blood picture shows megaloblastic anemia. Endoscopy showed idiopathic atrophy of the gastric mucosa. What is the cause of anemia?

Ans. Lack of intrinsic factor (See page 39).

7. An adult female is on treatment for iron deficiency anemia. What are the possible hematological tests to be done for the therapeutic prognosis?

Ans. Reticulocyte count,Hb level, iron profile, hematocrit.

8. Find out the absolute number of neutrophils, eosinophils and lymphocytes from the following blood count:

- **TLC (total leukocyte count): 9000/mm^3**
- **DLC count is as mentioned below:**
  - **Neutrophil: 56%**
  - **Monocyte: 7%**
  - **Eosinophil: 2%**
  - **Basophil: 1%**
  - **Lymphocyte: 36%**

Comment on the blood picture. Mention the physiological causes of leukocytosis.

Ans. Normal blood picture. Absolute counts: Neutrophil: 5040; Eosinophils: 180; Lymphocytes: 3240; Monocytes: 630; Basophils: 90 (See page 29).

9. A 28-year-old pregnant woman is Rh negative and her husband is Rh positive. What could be the possible consequences following:

- **1st pregnancy**
- **2nd pregnancy**
- **Subsequent pregnancies**

Ans. See page 65.

10. What are the hematological investigations done in a patient with iron deficiency anemia to confirm the diagnosis?

Ans. Peripheral smear, hematocrit, hemoglobin and serum ferritin.

7.2: SAMPLE PROBLEM SOLVING IN CLINICAL PRACTICALS

1. The hemodynamic parameters of a person are as mentioned below:

- **Left ventricular pressure: 120/zero mm Hg**
- **Left atrial pressure: 8/zero mm Hg**
- **Aortic pressure: 120/80 mm Hg**

Find out all the components of blood pressure and comment on the findings.

Ans. Systolic BP: 120 mm Hg, Diastolic BP: 80 mm Hg, Pulse pressure: 40 mm Hg, Mean pressure: 93 mm Hg.
Normal parameters.

2. The cardiovascular parameters recorded in a 20-year-old male subject during an exercise test is as follows:

		Heart rate (bpm)	*Systemic BP (mm Hg)*
a.	At rest	60	110/77
b.	Mild exercise	80	120/70
c.	Moderate exercise	108	130/76
d.	Severe exercise	140	144/84
e.	Very severe exercise	150	160/88

- **What is the WHO criteria of grading of exercise?**
  See page 141
- **Comment on the physical status of the person.**
  The subject has good exercise tolerance and is physically fit.
- **Give suitable explanations for the above cardiovascular changes.**
  See page 142
- **Give two major contraindications for exercise testing.**
  Two major contradictions for exercise testing are:
  1. Recent acute myocardial infarction.
  2. Recent history of unstable angina.

3. Calculate the pulmonary and alveolar ventilation in a person whose respiratory rate is 18 and the tidal volume is 300 mL?

Ans. Pulmonary ventilation is 5400 mL
Alveolar ventilation is 2700 mL.

4. Using the ECG tracing given below calculate the following parameters and comment on the findings.

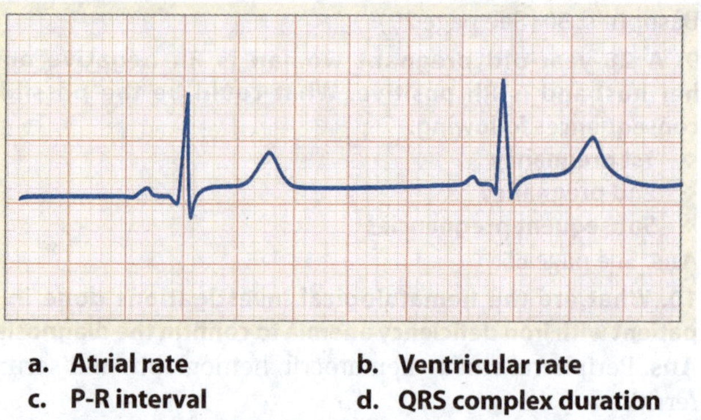

a. Atrial rate **b. Ventricular rate**
c. P-R interval **d. QRS complex duration**

Ans. a. 52/min b. 52/min c. 0.1 6 sec d. 0.06 sec.
This ECG is within normal limits.

5. Using the ECG calculate the mean QRS vector. What is the normal direction of right and left axis deviation and what do they represent?

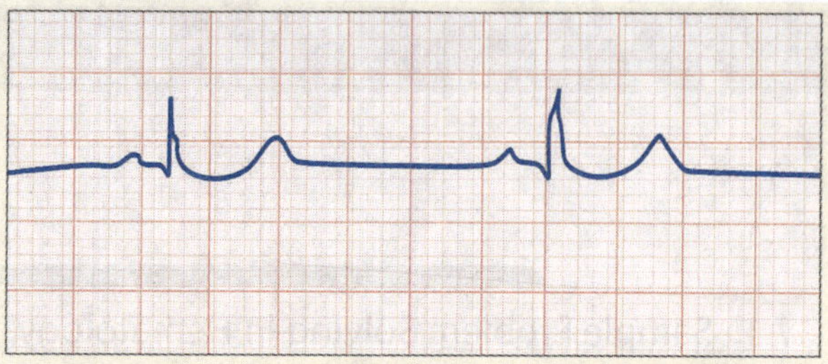

I

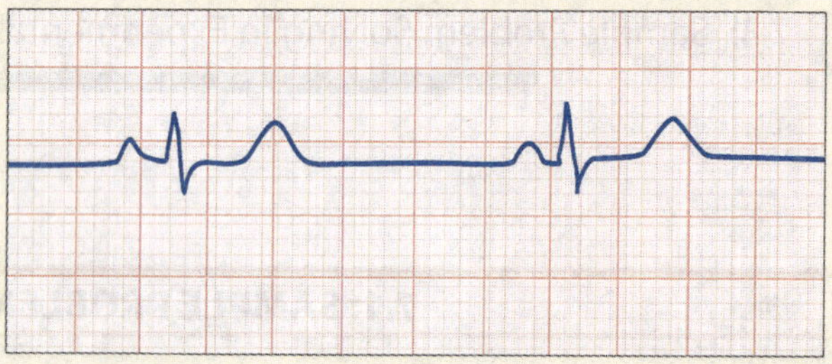

II

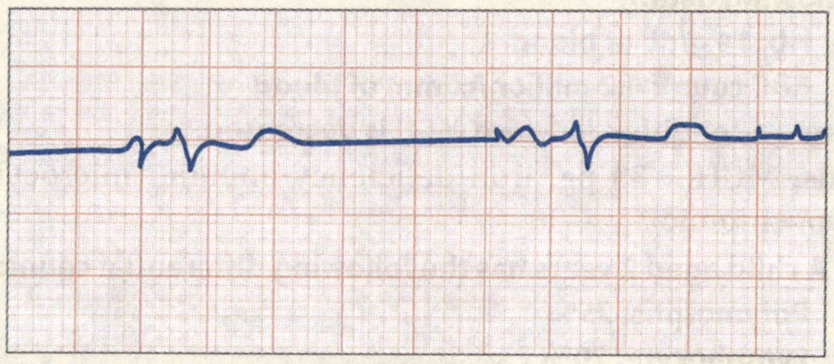

III

Ans. 20 degrees (See page 147).

6. Identify A. Define and give the normal range of vital capacity. Define FEV1. Calculate the inspiratory capacity from the graph.

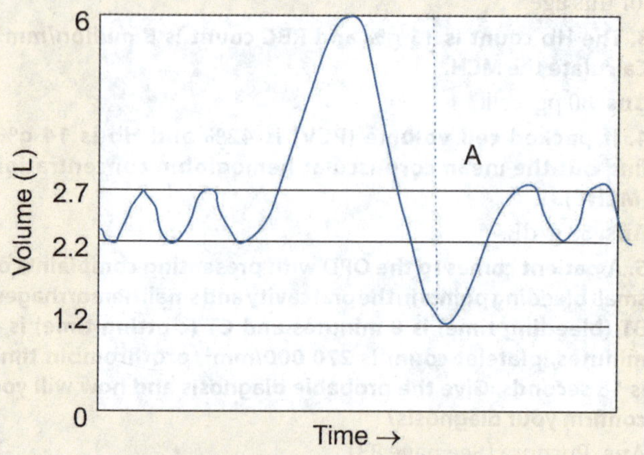

Ans. "A" is vital capacity (See page 110 and 115).
Inspiratory capacity is 3.8 L

7. Calculate the vital capacity and functional residual capacity from the diagram given below.

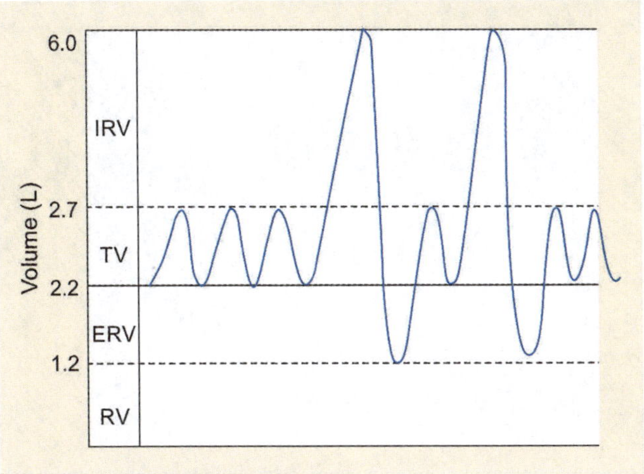

Ans. Vital capacity is 4.8L. Functional residual capacity is 2.2L.

7.3: SAMPLE PROBLEM SOLVING IN EXPERIMENTAL (AMPHIBIAN) PRACTICALS

1. Given that the tuning fork frequency is 100 Hz, calculate the duration of the various phases in the graph below.

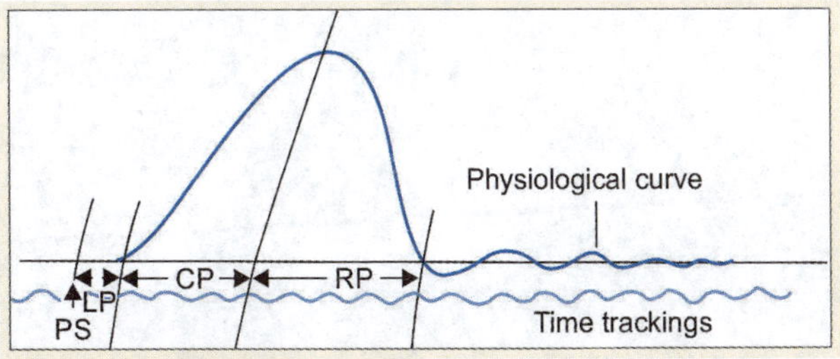

Ans. See page 262.

2. If the length of the nerve is 6 cm, calculate the conduction velocity from the given graph. Tuning fork frequency is 100 Hz.

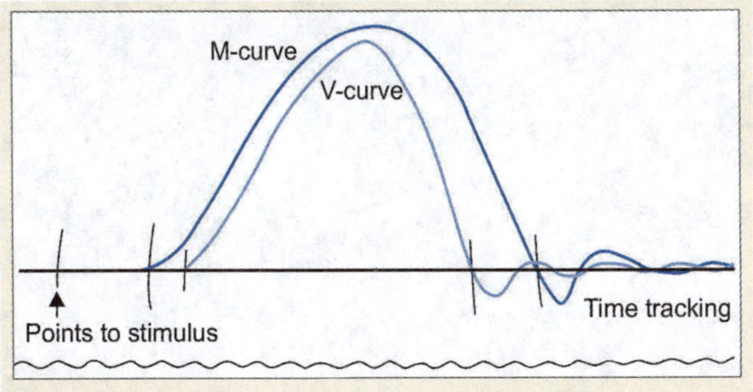

Ans. 6 m/s.

3. Identify the event that is taking place at point A. Give its causes.

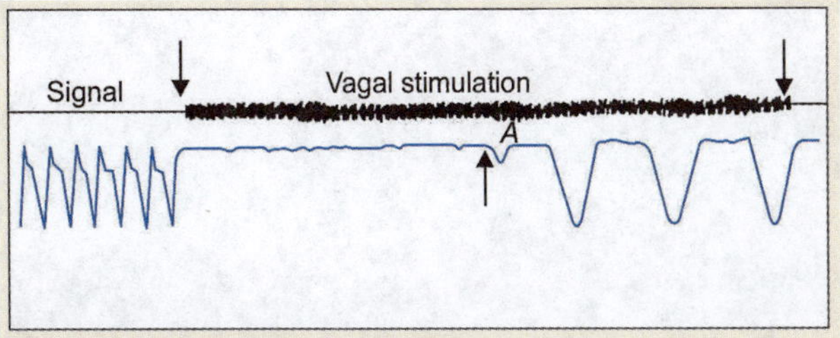

Ans. Vagal escape (See page 287).

4. In the graph given below, what does the arrow represent?

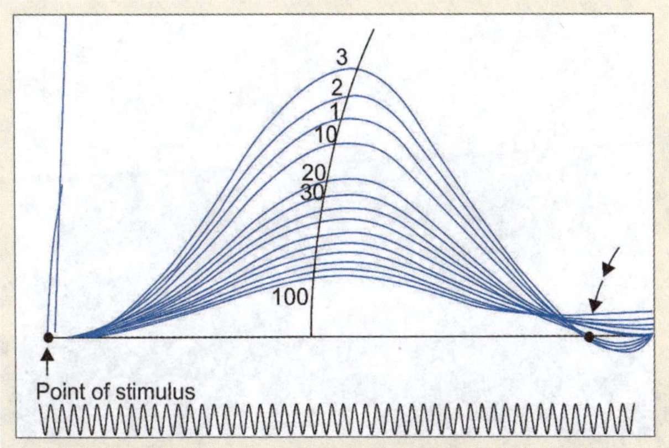

Ans. See page 275.

5. Identify the graph. What is compensatory pause?

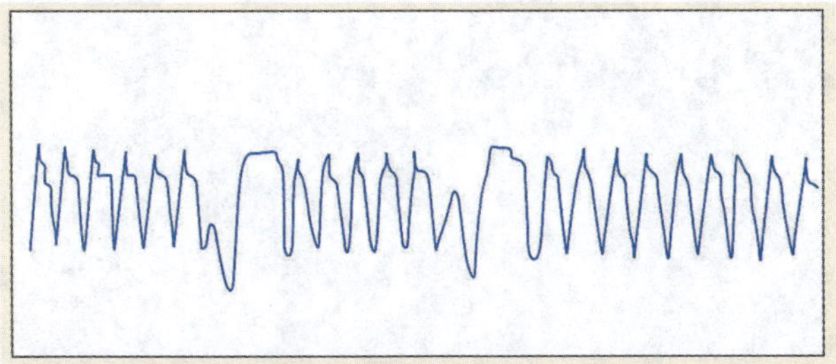

Ans. Extrasystole and compensatory pause (See page 283).

Appendix

UNITS AND MEASURES EMPLOYED IN PHYSIOLOGY

INTRODUCTION

The international system of units (SI Units-system International d' Unites).

Examples of basic SI units **(Table 1)**:

Table 1: Characteristics of basic SI units.

Physical quantity	*Name of SI unit*	*Symbol of SI unit*
Length	meter	m
Mass	kilogram	kg
Amount of substance	mole	mol
Energy	joule	J
Pressure	pascal	Pa
Time	second	s (or, sec)
Electric current	ampere	A
Thermodynamic temperature	kelvin	K
Luminous intensity	candela	cd

DECIMAL, MULTIPLES AND SUBMULTIPLES OF THE SI UNITS (TABLE 2)

These are formed by the use of prefixes. The Greek prefixes (deca, hecto, kilo, myria) denote multiplication. The Latin prefixes (deci, centi, milli) denote division. [The METER (Fr, METRE), the unit of length is the ten-millionth part of a line drawn from the pole to the equator].

Table 2: Decimal, multiples and submultiples of the SI units.

Multiple	*Prefix*	*Symbol*	*Submultiple*	*Prefix*	*Symbol*
10^1	deca	da	10^{-1}	deci	d
10^2	hecto	h	10^{-2}	centi	c
10^3	kilo	k	10^{-3}	milli	m
10^6	mega	M	10^{-6}	micro	μ
10^9	giga	G	10^{-9}	nano	n
10^{12}	tera	T	10^{-12}	pico	p
10^{15}	peta	P	10^{-15}	femto	f
10^{18}	exa	E	10^{-18}	atto	a

Unit of volume: The SI unit of volume is the *cubic meter* (m^3). But because of its inconvenience the *liter (L)* and *deciliter (dL)* are used as the units of volume for most applications in physiology and biochemistry. The equivalents of *metric, United States,* and *English (Imperial)* measures are also shown.

1 m^3 = 1,000 liters • 1 dL = 100 mL
• 1 cubic inch = 16.39 mL
1 fl oz = 29.57 mL • 1 mL = 0.0352 oz
• 1 mm^3 (1 cmm) = 1 μL (microliter)
1 liter = 1.76 pints • 1 pint = 568 mL = 20 fl oz
1 liter = 1.06 US liq Quart •1 m^3 = 1.31 yd^3
• 1 US = 32 fl oz = 0.951 liq quart
1 US = 0.83 English • 1 gallon = 4.55 liters
1 m^3 = 275 bus (bushel) • 1 bus = 0.0364 m^3

Unit of amount of substance: The "Molar" (e.g. mol/L; mmol/L) is used for substances of defined chemical composition. It replaces the equivalent concentration (mEq/L) which is not part of the SI system for measurements of sodium, potassium, chloride and bicarbonate (the numerical value of these four measurements is unchanged because these ions are univalent).

Unit of weight (mass concentration): The SI unit is the *kilogram* (kg). 1 kg = 1,000 g (grams)
1 kg = 2.20 pounds (lb; avoirdupois) = 2.68 pounds (apothecaries')
1 lb = 453.6 g = 16 oz •1 oz = 28.35 g •1 grain = 65 mg
1 tonne = 1,000 kg = 0.984 ton = 2,204 lb
1 ton = 1,016 kg = 1.02 tonne = 2,244 lb

Unit of length: The SI unit is the *meter (m).*
1 Angstrom unit (Å) = 10^{-10} m = 0.1 nm • [1 micrometer (urn) = 10^{-6} m (micron, μ, is obsolete, and in its place, the unit μm is used)].
1 in (inch) = 2.54 cm
• 1 cm = 0.394 in
• 1 yd (yard) = 0.9144 m
1 meter = 39.37 in • 1 meter = 1.09144 yd
• 1 meter = 3.28 ft (feet)
1 km = 0.621 mile • 1 mile = 1.609 km
• 1 mile = 1,760 yd
1 nautical mile = 1.852 km = 1.14 mile = 6,080 ft Knot = Nautical miles per hour

Unit of area: The SI unit of area is the *square meter (m^2)*.

1 cm^2 = 0.155 $inch^2$
- 1 in^2 = 6.452 cm^2
- 1 ft^2 = 929 cm^2

1 m^2 = 10.8 ft^2
- 1 m^2 = 1.20 yd^2
- 1 yd^2 = 0.836 m^2

1 acre = 4,840 yd^2 = 4,047 m^2 = 0.4047 ha (hectare)

1 hectare = 2.471 acres
- 1 sq mile = 2.59 km^2 = 640 acres

Unit of pressure: The SI unit of pressure is the *pascal (Pa)*. This is the pressure exerted by 1 Newton force on an area of a square meter (1 Pa = 1 N m^{-2}).

1 cm water = 98.1 Pa
- 1 mm Hg = 1 torr = 133.3 Pa = 0.1333 kPa

1 kPa = 7.60 mm Hg = 10.1 cm H_2O
- 1 lb/in^2 = 6.894 kPa

1 millibar (mb) = 0.1 kPa
- 1 dyne/cm = 10^{-4} kPa
- 1 normal atmosphere = 1 bar = 760 mm Hg = 101.3 kPa.

Temperature: The SI temperature scale is the kelvin scale (K) but it is inconvenient to use in medicine. The *Celsius* (formerly centigrade) scale (°C) has been retained.

- To convert Celsius degrees to Fahrenheit, multiply with 9/5 and add 32.
- To convert Fahrenheit degrees to Celsius, substract 32 and multiply by 5/9.

°C	-40	-10	0	10	20	30	35	37	40	45	100
°F	-40	14	32	50	68	86	95	98.6	104	113	212

LABORATORY VALUES OF CLINICAL IMPORTANCE

The following laboratory values are some of those which have frequent clinical relevance. Values in SI units are shown in brackets after the values in traditional units.

Body Fluids and Other Mass Data

Body fluid, total volume: 50% (in obese) to 70% (lean) of body weight.

- Intracellular: 30–40% of body weight
- Extracellular: 20–30% of body weight

(Of about 40 liters of water in a 70 kg man, 14 liters are in ECF (3.5 liters in vascular, and 10.5 liters in interstitial fluid compartments) and 26 liters in ICF).

Blood (Total Volume)

- Males: 70 mL/kg body weight
- Females: 65 mL/kg body weight (7.5–8% bw).

Plasma Volume

- Males: 39 mL/kg body weight
- Females: 40 mL/kg body weight.

RBC Volume

- Males: 30 mL/kg body weight
- Females: 25 mL/kg body weight.

Blood—Reference Intervals

Arterial Gases

- $PaCO_2$: 35–45 mm Hg
- PaO_2: 80–100 mm Hg at sea level.

Arterial Oxygen Saturation (At Rest)

- Sea level: 97%
- 5,000 ft: 90%
- 15,000 ft: 75%.

Adult blood contains 0.3 mL O_2 in physical solution and about 19 mL/dL in chemical combination with hemoglobin.

Carbon Dioxide Content, Plasma (Sea Level): 50–70 volumes/dL (21–28 mmol/liter).

Carboxyhemoglobin

- Nonsmokers: 0–2.3%
- Smokers: 2.1–4.2%.

Bleeding Time

- Duke method (finger, ear lobe): <5 minutes
- Ivy method (5-mm wound): <9 minutes
- Simplate: <7 minutes.

Coagulation Time

- Capillary blood: 2–5 min
- Venous blood (Lee and White): 5–15 min.

Erythrocyte sedimentation rate (ESR), mm 1st hour:

Westergren:
- Males: 0–15
- Females: 0–20.

Wintrobe:
- Males: 0–9
- Females: 0–20 (Increases with age).

Fragility of red cells: Hemolysis begins at 0.45% NaCl; complete at 0.35% NaCl solution.

Hematocrit (Hct; packed cell volume, (PCV)
- Men: 40–52%
- Women: 37–47%

[(SI: Men: 0.4–0.52 L/L, Women: 0.37–0.47 L/L)].

Mean corpuscular (cell) volume (MCV): 75–94 μm^3 (75–94 fl).

Mean corpuscular hemoglobin (MCH): 27–32 pg

Mean corpuscular hemoglobin concentration (MCHC): 30–36% (SI: 30–36 g/L).

Osmolality (serum): 275–295 mOsm/kg water.

Red cell count:
- Males: 4.5–6.5 million/mm^3 (SI: 4.5–6.5 × 10^{12}/L)
- Females: 4.0–5.5 million/mm^3 (SI: 4.0–5.5 × 10^{12}/L).

Hemoglobin

- Males: 13.5–18 g/dL
- Females: 11.5–16 g/dL.

White cell count (WCC): 4,000–11,000/mm^3 (SI: 4.0–11.0 × 10^9/L)

- Neutrophils: 40–75% WCC (2.0–7.5 × 10^9/L)
- Eosinophils: 1–6% WCC (0.04–0.44 × 10^9/L)
- Lymphocytes: 20–45% WCC (1.3–3.5 × 10^9/L)
- Basophils: 0.0–1.0% WCC (0.0–0.10 × 10^9/L)
- Monocytes: 2–10% WCC (0.2–0.8 × 10^9/L).

Platelet count: 150,000–400,000/mm^3 (SI: 150.0–400.0 × 10^9/L).

Lifespan: 8–10 days.

CARDIOVASCULAR SYSTEM

Cardiac output (Fick): 4.5–6 liters/min (cardiac index: 2.5–3.6 liters/min/m^2 BSA).

Capillary pressure (systemic):

- Arterial end: 32 mm Hg
- Venous end: 12 mm Hg
- Mean: 20 mm Hg.

Pulmonary capillaries (mean):

8 mm Hg (osmotic pressure of blood: 25 mm Hg; no tissue fluid formed).

Cardiac output (Fick): 4.5 liters/min.

(Cardiac index: 2.5–3.6 liters/min/m^2 BSA).

Coronary Artery blood flow: 50–120 mL/100 g left ventricle (Represents total left ventricular flow of about 115 mL/min in a 70 kg man).

Cerebral artery blood flow (total): 750 mL/min (50–60 mL/100 g tissue/min).

Cardiac rate:

- Infants: 130 beats/min
- Men: 70–72 beats/min
- Women: 78–80 beats/min

Renal blood flow: 1,300 mL/min.

Hepatic (mean flow), total: 1.0 L/min.

BRAIN

Nerve cells (neurons): Total number in human nervous system: >100 billion. **Growth:** Rate of growth reaches maximum early in life. By 6 months, the brain doubles in size; by 3 years, it triples; at 6 years, the brain is 95% of mature size with remaining growth achieved in about equal yearly increments of 10 g until age 20. Some replacement of damaged neurons continues later in life.

BIOCHEMISTRY

Reference Values (S: Serum; P: Plasma)

(Values in SI units are given in brackets after the values in traditional units)

Aminotransferases (S):

- **Aspartate-aminotransferase (AST, SGOT):** 10–14 Karmen units/mL; 6–18 IU/L (100–300 mmol/L).
- **Alanine-aminotransferase (ALT, SGPT):** 10–40 Karmen units/mL; 3–26 IU/L (50–430 mmol/L).

Amylase (S): 60–180 Somogyi units/dL (13–53 nmol/L).

Ammonia (whole blood): 80–110 mg/dL (45–65 mmol/L).

Bicarbonate (S or P): 24–30 mEq/L (24–30 mmol/L).

Bilirubin (total, S or P): 0.3–1 mg/dL (5–17 mmol/L) (About half is direct).

Calcium, total (S): 8.5–10.5 mg/dL (2.12–2.62 mmol/L) (varies with protein concentration).

Chloride (S): 350–375 mg/dL; 95–105 mEq/L (95–105 mmol/L).

Cholesterol (S): 140–300 mg/dL (3.6–7.8 mmol/L).

Fibrinogen (P): 150–400 mg/dL (1.5–4 g/L).

Glucose, normal, fasting (P): 80–90 mg/dL (4.4–4.9 mmol/L), Upper limit: 110 mg/dL (6 mmol/L).

2-hour postprandial (or after drinking 75 g glucose (50 g in children under 14 years of age).

Normal: 140 mg/dL (7.8 mmol/L). No value exceeds in renal threshold of 180 mg/dL (9.9 mmol/L).

Impaired glucose tolerance: 140–200 mg/dL (7.811.1 mmol/L).

Diabetes mellitus: >200 mg/dL (>11.1 mmol/L on more than one occasion).

Two fasting levels >145 mg/dL confirm the diagnosis of diabetes mellitus.

Immunoglobulins (S):

- **IgA:** 90–350 mg/dL
- **IgD:** 0–8 mg/dL
- **IgE:** <0.025 mg/dL
- **IgG:** 800–1,500 mg/dL
- **IgM:** 45–150 mg/dL (SI units in g/L).

Magnesium (S or P): 2–3 mg/dL (0.75–1.05 mmol/L).

Nonprotein nitrogen (NPN) (S): 20–30 mg/dL (14–21 mmol/L).

Osmolality (P): 285–295 mosm/kg of serum water.

Phosphate (as inorganic P) (P): 2.5–4.5 mg/dL (0.8–1.45 mmol/L).

Phosphatase, acid, serum: 0.2–1.8 IU (3–30 nmol/L).

Phosphatase, alkaline, serum: 21–91 IU at 37°C (0.4–1.5 mmol/L).

Potassium (S): 14–20 mg/dL (3.5–5.0 mmol/L).

Proteins, total, serum: 5.5–8.0 g/dL (55–80 g/L).

Protein fractions:

- **Albumin:** 3.5–5 g/dL
- **Globulin:** 2–3.5 g/dL
- **Alpha$_1$:** 0.2–0.4 g/dL
- **Alpha$_2$:** 0.5–0.9 g/dL
- **Beta:** 0.6–1.1 g/dL
- **Gamma:** 0.7–1.7 g/dL.

SGOT, SGPT: See aminotransferases.

Sodium (S): 310–340 mg/dL (136–145 mEq/L) (135–145 mmol/L).

Triglycerides, as triolin (S): 25–150 mg/dL (0.28–1.69 mmol/L).

Thyroid binding globulin (TBG) (P): 7–17 mg/L.

Thyroxine (T_4) (P): 70–140 nmol/L.

Thyroxine (free) plasma: 9–22 pmol/L.

Triiodothyronine (T_3), plasma: 1.2–3.0 nmol/L.

Urea (urea nitrogen) (S): 10–20 mg/dL (3.6–7.1 mmol/L).

Uric acid (urate) (S or P): 2–7 mg/dL (0.15–0.48 mmol/L) (slightly less in females).

Xylose (B): 5–50 mg/dL (0.33–3.33 mmol/L).

Zinc (S): 50–150 mg/dL (7.65–22.95 umol/L).

Nomogram for determination of body surface area from height and weight (Adults) (Fig. 1)

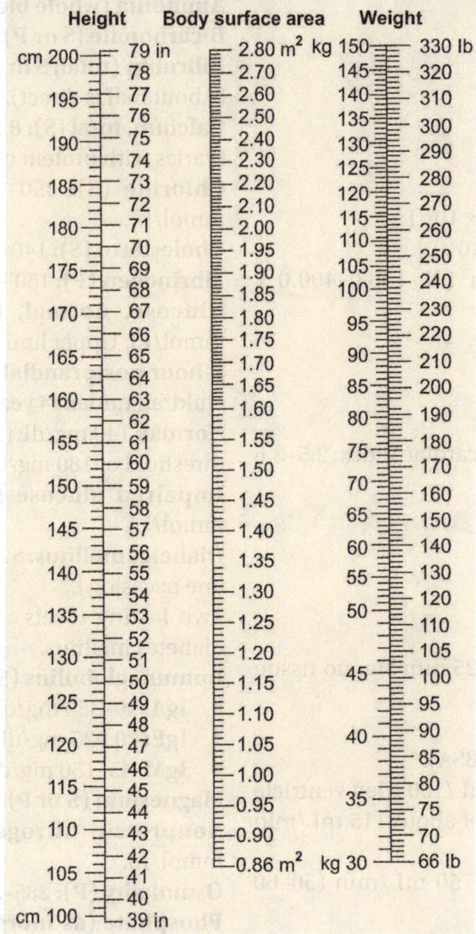

FIG. 1: Nomogram for determination of body surface area from height and weight (adults).

Body mass index (BMI) chart as per WHO Guidelines (Fig. 2)

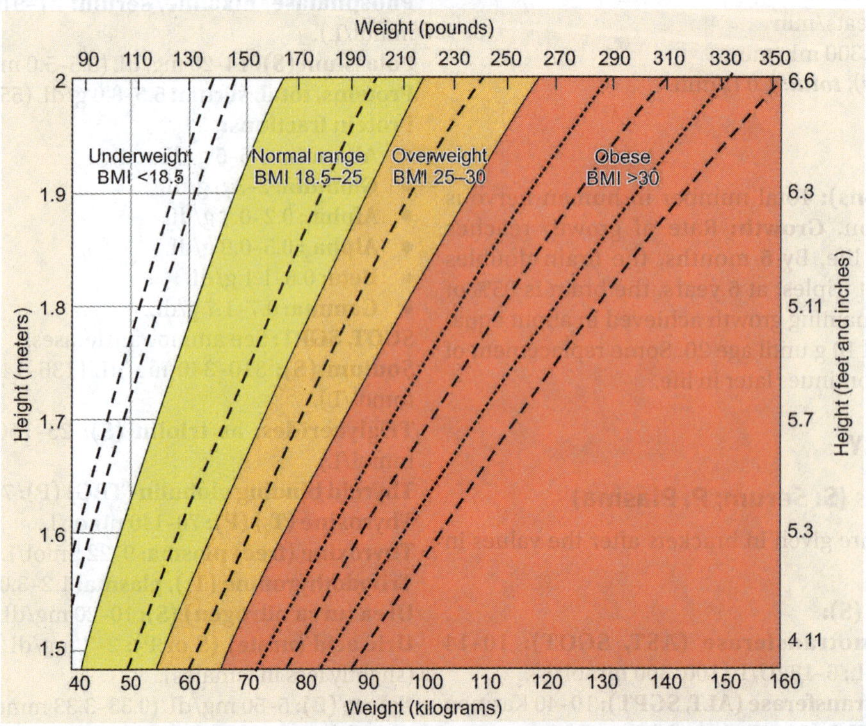

FIG. 2: Body mass index (BMI) chart: WHO guidelines.

Index

Page numbers followed by *f* refer to figure, *fc* refer flowchart, and *t* refer to table.

L

M

N

T